THE DIET BIBLE

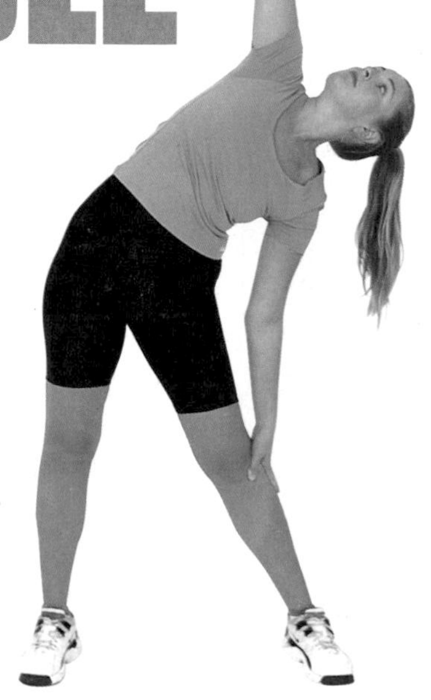

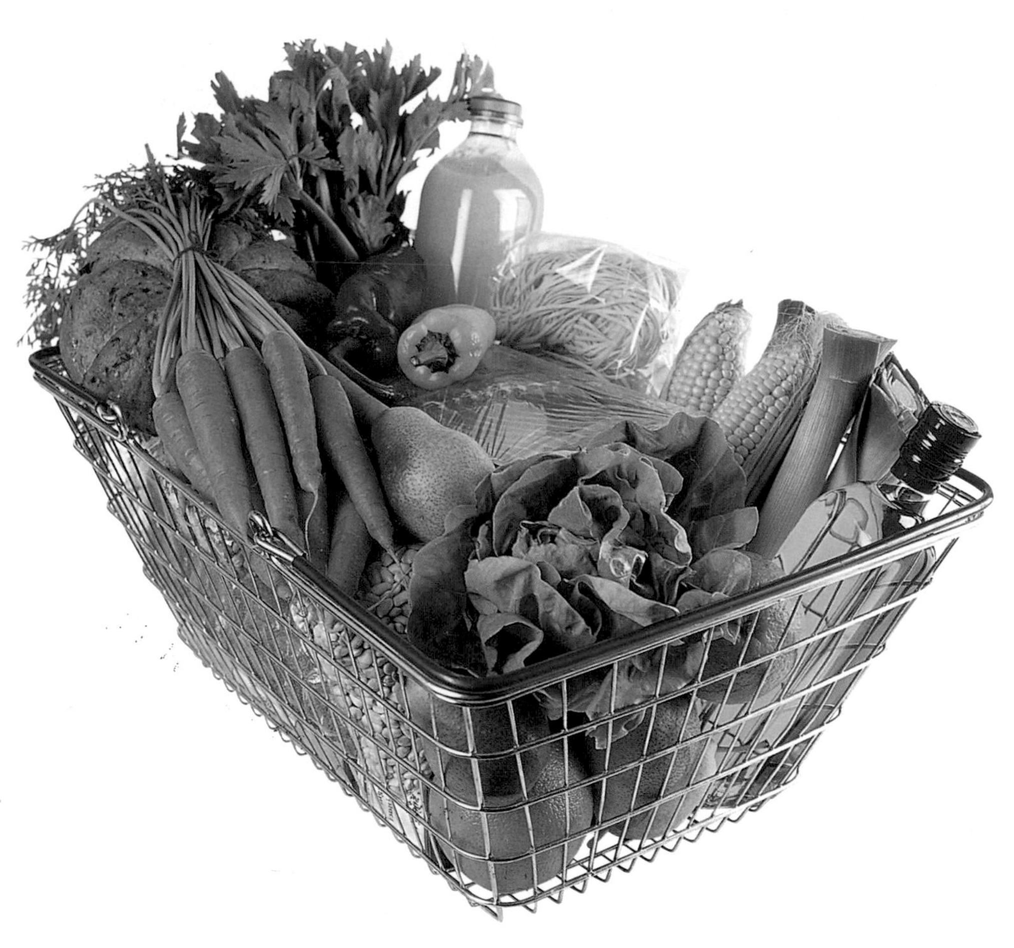

THE DIET BIBLE

covers over 50 diets and all the secrets of successful slimming and weight control

JUDITH WILLS

QUADRILLE

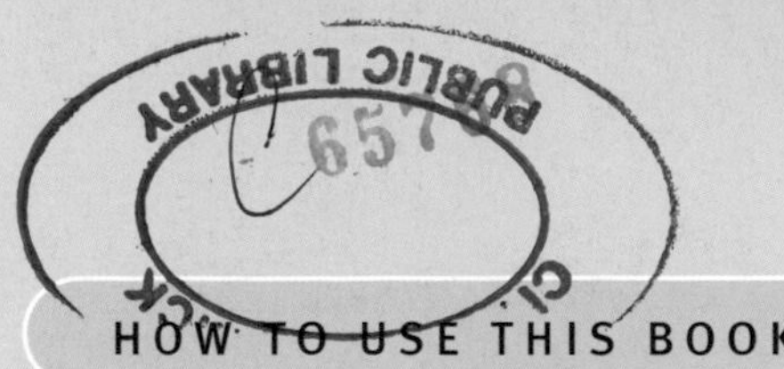

HOW TO USE THIS BOOK

There are five ways to use the book:

1 *Via the contents page*: simply look at the contents page opposite, where you will find the 10 sections that form the major part of the book listed. Find the section that matches the topic in which you are most interested (e.g. For women only), turn to that section and browse. The contents page also lists major features that appear in each section, with their page number. These provide background or back-up information to the questions.

2 *Via the index*: if you have a very specific topic in mind – e.g. 'weight gain in mid-life' – then pick out the main word or words in your topic and look them up in the index at the back of the book. In this instance you would probably look up 'weight gain'. There are several entries for 'weight gain'. Skim down them until you find 'weight gain, mid-life'. Look up the page number(s) listed and you will find all the main entries in the book for that topic. Numbers in bold illustrate a main feature entry – there are over 30 major features on a variety of topics in the book. Other words in your topic or query may also be in the index in a similar way and they may supply other ways to reach the answer to your query.

3 *Via the cross-references*: at the end of every answer to a question in the book you will find a list of cross-references that you can look up for further related information on the topic, or on linking topics. The questions are listed by number only – all questions in the book appear in numerical order. The features are also listed by number in the same way.

4 *Via the A–Z*: the second part of the book, beginning on page 240, is in the form of an A–Z listing of diet and fitness products, methods, programmes and facilities. If there is a particular named diet or product (e.g. The Atkins Diet, or fat substitutes) that you want to know about, just look it up. Contact details are given for most entries and again there are cross-references to other entries.

5 *Via the List of Questions*: on pages 7–9 you will find a complete list of all the questions in the book in numerical order. Check through the list relating to the section that most interests you and find the question nearest to the one you want to ask.

A Food Value Chart, listing over 300 foods with their calorie, fat and other nutritional values, appears on pages 280–83 to complete the information in *The Diet Bible*.

If there is any question you would like to ask that doesn't appear in the book, do write to me c/o Quadrille Publishing, telling me what it is, or visit my website at www.thedietbible.co.uk. In the next edition we will do our best to rectify the matter!

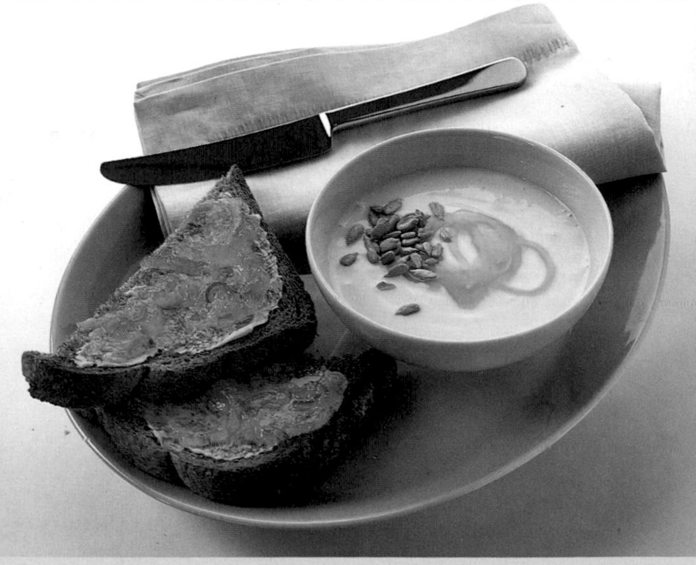

contents

Introduction

For the first time in the history of humankind, more people are overweight in the world than underweight, according to the World Health Authority. Obesity is the second largest cause of death in the USA (with similar statistics elsewhere) and overweight and obesity affect, cause or make worse over 30 medical conditions – many serious and life-threatening. Childhood obesity is increasing at an alarming rate and so, unless something is done, the situation is almost bound to get worse in the long term.

Obesity is a social and medical problem, and beating it is high up on the agendas of governments across the world. At a personal level, most people who are overweight would prefer not to be – because it is well documented that fatness causes a variety of negative effects apart from ill-health, including: teasing and isolation in children; a less active sexual life and less chance of relationship fulfilment; poorer employment and promotion opportunities; and higher risk of depression and emotional problems.

Americans spend $23 billion annually on weight-reducing products, programmes and services. It has been estimated that 30% of females and 20% of males in the UK, and 40% of females and 24% of males in the USA are trying to lose weight at any one time. In the long term, however, these efforts fail.

The Diet Bible doesn't pretend to offer new solutions to the global weight problem, but what I have tried to do is put together a resource in which I hope you will find not only all the facts, figures and practicalities you need to help you – and your family – reach and maintain a sensible weight, but also plenty of insight and encouragement as well. As far as I know, *The Diet Bible* is the first and only comprehensive collection of impartial information on diet, weight and fitness. My aim was for you to be able to find the answer to any question you may have on the subject quickly and easily – and, I hope, to find out more than you thought you wanted to know! It's a dip-in book as much as a reference book. *Judith Wills, October 2001*

LIST OF QUESTIONS

1 What does a body's total weight consist of and in what proportions?
2 What is the difference between surplus weight and surplus fat?
3 What is the basic mechanism that controls my body weight?
4 Does the metabolic rate vary from person to person?
5 Do fat people have slow metabolic rate?
6 Can I increase my own metabolic rate?
7 Could weight be due to faulty genes?
8 Any other influences on body weight?
9 Is it true that everyone's weight has a natural 'set point'?
10 Is weight fluctuation through life normal?
11 Are there any foods or drinks that can increase my metabolic rate?
12 What supplements can I take to speed up my metabolism?
13 Is there a foolproof formula for speeding up my metabolic rate?
14 Do emotional or psychological factors affect how I metabolize food?
15 Does how or when I eat – rather than what – affect my metabolism?
16 Can illness affect my metabolism?
17 Could my weight problem be due to 'sluggish' glands?
18 What is 'the energy equation'?
19 If I eat more calories than I use up, how quickly will I put on weight?
20 Can I put on weight without eating more?
21 Why do I never lose weight even though I hardly eat a thing?
22 Why do some people eat a lot more than me and yet stay slim?
23 Can a big appetite be controlled?
24 Why is weight easier to gain than lose?
25 How can I put on weight if too thin?
26 What's wrong with being overweight?
27 As you get older is weight gain natural or even desirable?
28 What is the definition of normal or ideal weight?
29 What are the definitions of under- and overweight?
30 What is 'body-fat percentage' and how does it relate to my weight?
31 Is there any very quick and easy way to tell if I am overweight?
32 Can dieting slow my metabolic rate?
33 Does dieting make us fat?
34 Will my percentage of body fat increase each time I diet?
35 Can I lose weight without dieting?
36 What's the best way to lose weight?
37 Is it good to take slimming pills?
38 Are there any operations that I can have to make me lose weight?
39 Why do so many people put weight back on after they have dieted?
40 How can I avoid regaining weight?
41 What factors affect my body shape?
42 Can a child change shape by doing anything specific while still growing?
43 As an adult, is the bone structure I have the bone structure I'm stuck with?
44 I'm very slim and fine-boned – how can I look more muscular and strong?
45 However much I diet and exercise, I seem to remain 'soft', with no muscle definition – is there any cure?
46 I am female, with bulky arm and leg muscles – even though I do hardly any exercise. How can I get rid of them?
47 What about spot-reduction – can I choose where I lose fat via exercise?
48 I'm not overweight but my stomach sticks out – what can I do about it?
49 I'm a flat-chested female – what foods or exercise will give me a bigger bust?
50 I've slimmed down to a weight I love, but I hate my flabby bum. Any ideas?
51 I have a short waist which makes me look out of proportion – can I alter this?
52 Are there any instant ways of changing my shape?
53 Is it true that a pear shape is the hardest shape of all to change?
54 Can I spot-reduce hips and thighs?
55 Is it true that overweight mostly on the lower body is perfectly healthy?
56 Why is an apple shape unhealthy?
57 Can I lose a big stomach and flabby waist without my legs getting thinner?
58 What's the best way to get a firm, flat stomach?
59 My bust is too big – can I reduce it through diet and exercise?
60 How can I improve the look of my thin and weak-looking arms and legs?
61 My face is fat and yet I'm quite slim – is there anything I can do about this?
62 How long will it take to exercise my body into a better shape?
63 I have a month to get in shape before a holiday – what can I achieve?
64 Would you recommend a salon wrap or similar to lose weight in a hurry?
65 What is the best home toning programme I can do in 20 minutes?
66 Which are the best and worst exercises for building muscle tone?
67 What home exercise equipment do you recommend for general toning?
68 Now I'm slimmer, how can I exercise away skin left from when I was very fat?
69 The diet's going fine, but can I shape up without spending any money?
70 What is the best exercise for making myself look taller and slimmer?
71 Can you recommend an easy exercise programme to limber up before and after the gym?
72 What changes in body shape and appearance are natural as you age?
73 Can I reverse age-related body shape changes through exercise?
74 What are calories?
75 In what foods are calories found?
76 What happens to food in the body?
77 What happens if I don't eat?
78 What happens if I eat more than I need?
79 What types of calories tend to put most weight on?
80 Do carbohydrate foods encourage weight gain?
81 Is sugar so bad for you?
82 Should I use artificial sweeteners?
83 Can a high-carbohydrate, high-fibre diet help me lose weight?
84 What is the Glycaemic Index?
85 What are the best foods for controlling hunger?
86 How can I avoid feeling weak and dizzy on a slimming diet?
87 Do I need to feel hunger pangs in order to lose weight?
88 Does a high-protein diet have any special benefits for getting/keeping slim?
89 Does fat make you fat?
90 Is a low-fat diet always the best and healthiest way to slim?
91 What exactly is food combining and is it a good system for weight loss?
92 Is eating nothing but raw food a good dieting idea?
93 Does a diet high in fruit and vegetables help weight loss?
94 I dislike most fruits and vegetables – how am I ever going to lose weight?
95 Is regular snacking between meals a good or bad idea?
96 How many meals should I eat a day for optimum weight loss?
97 Is just one meal a day the best way to control calorie intake?
98 How important is breakfast in a good slimming campaign?
99 Is it true you should breakfast like a king and dine like a pauper?
100 Does food eaten late convert straight to body fat while you sleep?
101 What are the best drinks to choose on a slimming diet, and why?
102 There are so many diets – how do I pick the right one?
103 Is there 'the perfect diet'?
104 How many cals/day do most people need to reduce to for weight loss?
105 What is a crash diet?
106 Are crash diets such a bad idea?
107 Is fasting a good way to lose weight?
108 What is the least number of calories I can eat to slim and stay healthy long-term?
109 What are the pros and cons of very-low-cal, liquid-only diets?
110 Can you really block calories in food so that they are not absorbed?
111 Is it true that there are foods which contain 'negative calories'?
112 Can I lose weight without drastic diet changes or calorie counting?
113 What is the most reliable and easy way to slim and maintain weight loss?
114 Could a food allergy be causing my inability to lose weight?
115 Does avoiding wheat products help you lose weight?
116 Is it a good idea to avoid dairy produce when slimming?
117 Are there disadvantages to diets restricted to just a few types of food?
118 I enjoy fast food, like burgers and chips. Is it really necessary to cut these out to lose weight and keep it off?
119 I love chocolate – can I eat is as part of a slimming diet?
120 I have a sweet tooth and can't live without desserts – any suggestions?
121 I adore cheese – how can my diet cope with its calories?
122 What are the best (quick and/or easy) cooking methods for slimmers?
123 I know I should lose weight – but how do I get motivated?
124 I've lost weight before and it all returns – what's the point?
125 Everyone tells me that diets don't work – so why bother?
126 Everyone tells me that I look just fine as I am – so why should I slim?
127 I'd like to lose weight but my family don't want me to – what do I do?
128 We live in a food-dominated society – how can I slim?
129 Food is my main pleasure – why should I deny myself?
130 Isn't it true that overweight people are just basically greedy and lazy?
131 Is there any real answer to the fact that diet food is very, very boring?
132 Can you define compulsive eating?
133 Can you recommend a strategy to beat comfort eating on carbohydrates?
134 I eat when bored – most evenings and weekends – what's the answer?

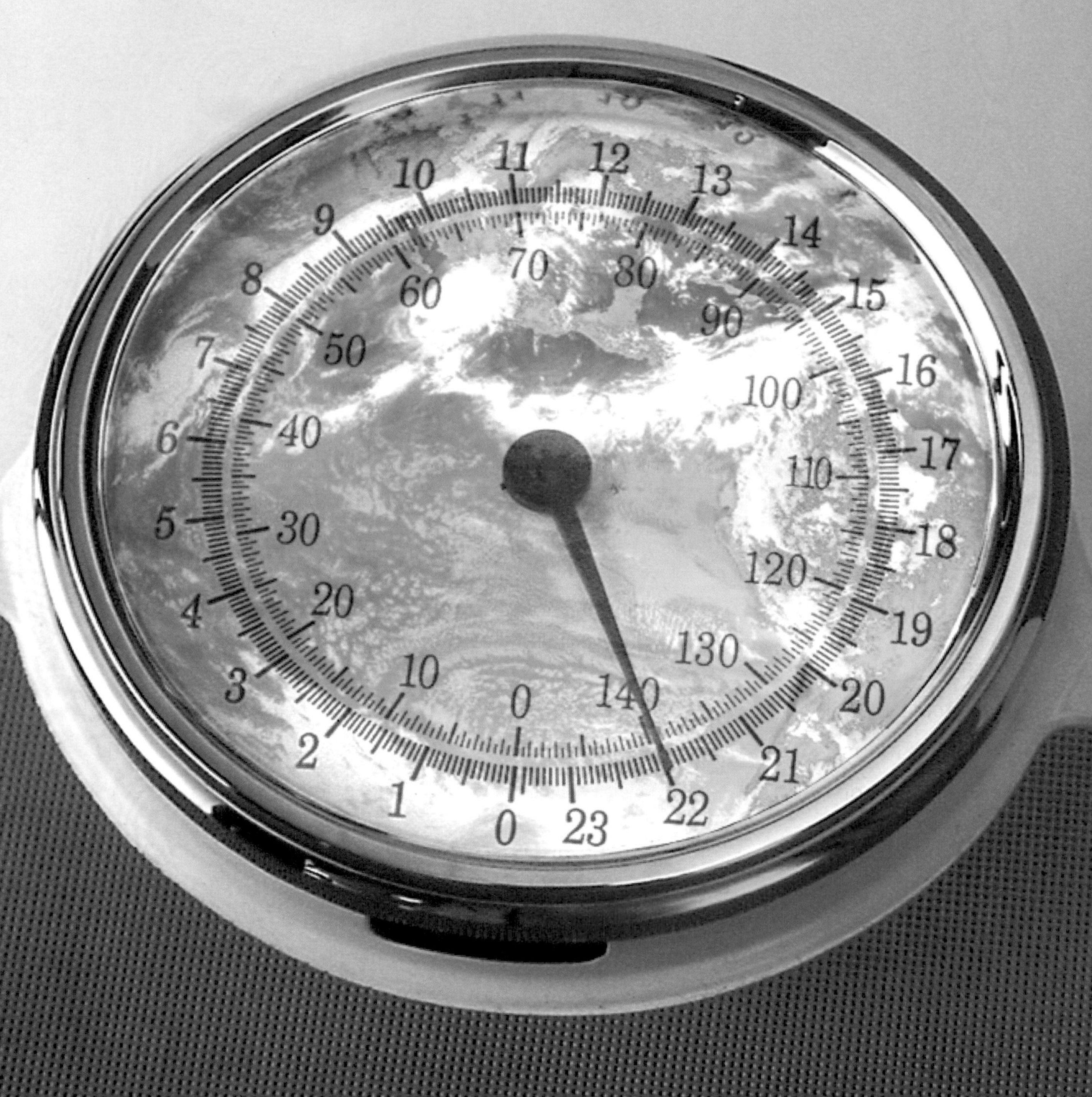

Section One

Your body, your weight

For the first time in history, more people in the world are now officially overweight or obese than are of normal weight or too thin. Despite the fact that most overweight people seem to spend a great deal of time worrying about their weight problems, it is still an epidemic that is escalating out of control. In America, 55% of the adult population are now overweight or obese, according to the American Obesity Society, and it is estimated that in 20 years' time, everyone in America will be overweight if nothing is done to reverse the trend. In the UK, there is a similar picture – 53% of English women and 63% of men are overweight or obese, according to the National Audit Office's latest census, and the number of obese people has tripled in 20 years.

This obvious inability to control our weight isn't through lack of interest on our part. It has been estimated that 30% of females and 20% of males in the UK and 40% of females and 24% of males in the USA are attempting to lose weight at any given time. In the Western world, weight control is a multi-billion-dollar industry. We are desperate to lose weight – but nothing's working, and lack of knowledge could be one main key. There are almost as many misconceptions about weight control as there are overweight people.

So in this section we aim to separate fact from fiction. From metabolism to appetite, from weight assessment to the best ways to lose weight – here you'll find all the answers to all the questions you've ever asked about your size.

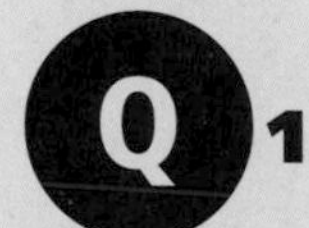

What does a body's total weight consist of and what proportions of fat, muscle and bone are there?

In a healthy male of average weight, the skeleton makes up 15% of total body weight, muscle 45%, and fat about 15%. In a similar female, the skeleton makes up 12% of total body weight, muscle about 35% and fat around 27%. For both sexes, the remainder is other matter, including skin, connective tissue, tendons, blood plasma, organs, hair, glands and so on.

The average body contains up to 70% of its total weight as water. Muscle is made of about 75% water, 20% protein and the rest is an assortment of minerals and other matter. Even body fat and bones are 50% water.

Talking of bones, as you will see, the average person's skeletal structure is quite light. A woman of 10 stone (64kg) would have about 17lb (7.75kg) of bone weight, while a man of 12 stone (77kg) would have about 25 lb (11.5kg) bone weight. Even people with larger or denser-than-average bones will, therefore, find that the old excuse of 'heavy bones' doesn't really wash!

See also:

- ▶ Question: 2.
- ▶ Features: 3, 4.

What is the difference between surplus weight and surplus fat, and how can I tell which is which?

When people become overweight or obese, their body-fat percentage increases, while changes in muscle and bone mass are usually relatively small. Weight increase due to altered bone mass is highly unlikely – even a 10% increase in bone mass would account for only an extra 2–3 lb (1–1.5kg) of body weight.

Muscle weighs more than fat and bone, and can also be increased quite drastically over time by means of exercise and good nutrition. So, somebody with a high muscle mass (for example, a weightlifter or field-sportsperson) could weigh much more than average, meaning that they would be overweight under the Body Mass Index classifications (see pages 28–9), while having no more body fat than an average person.

In this case, a Waist Circumference Test (see page 29) or a Body Fat Monitoring Test (see the A–Z) is a much more reliable indication of body fat; and if body fat percentage turns out to be low, then there is no need to lose weight. It is indeed highly unlikely that your surplus weight can be accounted for by increased muscle mass without you knowing about it – and a look in the mirror will obviously show muscle definition and tone, not flab.

Occasionally, fluid retention can account for surplus weight. Several conditions (such as premenstrual syndrome in women) and diseases (such as heart disease) can mean that the body retains more fluid than usual. This is often apparent (e.g., a swollen face, stomach, ankles). If you feel that it may be fluid, you should see your doctor. For 99% of us, however, surplus weight usually equals surplus fat.

See also:

- ▶ Questions: 3, 26, 31, 41–73, 300–306.
- ▶ Features: 3, 4, 21.
- ▶ Key index entries: body-fat percentage, body mass index, waist circumference.

FAT FACT

An average person has something in the region of 30 billion fat cells in their body, while a severely obese person may well have over about 300 billion.

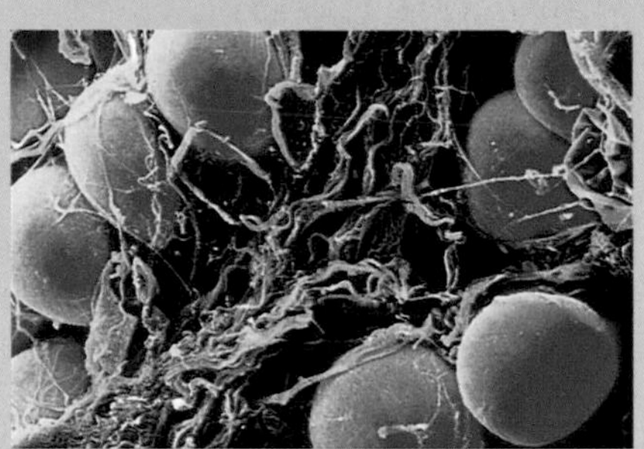

What is the basic mechanism that controls my body weight?

Your weight – particularly the amount of fat your body stores – is a reflection of the balance between your energy intake and energy expenditure. Energy intake is everything you eat or drink that contains calories (kilocalories) – units of energy – and energy expenditure is the amount of calories that your body burns up for fuel in living and working.

Energy expenditure can be divided into three categories. The first is your basal metabolic rate (BMR), which is the amount of calories you burn up in a given time just existing – i.e., lying down doing absolutely nothing. This accounts for approximately 60% of energy used in an average person. The second category is the amount of energy you use in activity – moving, talking, and so on – which accounts for an average of 30% of calories used. Lastly there is dietary thermogenesis, described as meal-induced heat production, which is the calories used up in eating, digesting, absorbing and using food. This accounts, surprisingly enough, for about 10% of our use of calories.

All these factors are variable – as, of course, is the amount we eat (i.e., the amount of energy with which we provide the body). If energy input and energy output remain in balance, our body weight remains stable. If energy input is higher, then the surplus energy eaten as food and not required by the body is then stored as body fat. If energy output is higher than energy input, the body fat stores are mobilized and converted back into energy – and, if this happens over a period of time, we lose body fat and therefore weight. The amount of your energy output over a period of time is known as your metabolic rate.

See also:

- ▶ Questions: 4–40.
- ▶ Features: 1, 2, 4, 28–30.
- ▶ A–Z entries: exercise classes, Metabolism Booster Diets, weighted workouts.
- ▶ Key index entries: BMR, calories, energy, metabolic rate.

4

Does the metabolic rate vary from person to person?

The rate at which the body burns up calories – at rest, during physical activity and via dietary thermogenesis (see the answer to the previous question) – can vary considerably with factors such as your gender, age and weight, your fitness, your body composition, the duration of and intensity at which you carry out work, and the type of food you eat. There are also other factors at work – genetic, hormonal and so on. The World Health Organization estimates that basal metabolic rate (BMR) alone can vary by as much as 25% up or down between individuals of similar weight. Add to that all the other variables, and you can see why to maintain their body weight in status quo some people have to eat a little and some a great deal. To find out your own metabolic rate, do the assessment in the feature overleaf.

See also:

- ▶ Questions: 3, 5–8.
- ▶ Features: 1, 2.
- ▶ Key index entries: BMR, body composition.

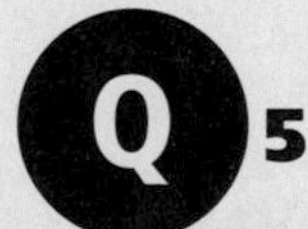

5

Is it true that fat people have a slow metabolic rate?

Emphatically no – in fact, quite the reverse! All other factors being equal, the heavier you are, the higher your metabolic rate will be. This is because a heavy body uses more energy both at BMR level and to move itself around (imagine the surplus fat as a block of concrete on your back and you will see why); because fat-free mass (metabolically active muscle and other tissue) also generally increases with weight, and because dietary thermogenesis increases. This is why when fat people lose lots of weight their new metabolic rate will be considerably lower than it was when they were still fat.

See also:

- ▶ Questions: 7–17.
- ▶ Features: 1, 2.
- ▶ A–Z entry: Metabolism Booster Diets.
- ▶ Key index entries: BMR, body fat composition, metabolic rate,.

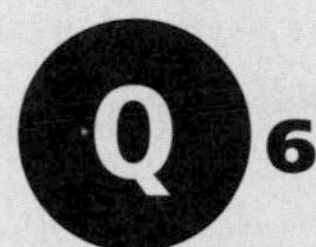

6

Can I do anything to increase my own metabolic rate?

Yes, quite a lot. Certain factors you can't alter – such as height, age, genetic and hormonal influences – but the rest you can.

You can alter your basal metabolic rate (BMR) by increasing the amount of lean tissue (muscle) your body contains, as muscle uses up more calories than other body tissue, even when resting. You can alter the amount of activity you do to burn up extra calories – the average is 30%, but many sedentary people use only about 15% more calories than their BMR in activity, while 50% or more of the metabolic rate of very active people may be accounted for by their activity.

You can also alter dietary thermogenesis by tweaking your food intake, and so on. However, if you are losing weight it is harder to increase your overall metabolic rate as you do so, because the reduction in weight will also naturally reduce your BMR at the same time (see the answer to the previous question).

See also:

- ▶ Questions: 3–5, 7–17, 333, 357.
- ▶ Features: 1, 2, 4, 28–30.
- ▶ A–Z entries: Body Clock Diet, exercise classes, Metabolism Booster Diets.
- ▶ Key index entries: BMR, high-protein diets, lean tissue, protein.

Assessing your own metabolic rate

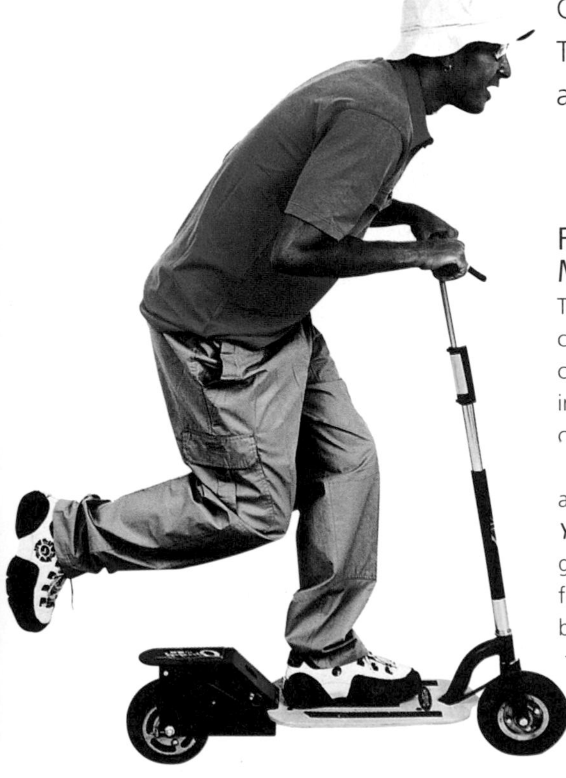

Get a rough idea of your current metabolic rate using these assessments. They're only a guide, though, as they involve major factors but can't take account of genetic, hormonal and other influences.

First work out your Basal Metabolic Rate

This is the 'bottom line' number of calories you need daily for your body to carry out basic involuntary functions, including breathing and the work of the cells in maintenance and repair.

The factors that most influence BMR are your sex, age, weight and height.

Your sex: because males tend to have a greater muscle mass (lean tissue) than females (and females have more fat), and because muscle burns up more calories than fat, men have a higher BMR.

Your age: after adolescence, when BMR is at its peak, it tends to decline slowly with age, unless lean body mass (muscle) is maintained.

Your weight: the heavier you are, the higher your BMR. By knowing your height and weight, it is possible to work out your Body Surface Area (BSA), which then gives a guide to your own personal BMR.

CHART 1

Hourly BMRs for men and women by age

Age	Men	Women
20	39	37
25	38	36
30	37	36
35	37	36
40	37	36
45	37	36
50	37	35
55	36	35
60	35	33
65	35	33
70	34	32
75	34	32
80	33	32

Working out your BMR

So, first work out your BMR for your sex and age using the age nearest your own on Chart 1, then find out your BSA factor, using Chart 2 (using the height and weight nearest to your own).

Then, using a calculator, multiply your Chart 1 result by your Chart 2 result. This is your hourly BMR. To get your daily BMR, multiply this by 24. To get your BMR per minute, divide the hourly BMR by 60.

Write your daily, hourly and per-minute BMR in the spaces provided.

Example: female aged 40, height 5ft 4in (1.6m), weight 140lb (64kg).
Hourly BMR: 36; BSA Factor: 1.7
Your personal hourly BMR (36 x 1.7): 61.2
Daily BMR (61.2 x 24): 1,469
BMR per minute (61.2 divided by 60): 1.02

YOUR BMR

Daily	Hourly	Per minute
_____	________	__________

Now calculate your Physical Activity Level

This is an estimate of the total calories you burn each day through activity of all kinds. Everything except sleep burns up calories at a rate greater than your BMR.

To simplify calculations, Physical Activity Level (PAL) factors have been devised according to your own estimate of your levels of activity. A PAL of 1.4, for example, means you burn up 1.4 times your BMR in activity through the day (this figure includes the BMR as well). The official PAL table starts at a factor of 1.4, but I have added a lower factor of 1.3, which I believe is much needed. To help you decide which level is right for you, see the examples opposite.

Once you've done this, simply multiply your BMR by your PAL factor to find out approximately how many calories you burn in a day. This is your total daily energy expenditure (excluding dietary-induced thermogenesis) and is the total that you can use to estimate how many calories a day you need in order to maintain your current weight. It is also the figure that you will need when assessing how many calories a day you need to eat in order to lose weight – for more on this, see the rest of Section One and Section Three – particularly Qs 36 and 104.

Write your total in the BOX here:

Example of calculating your approx total daily energy expenditure:

Daily BMR = 1,512; Daily PAL level = 1.4

Total Daily Energy Expenditure (1,512 x 1.4): 2,117 calories.

Your level of daily activity	PAL Factor
Very light: (most of day sitting at work or at home, a little slow walking, some standing and light household chores)	1.3
Light: (mostly sedentary, standing or slow walking, but including about 2 hours a day of further activity – e.g. gardening,heavy housework, brisk walking)	1.4
Moderate: (some occupational walking rather than just sedentary work, plus a little vigorous additional exercise, e.g. dancing, swimming	1.6 (women) 1.7 (men)
Heavy: (high levels of activity, both at work and in leisure hours	1.8 (women) 1.9 (men)

CHART 2

Body Surface Area Factor by Height and Weight

4ft 10in (1.45m)
- 70lb (32kg) – 1.1
- 80lb (36kg) – 1.2
- 100lb (45g) – 1.3
- 120lb (55kg) – 1.4
- 140lb (64kg) – 1.5
- 160lb (73kg) – 1.6
- 180lb (82kg) – 1.7
- 200lb (91kg) – 1.8

5ft 0in (1.5m)
- 80lb (36kg) – 1.2
- 100lb (45kg) – 1.3
- 120lb (55kg) – 1.5
- 140lb (64kg) – 1.6
- 160lb (73kg) – 1.7
- 180lb (82kg) – 1.8
- 200lb (91kg) – 1.9
- 220lb (100kg) – 2.0

5ft 2in (1.55m)
- 80lb (36kg) – 1.3
- 100lb (45kg) – 1.4
- 120lb (55kg) – 1.5
- 140lb (64kg) – 1.6
- 160lb (73kg) – 1.7
- 180lb (82kg) – 1.8
- 200lb (91kg) – 1.9
- 220lb (100kg) – 2.0

5ft 4in (1.6m)
- 100lb (45kg) – 1.4
- 120lb (55kg) – 1.6
- 140lb (64kg) – 1.7
- 160lb (73kg) – 1.8
- 180lb (82kg) – 1.9
- 200lb (91kg) – 2.0
- 220lb (100kg) – 2.1
- 240lb (109kg) – 2.2

5ft 6in (1.65m)
- 100lb (45kg) – 1.5
- 120lb (55kg) – 1.6
- 140lb (64kg) – 1.7
- 160lb (73kg) – 1.8
- 180lb (82kg) – 1.9
- 200lb (91kg) – 2.0
- 220lb (100kg) – 2.1
- 240lb (109kg) – 2.2

5ft 8in (1.7m)
- 120lb (55kg) – 1.6
- 140lb (64kg) – 1.7
- 160lb (73kg) – 1.8
- 180lb (82kg) – 1.9
- 200lb (91kg) – 2.0
- 220lb (100kg) – 2.1
- 240lb (109kg) – 2.2
- 260lb (117kg)– 2.3

5ft 10in (1.75m)
- 120lb (55kg) – 1.7
- 140lb (64kg) – 1.8
- 160lb (73kg) – 1.9
- 180lb (82kg) – 2.0
- 200lb (91kg) – 2.1
- 220lb (100kg) – 2.2
- 240lb (109kg) – 2.3
- 260lb (117kg) – 2.3
- 280lb (127kg) – 2.4

6ft 0in (1.8m)
- 120lb (55kg) – 1.7
- 140lb (64kg) – 1.8
- 160lb (73kg) – 1.9
- 180lb (82kg) – 2.0
- 200lb (91kg) – 2.1
- 220lb (100kg) – 2.2
- 240lb (109kg) – 2.3
- 260lb (117kg) – 2.4
- 280lb (127kg) – 2.5

6ft 2in (1.85m)
- 140lb (64kg) – 1.8
- 160lb (73kg) – 1.9
- 180lb (82kg) – 2.0
- 200lb (91kg) – 2.1
- 220lb (100kg) – 2.2
- 240lb (109kg) – 2.3
- 260lb (117kg) – 2.4
- 280lb (127kg) – 2.5
- 300lb (136kg) – 2.6

6ft 4in (1.9m)
- 160lb (73kg) – 2.0
- 180lb (82kg) – 2.1
- 200lb (91kg) – 2.2
- 220lb (100kg) – 2.3
- 240lb (109kg) – 2.4
- 260lb (117kg) – 2.5
- 280lb (127kg) – 2.6
- 300lb (136kg) – 2.6
- 320lb (145kg) – 2.7

Example of a woman with a BMR of 1,512 and a PAL of 1.3.

9 hours in bed (567 cals); 8 hours sitting at work (672 cals); 3 hours sitting at home, reading, eating (216 cals); I hour standing on train (108 cals); 30 minutes slow walking to commute (78 cals); I hour light gardening (132 cals); 1½ hours cooking, washing, dressing (189 cals). Total calories burnt = 1,962.

PAL (total cals divided by BMR) = 1.3.

Example of a man with a BMR of 1,750 and a PAL of 1.7.

8 hours in bed (583 cals); at work, 6 hours sitting and 2 hours standing (912 cals); 2 hours commuting (200 cals); half-hour jogging (274 cals); 3 hours sitting at home watching TV, etc. (263 cals); 2 hours heavy gardening (657 cals); 30 minutes dressing, etc. (90 cals). Total calories burnt = 2,979.

PAL (total cals divided by BMR) = 1.7.

NOTES

■ You can get an even more accurate assessment of BMR if you know your body fat composition (see Q30 and Body Fat Monitors in the A–Z), and therefore your fat-free mass (total body weight minus weight of fat). The formula is BMR = (21.6 x fat-free mass in kg) plus 370.

■ To work out a more accurate assessment of how many calories you burn in your own daily activities, turn to Feature 28.

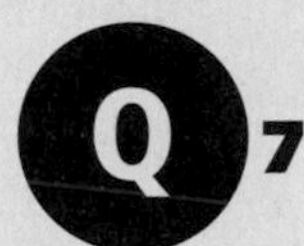

Q7

Could my weight be due to faulty genes?

The wide-ranging report on obesity published in 2000 by the World Health Organization concluded that 'while it is possible that single or multiple gene effects may cause overweight and obesity directly, and indeed do so in some individuals, this does not appear to be the case in the majority of people'.

However, the consensus of expert opinion is that your genes can have at least some influence on your susceptibility to be overweight. An overview of all the studies on the genetic influence suggests that 25–40% of cases of obesity have a hereditary factor and that intra-abdominal fat appears to have a genetic link of up to 60%. One study of twins concluded that 60% of body fat is determined by genetics.

If one of your parents is overweight, you may have inherited that parent's 'fat genes'. If both your parents are overweight, it may be that you are very unlucky and they both have faulty fat genes – but it is probably more likely that, as a family, you eat too many calories and don't take enough exercise to maintain energy balance. As one US researcher remarked, the human gene pool cannot possibly have altered so much in the last 30 years to account for the vast rise in the incidence of obesity; and, as another researcher remarks, 'You don't get fat in a famine.' Whatever the reasons, one estimate is that a child with two fat parents has a 70% chance of growing up obese.

Even if you have inherited a tendency to put on weight, it doesn't mean that you cannot lose weight or maintain a reasonable weight but that, for example, you may be more likely than someone without 'fat genes' to put on weight, given the same amount of food.

A few specific examples of how your genes may influence your weight:

- By giving you a BMR lower than average.
- By giving you a high percentage of body fat and a low percentage of lean tissue (muscle), which would predispose you to needing fewer calories than average for your height and weight.
- By giving you a larger than average appetite (see Q23).
- By giving you a blunted thermic response to food, meaning that your dietary-induced thermogenesis will be lower than average, causing a higher number of calories to be stored rather than burnt.

Research is being carried out in all these areas and, in future, it may be possible to reprogramme gene defects so that such people don't get fat. Meanwhile, the message is that by maintaining a suitable energy balance (calories in versus calories out), the majority of people can maintain a reasonable body weight.

See also:

- Questions: 22–3, 41.
- Feature: 4
- A–Z entries: Eat Right 4 Your Type, Metabolism Booster Diets.
- Key index entries: appetite, dietary-induced thermogenesis, genes, hormones, intra-abdominal fat.

DIET MYTH

'My genes are making me fat.'

Everyone is dealt a particular pack of genetic cards – but it is up to you how you play them. Some people's genes do seem to predispose them to overweight – but still a reasonable weight can be maintained with care.

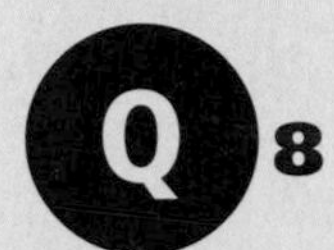

Q8

Are there any other influences on body weight?

The body processes that regulate weight are many and diverse, and orchestrated by our hormones. As US obesity specialist Jules Hirsch wrote in the *British Medical Journal*, 'The balance of food intake and energy expenditure that maintains constant energy storage is determined by the metabolism of muscle, liver, pancreas and intestine. The balance is regulated by the adrenal and sex steroids as well as adipose tissue itself, which together create a complex set of signals ... affecting energy dissipation and food intake. Hovering over this complex system are potent psychosocial and behavioural factors.' He concludes by remarking on the 'incredible intricacy and complexity of the system that maintains a fixed level of energy storage'.

So your answer is yes, there are other influences – and researchers are only really beginning to unravel the whole complicated system! However, you needn't worry about it too much. All you really need to know is whether or not you are managing your own energy balance successfully enough to maintain a reasonable weight.

See also:

- Questions: 1–7, 9–40, 333, 357.
- Feature: 2
- Key index entries: energy, hormones, metabolism.

FAT FACT

A few ethnic groups seem particularly prone to gain weight, especially when faced with a Western diet and lifestyle. For example, South Asians are more susceptible to intro-abdominal fat than the average.

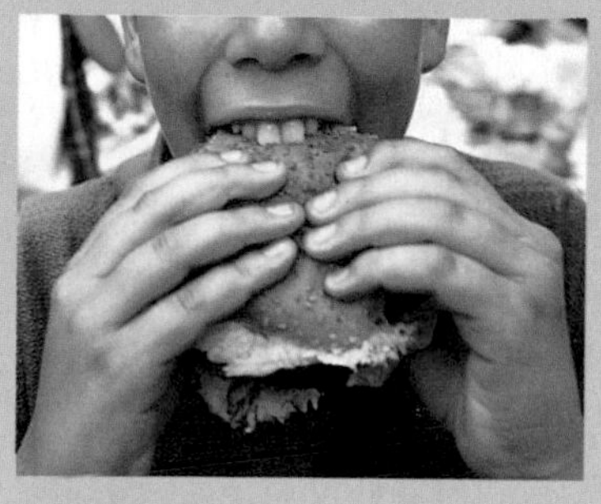

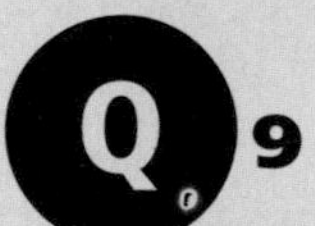

Is it true that everyone's weight has a natural 'set point'?

The set point theory says that your body has a natural 'correct' weight which it tries hard to keep, even against the odds. For example, if you think you're overweight but your body thinks it is happy with its weight, if you try to diet below it your body will do all it can to revert back to the set point. This would explain why 95% of slimmers put their weight back on again – because the weight they've been aiming for is too low for their personal metabolism to maintain.

Sadly, the 'set point' falls down somewhat if you apply it in reverse – i.e., if you pile on pounds through overeating, the body doesn't seem so keen to return to a lower weight, with the result that most of us tend to gain weight gradually as we age. (Proponents argue that the set point resets itself upwards as we age.)

Research confirms that, in the majority of people, the body probably exerts a stronger defence against a low calorie intake and weight loss than it does against a high calorie intake and weight gain: i.e., it protects stored body fat to some degree. Drastic restriction of calories can suppress the metabolic rate by up to 45%, and it is thought this mechanism evolved as a defence against starvation.

However, the set point theory IS still a debated theory rather than a concrete fact and, even if it is confirmed, the consensus of opinion is that regular exercise can alter it by increasing lean tissue, raising BMR and facilitating fat breakdown.

See also:

- Questions: 3–8, 10–40.
- Features: 1, 2.
- A-Z entry: Metabolism Booster Diets.
- Key index entries: BMR, metabolism, weight and ageing.

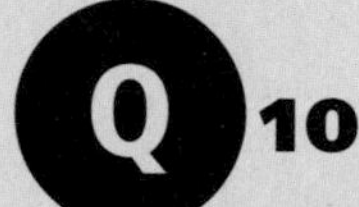

Is weight fluctuation throughout life normal?

There are not many people who stay at exactly the same weight throughout their adult lives, so yes, fluctuation is normal rather than the exception. Weight can be lost through illness, by loss of appetite, through reduced food intake at busy times or through periods of increased activity, for example. Weight may increase due to other sets of circumstances, such as holidays, celebrations and so on.

Apart from these periodic – and usually short-lived – changes, which shouldn't concern you unduly, the average pattern of weight gain and loss is as follows: weight tends to be lowest during the teens and early 20s, when calorie needs are greatest, then static in the later 20s and early 30s, gradually increasing in middle age up until around 65, when many people slowly begin to lose weight again into old age. This is an average pattern – which means you don't have to follow it.

See also:

- Questions: 6–9; 11–28, 72.
- Feature: 2.
- Key index entries: energy equation, weight and ageing.

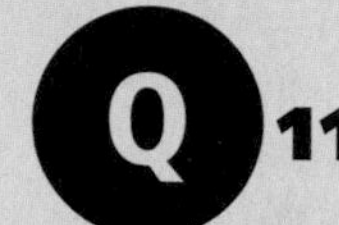

Are there any foods or drinks that can increase my metabolic rate?

Yes, there are several foods and drinks that appear to increase the metabolic rate.

Protein foods have a higher than average dietary thermogenic effect – as we saw in Q3, eating food produces heat, which equals calorie usage of around 10% of total energy expenditure. The effect of eating pure protein, however, produces a higher thermogenic effect – up to 25% of such a meal's calories may be burnt off due to thermogenesis.

In theory, this means that a diet consisting of high levels of protein would result in considerable speeding up of the metabolism. In practice, however, this isn't such a good idea, as a high-protein diet can stress the kidneys and liver, is linked with loss of bone calcium and may also be linked to higher blood pressure levels. In addition, high-protein eating is not a balanced diet and therefore nutrients present in other food groups may be in shortfall.

Some protein foods – particularly red meat and dairy produce – contain a fatty acid called conjugated linoleic acid (CLA), which has been shown to increase lean tissue in the body and may therefore increase metabolic rate. Detailed information about CLA appears in the A–Z.

Spices, particularly chilli, appear to raise the metabolic rate by up to 50%–

an effect that lasts for up to three hours after the spice-rich meal. This appears to be because the heart rate increases when spices are eaten. Several clinical research studies have found evidence of this effect. Spices are also good for the health in a variety of ways, so this is one metabolism-boosting trick you can use without guilt.

Caffeine-containing drinks increase the metabolism by arousing the nervous system's flight response and levels of adrenaline (epinephrine), increasing heart rate and 'fidget factor'. Caffeine equivalent to 2.5 cups of coffee can also increase endurance during moderate exercise. Coffee and colas are two of the drinks highest in caffeine. However, more than three or four cups of high-caffeine coffee a day is not recommended, because of possible adverse effects on health. Caffeine is also found in chocolate, tea and a range of manufactured drinks, including some sports drinks.

Interestingly, green tea also appears to stimulate the metabolism without increasing the heart rate. A Swiss study found that people who took extract of green tea burned significantly more calories than people who didn't. The phytochemical flavonoids in green tea seem to affect the 'energy' hormone noradrenaline (norepinephrine) in the body, which then speeds the process of fat oxidation.

If you have an iodine deficiency which may result in poor functioning of your thyroid gland, production of the hormone thyroxine may be low. This may lower your metabolic rate, and a diet rich in seagreens such as dulse, kombu or wakame, seafood and milk can raise your iodine levels and improve thyroid function and metabolism. If your thyroid function is normal, however, these foods won't help. (A blood test via your doctor can easily check whether your thyroid function is normal or not.)

See also:

- Questions: 12, 14–15, 79–90.
- Features: 2, 9.
- A–Z entries: caffeine, CLA,
- Key index entries: high-protein diets. iodine, metabolic rate, seagreens, thyroid.

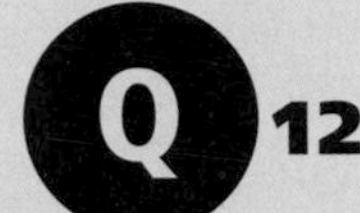

12

What supplements can I take to speed up my metabolism?

CLA capsules (explained in detail in the A–Z and also mentioned in the previous question) appear to increase the metabolic rate by increasing lean tissue. As far as we know, they are perfectly safe to take although quite expensive.

If your levels of body iodine are low, your thyroid function may be impaired, which can, in turn, reduce metabolic rate, and you may benefit from iodine-rich supplements such as kelp (or there are several multi-ingredient, so-called thyroid-boosting supplements available, which may include l-tyrosine, an amino acid that helps produce thyroxine). If you are not deficient, however, these supplements won't boost thyroid function, and dosing yourself without knowing whether or not you are deficient is probably unwise, as overdosing can be toxic and can actually suppress thyroid function (see Q17 for more on the thyroid and the A–Z for more on herbal diet supplements).

Supplements of DHEA (dehydroepiandrosterone), a naturally occurring steroid hormone, are said, among other things, to increase lean tissue and reduce body fat; however, you should be cautious about taking these. DHEA is present in the body in quantity at adolescence, and levels diminish over time after the age of 30. There have been concerns over its long-term safety and for many people benefits may be small or non-existent, unless a blood test shows you are deficient. In the UK, it is available on prescription only, but in the USA it is sold as a food supplement.

One recent trial published in the *International Journal of Obesity* found that supplements of a Chinese herbal preparation, Ma Huang (containing a natural form of the stimulant ephedrine), worked to help volunteers lose weight without strict dieting and the researchers concluded that this herbal supplement had a less adverse effect on the blood pressure than the new prescription slimming drug sibutramine (Reductil).

Other supplements used as aids to slimming – amino acids including L-carnitine, caffeine (including guarana), chromium, co-enzyme Q10, creatine and Ma Huang – are discussed in the A–Z.

See also:

- Question: 11, 37.
- A-Z entries: caffeine, chromium, CLA, co-enzyme Q10, herbal diet supplements, sports supplements.
- Key index entries: amino acids, iodine, lean tissue, metabolic rate, supplements.

13

Is there a foolproof formula for speeding up my metabolic rate?

Yes – increase the amount of regular exercise that you do, so that you move up to a higher PAL level (see Feature 1). Recent North American research clearly demonstrated that high-intensity (i.e., hard!) exercise raised the heart rate, metabolic rate and energy expenditure for several hours. However, ideal exercise should include not just aerobic work to increase calorie and fat burning but also strength work to increase the amount of lean tissue in your body. For every extra pound of muscle that you can put on, your body uses an extra 50 or so calories a day. A recent study found that regular weight training boosts your BMR by about 15%.

See also:

- Questions: 6, 11–17, 333, 343, 350, 357–8.
- Features: 1, 2, 28, 29, 30.
- A–Z entries: exercise classes, exercise equipment, gyms, running, weighted workouts.
- Key index entries: aerobics, BMR, exercise.

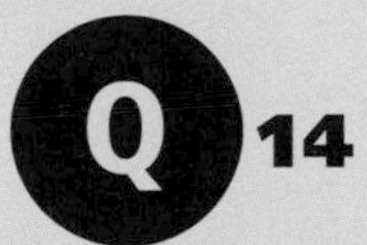

Q 14

Do emotional or psychological factors affect how I metabolize food?

It is well known that emotional factors influence our hormones, and vice versa. For example, one well-known hormone, adrenaline (epinephrine), is released when we are frightened, anxious or excited. Adrenaline speeds up metabolic rate.

If you are a very laid-back contented person, with little excitement in your life, you probably have fewer bursts of adrenaline (epinephrine) release and this could in theory predispose you to weight gain. All the slim and relaxed people in the world will disagree here, of course. Stress may make you more 'fidgety' and it has been shown that fidgeting can burn up many hundreds of calories in a day.

However, long-term, stress can also make you fat! The adrenal hormone cortisol, released when you're stressed, can increase fat storage in the abdominal area as, it seems, the deep fat in the stomach contains receptors that the cortisol prefers. Also, a surfeit of stress triggers cortisol to boost blood sugar levels (in preparation for 'fight or flight') which, if not used, are converted by insulin into fat for storage.

See also:

- Questions: 16, 22–3, 161–2.
- Feature: 2.
- Key index entries: adrenaline (epinephrine), blood-sugar levels, hormones, insulin, intra-abdominal fat.

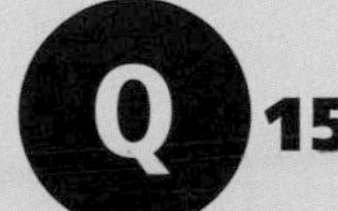

Q 15

Does how or when I eat – rather than what I eat – affect my metabolism?

There is support for the theory that consumption of small, regular meals will keeps your metabolism ticking over well and is a much better way to burn off the calories than, for example, one meal a day. Levels of the thyroid hormones that control your metabolic rate begin to drop within hours of your last meal – probably in response to the prospect of starvation (which was a likelihood when humans first evolved). Also, the thermogenic effect of dividing your calorie intake up over several meals might be slightly higher than if you have them all at one sitting.

One recent study done for the International Obesity Task Force found that obese people had a better chance of losing weight by eating little and often than by eating larger, less frequent meals. Another study concluded that an infrequent meal pattern is associated with a tendency towards obesity. Despite the fact that yet another study found that there was no difference in the metabolic rates of people who ate in a variety of different patterns, for most people I believe it is worth trying the 'little and often' method as other benefits are to be gained – hunger is better controlled and there may be less inclination to binge if meals are regular.

Eating in the hour or two after vigorous exercise may encourage the metabolism of food rather than its laying down as fat, as the metabolic rate is generally speeded up during this time. Similarly, moderate exercise (e.g. a walk) after eating may increase the body's natural thermogenic response to food and burn more calories.

It seems that there is good reason to eat slowly, though – one 2000 study in America found that obese people eat faster than slim people and have a greater tendency to central fat distribution (intra-abdominal fat).

There is no convincing evidence that eating food at any particular time of day (e.g. early in the morning) rather than at another time of day (e.g. in the evening) speeds up your metabolism, or for the idea that you should eat nothing except fruit before noon every day, which is a creed of Fit for Life and food combining.

See also:

- Questions: 14, 21, 23, 32, 36, 77, 87, 96–7, 100.
- Feature: 2.
- A–Z entries: Body-clock Diet, Fit for Life, food combining.
- Key index entries: BMR, eating patterns.

FAT FACT

US research confirms that people who fidget are more likely to be slim than people who don't.

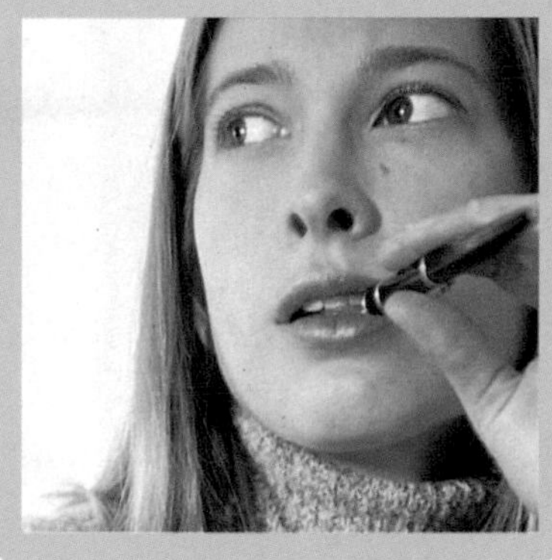

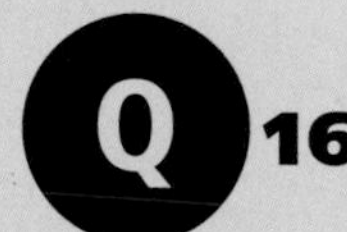

Q 16

Can illness affect my metabolism?

There are a few illnesses associated with weight gain. Diseases of the thyroid and/or pituitary gland, which control metabolism, can cause quite severe weight gain. Such diseases include hypothyroidism and thyroiditis. Tumours of the adrenal or pituitary glands may cause Cushing's disease, when overproduction of corticosteroids causes facial and abdominal weight gain amongst other symptoms. Corticosteroids given to treat a variety of medical conditions, including rheumatoid arthritis, may cause Cushing's syndrome.

Severe depression may also lower the metabolic rate, and indeed, some drugs (tricyclic) used to treat depression can also do so. Many types of long-term illness or incapacity may lower the metabolic rate, because such conditions often predispose to bed rest and/or lack of physical activity, which will reduce the body's lean tissue (muscle) and cause a corresponding drop in metabolic rate. Also, fewer calories are burnt up in activity, which will also cause weight gain if dietary calories aren't reduced.

Temporarily, high fever will raise the metabolic rate, as for every degree Celsius that the body temperature rises, there is a 10% rise in metabolic rate. In the later stages of cancer, rapid weight loss not accounted for by reduction in food intake is often present, and a raised metabolism may be the answer.

Several prescription drugs may cause weight gain – these include those already mentioned, plus sulphonylureas for non-insulin-dependent diabetes, beta-blockers for high blood pressure, cyproheptadines for allergies and hay fever, valproic acid and neuroleptics for epilepsy, phenothiazines for psychosis, pixotifen for migraine, and steroid-based contraceptives.

If you think that your weight gain may be due to illness or any drugs you are taking, you should talk to your doctor about this.

See also:

- Questions: 17, 20.
- Key index entries: glands, health and weight, illness, metabolic rate.

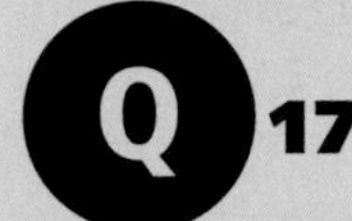

Q 17

Could my weight problem be due to 'sluggish glands'?

As we've seen in the answers to questions 8, 11 and 12, any malfunction of the thyroid glands, which help regulate metabolism, can cause weight gain if either of two hormones produced by these glands – thyroxine or T3 (triiodothyronine) – is insufficient. This is termed hypothyroidism. (Another dysfunction, hyperthyroidism, produces too much hormone and weight may then be lost due to this.)

This can come about in a variety of ways: if mild it may be corrected by increasing your intake of iodine, which is vital in the production of the thyroid hormones; if more severe, you may need artificial thyroid drugs.

If you think you have a thyroid problem (other symptoms may include cold hands and feet, feeling sluggish and lacking in energy, constipation, dry skin) you should talk to your doctor, who can arrange a blood test. If this is the problem and it is corrected, surplus weight should gradually go and your metabolic rate fairly quickly be restored to normal.

Problems with the adrenal glands may possibly also contribute to weight problems. Some specialists say that, with a permanently stressed life, these glands – which produce the stress hormones epinephrine (adrenaline) and norepinephrine (noradrenaline), and cortisol – get 'exhausted' and this can set off a chain of events that may produce weight gain. Again, you need to see your doctor if you have long-term stress and have gained weight disproportionately to the amount you eat.

By the way, interestingly, some foods seem to suppress the action of the thyroid – these are particularly soya beans and soya products, and also members of the brassica family including cabbage, cauliflower, spinach and Brussels sprouts.

Lastly, it is estimated that of all cases of obesity, only a maximum of 3% are actually caused by underactive thyroid, so don't be too surprised if this isn't your problem.

See also:

- Questions: 8, 11–12, 14, 16.
- A–Z entries: herbal diet supplements.
- Key index entries: adrenals, metabolic rate, stress, thyroid.

FAT FACT

Extreme temperatures – either very hot or very cold – can increase the metabolic rate by up to 20%.

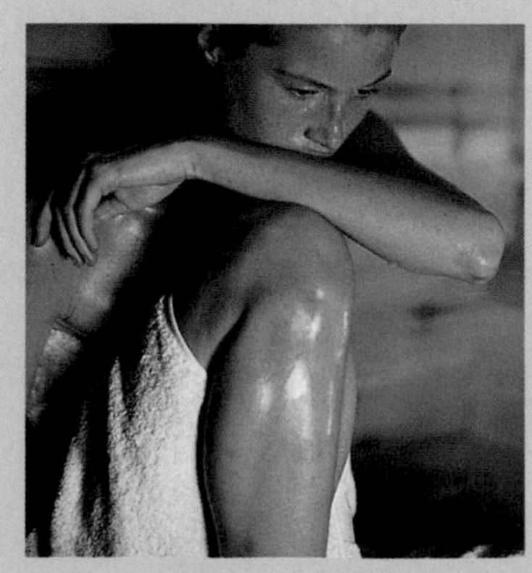

Q 18

What does 'the energy equation' mean?

The energy equation, or energy balance equation, is a way of expressing how your body balances its intake of energy (calories) with its expenditure of energy (calories).

The equation is thus:
Change in stored energy = energy intake – (minus) energy expenditure.
All this means is that:
- If energy intake equals energy expenditure then there will be no change in stored energy (body weight).
- If energy intake exceeds energy expenditure, then there will be an increase in stored energy (body weight gain). This is called a positive energy balance.
- If energy expenditure exceeds energy intake, then there will be a decrease in stored energy (body weight loss). This is called a negative energy balance.

Theoretically, weight gain or loss can be measured like this:
- 3,500 calories ingested in excess of energy expenditure means a 1lb (450g) weight gain.
- 3,500 calories burnt in energy expenditure in excess of energy intake means a 1lb (450g) weight loss.

As the body converts all surplus food (be it fat, carbohydrate or protein) to body fat, for 'stored energy' read 'fat'. Paradoxically, however, when weight is lost by creating a negative energy balance, some of the weight lost is lean tissue. Water losses and gains are not taken account of in the energy equation, as water is not stored energy (it is calorie-free).

In practice, due to other metabolic factors in humans, 3,500 calories burnt or eaten do not always equal 1lb (450g) of weight lost or gained. However, it is a reasonable blueprint and one upon which all weight-changing regimes rely.

See also:
- Questions: 19–20, 24.
- Key index entries: calories, energy, weight.

Q 19

If I eat more calories than I use up, how quickly will I put on weight?

Going back to the previous answer, eating 3,500 calories over and above that needed by the body to maintain its current weight will result in a gain of 1lb (450g). (To find out how many calories your body needs to maintain its current weight, you need to go back to Feature 1 – assessing your own metabolic rate.)

Example:
Your basal metabolic rate (BMR) is 1,512. Your PAL is 1.6. Therefore you need around 2,419 calories a day to maintain present weight.

If you eat 500 calories a day more than this every day for one week, without making any other changes, you will be giving your body 3,500 more calories than it needs (500 x 7 = 3,500), and you will, in theory, put on 1lb (450g) in weight.

So you see, it all depends on how much more you eat than you need. You would have a real job to put on 1lb a day because to eat an extra 3,500 calories a day on top of your normal needs would be quite hard. Not to say expensive. This gives the lie to people who say they put on half a stone when they go out for a meal. What really happens in this case is that much of the weight gained 'overnight' is in fact fluid retained by a meal high in carbohydrates and sodium. Most people generally overeat only slightly and thus put on weight very gradually.

See also:
- Questions: 18, 22, 24.
- Feature: 1
- Key index entries: BMR, calories, fluid retention.

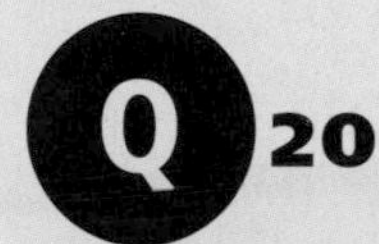

Q 20

Is it possible to put on weight without eating more?

Yes, it certainly is. A positive energy balance (weight gain, see Q18) can be achieved not just by increasing your energy input (eating more) but also by decreasing your energy output (doing less physical activity). Anyone who has been an active sportsperson and then gives up and puts on weight knows only too well the truth of this. As an example, if you give up one hour a day of, say, walking to and from work, but continue to eat in the same way, you would be expending about 200 calories a day less, which would equal 1,400 calories expenditure less a week – leading to a weight gain of about 1lb in 2½ weeks! And they say exercise doesn't help you lose weight!

Although reduced physical activity is the main cause of weight gain other than overeating, other variables may also be at play. For example, as you get older your metabolism slows down slightly, all other factors being equal, so that would cause a slow weight gain. Illness, depression, drugs and other factors may also be involved in any unexplained weight gain. If you feel you're gaining weight without a good reason, then do talk to your doctor.

See also:
- Questions: 16–18, 22, 24, 27.
- Features: 1, 2, 29.
- Key index entries: calories, hormones, metabolism, thyroid.

A day in the life of your metabolism

By altering your behaviour in small ways throughout the day, and paying attention to your natural body rhythms, you can increase your metabolic rate and calorie burn-up considerably, as well as lowering the total amount of calories eaten.

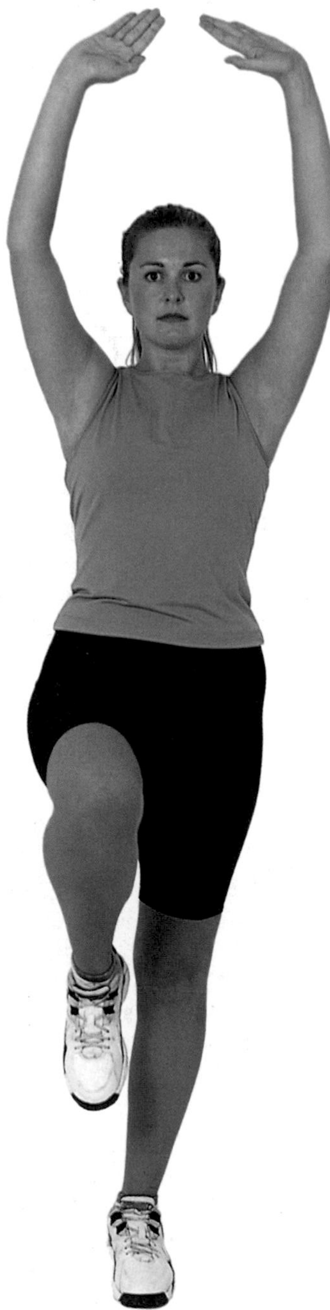

7am
Get up! Getting up an hour earlier than usual every day can burn off many extra calories, depending upon how you spend the time. Light household chores use up 2.2 times your basal metabolic rate (average extra 75 calories burnt on top of BMR per hour).

7.05am
Stand at an open window and breathe in deeply for a minute or two. This helps to waken your body and kick-start your metabolism.

8.00am
Have breakfast – a light meal including some protein, carbohydrate and fat (e.g. wholegrain cereal, semi-skimmed milk and some seeds) – the ideal combination to avoid hunger pangs later in the morning. A cup of coffee with your breakfast will increase alertness and boost metabolism. Don't rush your food – eat it slowly.

8.30am
Take 20–30 minutes light aerobic (cardiovascular) exercise (e.g. exercise bike, step video, or walk to work or the shops). This will help convert the carbohydrate in your breakfast to glycogen for your muscle stores and will give your metabolic rate, adrenaline (epinephrine) levels and mental alertness a boost as well as using about 3.5 times the calories of your normal BMR (average extra calories burnt up in 30 minutes = 55).

10am
Stand up as much as possible throughout the day if you have a sedentary job – e.g. when talking on the phone or to people. For every hour of standing rather than sitting, you can use up an extra 50 or so calories, depending on your BMR. Fidgeting, rather than sitting completely still, will also help to burn up calories so stretch, move your legs, wave your arms about!

11am
Take a 10-minute break and walk around or up and down stairs. Get some fresh air and eat a small healthy snack (e.g. an apple). The snack will help stave off hunger before lunch and increase your metabolic rate slightly.

12.45pm
Relax a little to prepare your digestive system for lunch – it will absorb food better if you are not tense. If at work, make easy phone calls or read mail.

1.00pm
Have a fairly high-protein lunch (chicken, meat, fish, pulses) between 1 and 2pm.

Protein raises the metabolic rate and there is some evidence that a high-protein, low-carb lunch will avoid the post-lunch tiredness slump that many people experience. Don't skip lunch – research shows if you eat now you tend to eat a healthier lunch than if you eat later, say at 3pm. A lunch will also help you avoid bingeing on sweet foods later.

Take time over eating your lunch – fast eating is linked with fat bellies!

1.30pm

Take 20–30 minutes of light aerobic exercise (e.g. a walk at a good pace). Research shows that the metabolism-boosting effect of eating is increased with exercise.

4pm

Have a small healthy snack, e.g. a pot of natural yoghurt or some dried apricots (see 11am).

5 or 6pm

Visit the gym. Research shows that for most people, this is the best time to work out, when muscle and core body temperature is at its highest and endurance levels are at their peak. Incorporate plenty of weight training, as 3–5 weight sessions a week, including up to 30 reps exercising all the major muscle groups, can increase metabolic rate by up to 15% over time.

7–8pm

Have your evening meal, including carbohydrates, protein and fat. Leaving it much later than this will make you inclined to eat more or binge on fatty, salty or sweet foods before your meal is ready. Begin to relax and wind down.

9pm

A session of easy yoga or stretching will help the body to de-stress and relax in preparation for bed, as your levels of adrenaline lower.

10–11pm

The best time to go to bed, as the body increases its output of melatonin, body temperature begins to drop and metabolic rate slows. As you sleep, lung function and breathing slow. Exercising when your body clock says it's time for sleep is counterproductive.

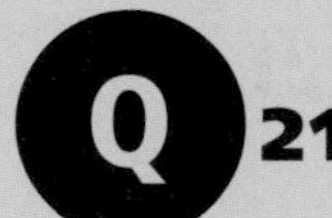

21

Why do I never lose weight even though I hardly eat a thing?

There could be several reasons. Firstly, you may already be at a reasonable body weight – people come in all shapes and sizes, largely governed by genetic make-up, and there is a wide range of weights within which you are still 'average'. If your genetics say you are your natural weight at, let's say, 10 stone, then you will find it hard to slim down to 8½. Maybe you are already thin – and then, of course, getting even thinner will be harder. So Rule 1 – aim for a reasonable weight. Check out your BMI in Feature 3.

If you really are overweight – but not obese – it could be your metabolic rate is lower than it could be, because you don't take enough exercise and have a small proportion of lean tissue (muscle), which would increase your metabolic rate – as we age, these problems may become more acute. Your metabolic rate may be genetically slower than average, for which there are dozens of causes being discovered and this is another reason to aim for a reasonable, not low, weight. As we age, our metabolic rate tends to slow (see Q27) and the WHO says menopause reduces the metabolic rate slightly.

If none of these seem to be your problem, it may be you're taking in more calories than you think you are. All the studies I can find that have tested slimmers under controlled scientific conditions, measuring actual calorie intake with their reported intake, have shown intake is underestimated by 12–25%. For example, one study published in 2000 by the *International Journal of Obesity* showed intake of the participants averaged 1,888 calories, but their reports averaged 1,576 – a difference of 16.5%. The worst 'guessers' underestimated by over 50%!

People tend to underestimate portion sizes, forget to count calories in drinks or foods nibbled while preparing meals, etc. Try measuring your food intake and keeping a food diary for a week or two, and see if this could be the case. You also need to be sure that you are creating a sufficient energy deficit to lose weight.

See also:

- Questions: 4, 22, 27–8, 104, 230, 333–8.
- Features: 1, 2, 3, 29, 30.
- A–Z entry: exercise classes.
- Key index entries: exercise, lean tissue, metabolism.

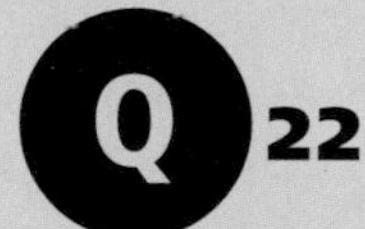

22

Why do some people eat a lot more than me and yet stay slim?

Your weight is basically controlled by the 'energy equation' (see Q18), which, in simple terms, means that to maintain your weight (be it slim, normal or overweight) you need, over a period of time, to balance your energy intake via your food and drink with the energy you expend. How much you can eat and drink without putting on weight depends on your metabolic rate – the rate at which you burn up calories, and this can vary tremendously from individual to individual. Some will have a high metabolic rate – for example, burning 3,500 cals/day (and be able to eat more without putting on weight) and others will have a slow one – for example, burning only 1,700 cals/day (and have to eat less to stay slim). Most of the previous questions in this section have explained variations in metabolic rate in more detail.

One interesting theory, shown in at least two studies, is that people who tend to put on weight easily have a blunted thermal response to eating. In some individuals, dietary induced thermogenesis (see Q3) can account for a rise in metabolic rate of 30% or so after eating, but in some fat people the rate is nearer 5%. This would mean that weight gain would be much more likely in the latter group and would vindicate at least some overweight people who claim they hardly eat a thing compared with others.

However, as we've seen, there is a lot you can do to alter your own metabolic rate. If it is naturally lower than average, however, you may never be skinny without resorting to unhealthy means.

It's also worth pointing out here that some research has shown that many thin people who seem to be eating a lot do actually eat less than overweight people – preferring low-fat salads, fruit and seafood, say, to chips, cheese and pork. They may be eating all the time, but are taking in a lot less calories than you would think. They may also burn up more calories through activity and 'fidgeting'. One test showed that 'fidgeting' helps to burn up to 800 calories daily. So it is by no means ALL a matter of genetics and metabolism.

See also:

- Questions: 3–21; 27.
- Features: 1, 2.
- Key index entries: dietary thermogenesis; genes, metabolism.

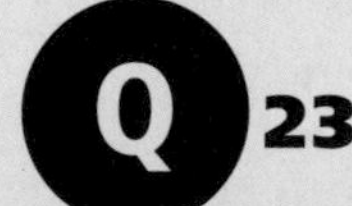

23

What causes a big appetite and can it be controlled?

Appetite – or hunger – is a basic survival mechanism controlled in the body by the hypothalamus, which ensures that we take in sustenance and thus stay alive. Many experts believe that a big appetite is a natural reminder of the not-too-distant past (in anthropological terms) when food was not easy to come by. When we did find it, we ate all we could as insurance against starvation – surplus stored as body fat would normally be used up for energy before the next meal became available. These days, of course, food is so plentiful in the West that we never get a chance to use our stored fat. However, appetite mechanisms haven't quite caught up with that yet.

That is one explanation. Other factors are also involved. One study on rodents showed they ate much more when given a choice of a variety of foods than when given a restricted range – the 'cafeteria effect'. No doubt many of us do the same – a good example is revival of 'appetite' after a savoury meal, when pudding appears – suddenly we're 'hungry' again! Anything new also has a similar effect. Food manufacturers exploit the 'new' and '50 varieties' themes to make us buy more.

You may also experience increased appetite when eating your special favourite foods. Habitual eating – eating a certain thing at a certain time – is also often mistaken for true appetite.

High levels of physical activity seem to increase the appetite in lean people – which is necessary to restore the energy balance – but in obese people who exercise this is not usually the case.

In women, appetite increases naturally via hormonal messages during latter pregnancy and in the pre-menstrual phase. Seasonal affective disorder (SAD) may also increase the appetite for carbohydrates, which help production of the 'happy' neurotransmitter, serotonin.

In fact, scientists are just beginning to unravel the chemicals, proteins and hormones in our bodies that can affect appetite and therefore weight. For over 10 years, they have known about the hormone leptin, a product of the 'ob' obesity gene. In rodents, lack of leptin increases appetite, but in humans leptin deficiency is rare – so giving extra leptin to obese people will rarely work. Indeed, obese people normally have high levels of leptin, as they have more adipose tissue than slim people, and the hormone is stored in body fat. However, it may be that obese people are resistant to leptin (as many are to insulin) and this may affect appetite and result in weight gain.

Meanwhile, there is interesting research on the body chemical dopamine, which, together with the other neurotransmitters, including serotonin and norepinephrine (noradrenaline), helps to regulate appetite and is linked with the 'pleasure factor' we find in food. Available dopamine seems to be reduced in people who are obese and who are compulsive eaters.

Perhaps in the future there will be drugs based on leptin and/or dopamine to help beat overeating. Meanwhile, scientists have found that exercise helps increase the body's sensitivity to both.

So what can be done about a big appetite that's making you overeat? Plenty. Research shows that eating slowly can help to moderate appetite, because the brain takes about 10 minutes to register full feelings – and a recent study showed that fast eating is linked with fat-bellied people! Fatty, sugary foods are worst, because they are eaten quicker than other foods.

Eating more frequently can also help control appetite by regulating blood sugar, and it's best if small frequent meals contain low Glycaemic Index foods (see Q84). Appetite may also be blunted by drinking a large glass of water before eating.

Appetite can be controlled by certain drugs currently available on prescription (see Q37) and some herbal diet supplements. At least three other appetite-controlling factors have been discovered – the nueropeptide GLP-1, the hormone orexin and the compound C75 – but research on these is still at an early stage.

See also:

- Questions: 36–7, 39, 79, 84, 89, 96, 129, 136, 138, 170, 201.
- Features: 9, 10, 12, 13.
- A–Z entries: herbal diet supplements, Overeaters Anonymous, slimming pills.
- Key index entries: appetite, eating habits, hunger.

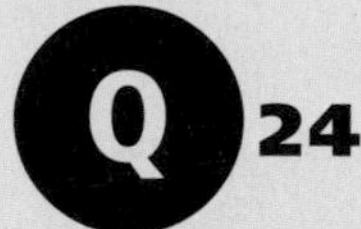

24

Why is weight easier to gain than lose?

This isn't true for all people – a surprisingly high number of adults find it very hard to put ON any weight, but admittedly the problem is more common in reverse. What appears to happen is that when you reduce calorie intake to produce a negative calorie balance, your body recognizes what is going on and, as a protection against starvation, reduces your metabolic rate to compensate. (If you read the answer to Q9, you will also see that there may be a 'set point' factor involved here too.) The reduced metabolic rate also makes sense because, after you've been losing weight for a while, your body weighs less and so will naturally have a lower BMR. (See Q6 and Feature 1.) And after crash-dieting, the body loses a proportionately high amount of lean tissue (muscle), which can also reduce the metabolic rate.

When a negative-energy diet (fewer calories eaten than expended) is followed, the normal pattern is that the body at first loses weight at the rate that would be expected (i.e., 1lb/450g weight lost for every 3,500 calories' deficit). Soon, though, weight loss slows down because the metabolic rate is slowing. Thus it seems harder to lose weight than it should be. The answer is to increase energy expenditure and lean muscle mass as discussed and perhaps (but not always) reduce calorie intake even more.

Regarding how easy it is to put ON weight, it sometimes seems that pounds come on overnight, but this is hardly the case. What happens is that if you suddenly eat a lot after a period of slimming, the body will retain more fluid and it is that extra fluid (often 3–5lb/1–2kg after a heavy meal) rather than body fat you've gained. Even a total blow-out meal would be unlikely to put on more than a pound of fat.

There are also psychological factors at work. It is easier to practise self-indulgence than self-denial. As long as you feel 'eating is nice' and 'dieting is horrid', you'll find it hard to lose weight and keep it off.

See also:

- Questions: 6, 9, 18, 20–3, 32–4, 39–40, 123–31.
- Features: 1, 2, 10, 11–15.
- A–Z entry: slimming clubs.
- Key index entries: eating habits, metabolic rate, set point theory.

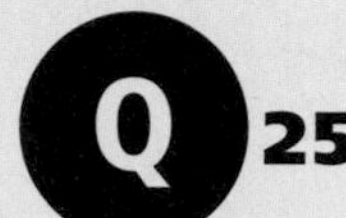

25

How can I put on weight if I am too thin?

Between 5 and 10% of the population are underweight or severely underweight and, for many of them, this is as perplexing as being overweight is for others. A fast genetically influenced metabolic rate plus, perhaps, a busy lifestyle and a penchant for exercise or 'fidgeting' can contribute. Illness, drugs, smoking – even a high caffeine intake – can all influence the metabolism and make weight-gain hard.

The good news is that the World Health Organization reports that thinness is not likely to be a health hazard for most people. Once thinness associated with smoking has been removed, borderline thin people are, according to results from the large American study of nurses, actually a healthy and long-lived bunch.

According to an overview of all conducted studies done by the American Institute of Nutrition, the optimum BMI for health is 18–25. However, specific problems may occur in thinness associated with very low body-fat percentage, for example inability to conceive in women, low nutrient intake (causing vitamin and mineral deficiencies, etc.), poor immune system due to lack of leptin production in the body, and osteoporosis. Fat is by no means a useless, inanimate substance.

Work out your BMI (Feature 3) and if you ARE too thin see a doctor, who should refer you to a dietitian. For advice on gaining muscle rather than fat see Section Ten. Generally, however (especially if, as many thin people find, you can't tolerate a large plateful of food), you should eat 'little and often', with balanced meals of about 30% fat, 50% carbs and 20% protein.

Between meals you could have fortified milk drinks of the kind used for athletes and convalescents and, in fact, high-calorie drinks, like milk shakes, smoothies and juices, are good ways to increase calorie and nutrient intake easily. Nuts and seeds also make good calorie-rich snacks or additions to salads. If you choose foods you genuinely enjoy, you may find you can also increase portion sizes without feeling overfaced. Appetite may be increased via relaxation methods coupled with gentle regular exercise, preferably in the fresh air.

Also consider ways to minimize energy output and thus reduce calorie deficit. Spend longer in bed; relax in front of the TV more. Look at your stress levels, as anxiety can increase stress hormone output (which can speed metabolic rate).

FAT FACT

Many illegal and potentially dangerous drugs, such as cocaine, amphetamines and ecstasy, can act to speed up the metabolic rate and/or dampen the appetite. Such drugs are, of course, absolutely not recommended under any circumstances for anyone as an aid to slimming.

If you are healthy, eating well, feel fit and have a BMI of at least 18 (if you don't smoke), and are having normal periods if you're female, then don't worry too much about your thinness – it really is better than having a BMI over 28 or so, especially if you're young (as energy needs are relatively high in the teens, maintaining a positive energy balance can be harder at this time). And, of course, you are the envy of millions who, rightly or wrongly, equate thinness with perfection.

See also:

- Questions: 29, 44, 153, 162–3, 216, 319, 330, 350, 361.
- Features: 3, 30.
- A–Z entries: exercise equipment, weighted workouts.
- Key index entries: body image, metabolism.

26

What is wrong with being overweight?

This all depends on the definition of 'overweight'. For any given weight and height, you can work out the corresponding BMI (Feature 3) and there are recognized guidelines on the BMI categories that pose health risks. A BMI index over 27.8 for men and 27.3 for women shows the first links with increased incidence of high blood pressure, diabetes and CHD, and these risks become greater as weight increases over BMI 28, and other health hazards also begin to be associated. The Nurses Study showed that, in overweight American female nurses, the relative risk of overall mortality increased in an almost exact line with the increased weight.

If you are healthy, fit and well, but a stone heavier than your sister, or than you'd like to be, and your BMI is within healthy limits, then it may be best to stop worrying about your weight and simply follow a lifestyle that ensures you don't put on too much more, so as to stop your BMI creeping to the 'at risk' range. Especially try to keep from developing an 'apple' shape, as central fat distribution is an indicator of increased risk of several conditions (see Section Nine and Feature 25).

Indeed, a reasonable covering of body fat has several advantages – it is insulating and protective, it secretes the hormone leptin which boosts the immune system, it may help mood, and it is essential for puberty and reproduction, and important in menopausal and older women.

That is not to say that true overweight is necessary for these normal functions, or that overweight should be taken lightly. The World Health Organization has declared obesity 'a chronic disease and a growing threat to health in countries all over the world'. In other words, gross overweight coupled with a lack of regular activity is a recipe for disaster if you wish to live a long healthy life. Sadly, moreover, everyone who is obese was once just mildly overweight – so it really is worth trying to stabilize weight at a pre-risk level.

See also:

- Questions: 29–31, 56, 247, 250, 300–306, 324.
- Features: 3, 21, 25.
- Key index entries: central fat distribution, waist circumference, weight and health.

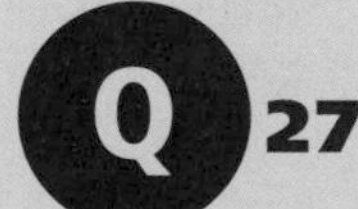

27

As you get older is weight gain natural or even desirable?

Gaining weight slowly or steadily as you get older is natural in the sense that it does occur in the majority of people in what the WHO terms 'industrialized societies'. The main reason for this weight gain is that, as we age, our muscle mass naturally declines through inactivity and the ageing process. Between the ages of 30 and 70, muscle strength and mass will decrease by an average of around 30% in most people – that's about 5lb (2.25kg) a decade for men, 3½lb (1.5kg) for women.

Our metabolic rate – the rate at which we burn calories – is dependent, to a large degree, upon our proportion of lean tissue (muscle) and, with the loss of this tissue, the result is a slowing of the metabolism. Hormonal changes – for example to the thyroid function, adrenal function and so on – can also slow down the metabolism. To counteract this, and maintain a steady weight, calorie intake would need to be gradually reduced as well. (As a rough guide, a reduction of around 100 calories a day for every decade over 30. This means that if you are say 60, you need 300 calories a day fewer than you did at 30, if you don't exercise and don't want to put on weight). In most people this doesn't happen and the result is a positive energy balance – extra fat stores on the body!

In theory, however, this process can be blunted. Research shows that, with regular

FAT FACT

An ingredient, P57, found in the South African succulent plant, hoodia, is thought to be a safe natural appetite suppressant, and pills containing it could be on sale over the counter within 2 years. Men of the Kung tribe used to nibble it while out hunting, to stave off hunger.

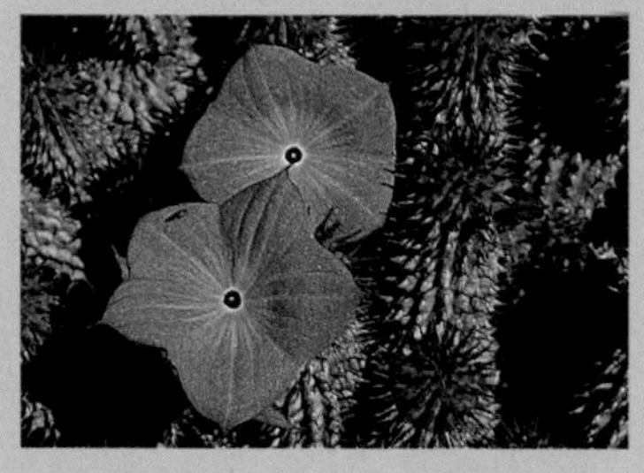

activity and weight training, lean tissue loss can be reduced by about half and cardiovascular (heart-lung) function can largely be maintained, which also helps maintain optimum metabolic rate. Hormonal changes may also be minimized with regular exercise. Regular activity in itself burns up extra calories but, if necessary, total calorie intake can be reduced slightly to maintain energy balance and prevent weight gain.

Research over 20 years on élite runners aged between 50 and 70 (about the fittest people for their age that you could find) shows that however hard you work, your body composition and shape will change with age – albeit much more slowly than average. In these athletes, their lean tissue decreased by an average of about 5½lb (half the normal average), their body fat percentage increased by 5% and their waist circumference by about 2 inches. (But they didn't put on any actual weight.)

This probably means that, for most of us taking reasonable exercise, we should regard moderate changes in shape and small increases in weight as natural as we age – the amount dependent upon how much exercise you do and how well you balance calorie intake with this expenditure. Huge increases in weight are not natural and are connected more with social and environmental factors – i.e., too much food and not enough activity.

And, yes, a reasonably small amount of weight gain may well be desirable as you get older if you were thin when younger – for example, thin people are more prone to osteoporosis in later life than are fatter people. Body fat stores may help to keep oestrogen levels in the body up, which in turn helps protect bones. As a guide, from 50 plus into old age, a BMI at the high end of desirable may be better than one at the low end. However, one recent study published in the *International Journal of Obesity* found that overweight pre-menopausal and menopausal women were more at risk of insulin resistance and impaired fasting glycaemia (predictors of diabetes) and suggested that in mid-life it is important to avoid gaining much weight – so, as you can see, little in the world of obesity research is ever simple!

To sum up: as we age, a small weight gain is natural and may even be good, whereas large gains are neither.

See also:

- Questions: 4, 6, 8, 10, 17, 72–3, 230-7, 247, 259, 303, 305, 364.
- Features: 1, 2, 3.
- Key index entries: ageing, andropause, hormones, lean tissue, menopause, metabolism.

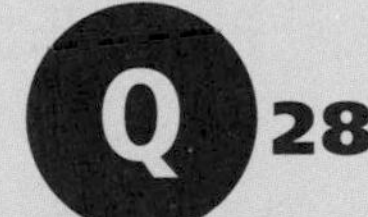

Q28

What is the definition of normal or ideal weight?

The basic classification of weight, from underweight through normal to overweight and obese, is Body Mass Index, explained in Feature 3. It is used worldwide, but figures may be interpreted differently by different organizations.

The World Health Organization, for example, describes normal weight as a BMI of 18.5–24.99. Some experts describe BMIs of 20–24.99 as normal; while 18–25 is associated with lowest risk of death (Q25). Others say that a BMI of up to 27 is acceptable, as the health risks don't really begin to show to a great extent until then.

There is obviously room for large differences in weight between people of the same height using the BMI. For example, someone 5ft 7in (1.66m) can weigh from as little as 114lb (52kg) to 154lb (70kg), and still be within the 18.5–24.99 limits.

Perhaps halfway between 20 and 25 could be considered 'perfect' – a BMI of 22.5 – an idea endorsed by the American Heart Association. A BMI of 22 has been cited by some as ideal for males. In another study, by the American Cancer Society, desirable BMIs for women were listed as 21.3–22.1 and 21.9–22.4 for men. Others feel such guidelines are too specific.

Another gauge of weight is your body-fat percentage, discussed in Q30.

In truth there is no such thing as a perfect weight for everyone at every time in their lives. Expert advice is that waist size should also be considered when deciding whether or not you are 'ideal' weight, as a disproportionately large midriff is an indicator of increased health risks.

See also:

- Questions: 27, 29–31, 56, 247, 250, 264, 324.
- Features: 3, 22, 25.
- Key index entries: Ashwell Shape Chart, body-fat percentage, Body Mass Index, central fat distribution, waist circumference, waist-to-hip ratio.

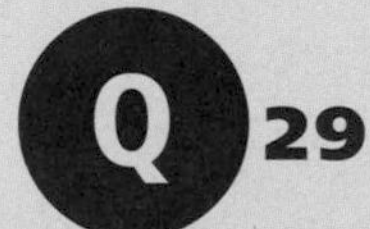

Q29

What are the definitions of under- and overweight?

If you read the previous question, you will quickly deduce that 'underweight' is considered to be a BMI of under 18.5 (or under 20, according to some), and 'overweight' a BMI of over 25. However these figures are not 100% reliable as a guide, as they take no account of body composition. For example, an athlete with a very high lean-tissue mass and low body-fat percentage might have a BMI over 25. Feature 3 helps you decide whether you are under-, ideal or overweight.

See also:

- Questions: 28, 30-1, 56, 250, 264, 324.
- Features: 3, 22.
- Key index entries: Ashwell Shape Chart, Body Mass Index, central fat distribution, waist circumference, waist-to-hip ratio.

Do you have a weight problem?

You may think you're overweight – but are you? Assess whether you're overweight or obese, using recognized international guidelines. Start here – first check your Body Mass Index (BMI).

The Body Mass Index is a formula used by health professionals throughout the world to assess an adult's body weight in relation to their height. It's a useful measure, because in most people it correlates highly with their body-fat percentage. However, body builders and some other sportspeople, pregnant or lactating women and very elderly, frail people shouldn't use it as a guide to overweight, and it shouldn't be used for children, who have their own calculations (see Section 8).

High BMI is linked to increased risk of death from all causes, including diabetes, cardiovascular diseases, high blood pressure and osteoarthritis (Feature 25 provides more on overweight and health problems).

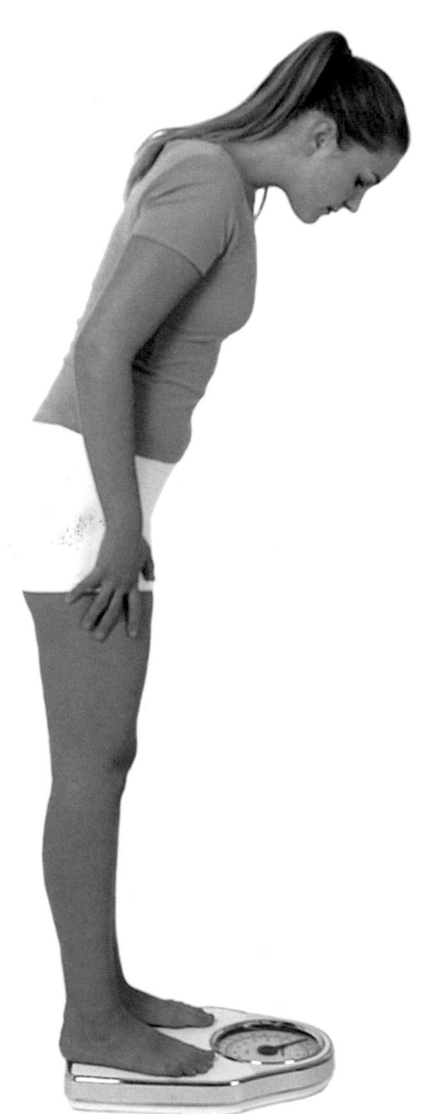

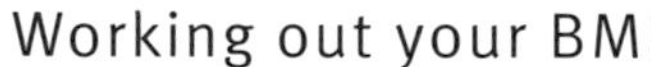

Working out your BMI

The calculation is simple: BMI = your weight in kilograms divided by your height in metres (squared) or:

$$\text{BMI} = \frac{\text{Weight (kg)}}{\text{Height (m)}^2}$$

- To get your weight in kilograms, divide your weight in pounds by 2.2.
- To get your height in metres, multiply your height in inches by 0.025.
- Squared height is your height multiplied by itself (e.g. 1.65 x 1.65 = 2.72). It is probably best to use a calculator to work this out.

Below is a table of weight for heights expressed as BMIs, which will save most people the trouble of working out the formula. If your own height and/or current weight isn't there, then you can use the formula as above.

BODY MASS INDEX CHART

Find your height and read down the column until you find the weight nearest yours, then read across for your approximate BMI.

Height (inches [metres])

60(1.5)	62(1.55)	64(1.6)	66(1.65)	68(1.7)	70(1.75)	72(1.8)	74(1.85)	**BMI**
Weight [(lb [kg])								
89(40)	95(43)	101(46)	108(49)	115(52)	121(55)	128(58)	135(62)	18
94(43)	100(46)	107(49)	114(52)	121(55)	128(58)	135(62)	143(65)	19
99(45)	105(48)	113(51)	120(54)	27(58)	135(61)	143(65)	150(68)	20
104(47)	111(50)	118(54)	126(57)	134(61)	141(64)	150(68)	158(72)	21
109(50)	116(53)	124(56)	132(60)	140(64)	148(67)	157(71)	166(75)	22
114(52)	121(55)	130(59)	138(63)	146(67)	155(70)	164(75)	173(79)	23
119(54)	127(57)	135(61)	144(65)	153(69)	162(73)	171(78)	181(82)	24
124(56)	132(60)	141(64)	150(68)	159(72)	168(77)	178(81)	188(86)	25
139(63)	148(67)	158(72)	167(76)	178(81)	188(86)	200(91)	210(96)	28
148(67)	158(72)	169(77)	180(82)	191(87)	202(92)	214(97)	226(103)	30
173(79)	185(84)	197(90)	210(95)	222(101)	236(107)	250(113)	263(120)	35
198(90)	211(96)	225(102)	240(109)	254(116)	270(122)	260(130)	301(137)	40

THE 10-SECOND TEST

By measuring your waist circumference you can get a strong indication of whether you are at health risk from your weight. Measure your waist in inches or centimetres without holding the tape too tightly or too loosely. As a guide, your waist measurement is the narrowest part of your trunk OR a spot approximately 1inch (2.5cm) above your belly button. Write your measurement down and check here:

Men

- Waist circumference over 94cm (37in) – indicates slight health risk; take care.
- Waist circumference over 102cm (40in) – indicates substantially increased risk.

Women

- Waist circumference over 80cm (31.5in) – indicates slight health risk; take care.
- Waist circumference over 88cm (34.5in) – indicates substantially increased risk.

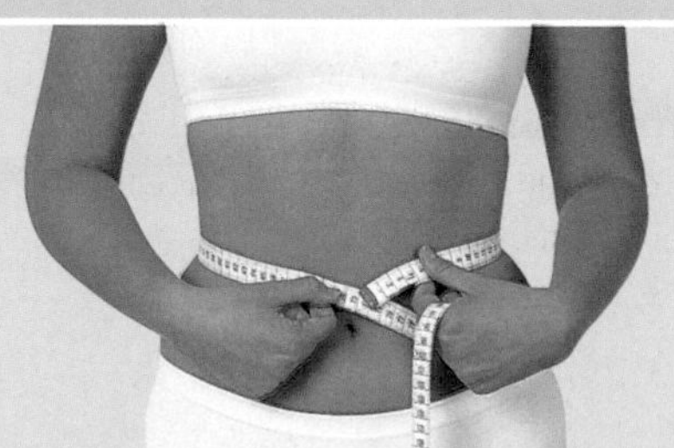

Waist measurements lower than these are classified as healthy.

NOTE: Abdominal fatness can also be gauged using the Ashwell Shape Chart (waist-to-height ratio) or the Waist-to-Hip Ratio. However, these are a little more complicated to use and research has shown that the basic waist circumference test shown here is equally, or more, accurate in deciding your health risks. For interest, both alternative methods are shown in Section 9 on page 213.

BMI under 18.5

Classification: *Underweight*

You do not need to lose any more weight and, although your risk of having health problems associated with obesity is very low, you may be at increased risk of other problems such as amenorrhoea in women (no menstrual periods), bone loss, nutrient deficiency and others (see Q319) – and the risks become greater the lower your BMI. Some experts say that this classification is too low and that underweight is a BMI under 20; but, when smokers are taken out of the equation, the classification seems sound.

BMI 18.5–24.99

Classification: *Normal range*

You do not need to lose weight or gain weight. You are within healthy weight guidelines and the risk of weight-related health problems is minimal. The 'ideal' BMI is between 22 and 23 for young adults. At the upper range of normal (around 24.99), if you feel you are overweight, do the waist circumference test above as an additional check. If you are at the upper end and have been gaining weight steadily at more than 5lb (2.25kg) per decade over age 25, it may be time to pay more attention to diet and exercise levels and aim to put no more on, or at least slow down the rate of increase.

BMI 25–29.99

Classification: *Overweight (pre-obese)*

From a BMI of 25 up to around 27, you have a slightly increased risk of health problems, and some experts feel that any weight between these BMIs should be called the 'caution zone' for overweight. By using the BMI with the waist circumference test above, you can get a clearer picture of whether or not you have cause for concern. Efforts should be made to ensure that your weight doesn't increase any more. From over 27 to 29.99, the risk of health problems becomes higher. In one study, a measurable increased incidence of high blood pressure, heart disease and diabetes was noted at 27.3 for women and 27.8 for men. Again, the waist circumference test gives you added information on your risk level. For many people within this category it would be advisable to lose weight to get your BMI down to at least 25–27.

BMI 30–34.99

Classification: *Obese Class 1*

You are officially 'obese' (very overweight) and at this level your risk of weight-related diseases increases considerably, especially if you have a large waist circumference (see the test above). Reducing your weight by even 5% or 10% would result in considerable health benefits.

BMI 35–40

Classification: *Obese Class 2*

Your risk of death and weight-related diseases and health problems increases considerably between these BMIs, with a risk defined as 'severe'. It is important to reduce your weight to a lower BMI.

BMI over 40

Classification: *Obese Class 3 (extreme obesity, morbid obesity)*

You have an extremely high risk of early death and weight-related diseases and health problems. At a BMI over 40, it is unusual not to have a medical condition associated with the obese condition. It is very important to reduce your weight to a lower BMI, and your doctor can refer you for specialist help and advice.

NOTE: Overweight and obesity can also be gauged using your percentage of body fat – but to determine this you need a body fat monitor (see A–Z). For definitions of obesity by body-fat percentage, see Q30.

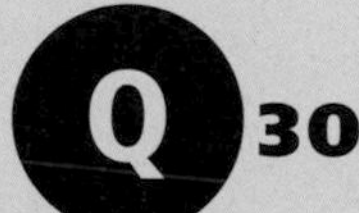

Q 30

What is 'body-fat percentage' and how does it relate to my weight?

Body-fat percentage is the percentage proportion of adipose (fat) tissue in your body by weight. Qs 1 and 2 give a detailed explanation. When people get fat, the increase in weight is nearly all accounted for by increase in fat mass – i.e., your body-fat percentage gets higher while lean tissue (muscle) mass remains fairly static.

For adult men, an average body fat percentage is 15–20%, (overweight would be over about 25% and obesity over about 30%), while for adult women an average is about 25–27% (overweight over about 30% and obesity over about 35%). In very overweight people, body-fat percentage can rise as high as 70%, and people with body fat over 55% are classed as 'morbidly obese'. In very fit people, body-fat percentages of around 10% for males and 20% for females are more normal. If body-fat percentage drops too low, health problems can occur – the critical lower limit for women is said to be 12–17%, depending on which expert view you take.

It is not possible to measure body fat percentage very accurately without professional equipment, however you can buy scales that include a body-fat calculator, or professional body-fat monitors.

For the average person, it is not vital to work out body-fat percentage, as your BMI and waist measurement as described in Feature 3 will do a satisfactory job of deciding if you are overweight.

See also:

- ▶ Questions: 1–6, 31–34, 45, 56, 247, 250, 319, 324.
- ▶ Features: 3, 4.
- ▶ A–Z entry: Body Fat Monitors.
- ▶ Key index entries: Ashwell Shape Chart, Body Mass Index, central fat distribution.

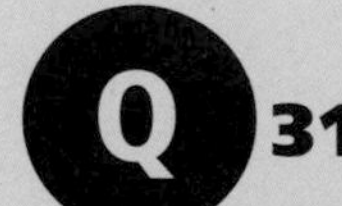

Q 31

Is there any very quick and easy way to tell if I am overweight?

The 10-second test: you get a very good indication of whether you're health-risk-related overweight by measuring your waist. If over 34.5in (88cm) for females or 40in (102cm) for males, then you're almost certainly overweight.

You can also try the 'pinch test' – if you can pinch a fold of flesh around your midriff at least 1 inch (2.5cm) thick, you're probably overweight (not exactly scientific).

Another quick rule-of-thumb is if you were at an ideal weight (BMI 22–23) at age 25, add 5lb (2.25kg) for every decade and you can assume you're not overweight. For example, at 55 you could be 15lb (6.75kg) heavier than at 25, and consider your weight as within bounds.

See also:

- ▶ Questions: 28-30, 56, 247, 250, 324.
- ▶ Feature: 3.
- ▶ A-Z entry: Body Fat Monitors.
- ▶ Key index entries: Ashwell Shape Chart, Body Mass Index, central fat distribution, waist circumference, waist-to-hip ratio.

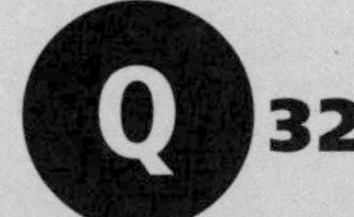

Q 32

Can dieting slow my metabolic rate?

Yes. If you lose weight, your metabolic rate will naturally slow down. This is mostly because when your body weighs less it has less work to do (carrying its new, lighter weight around) and so uses fewer calories.

This means if, say, you'd weighed 12 stone and now weigh 10, all other factors (e.g. activity levels) being equal, you'll need to eat less to maintain the new weight.

This is not, in essence, because dieting has adversely affected your metabolism, but because you weigh less. Research found people who had dieted down to a particular weight had similar metabolic rates to people of the same (lower) weight who had never dieted. (If you put on weight again, your metabolic rate will rise again.)

There may also be other factors at work here, tending to put the brakes on your metabolism – as we saw in Q24, the WHO says that the body seems to want to defend a high weight against weight loss more readily than it does a low weight against gain, so that a 3,500-calorie reduction in your food intake doesn't necessarily always translate itself to 1lb of fat lost – which is the equation in theory. This means that weight loss will progressively become harder as metabolic rate appears to slow down more than might be predicted from the weight loss.

People who take up regular physical activity, including aerobic work and some strength training, will find dieting doesn't tend to alter the metabolism so much. Regular aerobic exercise can increase your metabolic rate a little for several hours after exercise, as well as burning up extra calories during the course of the exercise. Weight training will also help to avoid the loss of lean tissue (muscle) for the dieter, and may even add some. Lean tissue is heavier and uses up more calories than other tissue (e.g. fat) and so a good proportion of lean tissue to fat in the body is essential to maintain a good metabolic rate. Crash or very-low-cal diets tend to lose a fairly high proportion of muscle as well as fat, whereas moderate energy restriction loses proportionately more fat, which is why steady slimming is best.

See also:

- ▶ Questions: 21, 24, 33–34, 39–40, 106, 205–7.
- ▶ Features: 1, 2.
- ▶ A–Z entries: crash diets, metabolism-booster diets.
- ▶ Key index entries: dieting, metabolism.

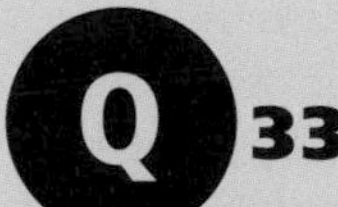

Q 33

Does dieting make us fat?

No – this is a very simplistic statement with a tiny grain of truth in it. If long-term calorie reduction made people fat, then people in famines throughout the world would be fat, not bone-thin. When you look at the evidence, it is obvious that if you don't get enough to eat, you will lose weight, not gain it.

If you create for your body a long-term energy deficit, expending more energy than you ingest in the form of calories, then you will definitely lose weight. It's always best if conscious 'dieting' is combined with regular exercise of various types and if the dieting is done in a steady manner on a suitable balanced diet.

There is some evidence that seems to show that repeated bouts of 'yo-yo' dieting may make it progressively harder to lose weight, but this is probably to do with the fact that repeated dieting tends to deplete lean tissue (muscle) and each time weight is regained the lost lean tissue isn't replaced unless muscle-building exercise is done. Over time this would mean that the metabolic rate would be reduced, as lean tissue is more metabolically active than fat. Severe crash-dieting may also deplete more lean tissue than slow dieting.

The answer is to avoid yo-yo- and crash-dieting – which are depressing anyway – and to get plenty of muscle-enhancing exercise, whether slimming or attempting to maintain your weight.

See also:

- ▶ Questions: 32, 34, 36, 39–40, 106, 125, 205–7, 333, 357.
- ▶ Feature: 2.
- ▶ A–Z entry: metabolism-booster diets.
- ▶ Key index entries: dieting, energy equation, exercise, metabolism.

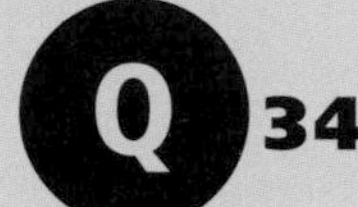

Q 34

Will my percentage of body fat increase each time I diet?

When you diet to lose weight you should decrease your percentage of body fat. However, the question implies that you are a yo-yo (sometimes called 'weight cycling') dieter and it is probably true that, with repeated bouts of yo-yoing, every time you return to a high weight, your percentage of total fat may have increased a little.

This is because, when you lose weight, some of the weight loss is lean tissue (particularly if you crash-diet) and, when you put weight back on, lean tissue isn't replaced. So you'll be your old weight, but have less lean tissue and thus may have a slightly higher percentage of body fat. Compared with the last time you were at this same high weight, your overall resting metabolism will have decreased slightly because of the lower proportion of lean tissue (see previous question). So this time it may be a little harder to lose weight.

Avoid yo-yo- and crash-dieting, and always exercise when slimming to retain as much lean tissue (muscle) as you can.

See also:

- ▶ Questions: 21, 24, 30, 32–3, 106, 205–7.
- ▶ Features: 1, 2.
- ▶ Key index entries: diets, energy equation, exercise, metabolism.

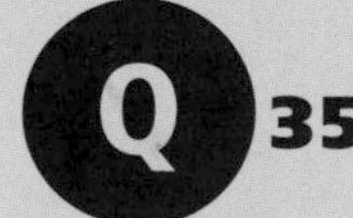

Q 35

Can I lose weight without dieting?

You can create a small long-term calorie deficit or negative energy balance by increasing the amount of exercise you do to 'burn up' calories, and this will be enough alone to help you lose weight slowly over time, all other factors being equal (e.g. as long as you don't begin to eat more). One group in a study who didn't diet but increased exercise levels lost about 6lb (2.75kg) over a year.

The amount you could lose like this would be about 1lb (0.5kg) for every 3,500 calories you burn up over and above your current rate. To burn an extra 3,500 calories over a week, i.e., 500 a day, would be possible but not easy (see the charts on pages 228–9). However, even an extra 200 calories burnt every day would produce weight loss over time.

The only other ways to lose body fat without 'dieting' (i.e., reducing your calorie intake to create a negative energy balance) are to have surgery such as liposuction or to take pills to speed up the metabolic rate. Some prescription slimming pills will do this, but others still require you to eat less and help by reducing appetite. Qs 37 and 38 discuss these options too. You can lose weight that is body fluid by taking diuretics, but these should only be taken under medical advice, and is pointless if you are trying to lose fat.

However, if by 'dieting' you mean 'following a set or crash diet', then it is perfectly possible to lose weight by altering your eating patterns, rather than 'going on a diet'. Several studies have shown that a healthy low-fat, high-carbohydrate diet of around 1,500 calories a day (much higher than in many diets) produces the best long-term weight loss, and that crash-dieting is, indeed, a waste of time. So, if you don't like the word diet, don't use it.

See also:

- ▶ Questions: 18, 36–8, 48, 87, 103–4, 113.
- ▶ Features: 9, 10, 29, 30.
- ▶ A–Z entries: cycling, diuretic diets, diuretics, exercise classes, herbal slimming pills, laxatives, running, slimming pills, sports supplements, slimming surgery, swimming, walking.
- ▶ Key index entries: eating patterns, exercise.

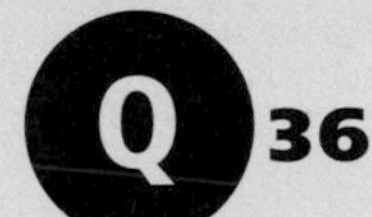

What is the best way to lose weight?

By both reducing your calorie intake a little (for most people around 500 calories fewer a day is a good average to aim for) and increasing your energy output (activity) on a regular basis.

There is probably no such thing as an absolute best for the way either to reduce calories or to exercise – both will vary according to your tastes, weight, means, health – and many other factors. The answers for you, personally, should become more apparent if you read through this book, which aims to look at all the options and provide unbiased advice.

In general terms, however, it seems that the most successful long-term weight-loss programmes involve reduction in total fat and simple carbohydrate intake, thus reducing total calorie intake, and eating regular meals containing plenty of fruit and veg at a slow speed. It also seems the most popular and easy way to increase energy output is regular walking.

See also:

- Questions: 79–122, 142, 145–8, 159–197, 217, 262, 266, 309–10, 321–3, 334–65.
- Features: 2, 8–16, 20, 23, 28–30.
- A–Z entries: individual named diets (e.g. Atkins Diet), slimming clubs.
- Key index entries: dieting, exercise, weight maintenance.

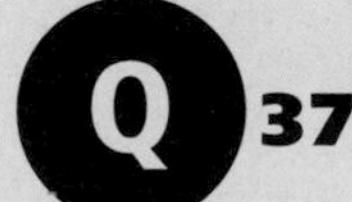

Is it a good idea to take slimming pills?

The World Health Organization describes approved prescription slimming pills as 'an adjunct to other weight-loss therapies and a way of helping to maintain body weight over time'. However, the WHO also points out that these drugs are best used in conjunction with diet and lifestyle management, and that when weight-management drugs are discontinued weight regain occurs.

It should go without saying that prescription slimming pills should be used under medical supervision. Current criteria in the UK are that intervention with drugs should only be applied after a minimum of 3 months of 'lifestyle intervention' and if a weight loss of 10% has already been achieved. However, these guidelines are not always followed. Normally you shouldn't be given a prescription for slimming drugs unless you have a BMI of at least 30 or have health problems associated with your weight.

Two drugs are most likely to be prescribed. One is orlistat (brand name Xenical), which works by blocking the absorption of about one-third of the fat in your food. Patients are required to follow a low-fat diet anyway (otherwise complications such as 'leaky bowel' may occur). The guideline for prescribing orlistat in the UK is that you should have lost 2.5kg (5½lb) in the previous month by diet and exercise, be between 18 and 75, and have a BMI of at least 28. There are other criteria for longer use.

The other drug is sibutramine (Meridia in the US and Reductil in Germany and the UK), which acts by both inhibiting appetite and stimulating metabolic rate. Possible side effects include unwanted increase in blood pressure, and, as it is fairly new, the long-term effects are uncertain.

Phentermine is another drug which stimulates the central nervous system and is used as an appetite suppressant.

Do I think slimming drugs are a good idea? I wouldn't presume to judge, but certainly the message seems to be that they are only to be considered for a small proportion of overweight people. The decision on whether you are a suitable patient is best left to a doctor or specialist who knows you. For that reason, I wouldn't recommend you visit a private doctor who has never met you before; private slimming clinics across the world offer pills at a price – which could include your health.

However, scientists in many countries are working hard to find a slimming pill that is safe and effective – recently there have been reported an injection that kills fat cells; a gene which stops mice making fat cells; and the uncoupling protein 'UPC-3', which can turn surplus calories directly into heat rather than body fat. A variety of non-prescription slimming pills with varying degrees of usefulness are sold.

See also:

- Questions: 12, 23, 35.
- A–Z entries: diuretics, herbal diet supplements, laxatives, slimming pills, sports supplements.

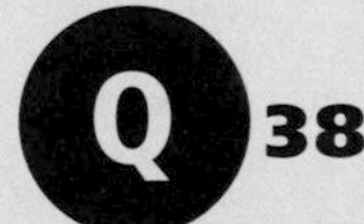

Are there any operations that I can have to make me lose weight?

Perhaps the best-known operation is now liposuction – a process that 'sucks' the fat from your body through a tube. It is the only operation, as far as I know, that actually removes your body fat – but it is usually not such a 'minor' operation as some people would have you believe.

Other operations rely upon reducing the amount that you can eat, or by preventing the absorption of foods, or a combination of the two. All of these operations are available privately, but may also be available in the UK via the NHS if you are a suitable case. However, they are not to be undertaken as anything except a last resort for the obese, as they have life-changing consequences, not all positive.

One other type of operation is an abdominoplasty, which is really for the post-obese person who has a lot of loose 'spare' skin hanging around. The operation cuts away the loose flesh. See your GP for a discussion about your options regarding surgery.

See also:

- ▶ Questions: 48, 59, 61, 68.
- ▶ A–Z entry: slimming surgery.

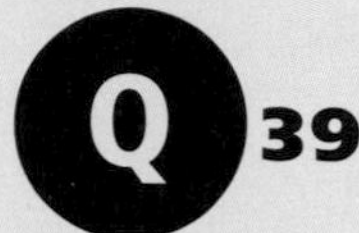

39

Why do so many people put weight back on after they have dieted?

All the research agrees with you – that the majority of slimmers do regain their lost weight. About 10% of slimmers will have retained their new slim weight after 9 months; only about 5% after several years. Some research (but not all) says that after 5 years almost everyone returns to, or goes higher than, their starting weight.

The main reason is usually that calorie intake gradually creeps up and, because, as we've seen (in Qs 5, 24, 32, 33 and 34), a slim person has a slower metabolic rate than a fat person, calorie intake needs to be restricted permanently if the new weight is to remain. This should not mean that a newly-slim person should have to remain on a 'slimming-level' diet for life, but certainly that a calorie intake lower than pre-diet levels is needed. Many people find it hard to continue with this more restrained way of eating.

The best way to keep weight off permanently is to take more exercise, but again many slimmers are reluctant to do this. In other words, ex-slimmers find that their lifestyle just isn't conducive to the permanent changes necessary for permanent weight loss. However, there is some brighter news. A very recent American study of ex-WeightWatchers slimmers found that 5 years later over 70% were still below their original weight and nearly 20% were within 5lb (2kg) of their original goal weight. Again in America, the National Weight Control Registry recruited 784 people who had maintained at least a 30lb (13.5kg) weight loss for an average of 5½ years. Most had a genetic background (e.g. fat parents) which might be assumed to predispose them to overweight, and, indeed, many had been overweight since childhood, but still managed to keep the weight off.

See also:

- ▶ Questions: 5, 18, 20, 22, 24, 27, 32–4, 40.
- ▶ Features: 1, 2, 9–13.
- ▶ Key index entries: eating patterns and habits, metabolism, set point theory, weight maintenance.

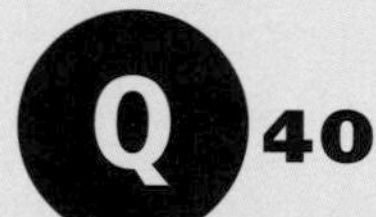

40

How can I avoid regaining all the weight I've lost?

First of all, let's hope that you have settled on a reasonable 'target' weight, which is always easier to maintain than one that is too low. For young adults, a target BMI of around 22 to 23 is as low as you want to go – but 25 would be fine if your starting level was higher than 28, especially if you are over 40. For older adults, a target BMI of around 24–25 is often reasonable. Use your common sense. If you go too low, you will need to reduce your regular calorie intake down low as well, and this may be too hard to do (see previous question).

Secondly, let's hope that you dieted slowly so that you didn't lose too much lean tissue (muscle). The more muscle you have on your body, the more calories you will burn up every day rather than storing them as fat. Research shows that very fast (crash) dieting does lose more lean tissue than slow dieting.

Thirdly, you need to eat a healthy balanced diet and keep the total fat content fairly low, while filling your plate with more of the complex carbohydrates, vegetables, fruits and low-fat proteins. You need to eat regular smallish meals and snacks – portion control is a simple method of watching total calorie intake. If you look at the Diet Bible Basic Diet (Feature 9), you will see how to use it as a blueprint for a weight maintenance plan. Other features in the book will give you plenty of ideas for meals.

Fourthly, look at your lifestyle and try to adjust it so that you are less inclined to overeat (see Sections 4 and 5).

Last, but definitely not least, you need to take regular exercise – preferably both aerobic (e.g. walking, cycling) and weight training (e.g. with free weights or at a gym). The people mentioned in the last paragraph of the previous question, who kept their weight off for at least 5 years, almost all cited regular exercise, such as brisk walking, or dancing, sport or gym work, as the main reason.

See also:

- ▶ Questions: 32–4, 36, 39, 103–4, 106, 132–48, 168–93, 328–65.
- ▶ Features: 3, 9–16, 20, 28–30.
- ▶ A–Z entries: exercise classes, gyms, slimming clubs, walking, weighted workouts.
- ▶ Key index entries: exercise, metabolism, weight maintenance.

FAT FACT

An average man has about 26 billion fat cells, called adipocytes, in his body while a woman has around 35 billion. When people put on weight, the fat cells first actually increase in size, then later multiply in obesity.

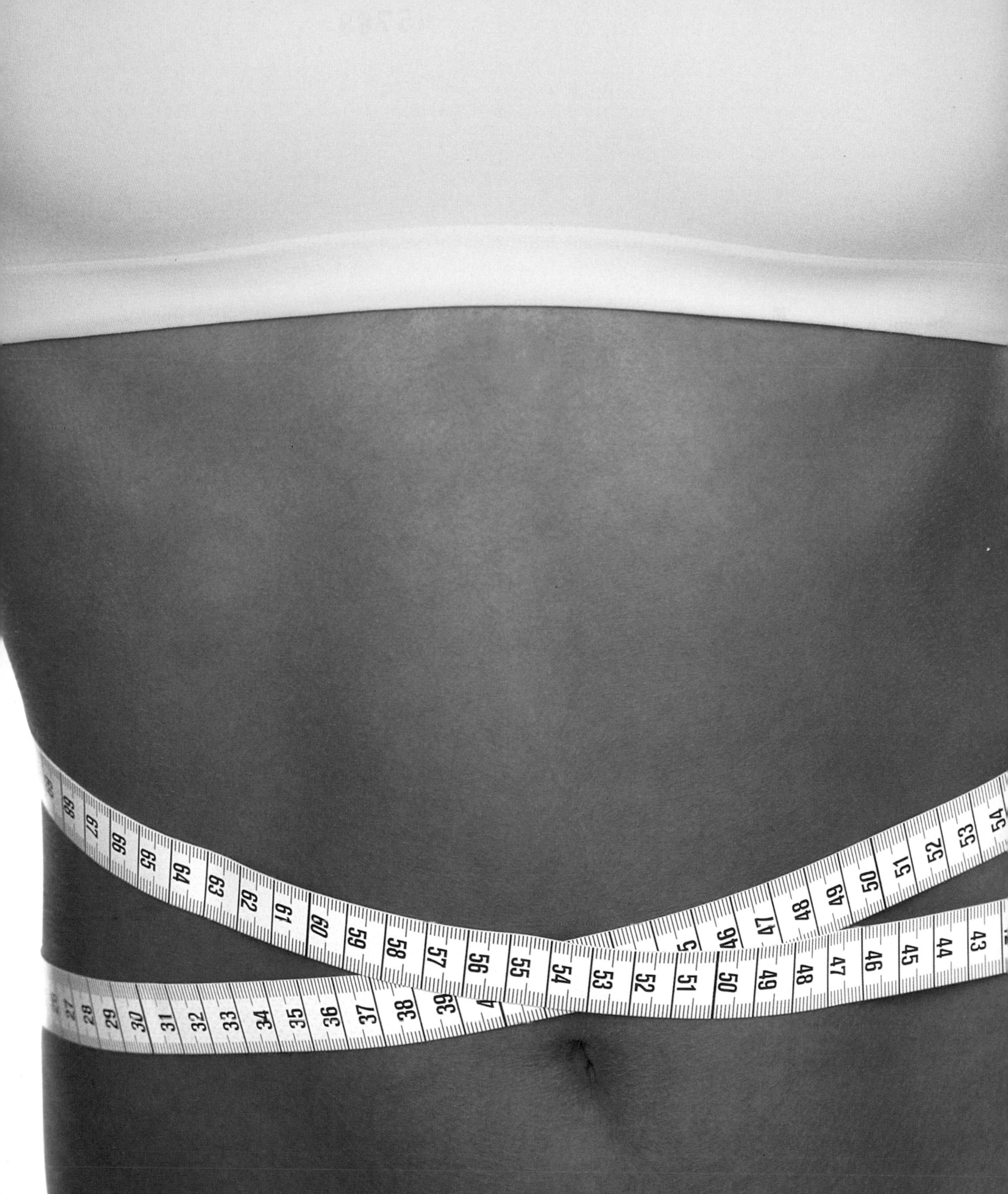

Section Two

Your body, your shape

When you're dissatisfied with your body, it is not always your weight that you hate, but your shape. Maybe the big hips, the big bust or bottom if you're female, perhaps the paunch or the skinny legs if you're male. Alternatively, you may feel out of proportion, not muscled enough, or too 'soft'-looking. It seems that whatever shape we are in, we're rarely satisfied.

In this section we look at why you are the shape you are, what can be done to change the parts you dislike – by means of diet, exercise, etc. – and what can't be done. We'll look at the three basic body shapes and help you decide which you are, and you'll also find out which body shapes are most appealing to both sexes.

Special features show easy ways to look better instantly and reveal how you can appear taller and slimmer by devoting just 10 minutes a day to toning up.

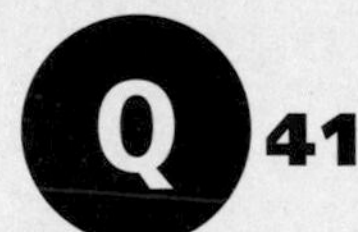

What factors affect my body shape?

Your shape is largely governed by your parents' genes – you take bits from both parents to make up your own unique self – but exactly how you will end up is, of course, a bit of a lottery! For example, if you have a father who is tall and thin and a mother who is short and plump, your genetic shape could be short and thin, or tall and plump, as well as tall and thin or short and plump. You could even end up neither short nor tall, and neither thin nor plump, because if you put short and tall together you get medium, and so on.

If you're lucky, you could take all the 'best bits' from each parent and end up completely gorgeous, even though neither of them is particularly handsome. That's why siblings can look so different – apart from identical twins, you each put your parents' genes into a different pattern. As you probably know, however, children from the same family usually do have many physical similarities and bear strong characteristics from one or other parent.

Other factors do come into the equation, though. Obviously, your gender has a large bearing upon your shape, because each sex is genetically programmed to have a predisposition to its own blueprint of muscle, bone, fat and so on. Males tend to have broader shoulders, wider necks, narrower hips and more muscled arms and legs – and tend to be taller with a lower percentage of body fat. Females tend to have higher body fat, deposited around the breasts, hips, bottom and thighs – with a lower percentage of muscle and tending to be shorter. Male and female hormones decide these sexual differences but, again, everyone has both male and female hormones in them and, depending upon the proportion of each that you have, your shape can be more or less mannish, more or less feminine.

Your shape can also be affected by your nutritional status in early life (see next question) and also, to quite a reasonable extent, by what and how much activity you do and have done. For example, look how different are the figures of a body builder, a gymnast, a marathon runner and a rugby player. Exercise has a quite tremendous power to help shape your body. Though, of course, people tend to choose the sport that fits in best with their original body blueprint – i.e., if you are tall, broad and powerful you are more likely to become a rugby player than a gymnast.

Weight is less of a factor in defining body shape than you may think, though being fat will accentuate shape. E.g., a fat pear-shaped woman looks more pear-shaped than a thin pear-shaped woman.

See also:

- ▶ Question: 7.
- ▶ Feature: 4.
- ▶ Key index entries: exercise, weight.

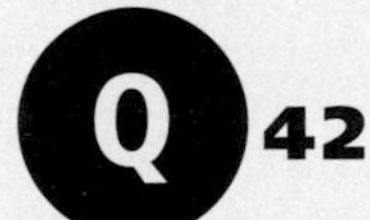

Can a child change their shape by doing anything specific while still growing?

Factors apart from heredity and sex can be altered somewhat. Bone structure can be optimized through good nutrition and enough sunlight. Strength can be encouraged with enough calories, protein, vitamins, minerals and essential fats. Both musculature and bone density can be enhanced via regular weight-bearing exercise, including walking, gym, and field sports. Exercise should also improve posture, which can affect shape. For more on feeding children, see Section 8.

See also:

- ▶ Questions: 216, 218, 224, 277.
- ▶ Feature: 2.
- ▶ Key index entries: child health, child's diet.

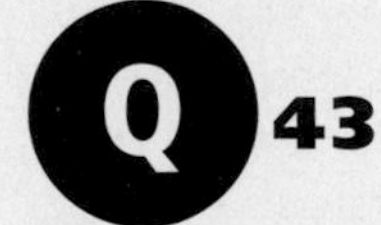

As an adult, is the bone structure I have the bone structure I'm stuck with?

Believe it or not, bones are not just static, solid, dry old bone, but living tissue which renews itself constantly. Bone mass isn't fully formed until your 30s, at what is called peak bone mass – and after that, unless you watch it, it is downhill all the way. So, in theory, you have quite a lot of control over the state of your bones.

Try to feed them well (with plenty of calcium-rich foods, like low-fat dairy produce, leafy greens, nuts, seeds, and with essential fatty acids in oily fish and a general good varied diet) and exercise well (with weight-bearing exercise for upper and lower body), from early in childhood, before peak bone mass is reached. After that, only good diet and exercise keep them at that peak. As we get older (especially after menopause and andropause), bone mass declines and gets harder and harder to retain. Again, good diet, exercise and perhaps other factors, such as hormone supplements, can help. Crash diets and maintaining too low a weight may both be bad for bone density.

See also:

- ▶ Features: 29, 30.
- ▶ A–Z entries: gyms, weighted workouts.
- ▶ Key index entries: andropause, healthy diet, menopause.

I'm very slim and fine-boned – how can I look more muscular and strong?

It sounds as if you are a true ectomorph (see Feature 4) and to change yourself into a burly mesomorph is not easy.

Trying to 'morph' from one category to another is hard, if not impossible – at least, without resorting to illegal drugs.

If you are a slim, delicate person, you can become a less slim and less delicate person through diet and exercise, but you have to be realistic. Daily attention to nutrition, weight training and levels of dedication would be called for.

Many people would envy you your shape (and, indeed, your capacity for calories that don't turn into fat) and my advice is to maximize your bone density (slim fine-boned people may suffer more at the hands of osteoporosis later in life) with weight-bearing exercise and a varied calcium-rich diet, build up a reasonable amount of body tone and strength with regular weight training and/or gym work and get on and enjoy life! If your self-esteem is low because of the way you see your body, other help is available.

See also:

- ▶ Questions: 25, 41.
- ▶ Features: 4, 30.
- ▶ A–Z entries: counselling, exercise classes, gyms, walking, weighted workouts.
- ▶ Key index entries: osteoporosis.

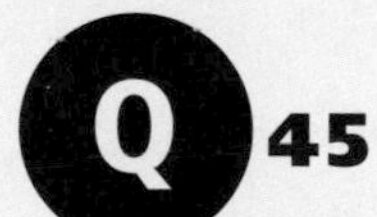

Q 45

However much I diet and exercise, I seem to remain 'soft', with no muscle definition – is there any cure?

You may be a natural endomorph type: these have a softer, more rounded look than other body types, with a higher proportion of body fat to muscle. Most people also become 'softer' with age (some call it flabby!) and you have to work harder as you age to maintain a well-toned appearance and/or increase muscle mass.

Also, you may be doing the wrong type of exercise – to see much difference you need to work out about 4 times a week with weights (or daily, using different major muscle groups on alternate days), gradually increasing weights used and reps – and you can't hurry it. Perhaps you haven't been working out for long enough. Give it a year (take a 'before' photo of yourself, so you have something to compare with – you will get a pleasant surprise if you've been working out with dedication). If you manage to increase muscle mass, this will increase your metabolic rate and you should also find slimming and/or weight maintenance easier. If you're still carrying too much subcutaneous (under-skin) and abdominal body fat, though, you won't be able to see the muscles even if they're there.

See also:

- ▶ Questions: 36, 41, 62, 65.
- ▶ Feature: 4.
- ▶ A–Z entries: gyms, weighted workouts.
- ▶ Key index entries: exercise, metabolism.

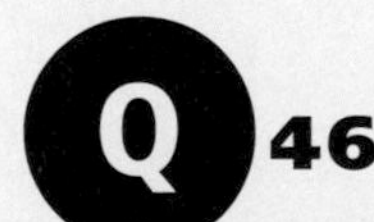

Q 46

I am female, with bulky arm and leg muscles – even though I do hardly any exercise. How can I get rid of them?

You sound like a classic mesomorph, and you are going to find it nearly impossible to turn yourself into a thin ectomorph or a rounded endomorph. However, some people with these body types would probably give a lot to be more like you. You can probably eat more or less what you want without getting fat and you are, no doubt, strong and fit as well, with good bone mass – all positives. What you may be able to do is streamline yourself with stretching exercises and/or yoga.

See also:

- ▶ Questions: 41, 47, 70.
- ▶ Feature: 4.
- ▶ A–Z entries: exercise classes, yoga.

Q 47

What about spot-reduction – can I choose where I lose fat via exercise?

Not really. It has been said that you can lose fat in specific places by working the muscles over them (the idea being that the muscle somehow burns extra fat in that place, or perhaps 'melts' it). However, research shows that this isn't the case. A study (reported in the excellent book *Exercise Physiology* by US professors McArdle, Katch and Katch) measured subcutaneous fat in either arm of tennis players and found that the fat underneath the playing arm (which was more muscular than the non-playing arm) was exactly the same as that under the non-playing arm. Body fat can only really be reduced by creating an energy deficit (see Q18) and using up stored fat this way – you can't dictate from where you want fat to go.

Research shows that fat tends to go first from the face, bust and abdomen – and, indeed, that the intra-abdominal adipose tissue is easier to mobilize than that elsewhere in the body, particularly of the hips and thighs. Hence, if you have a fat middle, it may appear that you are spot-reducing because, on a diet, this area will show the most marked changes initially. In reality, though, it isn't the case.

However, toning exercises can improve your appearance in specific areas by bulking, streamlining or flattening the area where the muscle is worked, giving you a better shape. This achieves a similar effect to spot-reducing and may be where the original misconception came from.

See also:

- ▶ Questions: 18, 41, 48, 52-4, 57, 59, 61, 64.
- ▶ Features: 4, 5, 6.
- ▶ A–Z entries: exercise classes, exercise equipment, gyms.
- ▶ Key index entries: exercise, weight loss.

Typing your body

People come in all shapes and sizes and it is unrealistic to try to conform to a shape far from your natural one. Broadly speaking, bodies can be categorized into one of three basic shapes. Some people are very true to type, but most of us may be near to one type but take some characteristics from another. Whichever you are nearest to, it is best to work 'with' it rather than 'against' it.

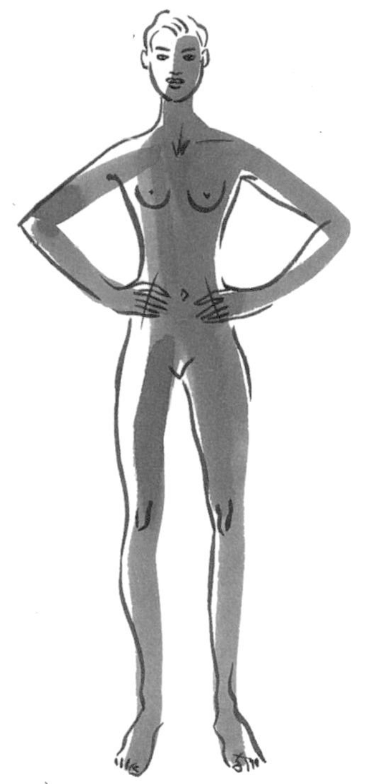

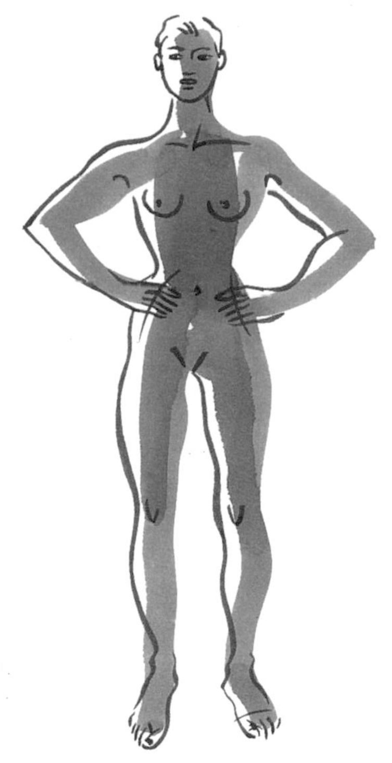

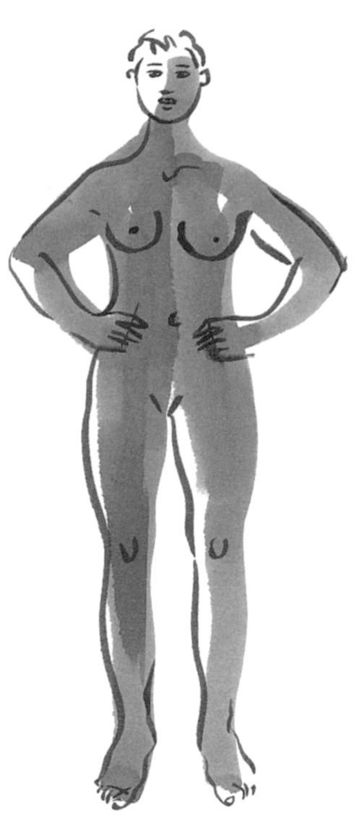

Ectomorph

The ectomorph body is tall and thin, looks 'narrow' and, usually, delicate. This type of person will probably find it hard to put on weight because of a high metabolic rate. Muscle profile may be low or moderate and can be improved with weight training. Body fat content will be lower than average and contours are sharp and angular. The ectomorph is suited to long-distance running, basketball and a variety of other sports in which limb length and light weight are advantages. In later life, an ectomorph may be predisposed to putting on weight around the abdomen.

Mesomorph

The mesomorph is well built, with well-muscled arms and legs and a general appearance of power. Mesomorph men are the closest body type to the classic 'V' shape, with powerful shoulders and chest, and slim midriff. Mesomorphs have a higher muscle-to-body-fat ratio than most and will be suited to sprinting, football, gymnastics and many other activities. Mesomorphs can eat plenty, as they usually like to keep active and their high proportion of lean tissue means their metabolic rate will be high. In later life they may do less sport and put on body fat.

Endomorph

The endomorph body is rounded, with a soft appearance. There is a higher-than-average body-fat percentage and muscle mass may be proportionately low. They may find that excess body fat accumulates easily and this may be compounded by a lack of interest in, or aptitude for, physical exercise. The endomorph will never be an ectomorph, but it is possible – with determination – to put on lean tissue, maintain weight at a healthy level and enjoy several forms of activity, such as walking or swimming. The endomorph should take care to avoid putting on too much weight, especially in mid-life.

Aren't endomorphs just fat ectomorphs or out-of-condition mesomorphs?

No, it's not as simple as that. If you were to visit a maternity unit and stay for a week, you would quickly see that when babies are born they really do all have their own shapes and sizes, even within the same family. Have a look at photos of yourself soon after birth (those ones on the rug with no clothes on!) and you should be able to spot your basic type from that. Sure, some mesomorphs can adopt endo-characteristics and some ectos may, in time, put on weight, but your basic type is what you were born with and what, mostly, you will stay with.

ANDROIDS & GYNOIDS

No, these aren't men from space, but two differing body shapes that may come into either of the 'big three' categories above.

Androids are an apple-shape, with most of their weight concentrated on the top half of the body, especially around the abdomen. Likely link: endomorphs, older ectomorphs and mesomorphs, especially males.
Gynoids are pear-shaped, with large hips, bottom and thighs, and proportionately small shoulders, chest and waist. Likely link: can occur in all three groups, especially females.

Of course, some people are neither particularly android nor particularly gynoid, but if you are an apple you can't turn into a pear, no matter how hard you diet or exercise, and if you are a pear you can't turn into an apple ditto.

Q 48

I'm not overweight but my stomach sticks out – what can I do about it?

You need to look for the likely cause. It could be that you suffer from abdominal bloating, which could be due to fluid retention. If you are female, this is most likely if your stomach grows large before a period, or if you tend to have fluid retained elsewhere (e.g. on the ankles or round the eyes). If so, see the diuretic diet in Feature 17. If you have no signs of this, it could be bloating through wind.

A diet very high in fibre, a poor balance of bacteria in the gut, stress, or other factors could cause this – and one main symptom will be that you do pass a lot of wind. A course of prebiotics (fructo-oligo-saccharides) and probiotics (acidophillus) should help this – any good health food shop will sell them. It may also be possible to pinpoint a food, or foods, that are causing the wind – possible culprits may be pulses, dried fruits, brassicas, yeasty foods, wheat, spices, coffee or alcohol. However, it may be that none of these foods are causing you problems and others may be to blame. In this case, eliminating the culprit(s) would be one solution, but strict elimination diets are only to be undertaken with professional guidance – see your doctor for referral.

One other dietary cause could be constipation, in which case the pre- and probiotics will also help, as will a diet high in citrus fruits and water. (Sadly, some high-fibre foods, such as pulses, dried fruits and brassicas, will prevent constipation but can make wind worse, so you have to be cautious here if you have both problems.)

Having ruled out all these causes, you are left with a) lack of abdominal muscle tone or b) poor posture – or a combination of both – as the likely causes. The majority of adults suffer from one or both problems to some extent. Feature 5 helps with posture and Features 6 and 24 provide abdominal toning exercises.

However, if you have an apple shape, as discussed on the left (and many apple-shaped people do have thin arms and legs and therefore don't consider themselves overweight), you should measure your waist and check Feature 3 to see if you are 'at risk' from a large middle. In this case, you may need to combine diet and exercise to gain a better shape and reduce health risks.

See also:
- Questions: 26, 28, 38, 56–7, 114, 203, 246–50, 324
- Features: 3, 4, 5, 6, 21.
- A–Z entry: slimming surgery.

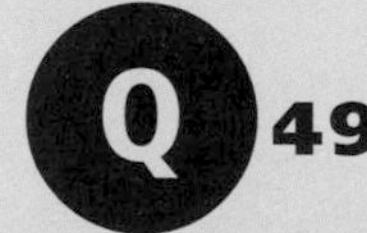

Q 49

I'm a flat-chested female – what foods or exercise will give me a bigger bust without putting weight on the rest of my body?

The bad news first – you can't really eat to put weight on your bust and nowhere else, just as you can't cut down on food and hope to lose weight from just one area. If you gained weight all over, you would put weight on your bust, but even then there is no telling whether it would be a little or a lot – and if you're pear-shaped it is more likely to end up on your hips and thighs.

However, there is still plenty you can do. You can improve your posture as per Feature 5, which will make your bust seem bigger and give you a better outline. Yoga will also help. You can also do chest exercises, such as push-ups and using a pec dec at the gym. These strengthen the pectoral muscles that lie beneath the breasts and will help 'uplift' them. A good well-designed, uplifting and cleavage-enhancing bra will complete the illusion.

You may also find that pregnancy and motherhood increase the size of your bust (however, I have to say that, with some women, the bust size actually decreases, though this IS less common) and, as you get older, the breasts often naturally increase in size.

See also:

- Question: 52.
- Features: 5, 6, 30.
- A–Z entries: exercise classes, gyms, weighted workouts, yoga.

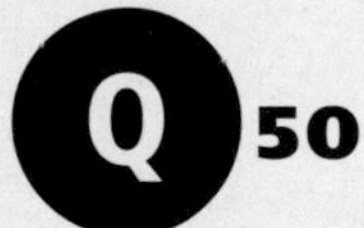

I've slimmed down to a weight I love, but I hate my bum – it is flat and shapeless. Any ideas?

You can improve a flat bum through both posture (see Feature 4) – standing correctly will immediately tighten and raise the bum – and regular 'gluteal' exercise, which will improve the size and shape of the buttocks a lot. Parallel squats and leg lifts will help (see Feature 6). A low-cost step platform is a good home investment for the glutes (as long as you use it!). At the gym, the step machine, the exercise bikes and the seated leg press will help. Stepping exercise classes are good. Outdoors, uphill walking, skiing and cycling are good. Other sports that give you a good bum are dancing, ice skating and gymnastics. To see improvement, you need to do whatever combination of these that you choose regularly.

I've also heard of bottom implants from the USA – like breast implants but larger. Before you consider this, however, remember that for many women a small bottom is the Holy Grail... and clothes do hang better if you have a slim behind!

See also:

- Question: 41.
- Features: 4, 5, 6
- A–Z entries: exercise classes, exercise equipment, gyms, weighted workouts.

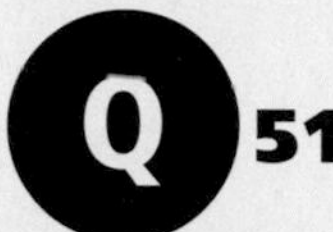

I have a short waist which makes me look out of proportion – can I alter this?

You can only really do this in three ways: one, through posture improvement – 'standing tall' can make the space between ribcage and hips appear longer; two, through stretching exercises such as the long body stretch and the waist stretch described in Features 5 and 7; and three, through yoga. Many yoga poses elongate or trim the waist (and losing an inch or two round here will also help create an illusion of more length). Indeed, any good body-conditioning class or session at home will improve the visual appeal of your body over time and help the overall balance.

See also:

- Questions: 41, 52, 62, 70.
- Features: 5, 6, 7.
- A–Z entries: Alexander Technique, exercise classes, Pilates, yoga.
- Key index entries: body image, exercise, posture.

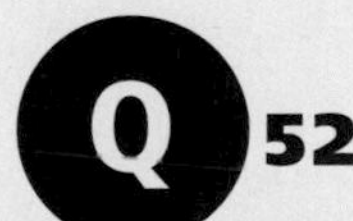

Are there any instant ways of changing my shape?

The best 'instant' way is by standing correctly – poor posture has a lot to answer for in terms of round shoulders, double chins, fat bellies, flat bottoms and knock knees (for example)! Feature 5 will explain how you can improve your look immediately and also provides exercises to help your posture long-term.

I suppose you could change some facets of your shape (e.g. fat stomach, big thighs) through liposuction – sometimes a painful process. It's not exactly instant but it does involve little effort on your part (apart from the work involved in earning the money to pay for it). For a special occasion, you could also try a salon wrap for a quick but short-lived minor change in your body measurements.

See also:

- Questions: 41, 62, 64.
- Feature: 5.
- A–Z entries: salon wraps, surgery.

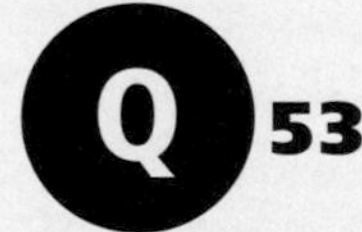

Is it true that a pear shape is the hardest shape of all to change?

This is a typically female shape, because the oestrogen hormones present in highest quantities in females predispose to laying down fat in the hip, thigh and bottom areas. This fat seems to be hardest of all body fat to 'mobilize' when an energy deficit is created (fewer calories taken in than are expended in energy) and it is thought that this evolved so that the female had plenty of fat stores to cope with pregnancy and breastfeeding in times of famine. In the Western world today, however, we rarely get famines, only feasts. In both men and women, studies have concluded that fat comes off the body from the top downwards, so this dispiriting aspect for a pear can also make it seem as if the fat never moves off the hips and thighs.

Hence, in essence, the pear shape IS hardest to change. Not all women are pear-shaped and, indeed, some men are pear-shaped – but if you are, you are basically stuck with it. Even if you manage to lose weight and lose inches, you will still be a slimmed-down pear shape, as your top half will have slimmed down too. It's not possible to find any diet or exercise plan that will get rid of the fat just off your lower body. However, you can tone up large hips, thighs and bottom with exercise and this can improve the appearance of a pear. Some people resort to liposuction, which has its drawbacks.

See also:

- ▶ Questions: 18, 54–5, 62.
- ▶ Features: 4, 6.
- ▶ A–Z entries: The Hip and Thigh Diet, slimming surgery.
- ▶ Key index entries: body shape, diets, pear shape.

54

Can I spot-reduce my hips and thighs by dieting?

No. When you create an energy deficit, by eating less and/or increasing exercise output, in general terms you will lose weight from all over. People who follow 'hip and thigh'-type diets also lose inches from their waist, bust and so on. In fact a 'hip and thigh'-type diet will probably seem to have more of an effect on the stomach at first, because body fat apparently shifts first from the face, bust (or chest) and stomach and last from the hips and thighs (see the answer to the previous question). People wanting to spot-reduce their stomachs will appear to have more success because of this – and research does show that abdominal fat is easier to shift. Not fair for the pear-shaped person, but see Q55 if you want to be cheered up.

See also:

- ▶ Questions: 54–5.
- ▶ Feature: 4.
- ▶ A–Z entry: The Hip and Thigh Diet.
- ▶ Key index entries: body shape, pear shape.

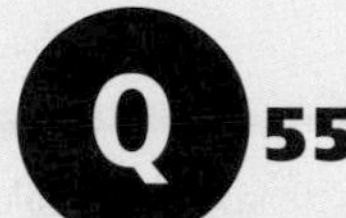

55

Is it true that if overweight is mostly on the lower half of the body it is perfectly healthy?

Nearly right. Very many research studies show that surplus weight concentrated around the abdomen (intra-abdominal fat, central fat distribution) is much more of a health risk than evenly distributed general overweight; also that heavy hips and thighs in women are normal, not a weight 'problem' (see Q53). It is because of this that some health professionals are now beginning to pay more attention to the Waist Circumference Test when judging overweight than to the Body Mass Index.

So, if you have a lot of weight on your hips and thighs but an average waist circumference (see Feature 3) – even if your Body Mass Index says that you are overweight – then you're probably not overweight at all! It is only if your waist is 'at risk' too, and/or your BMI is much over the normal range (again see Feature 3), that you may indeed be an overweight and at-risk pear.

To make sense of all these terms and figures you will need to refer back to previous questions and features as listed in the cross-references.

See also:

- ▶ Questions: 53–4, 102.
- ▶ Features: 3, 4, 9.
- ▶ Key index entries: BMI, intra-abdominal fat, waist circumference, waist-to-hip ratio.

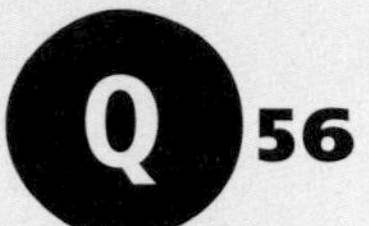

56

What is an apple shape and why is it unhealthy?

An apple-shaped person is one who has a tendency to store fat around the trunk (abdomen, bust) and upper arms (and who may have slim arms and legs), giving the shape of an apple – a small Cox or a large Bramley, depending upon how much fat is there. It has been found that this body shape has a higher link with several health problems, including diabetes and CHD (coronary heart disease), than other shapes (e.g. pear shape).

Indeed, even if the scales – or your Body Mass Index – don't say that you are overweight, but you have enough of an apple shape to give you a waist measurement over 37in (94cm) for men or 31½in (80cm) for women, then you have an increased health risk. Feature 3 gives much more information on all of this area.

So, if you are an apple, it is important to make lifestyle, eating and exercise changes to get your middle under control. As a bonus, you will also look a nicer shape. The good news is that intra-abdominal fat seems to be more co-operative in disappearing than lower-body fat.

See also:

- ▶ Questions: 26, 48, 57, 62, 102, 247–50, 324.
- ▶ Features: 3–4, 6, 9, 25, 29.
- ▶ Key index entries: BMI, intra-abdominal fat, waist circumference, weight and health.

How to lose pounds instantly

What a great idea – making bits of your body disappear, or look better, by simply standing or sitting correctly! You can look half a stone lighter in seconds – just by adjusting your body alignment. This could be the only 'instant miracle' you'll find in this book. Good posture is not only important for your shape, though, it can also help you feel better.

Poor posture can contribute to several of the body problems that people dislike most – a double chin, a droopy bust, a fat belly or a 'dropped' bottom, for example.

Mostly, poor posture comes along over time, encouraged by poor lifestyle habits – slouching in chairs, hunching over desks, not taking enough exercise, and many other factors. With the unpleasing body outline can come health problems too – poor body alignment is associated with headaches, neck pain, backache, and general aches and pains, as well as tiredness and lack of energy.

The illustrations on the right show the various benefits of standing correctly – follow the instructions and try to achieve the same stance yourself, in front of a mirror, and see how much better you look.

Of course, over years of incorrect use, the muscles that govern posture can become either too short, stiff and tight, or too long and weak – so if you find the right posture difficult, you definitely need exercises to help you get your muscles back into shape. Your abdominals, lower back, shoulders and gluteals probably need strengthening, and your chest, hamstrings and hip flexors may need stretching/suppling. Features 6 and 7 will help you to achieve this, and will, I'm afraid, take some weeks... there are no short cuts to strength and suppleness!

Also use the following tips – as, however diligently you do a daily 15 minutes or so of posture-improving exercise, if you spend the other 23¾ hours a day slouching around, you are unlikely to see the full benefit. Good posture is a 24-hour thing; get into the habit of it.

FINDING THE PERFECT PELVIC POSTURE

Experts say that the basis of all good posture is the correct tilt of the pelvis. The pelvis is the large bone structure connecting the lower spine with the legs and it consists of the ilium (hip-bone), pubis (pubic bone) and ischium bones.

If the pelvis is tipped too far forward, the stomach will stick out and the lower back have too great a concave curve and the spine be thrown out of alignment (1). If the pelvis is tipped too far back, the lower spine will be too rigid and flat (3). If it is aligned correctly as in the central illustration (2), correct posture will naturally follow. This 'neutral' tilt of the pelvis should also be maintained while sitting.

Stand in front of a mirror and practise tilting your pelvis into the correct position, keeping the knees slightly relaxed – you'll feel your ribcage naturally 'opening' as you do so.

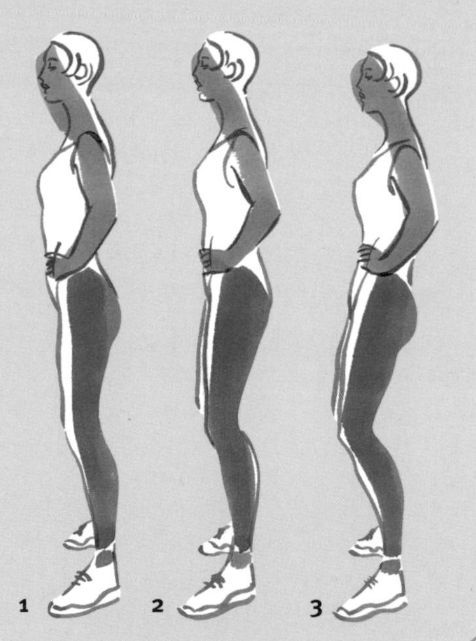

Other posture helpers

- Remember your posture as you stand – waiting for the kettle, cooking, chatting on the phone, standing in a queue. These hours really add up and can make a huge difference.
- Sit right, too – at work, in front of the TV, at the table, etc. Check now and then that your spine and pelvis are in neutral and your head well balanced on your spine, with no apparent muscle tension in the neck and shoulders.
- Yoga, Pilates and the Alexander Technique can all help you to gain better posture, as can many exercise classes, such as stretch and body conditioning (see A–Z).

1 With the upper body held in the correct position – shoulders relaxed and down, chest wide, neck balanced on the spine so that the ears line up with the shoulders – a double chin is minimized (and, indeed, can be prevented with regular good posture).

2 When the shoulders and spine are held correctly, the bustline becomes higher – good for a droopy or a small bust.

3 When the pelvis and spine are in perfect alignment and the bottom is tucked in, a 'pot belly' can virtually disappear – but it takes toned abdominal muscles to maintain this position for longer than a minute or so.

4 Correct posture can also lift the midriff area, making the waist seem smaller and the space between the lower rib and hipbone wider.

5 Strong abdominals and correct pelvic tilt uplift and 'tighten' the bottom by making the gluteal muscles work. This correct posture will also help to correct knock knees (inward-facing knees) and flat feet.

When correct posture is maintained, you may be up to an inch taller.

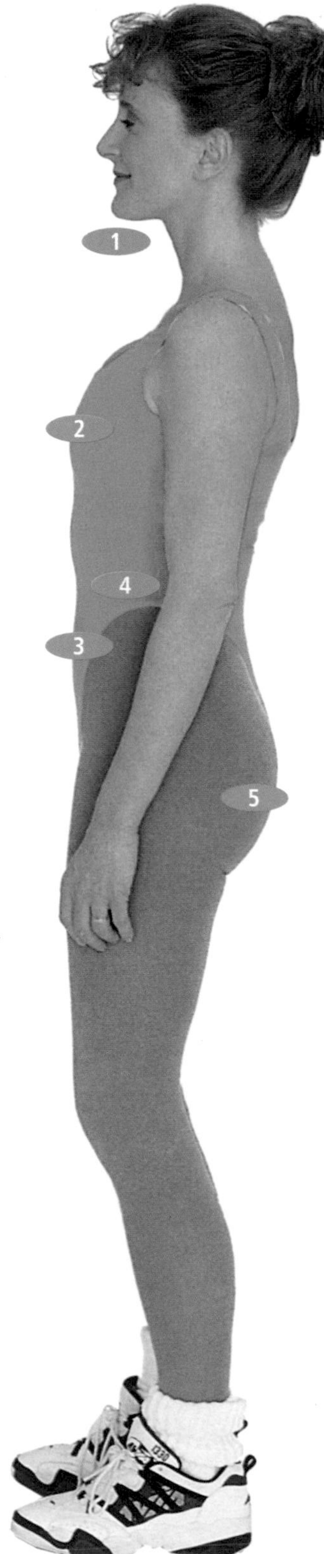

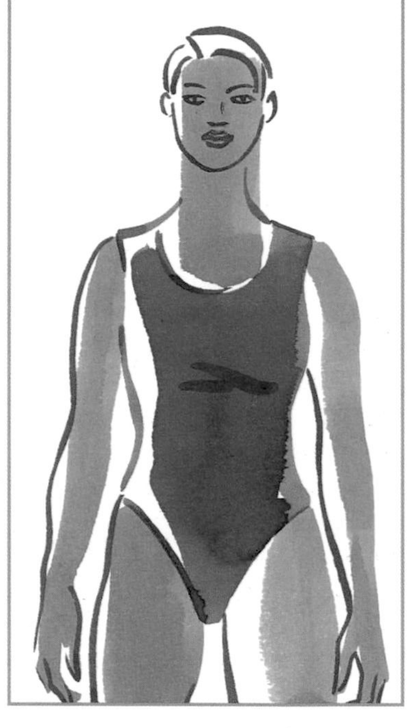

Front-on view of the upper body held in the correct position – shoulders relaxed and down, chest wide, neck balanced on the spine.

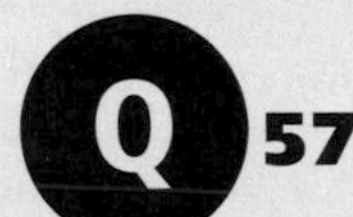

57

Can I lose my big stomach and flabby waist without my legs getting any thinner?

If you diet to lose weight (a good starting point might be Feature 9 or Q102), you will lose a little fat off your legs (and arms, and indeed elsewhere), but if you are the classic apple shape, with a round fat stomach and thin arms and legs, the fat loss on your limbs will hardly show compared with the amount of difference you'll notice on your middle. Apples are lucky in this way because the abdominal fat is usually not that hard to shift.

You should also combine the diet with exercise to trim your abdomen and add muscle – and therefore shape – to your limbs. The exercises in Features 6 and 21 will help. If you're out of condition, do this first and then you could move on to the weight training programme in Feature 30. Regular aerobic work, like cycling and/or rowing, will also help. At the end of all this, you should look more in proportion.

See also:

- Questions: 47, 56, 58, 102, 247.
- Features: 3, 4, 6, 9, 21, 29, 30.
- A–Z entries: exercise classes, exercise equipment, gyms.
- Key index entries: body shape, exercise.

58

What is the best way to get a firm, flat stomach?

Lose weight if you need to (e.g. on the plan in Feature 9) – no matter how terrific your stomach muscles, they won't show through layers of fat – and do lots of regular abdominal work for your muscles, exercising not only the rectus abdominis – the large 'six pack' muscle that runs the central length of your abdomen, but also the obliques, to either side, and the transversus abdominis, the 'core' muscles that lie across your abdominal region.

You only need a few different exercises to work all these areas, but you need to do them slowly and well. For some reason, many people hate doing abs exercises, and so skip them or do them in a half-hearted way. If stomach floor exercises make your neck hurt, use an abdominal cage, which can be quite cheap. Yoga and Pilates will also help tone and firm the abdomen.

The reason your stomach is often the first area to get slack if you don't pay attention is that it is an area of your body that doesn't get exercised much in the normal course of sedentary life. To target the abs during your normal day, try getting up from chairs without using your hands to help, walk uphill and downhill when you can (or stairs will do) and do the following exercise:

Sit in the correct pelvic tilt position (see Feature 5); draw in your abdomen, concentrating on the area below your belly button. Pull in as hard as you can, breathing normally, and hold for a count of 5. Relax and repeat whenever you remember. (You may not want to do this exercise if you have high blood pressure.)

Other stomach exercises are detailed in Feature 24 (this is mainly for men – but will work for women too) and Feature 6.

See also:

- Questions: 36, 48, 57, 62, 102.
- Features: 3, 5, 6, 9, 21.
- A–Z entry: exercise equipment.
- Key index entries: dieting, exercise, weight loss.

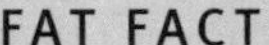

FAT FACT

What women like best in a man:
flat stomach, small bottom, muscular chest, well-shaped legs.

What men like best in a woman:
medium-sized breasts, round bottom, small waist, long legs.

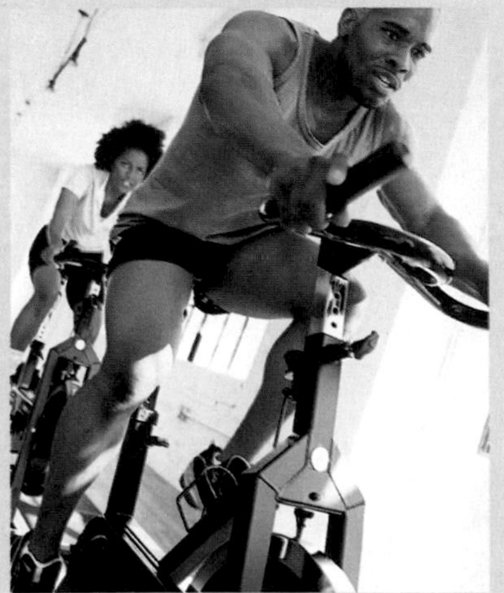

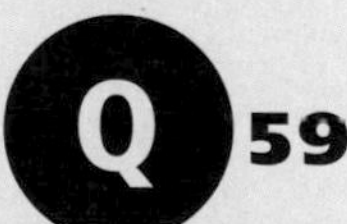

59

My bust is too big – can I reduce it through diet and exercise, without losing weight off the rest of my body?

As you'll see if you read the answers to Qs 47, 49, 54 and 57, the idea of spot-reducing or gaining fat on any one particular part of the body is a bit of a myth, with the exception that when you lose weight over time, it tends first to come off the face, bust and stomach. So I suppose if you lose a small amount of weight there is a chance that your bust will get smaller (along with your face and stomach) and, if you then stop at that point, the rest of your body will stay the same. However, this isn't an exact science. No exercise can reduce your bust, I'm afraid. If it is really very large and is causing you problems, I suggest you see your doctor and ask him to refer you to a specialist for further advice.

See also:

- Questions: 47, 49, 54, 57.
- Feature: 4.
- A–Z entry: slimming surgery.
- Key index entry: body image.

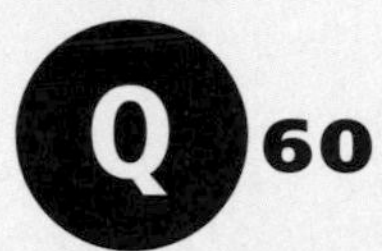

60

How can I improve the look of my thin and weak-looking arms and legs – the rest of me isn't too bad?

If you don't need to gain weight in the form of body fat, your only option is to gain lean tissue (muscle), and to do this you must do strength exercises for your arms and legs. This involves working against resistance, with weights or otherwise. Weights can be free weights or the kind you find at the machines in the gym. Resistance can be using your own body weight (e.g. in the classic push-up exercise) or someone else's. Various types of aerobic work (e.g. jogging for legs or rowing for arms) will also increase muscle strength and size in the limbs worked, by offering resistance of a different type. Training needs to be done regularly and with gradually increasing intensity (i.e., heavier weights, more repetitions, more resistance or longer work).

If you have thin arms and legs, it is possible that you are – or may become – an apple shape, in which case you may also consider doing training for your central body as well. You will find further information on all of this in various parts of this book.

See also:

- Questions: 41, 44, 56, 62.
- Features: 3, 4, 6, 28–30.
- A–Z entries: exercise classes, exercise equipment, gyms, weighted workouts.
- Key index entries: body shape, body image, intra-abdominal fat.

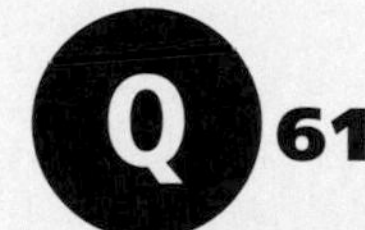

61

My face is fat and yet I am quite slim – is there anything I can do about this?

I am afraid, if your face is naturally round and full, even though you aren't overweight, you can't diet your face thin, and there aren't any facial exercises you could do to remove fat either (see the questions about spot-reducing: 47, 54 and 59). I have heard of people having liposuction on their face and even removing teeth to give themselves hollow cheeks, but this seems somewhat drastic. If you really don't like your cheeks, your make-up (if you happen to be female) and hairstyle can go a long way to disguising this. I'm also told that, as you age, the face is likely to thin down.

See also:

- Questions: 41, 47, 54, 59.
- Feature: 4.
- A–Z entry: slimming surgery.
- Key index entry: body image.

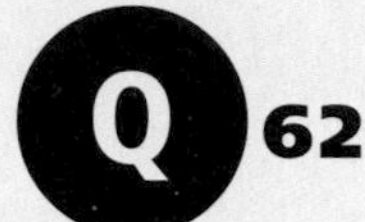

62

How long will it take to exercise my body into a better shape?

Unfit people beginning a regular strength and tone exercise programme may begin to see improvement within 2 to 3 weeks, especially around waist and stomach. Various trials have shown significant improvement in body shape can be achieved in 8–12 weeks, with lean tissue (muscle) increase up to 6½lb (3kg), and small decreases in body-fat percentage, through strength training alone.

Further reduction of body fat could be achieved with moderate calorie restriction and an increase in aerobic exercise, such as brisk walking or cycling. Combine all that with some work on your posture, and mobility exercises to improve flexibility, and you could certainly make a noticeable difference to your body shape in three months, whatever your age. People with an apple shape may notice even more difference.

How many hours a week you have to put in to achieve this will vary from person to person, but an hour a day would be plenty to achieve considerable improvements. If you are extremely unfit, you need to begin with light work and build up gradually, so it may take longer in terms of weeks, and you should see your doctor about beginning an exercise programme if you are ill, have any disability or haven't exercised in a long time.

Section 10 contains much more information on your weight and fitness.

See also:

- Questions: 53–8, 63, 65–7, 69, 72–3, 328–65.
- Features: 3, 4–7, 28–30.
- A–Z entries: exercise classes, exercise equipment, gyms.
- Key index entries: body shape, exercise, fitness.

10-minute tone

This simple home routine provides a workout for all your major muscle groups and will help you tone up in about 10 to 25 minutes, depending on how many sets you do.

General Instructions:

- Wear flexible, comfortable clothing and exercise in a warm area on a firm non-slip surface covered with a mat or thick towel.
- Don't exercise after a heavy meal.
- Take 3 minutes (already included in the total time for the routine) to do the warm-up thoroughly, as your muscles work better and more safely when warm.
- Carry out each move with concentration and effort, doing it in a slow and controlled way.
- Maintain good posture throughout the warm-up and exercises (see Feature 5).
- Repeat each exercise 8 or 10 times (or do fewer reps if the working muscle begins to shake). One batch of 8–10 repeats is called a set.
- As you get stronger, increase the number of sets you do to two, then finally to three, resting for 30 seconds between sets.
- When you have finished the routine, go to the stretching routine (Feature 7) and take 5 minutes to do the stretches there. This will help to prevent muscles from hurting the following day and will also help you become more supple.

How long will it all take?
One set plus warm up will take about 10 minutes
Two sets plus warm up will take about 18 minutes
Three sets plus warm up will take about 25 minutes
(Add another 5 minutes to these times for the cool-down stretches on pages 52–3.)

Warm-up (3 minutes)

- Circle both shoulders for 20 seconds and then march on the spot, starting slowly and then gradually raising your knees higher and pumping your arms more strongly. Do this for 2 minutes.
- Place the hands on the hips and, with the legs slightly apart, circle the hips clockwise then anticlockwise for 60 seconds.

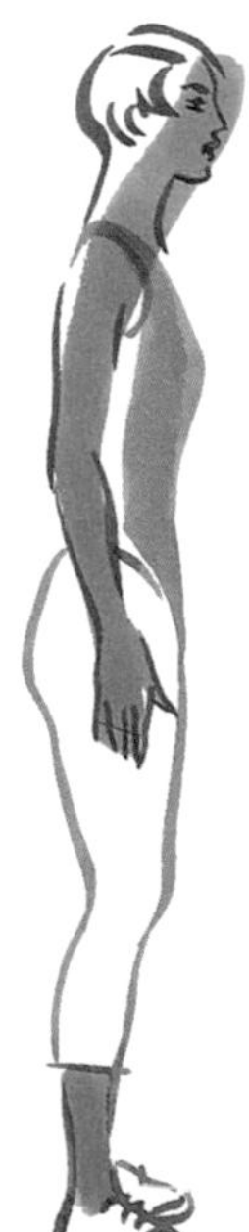

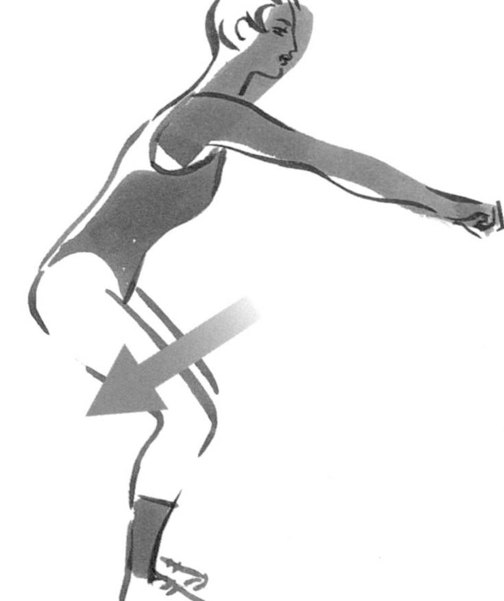

Squats (for bottom and thighs)

Stand with the feet hip-width apart and bend your knees until your thighs are approximately at a 45-degree angle to the floor, reaching your arms forward to aid balance as shown. Slowly return to the starting position.

In later weeks: as you get stronger, you can increase the difficulty of the exercise by squatting deeper, but go no further than when your thighs are parallel to the floor.

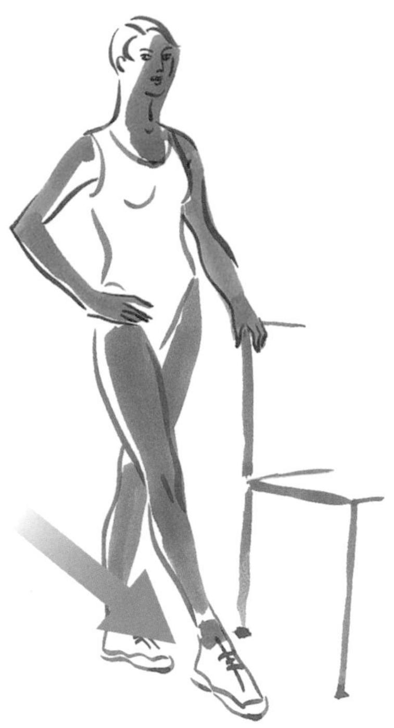

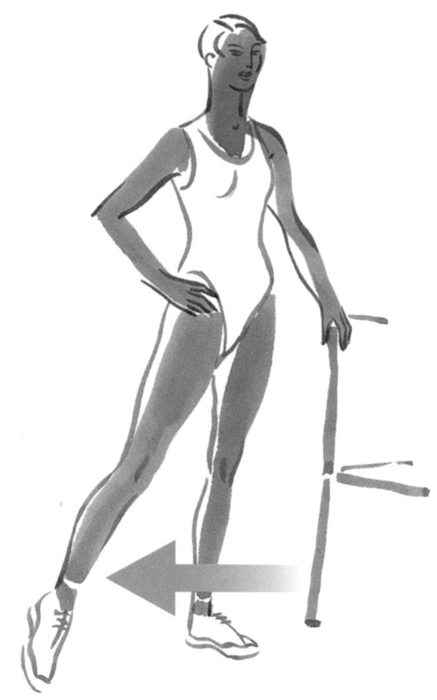

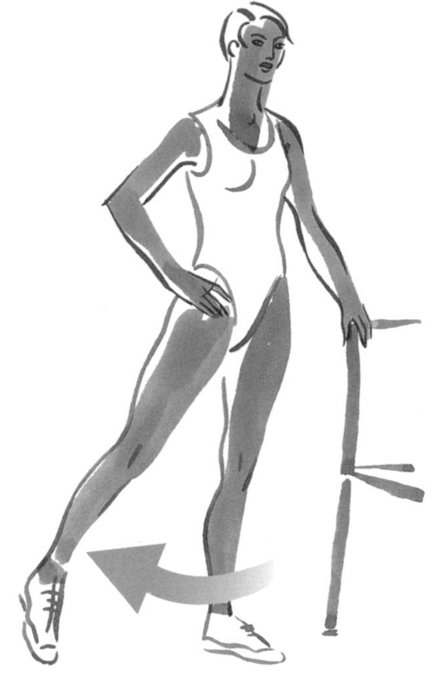

Outer thigh tone (for hips, outer thighs and bottom)

Stand (with your left hand lightly resting on the back of a chair if you like) with feet hip-width apart and place the right hand on your hip. Bring the right leg in front of you so that the pointed toe touches the floor; now sweep the right leg out, round and back in a smooth motion to as far behind you as the toe will go. Your toe can lightly touch the floor as you move. Bring the leg back to the starting position. Doing this once to right and once with the left leg counts as one repeat (but do all your repeats on the same leg before moving on).

In later weeks: if you feel like buying a set of exercise bands, you can increase the resistance by placing the bands round your ankles.

Side bends
(for obliques – sides of torso)

The sides of the waist are quite hard to tone up, so I have included an extra exercise for this area. Stand with the feet a little more than hip-width apart and place the left hand on the side of your head. Holding a 2lb (1kg) weight (or food can or filled plastic water bottle) in your right hand, bend down to your right as shown, then slowly return to upright. Doing this once to the right and once to the left counts as one repeat (but do all your repeats to the right first, then swap the weight over and exercise the other side).

In later weeks: increase the weight slowly if you can.

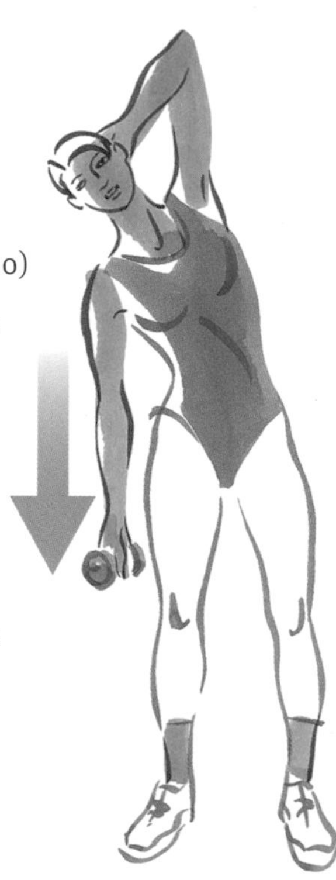

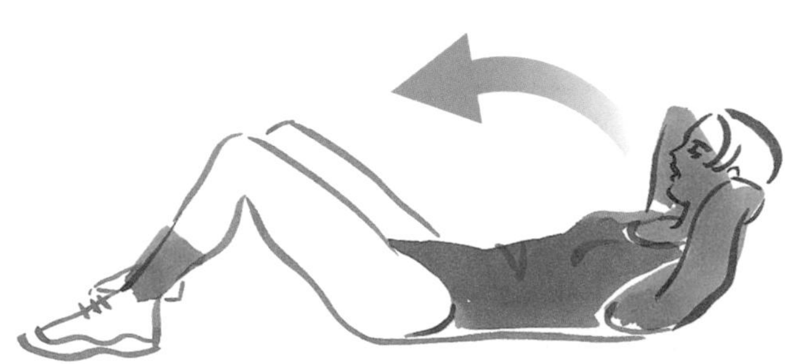

Crunches
(for rectus abdominis, i.e. front of stomach)

Lie on the mat with your knees bent, feet flat and spine relaxed, hands resting on the sides of your head. Breathe in and, as you exhale, curl up a few inches so that your head and neck are off the floor; then, as you breathe in, slowly return to the floor. If you have any neck problem, you could use an abdominal exerciser (see A–Z, exercise equipment).

Reverse curls (for transversus abdominis – i.e. core stomach muscles)

From the same starting position as the previous exercise, bring the knees into the chest with your ankles crossed and feet relaxed. Concentrate on the area of your stomach from belly button to pubic bone, and try to work the muscles in this area as you breathe in. Exhale and, still concentrating on this area, curl your hips towards your ribcage in a small controlled movement. Slowly return to the starting position.

In later weeks: you can bring your shoulders a little off the mat to meet your knees as you go.

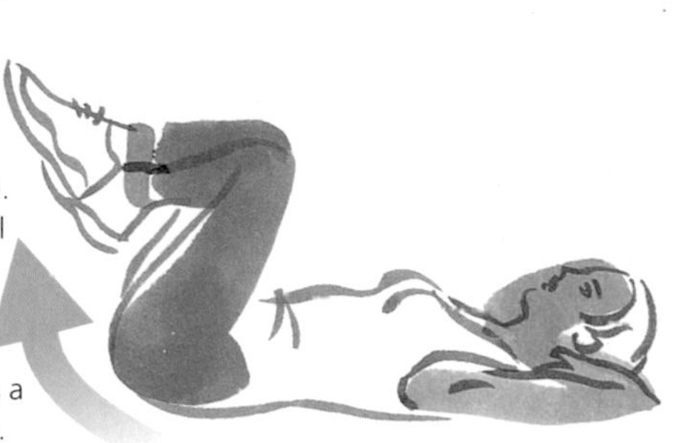

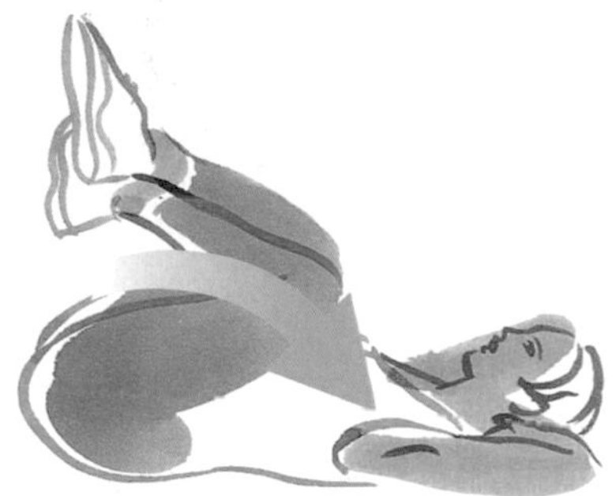

Diagonal crunches (for the oblique abdominal muscles/waist)

From the same starting position as the previous two exercises, as you exhale, take the right shoulder up, moving the right elbow towards the left knee and keeping your hips flat on the floor. Slowly return to the starting position. Doing this once with the right shoulder and once with the left is one repeat, but finish all your repeats on the right side before swapping to the left side.

In later weeks you will be able to come further up towards the knee.

Press-ups (for the chest and shoulders)

Turn over and kneel on all fours, with your thighs at right angles to the floor and with good posture. Wrists should be in line with the shoulders and fingers pointing forwards. Lower the chest slowly towards the floor as far as you can, then slowly return to the starting position.

In later weeks: move your hands and shoulders further forwards and lift your lower legs with ankles crossed, so that your lower body is supported on your knees (avoid this if you have joint problems).

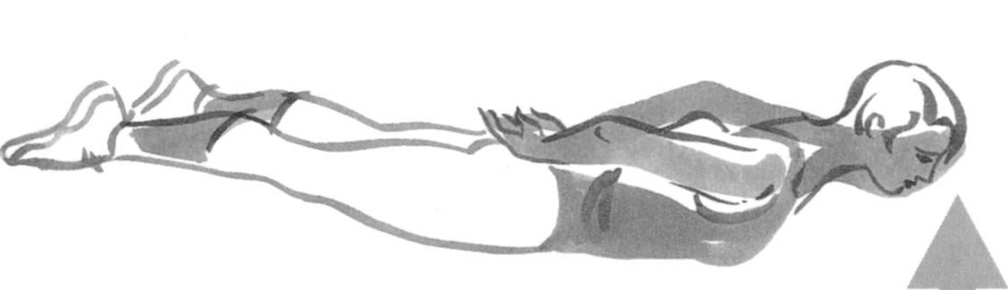

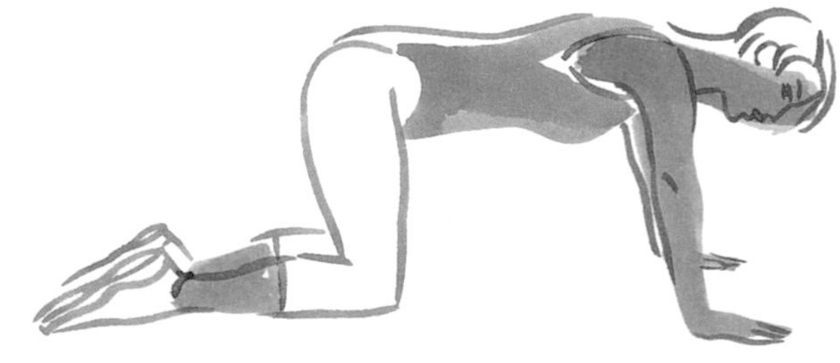

Back extensions (for the lower back)

Lie on your front, with the arms at your sides, hands resting on your bottom. Exhale and slowly raise your head and neck off the floor, looking towards the floor as you do so. Your hands will slide a little down your bottom. Slowly return to the starting position. In later weeks: alter the starting position so that you bring your right arm out in front of you, with your left arm bent and hand under head. When you raise your head and neck, also raise the right arm straight out in front of you. Do half your repeats on this arm, then the remainder with the left arm out in front of you.

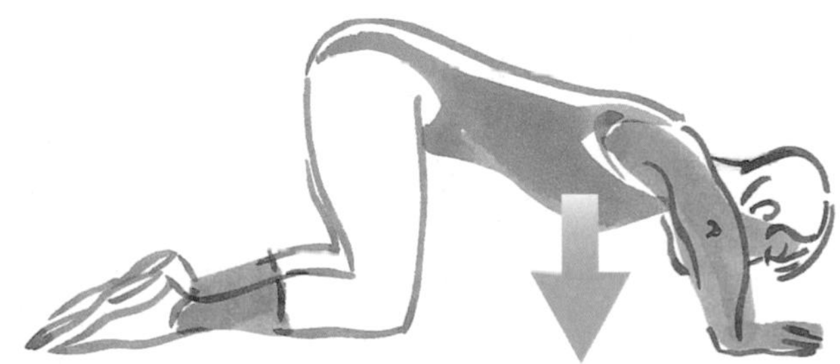

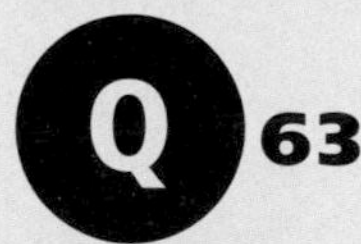

63

I have a month to get in shape before my holiday – what can I hope to achieve?

If you need to lose a little weight, you could probably lose about half a stone (3kg) without resorting to a crash-type diet. If you need to lose a lot more, you could probably lose a few pounds more. If you do regular weight-training and aerobic exercise (say, every other day), you could firm your stomach, slim down your waist a little, and improve posture and the appearance of your arms, legs and bottom.

How much is really up to you, your own body, how hard you work and so on. If you're really out of condition, however, you definitely shouldn't go 'mad' to try to get in shape – you could injure muscles or tendons, strain your back, you may feel exhausted, have headaches, and so on. Even if you only do very mild toning work, if you start today and do it regularly – at least 3 times a week – you'll definitely look and feel a bit better by your holiday. Don't forget to continue your programme during the holiday and when it is over.

See also:

- ▶ Questions: 52, 62, 65, 328-65.
- ▶ Features: 4–7, 9, 27–30.
- ▶ A–Z entries: exercise classes, exercise equipment, gyms.
- ▶ Key index entries: body shape, body image, exercise, slimming.

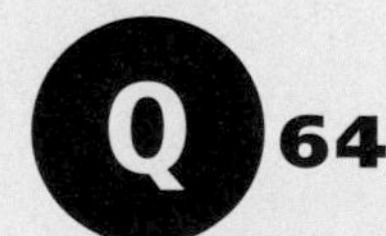

64

Do you recommend a salon wrap or similar treatment to help lose weight in a hurry?

What you will get from most salon wraps (discussed in more detail in the A–Z) is temporary inch loss from the wrapped areas. You will no doubt be measured at several strategic points before you are 'wrapped' and again afterwards, and the salon will add up the small losses and tell you that you have lost *x* number of inches altogether. This will probably sound more impressive than it actually is. However, you will probably find that the abdomen and waist area reduce the most, and this might be useful if you wanted to wear a special, slightly tight dress, for instance. Normally, after an evening of eating and drinking, most of the benefit of the wrap will disappear. It's only a temporary solution, as what has 'disappeared' is fluid not fat. No wrap can get rid of your fat for you; you need to create an energy deficit to do that.

See also:

- ▶ Question: 52.
- ▶ Feature: 5.
- ▶ A–Z entry: salon treatments.
- ▶ Key index entries: body shape, body image, exercise.

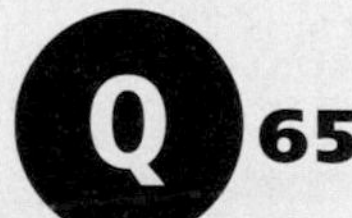

65

What's the best exercise programme for toning that I can do at home in about 20 minutes?

The programme in Feature 6 is a good all-round one for beginner or intermediate. It covers all the major muscle groups in from 10 minutes up. Combine it with the stretching programme in Feature 7 for safety and flexibility, and you will tone up sensibly over a period of a few months (although you'll look better after a few weeks). If you have time to do regular aerobic work, choose a type (or types) that combine an increase in your cardiovascular fitness with extra benefits for your muscle toning. Feature 28 shows which activities help which parts of your body most. For more advanced exercising, see Section 10.

See also:

- ▶ Questions: 66–73.
- ▶ Features: 4–7, 28–30.
- ▶ A–Z entry: exercise equipment.
- ▶ Key index entries: body shape, exercise.

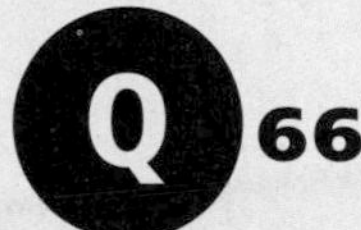

66

Which are the best and worst exercises for building muscle tone?

Assuming that a toned muscle is one with optimum strength and flexibility, then all exercise will help tone to some extent. Aerobic exercise tones the muscles being worked (e.g. legs in running, arms in rowing). Stretching exercise tones by conditioning, smoothing and elongating. Resistance (weight) training tones by altering the composition of the muscle and adding lean muscle mass (bulk).

If by 'building tone' you mean 'building muscle', then of the three only resistance/weight training puts on much lean tissue mass. One study showed that men who did an aerobic walking programme for 16 weeks added only about 1/2lb (0.25kg) of lean tissue during that time, whereas intense weight-training (combined with a high-protein diet) can add 1lb (0.5kg) a week or more.

One report says young men following a high-resistance training programme for a year can add 20% to body weight, most of which is lean tissue, and women can gain up to 75% of this amount. However, training on these levels is beyond the scope of this book and advice should be sought from a reputable gym.

See also:

- ▶ Questions: 41, 44–5, 62, 65, 67, 69, 356–8.
- ▶ Features: 4, 6, 30.
- ▶ A–Z entries: exercise equipment, gyms, weighted workouts.
- ▶ Key index entry: exercise.

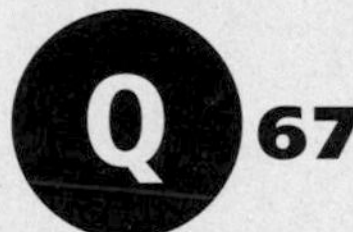

67

What home exercise equipment would you recommend for general toning?

I think the most useful pieces of equipment are a set of dumbbells (1, 2 and 3kg, plus a stand for them is useful) for toning upper body; a step platform for toning lower body; and perhaps a set of resistance bands (good for travel as they are so lightweight). An abdominal exerciser (cage) is a good idea as it saves strain on your neck when doing lying stomach exercises. More on all these is in the A–Z. However, you could get by without any of them, or spend a lot more.

See also:

- ▶ Questions: 65, 69.
- ▶ Feature: 6.
- ▶ A–Z entry: exercise equipment.

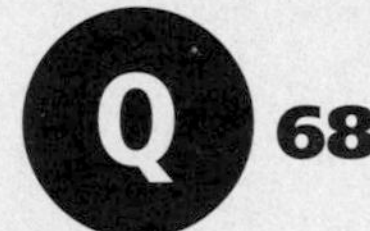

68

Now I have reached my target weight, how can I exercise away unsightly skin around my stomach and waist left from when I was very fat?

If you have lost a great deal of weight, these skinfolds can be very hard, if not impossible, to shift, especially if you were overweight for a long time and/or are older. It might be a good idea to see your doctor, as it is possible to remove the surplus skin via an operation called an abdominoplasty. You would be a good candidate as you are now down to target weight. You can also have the operation done privately. For more information, see Slimming Surgery in the A–Z.

See also:

- ▶ Questions: 57–8.
- ▶ A–Z entry: slimming surgery.

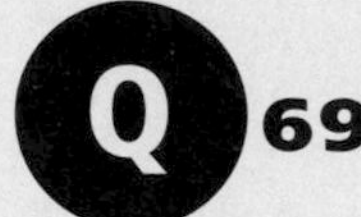

69

The diet's going fine, but can I shape up without spending any money?

You certainly don't need to join an expensive gym (or, indeed, any gym) or buy an expensive treadmill or multigym, for example. Just with regular walking (see Feature 29) and doing the toning programme in Feature 6, you will improve your fitness and appearance – assuming you are out of shape and unfit at the moment. This would cost you only a comfortable and supportive pair of walking shoes, trainers and suitable clothes for both programmes.

Quite often, however, people who start out doing a moderate and non-expensive programme get 'the bug' and end up buying all sorts of equipment. It is also true that a few fairly inexpensive and small pieces will help your programme. This is partly because, as your fitness improves, you need to work harder to keep improving (otherwise you 'plateau') and equipment can be a great help with resistance and aerobic exercise at home, as well as beating the boredom factor.

However, there are millions of once-used pieces of exercise equipment all over the world, gathering dust in cupboards under the stairs, and so it certainly is wise to think very carefully and choose very carefully before spending any money. As a rule, buying cheap equipment is a waste of money, not a saving, in the long run. The equipment section in the A–Z will help.

If you do decide to buy anything, my tip is to get a money box and put in it the money you're saving while slimming – say, on high-fat, high-cal junk foods or alcohol. Seeing this quickly mount up is a good motivation to stick to a reduced-calorie plan and, when you have enough, you can buy equipment without feeling guilty.

See also:

- ▶ Questions: 65, 67.
- ▶ Features: 5, 6, 7, 28–30.
- ▶ A–Z entry: exercise equipment.

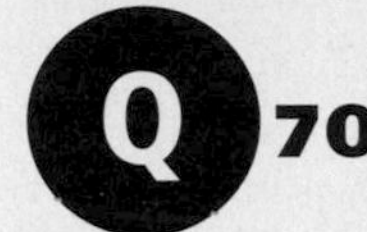

70

What is the best exercise for making myself look taller and slimmer?

Good posture is the best starting point – see Feature 5. Then any exercise that involves stretching will help you to look taller, as your muscles are streamlined. Examples are a stretching routine or class, yoga, Pilates and the Alexander Technique. Toning exercise will help you to look slimmer by flattening out the areas that most people don't like – a tummy bulge is a perfect example, so all the abdominal exercises in Feature 6 would help there.

See also:

- ▶ Questions: 41, 47–8, 51–2, 59, 62.
- ▶ Features: 4–7.
- ▶ A–Z entry: exercise classes.
- ▶ Key index entries: body shape, exercise.

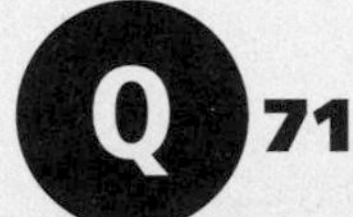

71

Can you recommend an easy exercise programme to limber up before and after the gym?

It really is essential to warm your body up properly before exercise and to cool down afterwards, and this is no doubt what you mean when you say you want to 'limber up'.

A warm-up literally warms up the major muscle groups to prepare them for exercise and helps to prevent strain and injury. It should also raise your heartbeat slightly. There is a short warm-up routine at the start of Feature 6. Before a vigorous gym routine, however, I would increase the time spent on this warm-up to 5 minutes – adding slow pedalling or slow treadmill will do.

A cool-down can consist of a couple of minutes resistance-free cycling on your gym exercise bike, or a little gentle marching on the spot to get your heart rate down slowly, followed by a stretching routine – stretching out all the major muscles and holding the stretches.

This stretching helps prevent muscle pain after your workout and is also the ideal time to 'supple up' your body as, after your gym routine, the muscles and tendons are more 'warm and willing'.

For stretches, do the whole of Feature 7, holding the stretches for 30 seconds each or longer. This is about as easy and simple a stretching programme as you'll get without skimping. Warm-up and cool-down should also be carried out before and after aerobic exercise – even a brisk walk.

See also:

▶ Features: 6, 7.
▶ Key index entry: exercise.

72

What changes in body shape and appearance are natural as you age?

Research has shown that, even in élite athletes who continue to exercise regularly throughout life, changes in body shape and composition do happen. Among élite runners studied over 20 years from the age of 50 to 70, the waist thickened by an average of 2 inches (5cm), body-fat percentage increased by an average of 5% and lean tissue (muscle) decreased by an average of 5½lb (1.5kg).

So, for people undertaking a less rigorous exercise regime as they get older – most of us – these changes could be expected to be sharply increased. That is, you will gain intra-abdominal fat and, possibly, extra fat elsewhere and you will lose muscle (on average, muscle strength decreases by 30% by age 70), meaning that you will look less toned up and fit.

Tests also show that if you don't do regular stretching and move each limb through its full range of movement, you will become less and less supple over time, because the connective tissue of the joints (tendons, ligaments and cartilage) stiffens. The result of this is a more awkward gait and general diminishing of movement typically associated with 'old age'.

Lastly, bone density diminishes with age (though this is blunted with regular resistance exercise) and the main effect of this on physical appearance is loss of height. In old age (70+), on average, people also tend to get thinner and lose body fat. However, before you get too depressed, there is a wealth of research to show that with regular exercise and good nutrition and posture, ALL these age-related symptoms can be greatly minimized and even, to a large extent, reversed – and it is never too late to start.

See also:

▶ Questions: 27, 41, 73.
▶ Features: 4–7, 28–30.

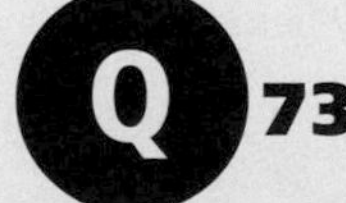

73

Can I reverse age-related body shape changes through exercise?

You can't reverse every last sign of ageing, but research does show that older people respond very well indeed to regular exercise – not just 'stopping the rot', but making amazing improvements to their shape and their amount of lean tissue (muscle); reducing their body fat percentage (and also greatly improving their cardio-respiratory fitness and overall health and chances of longevity). One typical study showed that men aged 60 to 72 doubled their muscle strength over 12 weeks of weight training. The consensus seems to be that in middle and old age you can have a body equivalent in fitness to someone 20 to 25 years younger with effort.

For older people as for the young, the best exercise is an all-round programme of resistance (strength) exercise, aerobic exercise and stretching – remembering to check with your doctor first and taking it very easy to start with. Most leisure centres provide exercise classes geared specifically for older ages. Good posture becomes even more important as you age.

See also:

▶ Questions: 72, 332.
▶ Features: 4–7, 28–30.
▶ A–Z entries: Alexander Technique, exercise classes, Pilates.
▶ Key index entries: body shape, exercise.

FAT FACT

Old people really do shrink. Due to bone loss and loss of fluid, shrinkage of 2 inches (5cm) is average. After the late 60s, body-fat percentage and Body Mass Index also usually fall.

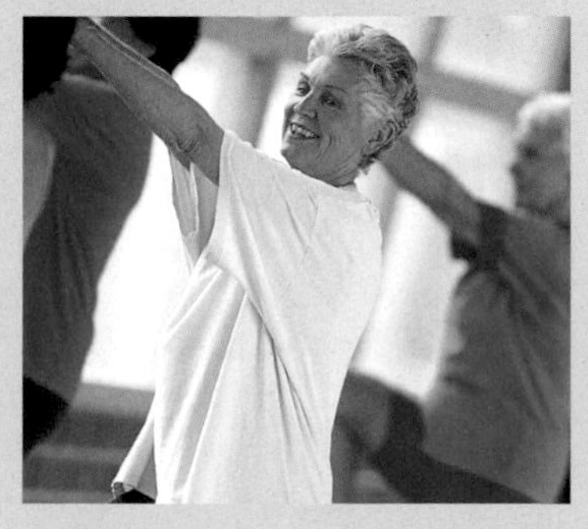

5-minute stretch

Use these few simple stretches to aid flexibility, as a cool-down after resistance work or aerobics, or try them at any time as an aid to helping you unwind and relax.

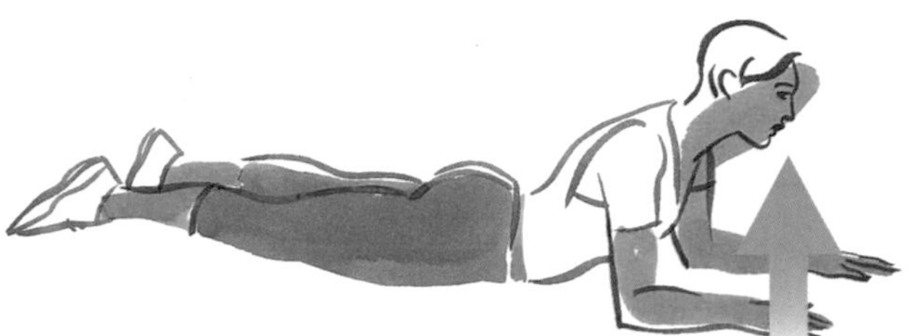

Abdominal stretch

Lie on your front, with the arms bent, palms under your shoulders, fingers pointing forward. Keeping your neck long and forearms in contact with the floor, raise your chest and shoulders until your upper arms are at right angles to the floor as shown. Hold, feeling a stretch through the front of your body.

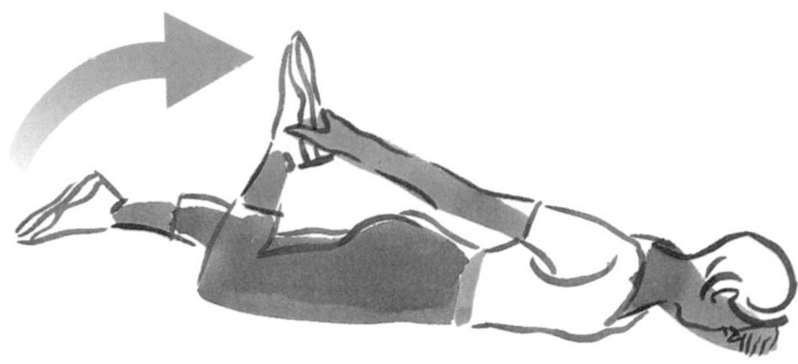

Quadriceps stretch

Lying on your front, bring your right foot towards your body and grasp the centre of the foot with your right hand to bring it in towards your right hip. Hold, feeling the stretch up the front of your right thigh. Repeat to the other side.

STRETCH TIPS

- Wear comfortable, stretchable clothing and do the stretches on a non-slip surface covered with a mat or thick towel.
- Do them when your body is warm (after other exercise is ideal).
- Hold each stretch for a minimum of 10 seconds, up to 30 seconds.
- Try to relax as you stretch, breathing calmly and deeply. You should find that after 10 to 15 seconds you can go further into the stretch.
- When stretching, you should feel a pleasant warm sensation in the muscle being stretched – you should not feel a 'burn'. Stop immediately if you do and try that stretch again tomorrow.
- Over time you will be able to do the stretches better – e.g. your legs will straighten out better in the hamstring stretch; your knees will get nearer the floor in the inner thigh stretch. That means you are getting more flexible and this will help your posture as well as helping protect you from exercise-related injury.
- Latest research finds that stretching as part of a warm-up may be a waste of time – it is no use either for improving performance or for preventing injury during exercise.

Back stretch

Kneel on all fours and arch your back like a cat. Hold, feeling a stretch through the lower and mid-back. Relax and lower your hips down to your heels, stretching your arms out forwards and feeling the stretch in your mid-back and shoulders. Hold.

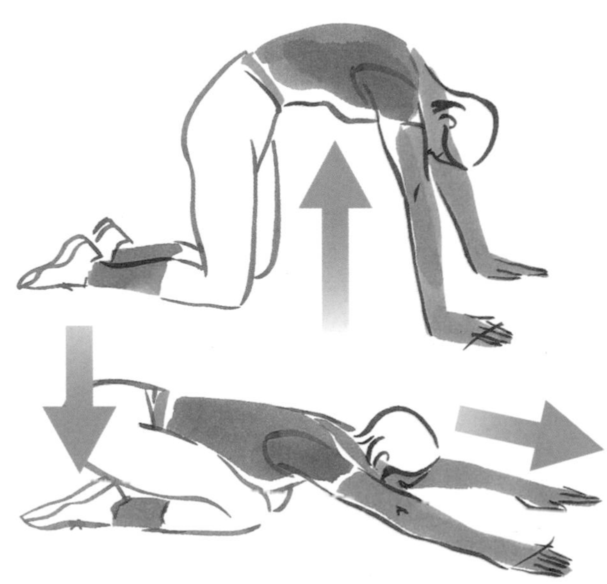

Hamstring stretch

Lie on your back with knees bent and feet flat on the floor. Clasp the back of the right calf with your hands and slowly bring your right leg in towards your chest, then slowly straighten your right leg as far as you can to feel a stretch at the back of the thigh. Hold. Return your foot to the floor and repeat to the other side.
NOTE: Many people have tight hamstrings and you may not be able to straighten your leg out much at first.

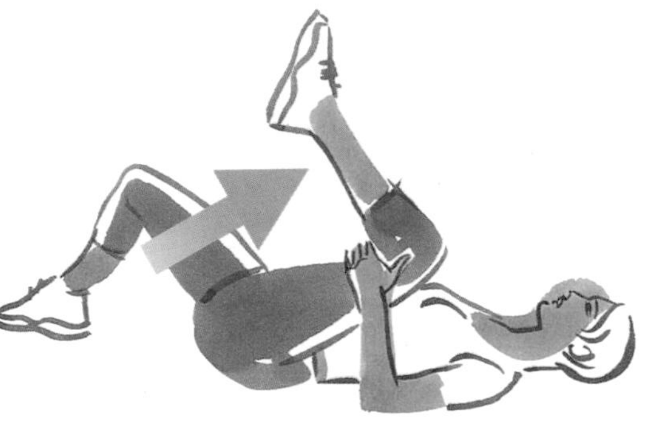

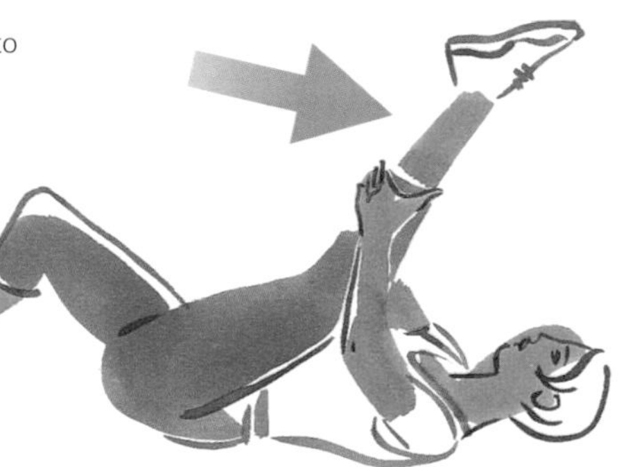

Chest stretch

Sit with your legs in a comfortable relaxed position with your back neutral (see page 42). Link your hands behind your back and, keeping your elbows bent, extend your arms behind you, pulling the shoulder blades together. Feel the stretch across your chest. Hold.

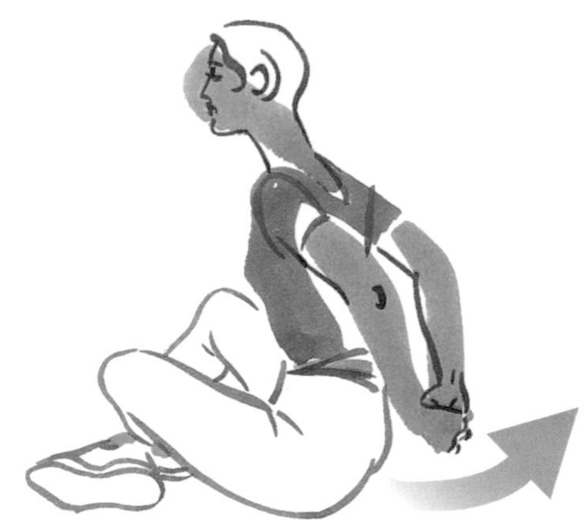

Outer thigh stretch

Sit with the left leg extended in front of you and with your right palm supporting you on the floor near your right hip. Take the right foot over your left leg and place it on the floor outside your left knee. Use your left arm or hand against the outer side of your right knee to move the right knee gently towards your body, feeling the stretch in the right buttock and thigh. Hold. Repeat to the other side.

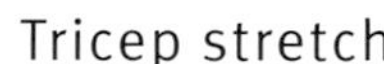

Tricep stretch

In the same sitting position as the Chest stretch, bend your left arm with the elbow close to your head and the left hand behind – and to the right of – your head. Using your right arm, apply gentle pressure on the upper arm near the elbow, moving it backwards until you feel a good stretch up the triceps (back of arm). Hold.

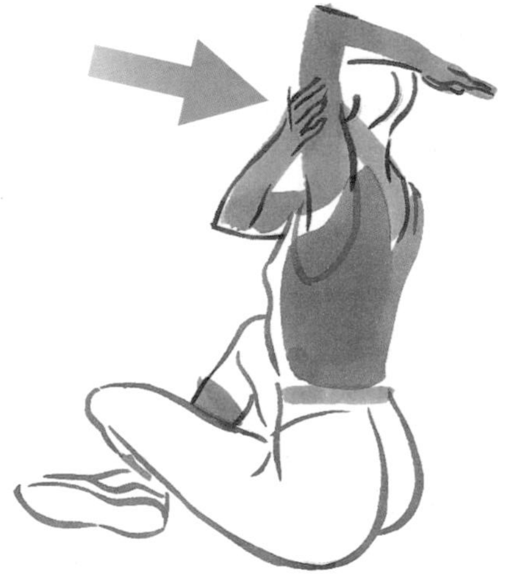

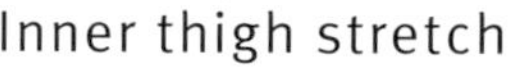

Inner thigh stretch

Sit with your legs bent, soles of your feet together and knees apart. Clasp the inner ankles with your hands and rest your forearms along your lower legs as shown. Press gently on the inner knees to ease them a little nearer the floor. When you have taken the press as far as is comfortable and feel the stretch in your inner thighs, hold.

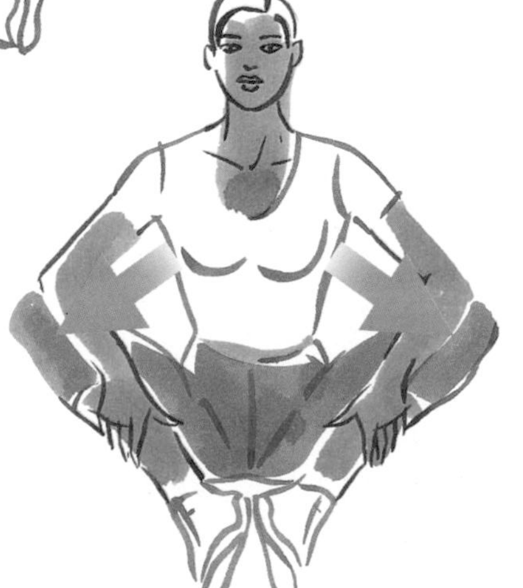

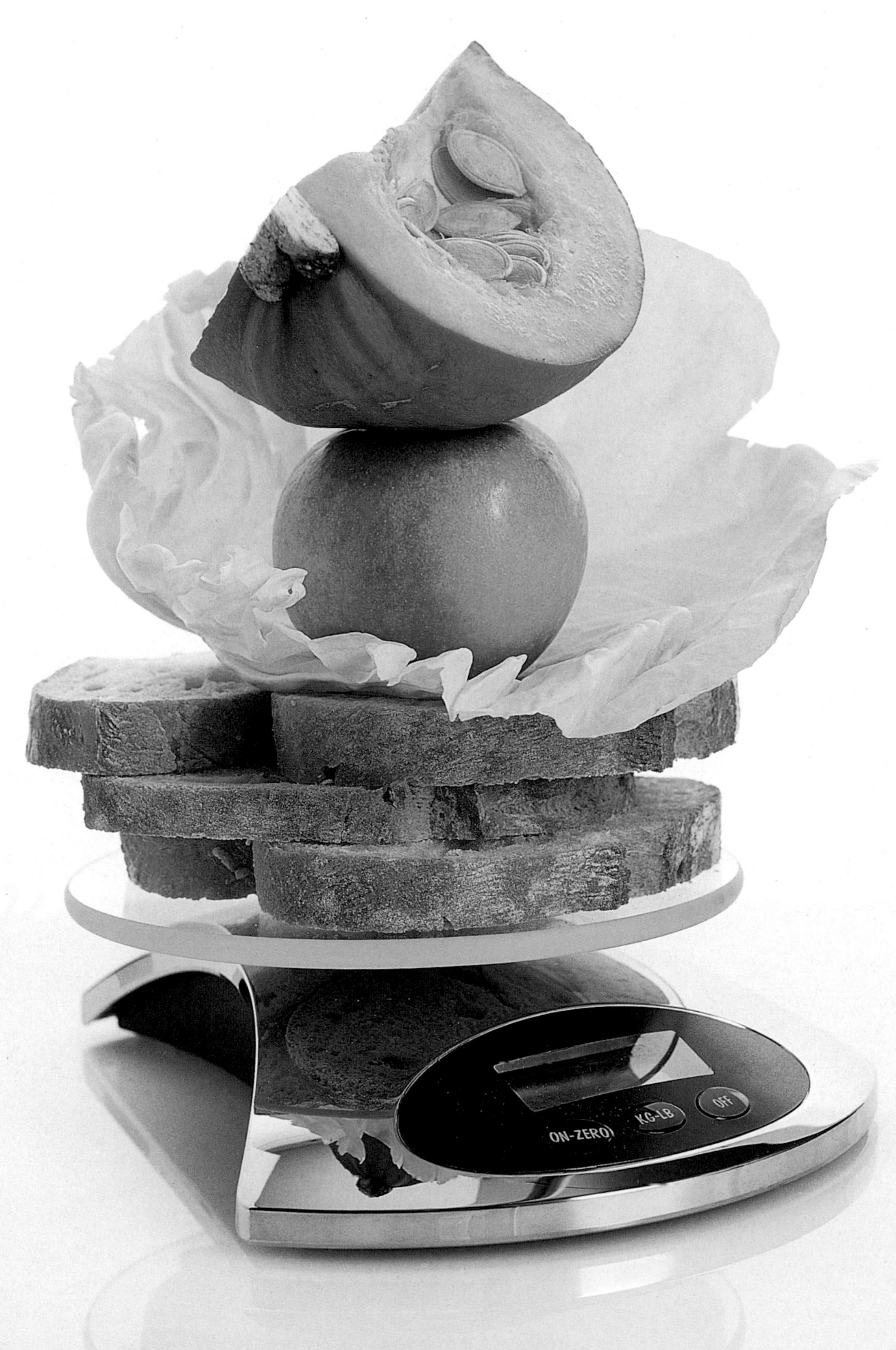
ON-ZERO
KG-LB
OFF

Section Three

Food, glorious food

It is nothing but a pity that in the minds of many slimmers, would-be slimmers, and even many people simply worrying about eating a more healthy diet, food is regarded as 'the enemy', and hence eating becomes a battleground.

Such a battle is hard to win, because we're not even always sure who the enemy is, or what strategies to employ. Which foods are the 'goodies'? Which are the 'baddies'? What will really work to get this problem licked? Fasting? Food combining? One meal a day? And, of course, we're fighting a foe that we really want to embrace (give in to the banquet, the binge), so determination is low. Hence those who do win the food – and weight – battle tend to be diet dictators, using iron will to stay in control.

Perhaps, then, for all those who worry about their weight, the answer is to get back to viewing food as part-pleasure, part-necessity, but never something against which to wage war. This section aims to banish the guilt and alter the seesaw of love and hate into something more balanced, via the facts and, hopefully, a large dose of common sense and reassurance.

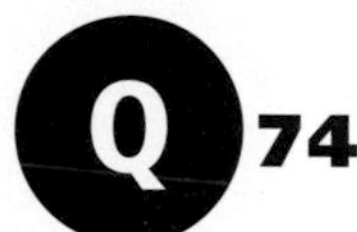

Q 74

What are calories?

Calories are a measurement of energy, like the energy in food and that expended by humans. One kilocalorie (generally simply referred to as a calorie in nutrition, and certainly in this book) is the energy it takes to raise the temperature of one kilo of water by 1°C. For example, a food item containing 200 calories has enough energy to raise the temperature of 200kg of water by 1°C, or 2kg of water at 0°C to 100°C (boiling point). Human energy intake and output are also sometimes measured in kilojoules (now the official measure in the EU). One (kilo)calorie equals 4.2 kilojoules (kJ). A megajoule is 1,000 kilojoules.

Calories in food are measured by burning it in a calorimeter and measuring heat released into a surrounding water bath. Similarly, human energy output can be measured in a large form of the calorimeter – an airtight room where heat given off by the person is measured and converted into calories 'burnt'.

By experiments like these we can measure the energy (calorie) cost of living and activity for anyone.

See also:

- ▶ Questions: 75–79, 104, 108, 110–11.
- ▶ A–Z entry: calorie counting.
- ▶ Key index entries: calories, energy, food value charts.

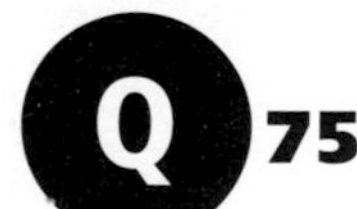

Q 75

In what types of food are calories found?

Almost everything that you eat or drink contains calories – with the notable exception of water. Some items, such as dried herbs, diet drinks and black tea (as examples), contain virtually no calories.

The four food groups that contain calories are carbohydrates, fat, protein (the 'macronutrients' – so called because they are the major nutrients) and alcohol. The food you eat can be made up from one or more of these food groups. Most foods contain at least two – e.g., a potato is mostly carbohydrate but also contains some fat and protein, and a beefsteak contains fat and protein but no carbs. Sugar is an exception – containing only carbohydrate – and pure oils are another exception – containing only fat.

The macronutrients each contain different quantities of calories. Carbohydrate contains 3.75 cals per gram; protein 4 and fat 9. Alcohol contains 7 calories per gram (most alcoholic drinks are a mixture of carbohydrate and alcohol).

See also:

- ▶ Questions: 74, 76–9, 104, 108, 110–11.
- ▶ Feature: 9.
- ▶ A–Z entry: calorie counting.
- ▶ Key index entries: alcohol, calories, carbohydrates, fat, food value charts, macronutrients, protein.

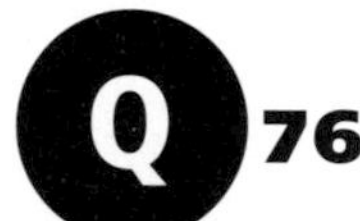

Q 76

What happens to food after I've eaten it?

The food is broken up in your mouth and mixed with saliva to help it travel down the oesophagus (a journey of about 3 seconds) to the stomach. In the stomach, the gastric juices (a mix of enzymes, mucus and hydrochloric acid), with the help of muscle contractions called peristalsis, break the food down into chyme – a semi-liquid state. Protein begins to be broken down into peptides. The only nutrients that can be absorbed into your bloodstream via the stomach are alcohol, which is why its intoxicating effects are apparent so quickly, a small amount of simple sugars, water and water-soluble vitamins and minerals.

After up to 5 hours in the stomach, the chyme is properly 'churned' and ready to move on. (Liquids that have been ingested will pass through the stomach quickly – sometimes in only minutes. Carbohydrate foods pass through the stomach quickest – around 2 hours – protein next and fatty foods slowest.) Now the chyme gradually passes through the three sections of the small intestine – the duodenum, the jejunum and the ileum – where it mixes with digestive juices and most absorption of nutrients takes place.

Enzymes (proteins that speed up chemical reactions in the body) finish the breakdown of protein into amino acids. Fats are broken down into glycerol and fatty acids. Carbohydrates are broken down into maltose, glucose, fructose and galactose. Now these macronutrients, together with micronutrients (vitamins, minerals) and water, can pass through the walls of the small intestine and are carried in the blood or lymph to where they are needed. This journey through the small intestine takes about 3 hours.

The simple sugars (the broken-down carbohydrates) are carried by the blood to the liver, after which they can either be sent to the cells as glucose for use as energy after further processing, or be converted into glycogen and stored in the liver or muscles, easily available when energy is required suddenly. The surplus is converted into fatty acids and stored in

> **FAT FACT**
>
> Research reported in *The Lancet* concludes that diminished sense of taste and smell decrease appetite – bland diet may help some people to slim.

the adipose tissue. (However, alcohol cannot be stored in the body and must be 'burnt' as energy.)

The amino acids (the broken-down protein) are also carried in the blood to the liver. From here they may be circulated and used to build or repair muscle and enzymes as needed. If the body requires extra energy (say, if not enough carbohydrate has been eaten to produce enough simple sugars for current needs), the amino acids can be converted into a form of simple sugar and used as energy. Surplus amino acids can also be converted into fatty acids and stored in the adipose tissue.

The fatty acids and glycerol (broken-down fat) are carried around the body in lymphatic fluid as triglycerides and join the blood, which may give it a milky appearance. When the circulating fat finds tissues needing energy, enzymes help it to be taken up by these cells. However, fat is not the body's favourite energy source for normal everyday use – glucose is, especially in unfit people. Unused blood fats are returned to the liver and then stored as adipose tissue, the body's major reservoir of energy. This can be converted back to usable energy at any later date via further chemical reactions, once the body perceives an energy deficit or during exercise. Fat cannot be converted into protein and only 5% of it (the glycerols) can be converted into glucose. However, dietary fat is more easily converted into body fat than either carbohydrate or protein.

Back in the intestines, the remaining unabsorbed matter is passed through the large intestine – the colon – which absorbs some of the water, and finally it is excreted as faeces. The journey through the large intestine takes, on average, 14 hours.

See also:

- Questions: 77-90.
- Feature: 8.
- Key index entries: anabolism, catabolism, digestion, metabolism.

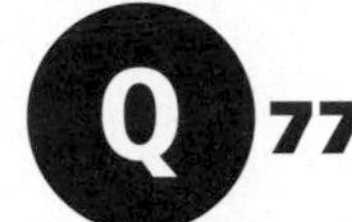

77

What happens in my body if I don't eat?

On water only and no food, your body takes about 2 days to use up both the food you've eaten and its glycogen stores. During this time you'll feel hungry and blood sugar levels will dip, which can leave you feeling weak, faint, dizzy and lacking in concentration. You'll lose several pounds, which is mostly fluid, as you'll also excrete extra urine. After 2 days, the body begins to rely completely on its own fuel for energy – its fat stores and lean tissue.

After 3 days on a fast, it is normally reported that hunger pangs cease and bad breath begins. This may have an odour of 'pear drops' or nail polish remover, and is due to the production of substances called ketones, which happens when fat is burnt in the absence of glucose. You begin to feel the 'fasting high' – full of energy and clear-headed, as well as calm. Your metabolism slows down to try to conserve energy and you may feel the cold more. You may also be constipated. Loss of water – together with minerals, including sodium and potassium – continues. Weight loss takes place at about 1 pound a day.

If the fast continues for more than a few days, it can place a strain on the heart and kidneys. Nutrient deficiencies start to become apparent (e.g. without vitamin C, gums may bleed). Bone loss may occur and periods may stop in women. Prolonged ketosis can be dangerous. Death from malnutrition and body malfunctions is likely within 60 days. Ketosis and fasting are discussed in detail in Qs 88 and 107.

See also:

- Questions: 76, 86–88, 97, 105–109.
- Feature: 9.
- A-Z entries: fasting, high-protein diets, low-carbohydrate diets, very-low-calorie diets.
- Key index entries: fasting, ketosis.

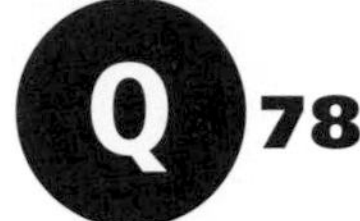

78

What happens if I eat more than I need?

Eat more protein than you need and excess can be converted into glucose for energy, if needed, and then into fat stored in adipose tissue. Eat more carbs than you need and excess is converted into fat or nonessential amino acids. Eat more fat than you need and excess is stored as body fat.

When you drink alcohol, it can't be stored and must be disposed of (via breath or urine) or used for energy. Alcohol metabolism takes precedence over carbohydrate metabolism and thus, if you drink to excess, more carbs will be stored as fat. So excess calories of any type can contribute towards making you fat.

See also:

- Questions: 18, 75–6, 79.
- Feature: 1.
- A–Z entry: calorie counting.
- Key index entries: calories, weight maintenance.

FAT FACT

In an average lifetime, the digestive system will process around a staggering 30,000kg of food.

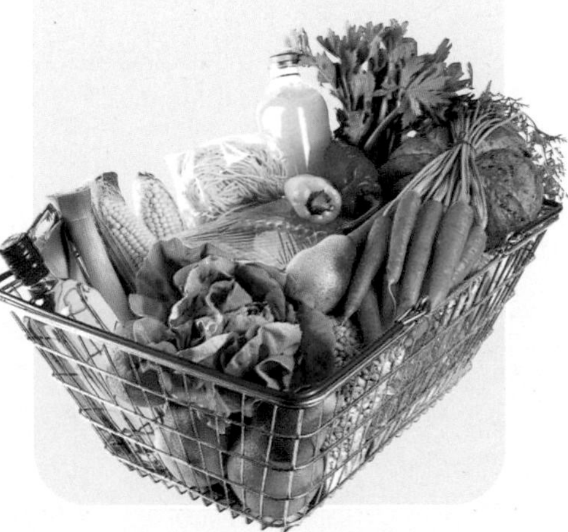

FAT FACTS

The stomach secretes 3 litres of gastric juice a day.

In a young adult, the average length of the small intestine is around 3 metres – in old age, it may well have stretched to about double that length.

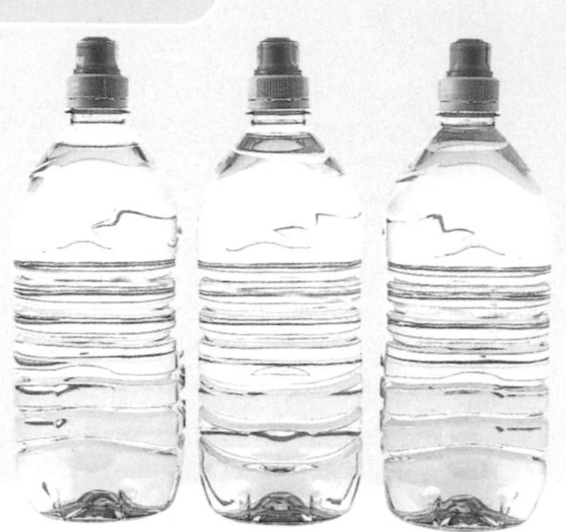

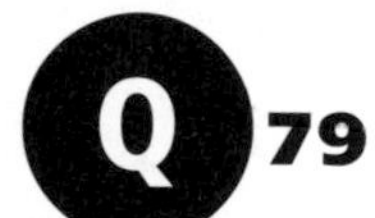

79

What types of calories tend to put on most weight?

Surplus calories from all types of food – fat, carbohydrate and protein – have the potential to be stored as body fat and thus will 'put weight on'. However, the consensus of opinion from experts seems to be that a diet high in fat calories may predispose you to weight gain. This is discussed in more detail in other questions.

See also:

- Questions: 18, 74–6, 80, 89.
- Features: 1, 8.
- Key index entries: calories, carbohydrate, fat, metabolism, protein.

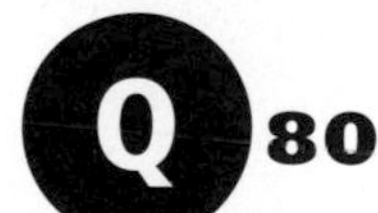

80

Do carbohydrate foods encourage weight gain?

All types of food calories eaten 'surplus to requirements' are stored as body fat and that applies to surplus carbohydrate foods as much as anything else. (A surplus is defined as taking in more calories than you expend in energy. To work out your own energy requirements you need to go back to Feature 1.)

Having said that, there may be a small scientific advantage in overeating on carbohydrates rather than fat, because fewer of the carbohydrate calories will end up as part of your body fat. This is because carbohydrate burns off about 25% of its calories in the 'effort' of turning itself into body fat for storage, whereas dietary fat is very efficient at turning itself into body fat and uses only about 3% of its calories in the process. Therefore, there will be a little less body fat gained from an excess carbohydrate intake of, say, 500 calories than an excess fat intake of 500 calories.

Carbohydrate consumption can, however, influence weight in other ways. First of all, for practical purposes, I am going to divide carbohydrates into two types. Type one consists of the simple and highly refined carbohydrates, like table sugar, sweets and white flour. Type two describes all the complex and 'natural' carbohydrates like pulses, whole grains, fruits and vegetables. (This isn't quite the same as the usual division of carbohydrates into 'simple carbohydrates' and 'complex carbohydrates', because the carbohydrate content of fresh fruits – with the exception of bananas – is in the form of sugars, which are simple carbohydrates, not complex. 'Complex' carbohydrates are contained in starchy foods and dietary fibre. Vegetables usually contain both starch and sugar.)

The simple, or highly refined, carbohydrates, like packet sugar and white flour, may be partly responsible for encouraging you to eat more calories than you need and thus put on weight. There are several reasons for this:

1 They are often combined with fat by food manufacturers into highly dense, high-calorie foods (sometimes called 'junk' foods), such as cakes, biscuits, confectionery, desserts, pies, etc. These are the foods that, research shows, are most likely to be 'binge' foods or 'comfort' foods. It is also shown that they usually 'slip down easily' and are therefore usually eaten quickly, so 'I'm full' signals don't come into play in time to prevent you eating more than you need.

2 Low-fat carbohydrate foods, such as white bread, fatless cakes, slimmers' biscuits and desserts, and much confectionery don't promote satiety – i.e., you don't feel full for long after you've eaten them. They may also cause blood-sugar levels to rise rapidly and then dip rapidly (see Q84). These effects may make you more inclined to eat more.

On the other hand, what I call the 'natural' carbohydrates – like whole grains (brown rice, porridge oats, whole-wheat pasta), root and other starchy vegetables (such as potatoes and yams) and pulses, along with fresh fruits and veg – have been shown to work in almost the opposite way. They slow down eating time, as they are high in bulk and need chewing. They are not dense – meaning that you get much more weight of food for your calories and it is actually hard to eat enough of them to get a surfeit of calories. They promote satiety by filling the stomach, taking longer to digest and keeping blood-sugar levels even – although some are less good at this than others (see Q84). They are also less usually eaten combined with high amounts of fat – although not always. Many fruits and veg, pulses and oats, barley and rye are good sources of soluble fibre, which helps to slow down the rate of sugar absorption and also lower blood LDL cholesterol levels.

A diet high in carbohydrates can increase fluid retention in the body – they tend to 'soak up' more fluid and hold on to it; hence you may feel more bloated and your stomach may look larger on such a diet. However, this isn't fat.

Researchers have pointed out in defence of the high-carbohydrate diet that in the UK during the last world war the national diet was high in carbohydrate (55%) and moderate in fat (33%), and that the population was slimmer and healthier than we are today.

The consensus seems to be that a diet high in 'natural' carbs doesn't encourage weight gain and, as a bonus, is also 'good for you' in terms of nutrients, fibre and possible protection against disease.

See also:

- Questions: 78–9, 81–90.
- Features: 9, 10.
- A–Z entry: low-fat diets.
- Key index entries: carbohydrates, Glycaemic Index, junk foods.

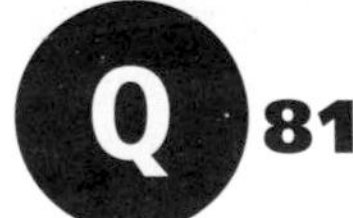

Is sugar so bad for you?

Dietary sugar can be divided into two categories. One is extrinsic – the types extracted from sugar cane or beet, honey, etc., and added to manufactured foods such as cakes, biscuits, desserts, confectionery or preserves, soft drinks and alcohol. The other is intrinsic – natural sugar found as part of the cellular structure of the plant, in foods such as fresh and dried fruit and vegetables. These fruits and veg make up an important and necessary part of a healthy diet and the sugar in them is more slowly absorbed, partly because of their soluble fibre content.

Extrinsic sugars can, as we saw in the previous question, lead to overeating, and the World Health Organization reported that a preference for sweet-fat mixtures has been observed in obese women and may be a factor in promoting excess energy consumption. Regular consumption of extrinsic sugar is a major cause of tooth decay. A high-sugar diet may promote insulin resistance, a condition where high blood-sugar levels mean that the hormone insulin (which helps cells to absorb the glucose) is released in higher-than-normal amounts, and over a long period of time this may blunt the response of insulin, which then needs to be produced in ever greater quantities. Type-2 diabetics have insulin resistance. However, other types of simple carbohydrates can also promote high blood-sugar levels. There is also some evidence that a high-sugar diet produces raised levels of a substance called glycosylated haemoglobin in the blood, high levels of which are associated with a greater risk of heart disease.

Sugar, in itself, contains no nutrients at all except calories. In addition, many commercially produced foods high in sugar are also low in nutrients (such as phytochemicals – minute plant compounds linked with good health) and fibre, and may be high in artificial additives and saturated or trans fats.

Although small amounts of sugary foods can be incorporated into any weight-maintenance diet or even a slimming diet, some people find it easier to avoid extrinsic sweet foods altogether and 're-educate' their palates. Brown sugar is not significantly different from white sugar in nutritional terms (and may be just coloured white sugar) and has a similar calorie value. Honey is also categorized as an extrinsic sugar. It has slightly fewer calories than sugar as it contains more water. Although good-quality natural honey is a well-known antiseptic, and may have other small health benefits, most mass-produced honey is no better than sugar.

It seems clear that extrinsic sugary foods do encourage surplus calorie consumption and contribute little, if anything, to the overall nutritional quality of your diet. The conclusion must be that if you are trying to cut calories, such sugar calories, together with saturated fat calories, should be the first to go.

See also:

- Questions: 80, 82–5, 97, 118–20, 139, 143, 185, 199.
- Features: 9, 12, 13.
- A–Z entries: Glycaemic Index diet, Sugar Busters.
- Key index entries: carbohydrates, sugar.

FAT FACT

When the nutrients from our food are metabolized within the cells for energy, this is called catabolism. When these nutrients are metabolized for use in growth and repair, the process is called anabolism.

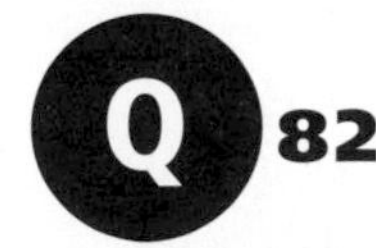

Should I use artificial sweeteners?

Intense artificial sweeteners such as aspartame, acesulfame-K and saccharin – used not only as tablet and granule sweeteners for drinks, cereals, etc., but also present in many commercial products, including diet drinks and many sweet diet products, are virtually calorie-free and, in theory, will help you to cut down on calories if you have a sweet tooth by replacing sugar in the diet.

However, in my opinion – and that of many experts – this is not as useful long-term as it might seem, as replacing one sweetener with another does nothing to re-educate your palate to enjoy less sweet tastes. There is also some evidence from one UK study that people who have a high intake of artificial sweeteners actually take in more calories overall than people who don't. It is thought that the sweeteners may upset normal appetite mechanisms (or simply don't provide enough satiety value).

Research in the USA shows that, in animals, the sweetener aspartame hinders production of serotonin (the brain's 'happy hormone'), which can suppress appetite. Lack of it may be linked to depression and binge eating, and lab animals fed aspartame actually became obese.

There is always much debate about the safety of artificial sweeteners – for example, even those deemed safe by one government are banned by another. Some, such as saccharin and cyclamates, have been linked with cancer in lab animals and there seems to be little international consensus on their long-term safety. Aspartame (brand name Nutrasweet) shouldn't be used by children with a phenylketorunia defect.

Another sweetener is sorbitol, which is related to sugar. It is a polyol (sugar alcohol) and often used in diabetic products as it is absorbed less rapidly into the blood than sugar. Sorbitol is a little less sweet than sugar, but not calorie-free – it has 2.4 cals per gram (or 12 a teaspoonful) compared with 3.94 cals per gram (or 20 a teaspoonful) for sugar. In large amounts it can be laxative. Mannitol and xylitol are two other similar polyol sweeteners.

Another sugar alternative is fructose – fruit sugar. This is not an 'artificial sweetener', as it is the sugar from fruit. Like sorbitol, it has a less marked effect on blood sugars. It contains about the same number of calories as sugar (sucrose) but is sweeter, so you need to use a little less. In large amounts, fructose may cause unwanted side effects. None of these sweeteners are necessary – even for diabetics – but may be useful for some.

So, should you use intense artificial sweeteners? Since we've been ingesting large amounts over the past 20 years or so, our collective weight has gone up, and sugar intake has hardly changed. There may be drawbacks and so there doesn't seem to be much point.

See also:

- ▶ Questions: 80–1, 84–6, 101.
- ▶ Feature: 13.
- ▶ A–Z entry: Glycaemic Index diets, Sugar Busters.

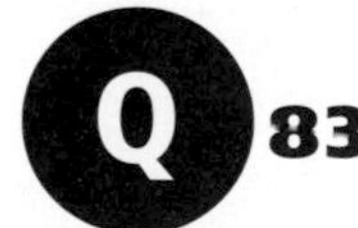

Can a high-carbohydrate, high-fibre diet help me lose weight?

Although the most important factor in a weight-reducing diet is lowering total calorie content far enough to create an energy deficit (see Q18), many international bodies with an interest in controlling obesity do encourage a diet rich in carbohydrates as a good way to lose weight and maintain the weight loss. However, the carbohydrate content of the diet needs to be mainly from natural or complex carbohydrates (see Q80 and the panel above), the fat content should be moderate or low, and overall calorie intake should be restricted.

The typical Western diet contains about 35–40% fat, 40–50% carbs and 15–20% protein. The US Department of Agriculture, in its recent paper on popular weight-loss diets (Jan 2001), says that 'low-fat diets containing a high proportion of complex carbohydrates, fruit and vegetables are naturally high in fiber and low in caloric density. Individuals consuming such diets consume fewer calories and lose weight.' The typical diet following these guidelines is, according to the USDA, 25% fat, 60% carb and 15% protein, with a daily total energy intake of about 1,450 calories.

Indeed, in one trial reported in the *International Journal of Obesity* in 1997, it was found that, over 14 days, moderate-fat, high-complex-carbohydrate reduction diets produce weight loss 'even when they are consumed *ad libitum*' (freely – i.e., calories weren't restricted). The most likely reason for this effect is that a high-

COMPLEX AND NATURAL CARBOHYDRATE FOODS

Complex and natural carbohydrate foods include all pulses, such as lentils, chickpeas, kidney beans, baked beans, cannellini beans; all whole grains including oats, rye, wheat, brown rice and foods made from those grains (e.g. whole-wheat pasta, rye bread, wholemeal bread, whole-grain breakfast cereals); starchy vegetables, e.g. potatoes, sweet potatoes, parsnips; all fresh, dried and frozen fruits or fruits canned in water; and all fresh and frozen vegetables or vegetables canned in water or brine.

Almost all these foods are good or excellent sources of dietary fibre, but among the highest are pulses, dried fruits, legumes such as peas and sweetcorn, pot barley. Some nuts and seeds are also good sources of fibre, but these are denser foods because of their fat content. The Food Value Charts at the back of the book give carbohydrate and fibre content of 200 foods.

complex-carb diet has a very high satiety value, so that a dieter has no inclination to overeat and can actually create a calorie deficit without feeling hungry. Such a diet will also naturally be high in insoluble and soluble fibre – incidentally, itself a complex carbohydrate. The World Health Organization, in its recent report 'Obesity', says fibre limits energy intake by lowering a food's density and allowing time for appetite-control signals to occur before large amounts of energy are consumed. Soluble fibre is particularly good at this.

So the answer seems to be yes, this IS a very good way to diet and to maintain weight loss for many people. It is also one of the healthiest, because it will naturally reduce overall and saturated fat content of the diet, and should contain more than adequate amounts of fibre, most vitamins and minerals, and plant chemicals. It will also maintain healthy bowel function and avoid the constipation that is the plague of many low-calorie diets. However, it could be short on some nutrients (e.g. iron, if meat is avoided, or calcium, if high-fat dairy produce is avoided).

The Basic Diet in Feature 9 is based on the moderate-fat, high-natural-carb way of eating, and is nutritionally sound.

See also:

- Questions: 79–81, 84–90.
- Features: 9–10.
- A–Z entries: Glycaemic Index diets, low-fat diets, The F-Plan.
- Key index entries: carbohydrates, fibre, food value charts, high-carbohydrate diets.

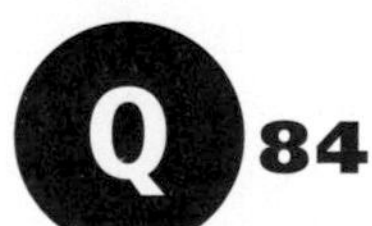

84

What is the Glycaemic Index?

The Glycaemic Index consists of a scale from 1 to 100, showing the rate at which carbohydrate foods are absorbed into the bloodstream. Glucose, which is absorbed most quickly, is rated 100. This index was designed originally to help professionals treat diabetics (because it is extremely important that they maintain controlled blood-sugar levels).

For non-diabetics, particularly those needing to follow a calorie-restricted diet or who have trouble maintaining weight, the Glycaemic Index has relevance, because foods which have a low or moderate GI rating tend to help us keep full for longer, as well as keeping the blood-sugar levels more constant.

The box below shows a selection of foods which have a low, medium or high GI rating. A quick look at it will turn up some surprises. Not all foods high in dietary fibre are low on the index, for one thing. For example, brown rice and wholemeal bread are high-GI foods, while yoghurt is a low-GI food.

What is interesting is that the same food may have a different GI according to how it is cooked (e.g. boiled potatoes are medium, while mashed or baked are high), or other factors – including the size of the particles in the food, and even the variety (e.g. basmati rice has a lower GI than ordinary white or brown rice).

THE GLYCAEMIC INDEX

Low-GI foods – 40 or less (slow-release, long-term energy – try to include plenty of these foods in your diet):

All pulses, including lentils, soya beans, kidney beans, chickpeas, butter beans, baked beans.
Barley (pearl or pot), whole-wheat pasta, whole rye grain.
Apples, dried apricots, peaches, cherries, grapefruit, plums, oranges, pears.
Avocados, courgettes, spinach, peppers, onions, mushrooms, leafy greens, leeks, green beans, broad beans, Brussels sprouts, mangetout, broccoli, cauliflower, tomatoes.
Yoghurt, milk, nuts.

Medium-GI foods – 41–60 (medium-release, medium-term energy)

Sweet potatoes, boiled potatoes, yams, raw carrots, sweetcorn, peas.
White pasta, oats, porridge, oatmeal biscuits, All Bran, noodles, popcorn.
Whole-grain rye bread (pumpernickel), pitta bread, buckwheat, bulgar, white and brown basmati rice.
Grapes, kiwi fruit, mangoes, beetroot, fresh dates, figs, slightly under-ripe bananas, apple and date bars.

High-GI foods – over 60 (fast-release, short-term energy. For slimmers, best eaten along with protein/fat/low-GI foods)

Glucose, sugar, honey, pineapple, raisins, watermelon, ripe bananas.
Baked potatoes, mashed potatoes, parsnips, cooked carrots, squash, swede.
Brown and white rice other than basmati, rye crispbreads, wholemeal bread, white bread, rice cakes, couscous, bread sticks.
Cornflakes, Bran Flakes, instant oat cereal, puffed cereal, wheat crackers, muffins, crumpets.
Orange squash, dried dates.

Yoghurt and milk are low on the GI index because, although they contain simple sugars (lactose), the protein and fat content bring the overall GI down to low. Adding protein and/or fat to a high-GI food will make it have a lower 'GI effect' and slow the rate of absorption. So, for slimmers, high-GI carbs should be eaten with some protein or fat (though eating *lots of* fat will not help a slimming diet). Protein and fat foods are not measured on the GI, but they are both slowly absorbed into the bloodstream.

Measurements of the Glycaemic Index of foods vary according to how and where the measuring was done, which is why I haven't given specific values for each food – but the list on page 61 gives a reasonable consensus of GI groupings for a range of common foods.

See also:

- ▶ Questions: 76, 80, 83, 85–7
- ▶ Feature: 9.
- ▶ A–Z entry: Glycaemic Index diets.
- ▶ Key index entries: blood-sugar levels, carbohydrates, digestion.

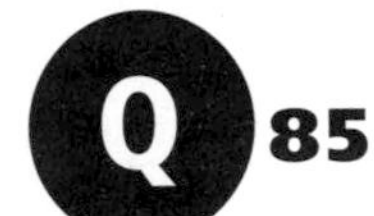

85

What are the best foods for controlling hunger?

Carbohydrate foods that are low or moderate on the GI (see the previous question) are best as they are absorbed slowly into the bloodstream and keep blood-sugar levels steady because they don't provoke a quick 'rush' of insulin.

Fresh fruits and veg are good, because they are relatively high in fibre and water and you get a lot of 'bulk' on your plate, which slows the rate of eating and allows the 'feeling full' mechanism to kick in before you eat too many calories. Foods especially high in soluble fibre are very good at keeping hunger at bay – examples are pulses, mangoes, dried apricots, Brussels sprouts, peas and spring greens.

Moderate amounts of fat and lean protein, both of which take longer to be absorbed into the blood than carbs, will help keep you feeling full for longer. This is probably one reason why most people are not successful long-term on diets that are very, very low in fat. You need some fat to keep you satisfied!

See also:

- ▶ Questions: 23, 36, 83–4, 86–90, 93, 95–9.
- ▶ Features: 9, 10.
- ▶ A–Z entries: calorie counting, Glycaemic Index diets, low-fat diets, hypoglycaemia.
- ▶ Key index entries: Glycaemic Index, hunger, satiety.

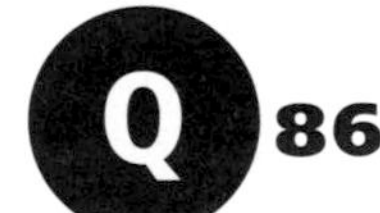

86

How can I avoid feeling weak, tired and dizzy on a slimming diet?

You need to eat regularly – having, say, three smallish meals and two small snacks a day, including foods low on the GI (see Q84). This will help keep your blood-sugar levels steady and prevent the 'dips' that accompany going for long periods without food. Weakness and dizziness are possible symptoms of low blood sugar. What happens then is that you are inclined to have a quick 'binge' on something high in simple sugars, e.g.chocolate, and, while this will raise blood sugar quickly, it will also dip quickly, leaving you feeling worse than before – and inclined to try yet another quick fix.

Ideal snacks to keep blood sugar even are a small handful of nuts and dried apricots, an apple and a few cherries, or a pot of low-fat yoghurt. Ideal lunches and suppers are basmati rice or new potatoes with plenty of fresh vegetables or salad and chicken, fish or lean meat.

Tiredness may or may not be a symptom of unsuitable low-calorie dieting. Many people on healthy reduced-calorie diets report having more energy than usual – probably because their previous eating patterns may have been high in simple carbohydrates (see Q80), which tend to be soporific. If you have only become tired since starting on a slimming diet, then you should make sure that it contains enough of the essential nutrients, including iron, B vitamins, vitamin C and so on. The plan in Feature 9 is nutrient-rich and is a good starting point for most. Perhaps you're trying to lose weight on too few calories – increase them slightly and you may feel better. No one should try to slim on a diet that contains fewer calories than their BMR (Feature 1) requires. If none of this applies, see your doctor for advice.

See also:

- ▶ Questions: 80, 84–5, 87, 95, 102–3 105–6, 108.
- ▶ Features: 1, 9.
- ▶ Key index entries: blood-sugar levels, Glycaemic Index, healthy eating.

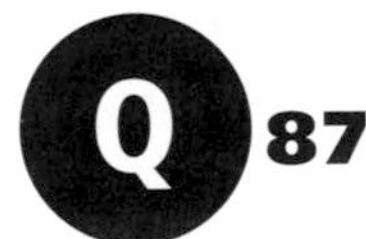

87

Do I need to feel hunger pangs in order to lose weight?

Not really. Hunger pangs are the normal stomach muscle contractions which help to 'mash up' food when you eat it (see Q76). When your stomach is empty, however, the contractions have nothing to do except churn up air – and this is the noise and sensation of 'pangs' you feel. At this stage your brain may also be quietly telling you that you need to eat because it is receiving signals from your body to that effect.

Obviously, if you follow a diet very low in calories, which involves eating fewer meals, or meals of the types of food that get quickly digested by your stomach and are low in bulk (like many of the typical ready-meals for dieters), then you will feel hunger pangs. This is a classic diet pattern that many slimmers have followed down the years but, as you will see if you read elsewhere in this section, this isn't a brilliant way to slim at all.

If you eat a diet reduced moderately in calories to no lower than your BMR requirements, that is high in natural and complex carbohydrates, including plenty of fresh veg and fruit and items low on the GI (Q84), with some lean protein and a little fat, and if you eat three times a day plus two between-meal snacks, then you can lose weight without ever feeling a proper hunger pang. You literally 'fool' the body into feeling full. One study showed that the average slimmer can cut calories by 450 a day on this type of diet without feeling hunger pangs, and this would be enough to lose nearly 1lb a week in weight. This type of diet is explained in more detail elsewhere in the section.

As the answer to Q83 explained, people who followed such a diet in one experiment actually didn't have to count calories at all – they ate all they wanted of the allowed foods every day and still lost weight! Taking extra exercise will also burn off calories and allow you to eat more – studies show that for most people, exercise doesn't increase hunger.

To sum up, diets that make you hungry are not going to help you succeed. (Interestingly, when people go on a total fast, they say that their hunger pangs disappear within three days or so – but that's a different story!)

See also:

- Questions: 80–86, 88–113.
- Features: 1, 9, 10.
- A–Z entries: Glycaemic Index diets, low-fat diets.
- Key index entries: BMR, Glycaemic Index, healthy slimming, high-carbohydrate diets, hunger.

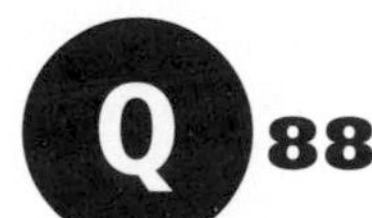

88

Does a diet high in protein have any special benefits for getting or keeping me slim?

A diet high in protein (30% or more of total calories as opposed to the 10–15% recommended for a balanced diet) will only help you to lose weight if the other macronutrients – carbohydrates, alcohol and fat – are reduced sufficiently to create an overall calorie deficit. It is this overall deficit that matters more than any combination – or exclusion – of the macronutrients, a fact confirmed by the US Department of Agriculture in their recent report on popular diets.

Most high-protein diets are actually reduced-calorie diets that contain a high proportion of protein, a very low proportion of carbohydrate (sometimes almost none at all) and varying amounts of fat – sometimes quite a lot. However, a high-protein, very-low-carbohydrate diet does have special properties that can make it seem easier to lose weight.

Initial weight loss will usually be high as, with a low-carbohydrate intake, the body's carbohydrate stores (glycogen) are depleted, and with them water. Also the very low carbohydrate and fibre content of the diet will naturally tend to reduce retained fluid in the body. Water loss, of course, is not fat loss and, once the low-carb diet is abandoned, the weight lost through fluid will return.

It has also been reported that a high-protein diet can increase dietary induced thermogenesis (DIT) – which means that it may help your metabolism to speed up and therefore create a greater calorie deficit than would be apparent with other types of diet. For more on DIT see Section 1. One estimate is that this increased thermogenesis could account for burning up 25% of the calories in a protein meal.

FAT FACT

Saturated fat is found in many different foods – not just meat and dairy produce. It is contained in small amounts in vegetables, grains and pulses, for example, and 'polyunsaturated' oils usually contain quite high percentages of saturates.

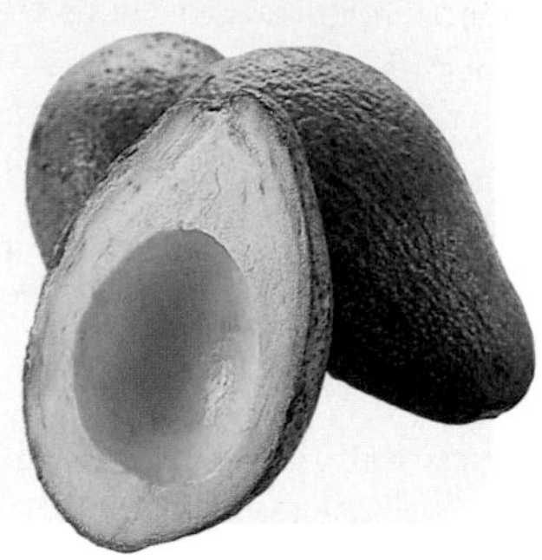

Lastly, a very-low-carb, high-protein diet produces ketones in the blood that are responsible for reducing appetite and hunger pangs. This makes such a diet relatively easy to stick to. These findings could explain why many people do find it easy to lose weight on a high-protein, low-carbohydrate diet.

Sadly, however, as with many things that seem too good to be true, there is a down side. High intake of protein – particularly animal protein like meat and dairy produce – is associated with various health problems. It can lead to excessive production of waste products – particularly urea – and place a strain on the kidneys (increasing likelihood of stones) and liver. Increased levels of uric acid in the blood can increase risk of gout. High protein intake is also linked with bone demineralization and may exacerbate osteoporosis.

There is also a small amount of evidence linking a high protein intake and high blood pressure. There may be constipation as the diet is low in fibre, and bad breath is a side effect of protein-induced ketosis. Lastly, high-protein diets may also be high in saturated fat, which is linked with many health problems, including increased risk of heart disease.

The other problem with a high-protein, low-carb diet is that it also can result in a shortfall of various important nutrients. These are discussed in more detail in the A–Z section under high-protein diets, where you will also find several popular high-protein diets listed.

To sum up: a calorie-reduced, high-protein diet may help you to lose weight but is not healthy and so is not to be recommended. The diet as outlined in Q83 will also stave off hunger and produce weight loss, while being healthy.

See also:

- ▶ Questions: 3, 79–90.
- ▶ Feature: 9.
- ▶ A–Z entries: Atkins Diet, diuretic diets.
- ▶ Key index entries: diuretics, high-protein diets, ketosis, protein.

FAT FACT

One fat – conjugated linoleic acid (CLA), which is found in meat and dairy produce – can actually help weight loss when supplements are taken. Sadly, it is nearly impossible to get enough CLA from a normal diet to give the benefits.

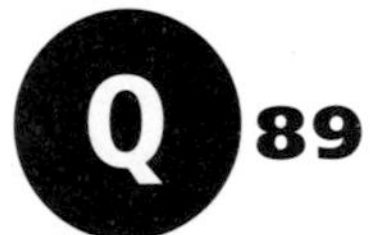

89

Does fat make you fat?

Any of the major nutrients – fat, carbohydrate or even protein – if eaten to excess (creating a positive energy balance, see Q18) can make you fat. On the other hand, some slimming diets (many of the high-protein, low carbohydrate ones) actually have a high fat content. So you can lose weight on fat. However, as the US Department of Health pointed out in its 2001 survey of popular diets, such diets work because they are self-limiting – there is only so much fat and protein you can eat in one sitting without carbohydrate.

Having said that, one of the most effective ways to keep your weight down is to reduce the fat content of your diet. Many international trials have come to this conclusion. One recent Spanish study of obese people found that their fat intake was far higher and carbohydrate intake far lower than recommended levels, and came to the conclusion that 'dietary intake, especially fat intake, seems to be the main factor contributing to obesity...'

A Canadian trial in 1998 found that 'significant positive correlations were found between the percentage of dietary energy as total fat, and body fatness... The high fat diet might lead over time to excess body fat deposition.' A US review of 28 different trials published in the *American Journal of Clinical Nutrition* in 1998 concluded that dietary fat plays a role in the development of obesity.

Another overview of trials on 1,728 individuals, conducted by the Research Department of Human Nutrition in Denmark in 2000 concluded that 'a reduction in dietary fat without restriction of total energy intake prevents weight gain in subjects of normal weight...' Take note: according to that last research, by reducing your fat intake you can still eat unrestricted calories and not put on weight!

But why does fat make you fat? As we saw in Q80, dietary fat is very efficient at storing itself as body fat (about 97% efficient), unlike carbohydrate and protein. And, of all the nutrients, fat is the most energy-dense at 9 cals per gram (carbohydrate is 3.75 and protein 4).

Fat also seems to be very palatable to humans, especially when combined with sugar or salt. It has good mouth-feel and 'slips down easily'. For this reason, and because it is cheap, it is a key ingredient in many commercial products which are easy to overeat. The World Health Organization says that 'sweetened foods of high fat content are expected to be conducive to high energy consumption'.

Research shows that high-fat, low-bulk foods (such as chocolate or cheese), probably because of the effect described, can make us eat to excess before the brain signals that we are full. The WHO says, 'The fat-induced appetite control signals are thought to be too weak, or too delayed, to prevent the rapid intake of the energy from a fatty meal. Episodic intakes of high-fat foods are therefore likely to overwhelm these signals...'

Studies show that the fat element of the diet can be taken away, or added, to a certain extent with no perceived difference in the satiety of the meal. A recent study found that it was possible to remove an average of 450 calories' worth of fat from the average high-fat main meal without it being noticed – enough to produce a weekly weight loss (at 7 such meals per week) of nearly 1lb.

Research shows that by reducing the fat content of meals, but keeping the overall bulk of the meal (via plenty of natural and complex carbohydrates and lean protein), people don't feel hungry and don't overeat. Therefore they don't get fat. As the WHO says in its 2001 report on obesity, fat appears to be the key macronutrient that undermines the body's weight-regulatory system.

See also:

- ▶ Questions: 79, 90, 103–4.
- ▶ Features: 8, 9.
- ▶ A–Z entry: Eat Fat, Get Thin.
- ▶ Key index entries: fat, high-protein diets, low-fat diets, macronutrients.

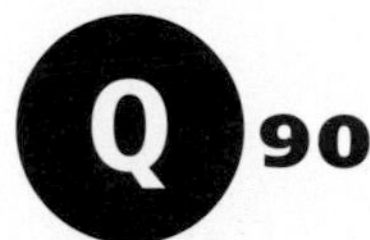

90

Is a low-fat diet always the best and healthiest way to slim?

As we saw in the answer to the previous question, fat tends to keep you fat, and the opposite also seems true – that low-fat eating can keep you slim. The consensus of professional opinion seems to be that a reduced-fat diet is best at helping people to lose weight and keep it off. The World Health Organization, having viewed all the evidence, says that modest energy-deficit diets (i.e. not crash) and *'ad libitum'* (eat freely) low-fat diets appear to have a better long-term outcome than very-low-calorie diets. They also say that low-fat, high-carbohydrate diets are superior in maintaining weight loss 2 years on, compared with standard calorie-counting diets.

Any diet which produces long-term weight loss in obese or very overweight people will probably bring health benefits, because overweight is linked with so many health problems (see Feature 25), and a moderate low-fat diet with a high intake of complex carbohydrates, fruit, vegetables and adequate lean protein is probably healthier than other types of calorie-reducing diet. Such diets have been shown to lower blood pressure and 'bad' LDL blood cholesterol, and may have a small effect in lowering the risk of heart disease.

However, there are very healthy fat-reduced diets and less healthy low-fat diets. The difference is in the types of fat allowed to remain in the diet on any reduced-fat regime and the amount of fat left. *Very* low-fat diets may actually *increase* the risk of heart disease. Not all fat is bad! A good slimming diet reduces the level of saturated and trans fats in the diet to a minimum, while retaining adequate amounts of omega-3s and omega-6s in the diet – the essential fatty acids (EFAs). Feature 8 will show how to do this.

These EFAs have, in recent years, been shown to be vitally important in maintaining good health and helping to prevent disease. They can lower LDL cholesterol and raise the 'good' HDL cholesterol, lower blood pressure, balance the immune system, help prevent stroke, improve brain function, help control PMS and breast pain, improve pain from arthritis, can help lift depression, and more.

To provide adequate essential fats in your diet, your low-fat programme should, in my opinion, go no lower than 20–25% fat and, for omega-3s, should incorporate regular oily fish (3–5 portions a week), nuts, pumpkin, flax and other seeds, leafy greens and oils from these items. People who dislike many of these, should take a daily fish oil supplement rich in omega-3s. For the omega-6s, small amounts of corn, sunflower or sesame seed oil will suffice.

These EFAs are better absorbed when saturated and trans fat intake is low. Small amounts of olive oil can also be used, as monounsaturated fatty acids help prevent colon cancer, may raise HDL cholesterol levels and certainly appear to have none of the negative effects of trans and saturated fats.

The Basic Diet in Feature 9 contains adequate amounts of beneficial fatty acids.

See also:

- Questions: 89, 103, 307, 311
- Features: 8, 9, 25.
- A–Z entries: low-fat diets, very-low-fat diets.
- Key index entries: fat, healthy eating.

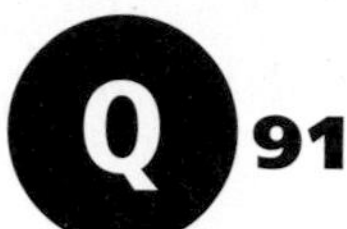

91

What exactly is food combining and is it a good system for weight loss?

Invented over 70 years ago by US doctor William Hay, this involves separating intake of carbohydrates (e.g., bread and potatoes) and proteins (like meat and dairy produce), so you never mix the two at the same meal. The theory (described in more detail in the A–Z entry) is, basically, nonsense.

However, the system also emphasizes whole fresh foods, and avoids refined foods. The overall content of the diet is thus probably healthier than the average Western diet, but lack of protein with carbohydrate meals can result in low blood sugar. Weight loss will almost certainly follow for anyone who is overweight and sticks to the regime. There is no 'magic' in the food combining aspect, though, to produce weight loss – it is simply the result of creating a calorie deficit. It is hard to eat a lot of calories on a diet that places so many restrictions upon how, when and what you eat. (Try unlimited pasta with no meat or egg sauce!)

There are easier ways to eat a healthy, slimming diet – why replace one set of eating fads with another? No doubt proponents will write in to argue the point.

See also:

- Questions: 76, 84, 102–3.
- Feature: 9.
- A–Z entries: Food Combining.
- Key index entries: blood sugar, energy equation.

FAT FACT

The brain is 60% fat and one of the constituents is DHA – the omega-3 essential fat found only in fish. This may show that the old wives' tale about fish being good for the brain really is true.

The fat in your food

Here's your potted guide to the fats in your food – which are good, which are less good, and how much you need of each in your diet.

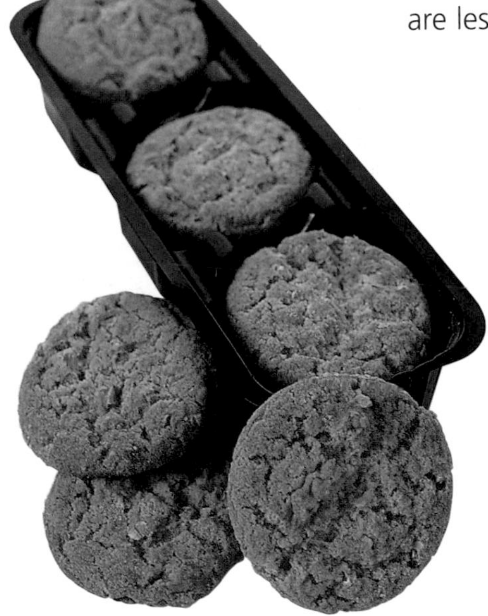

Fats to cut back on...

Saturated fatty acids: contain carbon atoms saturated with hydrogen atoms. Fats which are solid at room temperature contain the highest amounts of saturated fatty acids.

Examples of foods high in saturates: butter, lard, the fat in meat and cheese; the fat in milk, cream and many commercial bakes and desserts.

Health facts: a diet high in saturates can raise levels of LDL blood cholesterol and can 'block' the work of the essential fatty acids (see right). Foods high in saturated fat are the best sources of the fat-soluble vitamins A and D, and so a small amount is useful in the diet. Most of us eat much more than we need – in a healthy reduced-fat diet you need no more than about 5% of your daily calories from saturates.

Trans fats: unsaturated fatty acids which have been hardened or hydrogenated in the manufacturing of commercial foods such as margarine, cakes and biscuits. These trans fats are nutritionally similar to saturated fats or worse, as they raise blood LDL cholesterol levels and may also lower 'good' HDL cholesterol. There is no nutritional requirement for these trans fats in the diet, so they add needless calories and are best avoided.

Fats to watch your intake of...

Polyunsaturated fatty acids: contain carbon atoms joined together by more than one double bond and are liquid even when cool. They are more 'unstable' than other fats and likely to go rancid when stored in warmth or at length, and may 'oxidize', creating 'free radicals', which can harm health (see index) when used for cooking.

Examples of foods high in polyunsaturated fats: corn oil, safflower oil, sunflower oil. The fat in some nuts, most seeds and some fish is also mainly polyunsaturated.

Health facts: polyunsaturates lower blood LDL cholesterol but don't raise 'good' HDL cholesterol. A high intake of some polyunsaturates has been linked with increased risk of cancer and some other disorders. This may be because of the oxidization effect and increased free-radical production.

Highly polyunsaturated oils, such as corn, sunflower and safflower, are therefore best not used in high-temperature cooking. Plant oils tend to be good sources of the fat-soluble vitamin E, adequate intake of which is important for good health.

The polyunsaturated group of fats contains the *essential fatty acids*, linoleic acid (omega-6 group) and alpha-linolenic acid (omega-3 group). A regular intake of these is important for growth, smooth general body running and maintenance, for health protection and disease prevention. Most plant, nut and seed oils contain high amounts of the omega-6s and are best eaten cold or lightly cooked, while linseeds (flaxseeds), walnuts, pumpkin seeds and rapeseed oil are good sources of omega-3s. Spinach, broccoli and other dark leafy greens are also useful sources.

Also in the omega-3 groups are two

Can omega-3s help you slim?

There is some evidence that omega-3 fats help regulate the body's blood-sugar levels by increasing insulin sensitivity. This means that hunger can be kept at bay and may also mean less risk of both diabetes and obesity. There is also interesting evidence that a diet high in omega-6s and low in omega-3s causes mice to gain weight, and a diet high in omega-3s causes them to lose weight. Fatty-acids expert Udo Erasmus says that omega-3s increase our metabolic rate and energy levels; however, this needs more research.

A GUIDE TO HOW MUCH FAT YOU NEED

A moderate reduced-fat diet will contain around 25% of its total calories as fat. This is a rough guide to how much fat of each kind you would need to provide 25% of total calories on an average healthy slimming diet and an average maintenance diet for females. To work out a reasonable fat intake for other levels of calorie intake and other needs, see the panel below.

How much fat to have...	on a 1,500cal, 25% fat slimming diet	on a 2,000cal, 25% fat maintenance diet
Total fat	42g (25%)	55g (25%)
Saturated/ trans fats	8g (5%)	11g (5%)
Polyunsaturated fat	17g (10%)	22g (10%)
Monounsaturated fat	17g (10%)	22g (10%)

NOTES:

- More information on cholesterol in the diet appears in Q326 and Feature 27.
- All fat-containing foods are a mixture of the different types of fat– e.g. butter is 20% monounsaturated fat and sunflower oil is 12% saturated fat.
- Remember that all fat contains 9 calories per gram and even 'good' fats can be too much of a good thing if you eat them to excess. The Food Value Charts at the back of the book give total fat and saturated fat values for over 200 foods.
- Low-fat spreads can be useful to help reduce fat in the diet – there are many makes available, some high in polyunsaturates, some high in monounsaturates and others containing cholesterol-lowering esters. See Low-fat foods in the A–Z.

important fatty acids called EPA and DHA, found mainly in oily fish. These can help prevent blood clotting and are linked to lower risk of CHD and stroke, as well as improving brain function. EPA and DHA can be made in the body from alpha-linolenic acid, though this isn't an easy transformation.

Aim for a diet containing around 10% of total calories as polyunsaturates, with a good balance of omega-6s and omega-3s, and watch how you store the oils.

Monounsaturated fatty acids: contain carbon atoms joined to others by a double bond and are only partially saturated with hydrogen atoms. Fats high in monounsaturates tend to be liquid at room temperature but may solidify when cooled.

Examples of foods high in monounsaturates: olive oil, rapeseed oil, most nuts, and avocados. Monounsaturates appear to be 'good' fats, as they may lower LDL cholesterol and tend to raise the 'good' HDL cholesterol. Oils high in monounsaturates are best for use in cooking as they tend not to oxidize under heat.

SETTING YOUR OWN DIETARY FAT LEVEL

For people wanting to lose weight, no less than 20% total fat and no more than 30% total fat is recommended, with 25% seeming a good all-round level. Examples in the box above show how many grams of fat you will be eating on a typical 1,500 cals/day reducing diet. For example, at 42 g of total fat, you could divide this up as follows: 15g each for lunch and main meal, 8g for breakfast and 2g each for 2 snacks.

Some people will need to be eating slightly less, or more, than these calorie amounts, depending on their metabolic rate. Q104 explains how to work out how many calories a day you should be eating. Once you know this, it is easy to work out how many grams of fat you will need on 20%, 25% or 30% of total calories.

For example, 25% of a 1,750 calories a day diet is about 440 calories. Fat contains 9 cals/gram so you will need around 50 grams of total fat a day. Of this, estimate saturated fat at 5% of total calories, and mono- and polyunsaturated fats at 10% each of total calories.

For people on weight-maintenance diets: you will be eating more calories than on a slimming diet and therefore can have proportionately more fat. The box above shows how much fat you can eat on a 2,000 calories a day, 25% fat maintenance diet (typical for some women). 25% total fat is still a good level (see Q89), but you can increase fat to 30% if you like. Work out your total and individual daily fat grams by following the advice for slimmers earlier.

The fat content of foods is shown in the Food Value Charts at the back of the book. This is only a guide – there is no need to try to work out your daily fat intake to the last gram.

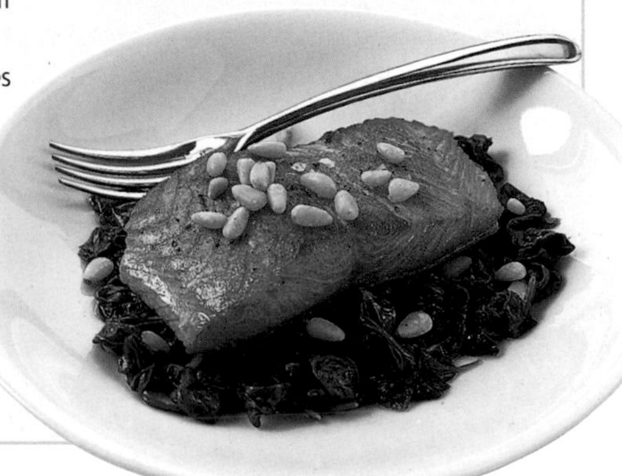

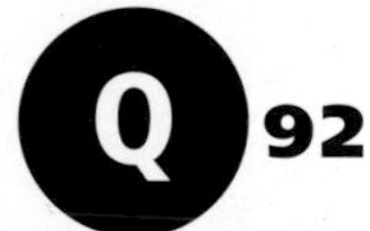

Q 92

Is eating nothing but raw food a good dieting idea?

A raw-food diet tends to consist almost exclusively of plant foods – vegetables, fruit, nuts and seeds. You could, in theory, also eat some raw fish or meat, but most raw-eaters tend to be completely vegan.

Because a raw diet is so high in fruit and salad items, it has a very low calorie-to-bulk ratio – this means that you get lots of stuff to chew on for very few calories, compared with the average Western diet. It is almost impossible to eat too many calories for your needs on such a regime and, if you are overweight, it follows that you would lose weight quite rapidly on such a plan. Also, hunger isn't nearly as much of a problem as you would think, as the very high fibre content of such diets tends to slow down the rate of eating and also helps the body's satiety (feeling full) mechanism to work well.

However, a raw-only diet isn't, perhaps, such a good idea as it would seem. For the average person it means a huge change in their diet habits, and generally research shows that most people cannot sustain radical diet changes. Also, it is not a varied or balanced diet (the protein and starch content will inevitably be low) and could lead to dietary deficiencies. Lastly, rapid weight loss isn't always such a good idea; almost all studies on the subject show that weight lost slowly is much more likely to stay off.

See also:

- ▶ Questions: 23, 83, 102, 105, 117.
- ▶ A–Z entries: crash diets, raw food diets.
- ▶ Key index entries: appetite control, balanced diet, rapid weight loss.

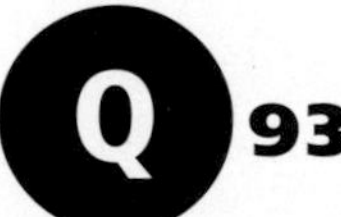

Q 93

Does a diet high in fruit and vegetables help weight loss?

Eating plenty of fruit and veg should certainly help your weight-loss campaign, for various reasons. One, they all contain a high ratio of bulk to calories. This is because of their high water content and, generally, low fat content. For example, apples are 88% water, carrots 90% and bananas 75%. Two, they offer plenty of 'bite'. Because of their high cellulose/ fibre content they help to make you feel full, even though they contain few calories. Raw or lightly cooked fruit and veg will also give 'crunch' factor. Because of this bulk and bite effect, it has been shown that, while an average 125g apple takes around 3 minutes to eat and contains just 60 calories or so, a small 25g milk chocolate bar containing 130 calories takes just 1 minute. As we've seen in previous questions, slow eating helps weight control and helps you feel more satisfied.

Fresh and dried fruits are both natural sources of sweetness, and make a good substitute for sweets and chocolate for those with a sweet tooth. Also, many fruits and veg are low on the Glycaemic Index (see Q84), with plenty of soluble fibre, and will help you feel full for longer and keep blood sugar levels even.

Lastly, fruits and vegetables provide a wealth of nutrients that may be hard to come by from other foods – for example, vitamin C, carotenoids, potassium, fibre and phytochemicals – and health organizations around the world recommend at least five portions a day of fruit and veg for health protection.

It would just be possible, I suppose, to eat enough fruit and veg actually to gain weight, but it would be very, very difficult and you would have to concentrate on the denser ones like roots and avocados.

FAT FACT

Starchy root vegetables, such as potatoes and yams, don't count towards your daily 'five a day' fruit and veg intake, but pulses, dried fruits, tomato sauce and fruit juices do.

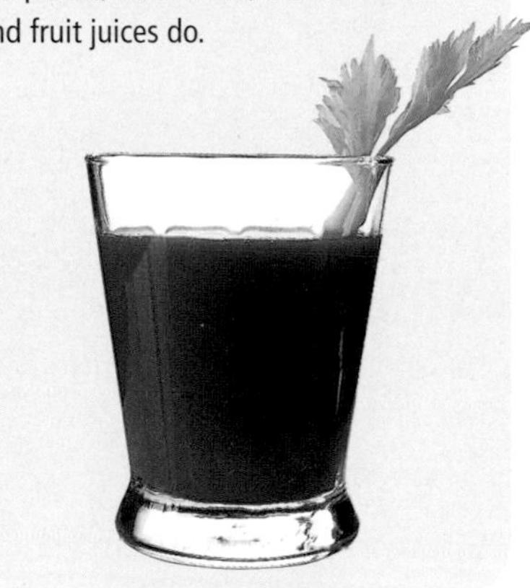

Eating five to seven portions of fruit and vegetables a day will, in my opinion, greatly enhance your chances of sticking to a reduced-calorie plan, losing the weight and keeping it off.

See also:

- ▶ Questions: 80, 83–4, 92, 94.
- ▶ Features: 9–10.
- ▶ A–Z entries: raw food diets, vegetarian diets, whole-food diets.
- ▶ Key index entries: food value charts, fruit, Glycaemic Index, soluble fibre, vegetables.

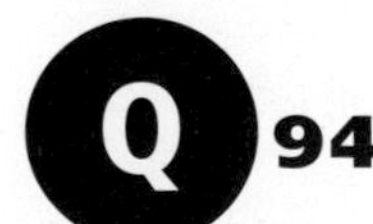

Q 94

I dislike most fruits and vegetables – how am I ever going to lose any weight?

Fruits and vegetables supply much needed vitamin C, phytochemicals, fibre and so forth in any diet, whether slimming or not, so it is a pity for your health's sake that you don't eat them.

You may consider a 500mg vitamin C supplement daily as a precaution (even though supplements are nowhere near as good as the 'real thing'). Fruits and veg also add much needed low-calorie bulk to the plate of any slimmer. Now there are three things to ponder on here:

1 Why do you dislike most fruits and vegetables? Is it because you perceive them as healthy and therefore not desirable? Read all of Section Four for insight into how you can alter this view and gain a genuine liking for healthier foods.

2 If it is because you really do dislike the taste or texture, then the keyword in your question is 'most'. If you dislike most fruits and veg, there must be some you do like. Concentrate on these and perhaps try new exotic varieties. Also concentrate on preparing fruit and veg in new ways. No one likes overcooked vegetables – attractively prepared, however, they are more appetizing. Buy the freshest, tastiest varieties you can afford – stale, dry apples and tasteless tomatoes don't appeal to anyone really.

3 Think about 'disguising' vegetables in puréed soups, puréed roots, juices, casseroles, pasta dishes, stir-fries and so on. Similarly with fruit, try them stewed, juiced, in smoothies, puréed on cereal and so on.

Lastly, remember that weight loss doesn't depend upon relying on any one particular food or food group. It depends upon creating an energy deficit by cutting down on your total calorie intake (and/or upping the amount of calories you burn). If you still decide NOT to eat fruit or vegetables, then it will be harder to lose weight without hunger – but it can be done.

See also:

- Questions: 18, 79, 131, 166, 307.
- Features: 11, 13.
- A–Z entry: calorie counting.
- Key index entry: healthy eating.

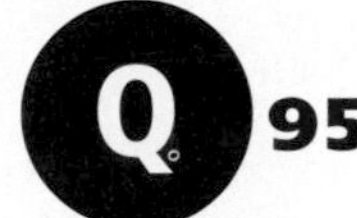

Is regular snacking between meals a good or bad idea?

It all depends upon your definition of the word 'snack'. Assuming you are trying to lose weight and/or stay healthy, regular snacks of high-fat and/or high-sugar items, such as crisps, pastries, cakes, biscuits, chocolates and sweets, are not a good idea. These will add many extra calories and grams of fat to your diet and research has shown that people tend to snack on these foods when they aren't hungry. The urge to eat these types of between-meal snacks can be controlled by a diet rich in foods low on the Glycaemic Index and with the help of the Retraining Programme outlined on pages 104–5.

However, healthy between-meal snacks can be an excellent idea for people trying to control calorie intake. This is because such snacks help to keep the blood-sugar levels constant, keep hunger at bay for few calories and help to avoid snacking on the less favourable items listed above.

Ideal snacks are low on the Glycaemic Index and also low – or fairly low – in calories and fat. A few examples of such items are apples, dried apricots, raw vegetables, natural low-fat yoghurt or a couple of spoonfuls of brown basmati rice. Even nuts and seeds can be eaten in moderation – one study published in the *International Journal of Obesity* found that snacking on peanuts, almonds or peanut butter between meals didn't result in increased weight gain because satiety value was high and the trial participants automatically adjusted their calorie intake so that they didn't gain weight. Nuts and seeds are high in fat but low in saturated fat. Other research shows that frequent eating helps people regulate their energy intake.

Between-meal snacks, however, should be small if you are trying to lose weight, as they will obviously count towards the day's total calorie intake. Alternatively, you could have larger snacks and smaller 'main meals'. Further information on the Glycaemic Index and a chart of GI food values appears on page 61.

See also:

- Questions: 15, 18, 23, 77, 84–6, 103, 201, 307.
- Features: 9, 13.
- A–Z entries: Glycaemic Index diets, metabolism booster diets.
- Key index entries: blood-sugar levels, food value charts, hypoglycaemia, metabolism.

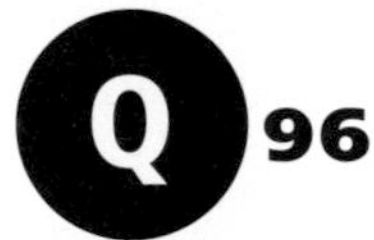

How many meals should I eat a day for optimum weight loss?

The consensus of opinion is that you should eat small, regular meals. An ideal pattern would be a breakfast, a mid-morning snack, a lunch, a late-afternoon snack and an evening meal. The ideal content of such meals is dealt with elsewhere in the book.

Eating regularly helps to keep your blood sugar levels even, keeps you feeling full, helps you cope better psychologically with eating fewer calories, and helps to avoid bingeing. Obviously you need to make sure that the meals and snacks you choose don't add up to more calories than you need for weight loss.

See also:

- Questions: 86, 95, 97, 104.
- Feature: 9.
- A–Z entry: calorie counting.
- Key index entries: calories, diets, food value charts, snacking.

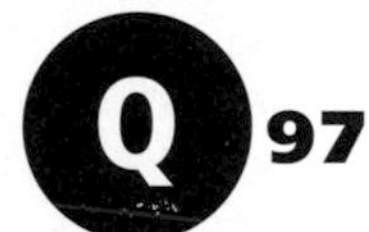

Q 97

Is just one meal a day the best way to control calorie intake?

A high percentage of people who try this method of calorie restriction find that they can only manage it for a short period of time – psychologically and physically, one meal a day doesn't suit us.

On such a system, blood-sugar levels are likely to be low for much of the day apart from the few hours after the meal. This can result in fatigue, dizziness, poor concentration and other problems described in more detail in Q86. Hunger pangs would be present for the first two weeks or so on such a regime (studies show that after this time they tend to disappear), which would be reason enough for most people to give up. The iron willpower needed to overcome these problems is tremendous, and unplanned bingeing is a probable consequence. Socially and at home, one meal a day may cause problems too. If a diet fits in with your lifestyle you're more likely to stick to it.

Lastly, research shows that eating frequently is better for the digestion and the metabolism, and can help to burn up calories. A single meal, followed by what is effectively a mini-fast for the rest of the day, may result in a drop in levels of the thyroid hormone T3, which otherwise helps to raise your metabolic rate.

Although calories are likely to be restricted naturally on such a plan (as there is a limit to how much you can eat at one sitting) there are other, easier and healthier, ways of eating and slimming.

See also:

- Questions: 15, 77, 87, 95, 102–3, 113, 143, 156, 169.
- Features: 2, 9.
- Key index entries: binge/starve syndrome, blood sugars, fasting, hunger pangs, metabolism.

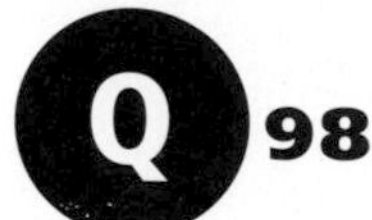

Q 98

How important is breakfast in a good slimming campaign?

There are studies which indicate that people who eat breakfast tend to be slimmer than people who don't. There are also studies which show that overall fat intake is lower and carbohydrate intake higher (a good way to eat) in people who have breakfast.

Unfortunately, there are also studies which show that people who don't eat breakfast take in fewer calories overall than people who do. In other words, the debate is still open. It is true that there are also a lot of overweight people who eat breakfast. However, the answers to the previous three questions should show you that regular eating is a key to successful weight loss, and of all the meals, breakfast is the one that it makes most sense not to skip.

This is because you have 'fasted' all night – for about 12 hours – and your blood-sugar levels are bound to be low. If you skip breakfast, you will find it much harder to resist sweet, starchy and fatty 'junk' snacks later in the morning, once you reach that sudden point when you've suddenly just GOT to have something to eat. Normally this coincides with coffee break, with disastrous consequences. If you have a breakfast containing some complex (preferably low on the Glycaemic Index) carbohydrate, some protein and a little fat, you will be unlikely to do this.

Breakfast is also a good time to pack in good nutrients, e.g. calcium (in yoghurt, milk), fibre and whole grains (in bread, cereal), essential fats (in nuts, seeds), vitamin C (in fruit) and soluble fibre (in fruit, oats). A well-designed breakfast need not take a lot of time to prepare or eat, won't supply too many calories or too much fat, and will keep you satisfied until your next meal – which should be a small, healthy, mid-morning snack. You should be able to get everything you need in a breakfast containing no more than 20% of your total day's calorie intake. If you prefer a larger breakfast, have a smaller lunch and/or evening meal to compensate.

See also:

- Questions: 96–7, 99, 104.
- Feature: 9.
- A–Z entry: calorie counting.
- Key index entries: blood-sugar levels, breakfast, calories, food value charts.

Q 99

Is it true you should breakfast like a king and dine like a pauper?

Assuming this means having a large breakfast and a very small evening meal, this is a reasonable way to eat for those whose body clock and social habits can stand it. The terms used in this old saying are probably somewhat exaggerated – breakfast need not be a sumptuous spread but, instead, a reasonably sized and well-balanced meal, containing some protein, carbohydrate and fat. Whole-grain cereal, semi-skimmed milk and fresh fruit would do very well.

Research shows that a breakfast like this helps restore blood-sugar levels after the night fast and helps brainpower and concentration throughout the morning. As far as your slimming diet goes, there is some small benefit to be gained from consuming at least some of your day's calorie allowance at breakfast time – a good read of Section One will prime you about food metabolism.

It is in the evening that most people tend to overeat and so, for overweight people, calories and fat at that time of day can happily be cut without detriment to health or stomach. Halving your portions of the high-density elements (meat, dairy, fat, starches) of your evening meal is a reliable way to save calories and may be easier on the digestion as you sleep. There is, however, no real truth in the idea that calories in the evening turn to fat during the night – a subject discussed in more detail in the next question. What matters most is the overall number of calories consumed over a period of time. For your health, several medium or small meals spaced throughout the day are probably optimum.

See also:

- ▶ Questions: 15, 98.
- ▶ Features: 2, 9.
- ▶ A–Z entry: calorie counting.
- ▶ Key index entries: breakfast, metabolism.

DIET MYTH

You shouldn't eat bananas when you're dieting.

False: an average banana contains about 90 calories – little more than a typical apple – only 2.5g starch and virtually no fat.

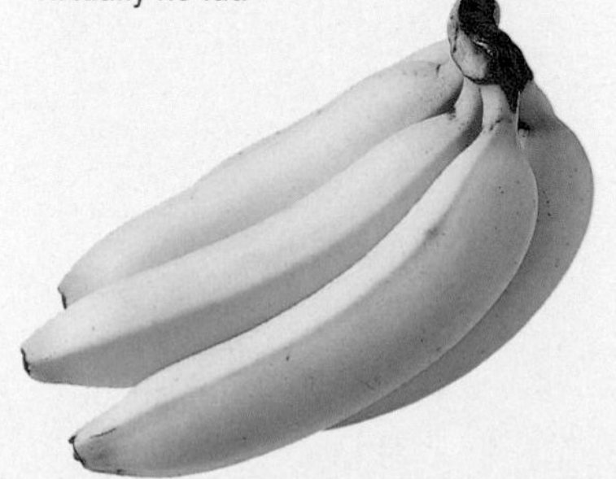

Does food eaten late in the evening convert straight to body fat while you sleep?

Oh, this really is one of those old wives' tales that sticks and sticks! As we saw in Q76, most of the food you eat takes a few hours to be broken down and absorbed before it can even begin to be used by the body for energy, or stored as fat. The next fact to remember is that we continue to burn calories even while we are asleep – quite a few of them. An average person may burn, let's say, 60 calories an hour for their basal metabolic rate (which is the rate you're burning calories when you are asleep). So, suppose you have your evening meal at 8, by 8 the next morning, you will have burnt up 12 x 60, or 720 calories, just lying there asleep or reading or whatever. (Indeed, one recent study published in the *International Journal of Obesity* found that feeding people a large meal in the evening increased their metabolic rate for several hours after the meal even as they slept.) Unless your evening meal contained more calories than that, then there won't have been any spare to be laid down as fat. Certainly on the Diet Bible Basic Diet it won't get a chance.

Even if food is converted into body fat, once you create a small energy deficit, by exercising or by taking in fewer calories than you need, the fat can quickly be converted back into ready energy. Obviously, if you eat a huge amount every evening, which tips your energy balance into the positive, in the long term you will put on weight. But it would be the same if you overate each lunchtime or breakfast instead. It is the overall amount of calories that you eat during the course of the day – or week – that is most important, not what time of day you eat them, or whether you go to bed afterwards.

Few people manage to balance their energy input and output exactly – eating only just exactly enough at each meal and no more to compensate precisely for the amount of calories they've burnt up since the last meal – or are going to burn up before the next meal. Who could be so clever – or would want to be so obsessive? Energy balancing is a long-term process, not a short-term thing.

See also:

- ▶ Questions: 18, 95–9, 104.
- ▶ Features: 2, 9.
- ▶ Key index entries: energy equation, metabolic rate.

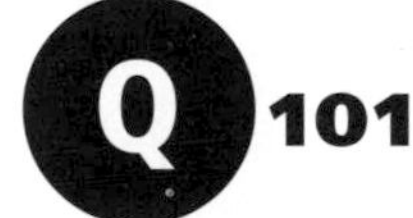

What are the best drinks to choose on a slimming diet, and why?

Boring as this may be going to sound, plain water really is the ideal drink for a weight-watcher. This is because water is calorie-free, contains no artificial additives, hydrates you and can even help to fill you up – a glass before a meal and one sipped during a meal will help to blunt the appetite a little. You could also go for water with a dash of real juice added, for an exciting change.

Now, here is some good news. For something hot, experts have decided that it is, after all, okay to choose tea. The latest trial results, revealed at the American College of Cardiology Conference in 2001, show that tea really is good for the cardiovascular system. It can help to prevent blood clots and open up the arteries in people with severe heart disease. It is also rich in antioxidants, which can also help prevent heart disease and perhaps cancers. Moreover, it is virtually calorie-free and, at 40mg caffeine for an average 200ml (7fl oz) serving, you could have 7 cups a day before getting near the recommended maximum caffeine intake of 300mg a day.

It has often been said that tea is diuretic and that it doesn't count towards the day's fluid intake. In fact, tea is only mildly diuretic and will only increase urine excretion by a small amount – nowhere near enough to cancel out the amount of liquid you ingest. One drawback: tea shouldn't be drunk with food, as it can hinder the absorption of minerals.

Green tea and redbush (roibosch) tea are both virtually calorie-free and contain antioxidants while being low in caffeine or actually caffeine-free, so they are both excellent drinks too. Redbush tea tastes similar to ordinary black tea. Herbal teas, such as rosehip, camomile or peppermint, are all low in calories at between 2 and 12 a cup, and are pleasant to drink (if you like them). Some may have mild health properties too (e.g. camomile will help you sleep; peppermint may aid digestion).

The chart on the left gives pros and cons of other drinks. Remember, though, that if it contains calories (some contain a lot), those count towards your day's energy intake.

See also:

- ▶ Questions: 11, 186–7.
- ▶ A-Z entries: caffeine, VLCDs.

PROS AND CONS OF COMMON DRINKS

Drink	Pros	Cons	Cals per 200ml (7fl oz)
Coffee	Low calorie; metabolism-boosting; increases alertness	High intake linked with mineral malabsorption, arthritis, high blood pressure/cholesterol	2 – 4
Fruit juice and smoothies	May be rich in vitamins minerals and phytochemicals; natural	Calorie-rich; can cause tooth decay; may be high on Glycaemic Index	70 – 200 approx
Vegetable juice	Rich in vitamins, minerals and phytochemicals; natural; low in calories	----	30 – 40 approx
Milk	Rich in calcium and some B vitamins	May be high in calories; may be high-fat; people may be intolerant	66 (skimmed) – 132 (whole)
Yoghurt drinks	Rich in calcium, some vitamins and minerals; may contain probiotics	May be high in sugar and additives	60 – 100
Low-calorie fizzy drinks, cordials and squashes	May be more palatable than water for some; low in calories	Contain artificial sweeteners; may contain artificial additives, caffeine	2 – 5
Squashes, cordials and fizzy drinks	----	Fairly or very high in calories; contain sugar/sweeteners; may contain artificial additives and caffeine.	50 – 100 approx
Health, sports and energy drinks	Some may be useful for sportspeople to restore blood-glucose levels	May be high in calories; may contain sugar; may contain various additives	Varies

Q 102

There are so many diets – how do I pick the right one?

That's what this book aims to help with. Qs 36 and 79–90 give the background to what makes an ideal slimming diet. Q103 discusses the 'perfect' diet and Q104 tells you how many calories you should be slimming on. From this you can build a picture of sensible and successful dieting.

Then, if you wish to see if a specific named diet fits in with these criteria, you can look it up in the A–Z, where all the pros and cons of each are listed, along with a total score. From this you can make a choice. Alternatively, you can use the information in this book to build your own diet, or use the diet in Feature 9.

See also:

- ▶ Questions: 36, 79–90, 103–4.
- ▶ Feature: 9.
- ▶ A–Z entries: calorie counting, low-fat diets.
- ▶ Key index entries: calories, diets, food value charts, healthy dieting, Top 20 Popular Diets.

Q 103

Is there such a thing as the perfect diet?

If you mean a perfect slimming diet, it is the one that gets you slim without pain, keeps you at your maintenance weight without pain – and that you like. Of course, that will vary somewhat from person to person, but various international bodies have decreed that the ideal diet for most people is one that:

- Reduces weight at a slow or moderate speed.
- Is low or moderately low in fat and proportionately high in carbohydrate.
- Is low in density and high in bulk – meaning lots of vegetables, salad and fruit, as well as enough starch and lean protein.
- Offers a high chance of compliance – i.e., you will stick to the diet. The consensus seems to be that this will be a diet that offers high satiety value, presents plenty of food on the plate and is not difficult to follow. The reduced-fat, high-carbohydrate diet wins on all counts – and it is a healthy way to eat.

As far as weight maintenance goes, again, the low-fat, high-carb diet wins. The World Health Organization reports that such a diet has been shown to be superior to a calorie-counting diet for maintaining weight two years later (after the initial diet).

Both for weight loss and for weight maintenance, the consensus is that regular exercise is a vital part of the equation. The Diet Bible Basic Diet in Feature 9 is a blueprint for the recommended eating pattern for success.

See also:

- ▶ Questions: 36, 79–122.
- ▶ Feature: 9.
- ▶ A–Z entries: Various diets explained.
- ▶ Key index entries: diets, healthy eating, weight control.

FAT FACT

If everybody in the UK who needed to lose a stone in weight actually did manage to do so, the roughly 17,000 billion uneaten calories that this represents would cost the food industry approximately £17 billion in lost revenue.

Q 104

How many calories a day do most people need to reduce to in order to lose weight?

The larger a daily energy deficit you create (see Q18) the more weight you will lose, but you could create a tiny (say 50 cals/day) deficit and lose it very slowly over time. The pros of a large deficit are rapid weight loss and the cons are hunger, nutrient deficiency and non-compliance. The pros of very slow weight loss are good compliance and higher nutrient intake, but few results – a compromise seems best.

Some experts recommend dieting at Basal Metabolic Rate (see Feature 1). Then whatever activity you do on top of this creates your calorie deficit – the more you do, the quicker you lose weight.

The World Health Organization says the lowest calorie limit for dieting (not under medical supervision) should be 1,200/day, but that most people tolerate best a daily deficit of between 500–600 calories and, from my experience of helping people lose weight, this is right. It will result in a weekly weight loss of a pound or a little more, which equals about 4 stones a year! This is also the level linked with your best chance of maintaining weight loss.

For most people, a daily deficit of 500–600 calories will not take them as low as just 1,200 cals. The US Department of Agriculture says that even in the absence of physical activity, diets of 1,400–1,500 cals/day result in weight loss for adults. If you want to see exactly how many cals/day you should be eating to create a 500–600 deficit, go to Feature 1 and work out your daily calorie output. Then simply deduct 500 (or 600) calories to give you your dieting rate to lose a pound a week.

This is a good check as you may not need to go as low as 1,200–1,500 cals/day. If you're very overweight, very tall, young, etc., and have a high metabolic rate, you'll need perhaps 2,000 cals/day at least, at first. Go too low, you'll feel hungry and deprived and won't stick to the diet. On the other hand, if you have a very low metabolic rate you may need to go a little lower than 1,400–1,500 to achieve 1lb a week loss. You may decide to increase activity levels to raise your energy output.

Lastly, if you decide to diet on the same level as your BMR, then eat that many calories a day. If you don't want to count calories, various plans do this for you (e.g. the Basic Diet overleaf), or see Q112.

While dieting, re-check your metabolic rate, as losing weight lowers BMR and you may need to lower calorie intake slightly. Also remember that exercise will help raise total energy output and let you eat more, or lose weight a little quicker. It will also conserve muscle, which helps minimize the metabolic slowing due to dieting.

See also:

- ▶ Questions: 3–6, 18, 32, 35, 74, 103, 108, 112.
- ▶ Feature: 9.
- ▶ A–Z entries: calorie counting, low-fat diets, etc.
- ▶ Key index entries: calories, dieting, energy, food value charts, metabolism.

The diet bible basic diet

A blueprint for weight loss and weight maintenance

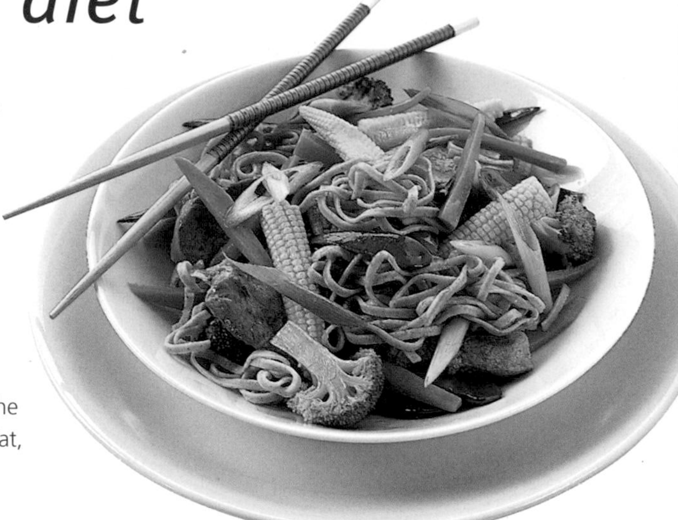

This seven-day diet contains approximately 25% fat (of which about 5% are saturates), 20% protein and 55% carbohydrate, and at least 18g fibre a day. The amounts given total approximately 1,500 calories a day, which is a suitable slimming level for many people.

The plan is intended as an example of how a healthy slimming diet looks – in subsequent weeks you can vary the menus to suit yourself, with the help of the Food Value Charts at the back of the book and the meal suggestions in other parts of the book, or simply follow the low-fat, high-carb route using the suggestions in Q112 and Feature 10.

Extras:

- Drink plenty of fluid every day – about 2 litres ($3\frac{1}{2}$ pints). Water, black and green tea, herbal tea, redbush tea are unlimited. Limit coffee to 3–4 medium-strength cups a day, which you shouldn't count towards your fluid intake.
- You have a 300ml ($\frac{1}{2}$ pint) skimmed milk allowance for use in tea and coffee or as a drink by itself.
- You can also have unlimited green salad items, leafy green vegetables, fresh or dried herbs and spices, vinegar, balsamic vinegar, lemon juice.
- Where vegetables are listed, have large portions.

Weight maintenance and differing dieting needs

The basic blueprint contains about 1,500 calories. If your own ideal slimming level is different (see Q104), simply decrease or increase portion sizes to suit. (For example, if you are slimming on 1,750 calories, you would need to increase portion sizes by about 15%.) For weight maintenance simply do the same (e.g. if your weight maintenance level is 2,000 calories a day, simply increase portion sizes by about 30%). Alternatively you could select 500 extra calories' a day worth of foods from the Food Value Charts at the back of the book, trying to keep the fat in the extra items to no more than 25% (14g fat). Alternatively, read the answer to Q113 and Feature 10 for further advice on menus for weight maintenance.

Day 1

Breakfast: 1 x 125ml tub of natural low-fat bio yoghurt topped with 1 segmented satsuma, 1 level tbsp pumpkin seeds, 15g ($\frac{1}{2}$oz) muesli oats and 50g ($1\frac{3}{4}$oz) dried ready-to-eat chopped apricots.
Snack: 1 small banana.
Lunch: 1 round whole-wheat pitta, 100g ($3\frac{1}{2}$oz) fresh tuna, grilled, 1 large mixed tomato and leaf salad dressed with 1 tablespoon olive oil; 1 apple.
Snack: 1 tbsp sunflower seeds.
Evening meal: 60g (2oz) (dry weight) whole-wheat pasta topped with 4 tbsp tomato sauce simmered with chopped courgette and green pepper until cooked, plus 1 tbsp grated Parmesan.
1 medium glass of dry white or red wine or fresh fruit juice.
100ml ($3\frac{1}{2}$fl oz) soft-serve vanilla ice-cream.

Day 2

Breakfast: 50g ($1\frac{3}{4}$oz) (medium portion) muesli topped with 1 kiwi fruit, chopped, 1 level tbsp flaxseeds and 3 tbsp skimmed milk (extra to allowance).
Snack: 1 apple.
Lunch: 550ml chilled-counter mixed bean and vegetable soup served with 1 large (30g/1oz) slice of dark rye or wholemeal bread; 1 individual tub of low-fat fruit fromage frais.
Snack: 1 level tbsp pumpkin seeds.
Evening meal: 100g ($3\frac{1}{2}$oz) lean fillet of pork, thinly sliced and stir-fried in $1\frac{1}{2}$ tsp sesame oil with 250g (9oz) mixed stir-fry vegetables (e.g. carrot, broccoli, spring onions, baby sweetcorn, mangetout); served on 40g ($1\frac{1}{2}$oz) (dry weight) whole-wheat egg thread noodles, reconstituted.
25g ($\frac{3}{4}$oz) chocolate of choice – preferably dark, organic.

Day 3

Breakfast: 1 medium bowlful of porridge made with equal parts skimmed milk and water, topped with a little extra milk, a good tsp of runny honey and 1 level tbsp flaxseeds.
Snack: 20g ($\frac{2}{3}$oz) no-need-to-soak dried apricots.
1 orange.

Lunch: 45g (1 1/2oz) (dry weight) pasta shapes, cooked and mixed with 50g (1 3/4oz) crumbled feta cheese, 2 medium tomatoes, chopped, some chopped cucumber and spring onions and I tablespoon ready-made good-quality pesto dressing, plus basil leaves if liked.
Snack: I plum.
I tbsp sunflower seeds.
Evening meal: 200g (7oz) cod fillets, baked or otherwise cooked without added fat and served in a sauce made by melting 7g (1/4 oz) butter until just turning brown and mixing with a few rinsed capers and a dash of balsamic or white wine vinegar; serve with a portion each of broccoli and mangetout and 200g (7oz) new potatoes.
I medium glass of dry red or white wine or fresh fruit juice.
I small banana.

Day 4

Breakfast: I medium slice (30g/1oz) wholemeal bread topped with I teaspoon of low-fat spread and I tsp low-sugar marmalade.
I x 125ml tub of low-fat natural bio yoghurt topped with I good tsp runny honey and 1 level dsp sunflower seeds.
Snack: I apple.
20g (2/3oz) shelled almonds (skins on).
Lunch: 575ml chilled-counter Mediterranean vegetable soup (e.g. red pepper and basil).
25g (3/4oz) Brie with I dark rye crispbread.
I small banana.
Snack: I pear.
20g (2/3oz) ready-to-eat dried apricots.
Evening meal: Breast of chicken fillet (no skin) coated in a mix of low-fat natural bio yoghurt and some mild curry powder, and baked until cooked through; served with 50g (1 3/4oz) (dry weight) basmati rice, boiled, a large dark green and herb leaf side salad; a side dish of bio yoghurt and chopped cucumber.
I medium glass of dry white or red wine or fresh fruit juice.

Day 5

Breakfast: Medium portion (50g/1 3/4oz) muesli topped with 20g (2/3oz) chopped ready-to-eat dried apricots, 1 level tbsp flaxseeds and I segmented orange plus 3 tbsp skimmed milk.
Snack: I apple.
Lunch: I medium egg, hard-boiled and 30g (1oz) extra-lean ham in 2 medium slices of wholemeal bread, spread with low-fat mayonnaise with unlimited salad items; mixed side salad of tomatoes, cucumber, red onion, leaves; I individual tub of diet fruit fromage frais.
Snack: I medium banana.
Evening meal: I large (250g/9oz) baking potato, baked and topped with 100g (3 1/2oz) good-quality ready-made ratatouille and 1 tbsp grated Parmesan cheese.
1 x 150g tub of Greek yoghurt with honey.

Day 6

Breakfast: 80g (2 3/4oz) mixed dried-fruit compote, simmered in water to cover for 1 hour until soft; and served with 100ml (3 1/2fl oz) low-fat natural bio yoghurt topped with I tbsp muesli.
Snack: I dark rye crispbread with I tsp Marmite.
Lunch: 85g (3oz) mackerel fillet (canned, thoroughly drained (drained weight))
I level tbsp dijonnaise mayo-mustard dressing.
Large mixed salad of leaves, herbs, tomato, cucumber; oil-free dressing to taste.
I medium wholemeal roll; I satsuma or nectarine.
Snack: I small banana.
Evening meal: 100g (3 1/2oz) beef fillet strips, 50g (1 3/4oz) each shredded spring greens, sliced tomatoes and mushrooms, all stir-fried in 1 scant tablespoon olive oil and served with 50g (1 3/4oz) (dry weight) tagliatelle, boiled (stir to combine).
I medium glass of dry white or red wine or fresh fruit juice.

Day 7

Breakfast: 1/2 pink grapefruit.
I medium bowlful of porridge made with equal parts skimmed milk and water; topped with a good teaspoonful runny honey, a little skimmed milk and I tsp flaxseeds.
Snack: I kiwi fruit.
20g (2/3oz) raisins.
Lunch: 40g (1 1/3oz) (dry weight) basmati rice, boiled, cooled and served with 100g (3 1/2oz) cooked chicken strips, I small segmented orange, chopped cucumber and 1/2 tbsp pine nuts, tossed in oil-free French dressing.
Snack: 2 dark rye crispbreads topped with Marmite.
Evening meal: 100g (3 1/2oz) salmon fillet topped with a mixture of 1 1/2 tsp olive oil blended with I garlic clove, a handful of fresh coriander leaves and some sea salt, grilled and served with 200g (7oz) boiled potatoes mashed with seasoning and 1 dsp olive oil, a portion of peas and a portion of spinach.
I medium glass of dry white or red wine or fresh fruit juice.

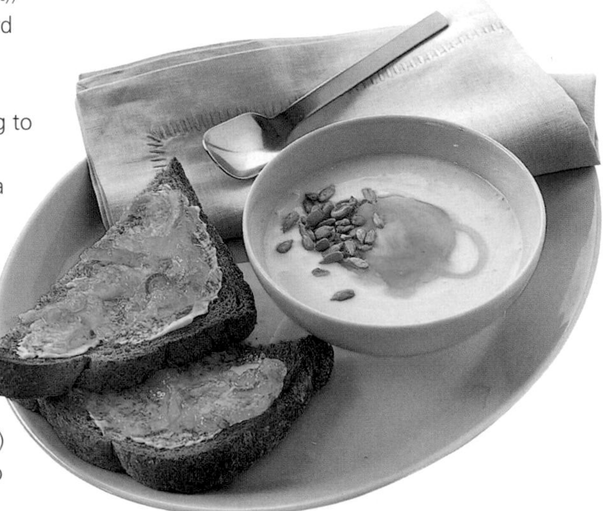

What is a crash diet?

A diet very low in calories (usually anything less than 1,000 calories a day) is described as a 'crash diet', often with a 'faddy' eating element to it – for example, nothing but eggs and milk, or cheese and tomatoes – which will result in rapid weight loss. Usually over 3lb (1.5kg) a week is promised.

See also:

- Questions: 106–9, 312.
- A–Z entry: crash diets.
- Key index entry: healthy slimming.

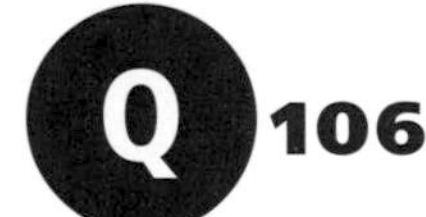

Are crash diets really such a bad idea?

Amongst health experts, crash diets are seen as a bad idea for most people as:

1 they encourage loss of more lean tissue (muscle) than diets which produce a slower weight loss on a higher calorie level.

2 they may be lacking in nutrients – both macronutrients such as fat, protein or carbohydrate, and micronutrients such as vitamins and minerals.

3 they don't encourage sensible eating habits and this means that after the crash diet is over weight is easily regained. In time, this can turn into a 'yo-yo' dieting habit, which is very demoralizing.

See also:

- Questions: 105, 107–9, 312.
- A–Z entry: crash diets.
- Key index entry: healthy slimming.

Q 107

Is fasting a good idea for weight loss – and how long can I fast?

If you go back to the answer to Q77, you will find there a detailed explanation of what happens to your body when you drink water but don't eat, right down to death after 60 or so days. After reading it, you will probably agree that fasting as a means of long-term weight loss isn't such a good idea, even though it is bound to produce good results while it lasts.

There are many advocates of fasting, and it is a well-recognized way of life in India. There are, however, inherent dangers in fasting and, no doubt, once the fast is over, the almost inevitable regaining of weight (see the answer to the previous question), so it does seem rather pointless.

Incidentally you may have heard of the female 'guru' in Australia who claims she never eats and 'lives on light'. Apparently followers of her regime have died and, in a monitored experiment, the lady herself became ill on her own regime after a week!

Having said all that, some people enjoy short regular periods of fasting – say, one day a week, or a two-day fast once a month, or a week's fast four times a year – and are none the worse for it. Used in such a way, it is possible that fasting might help keep weight stable. However, for most people, I am sure that a good detox diet is a better idea, and this is discussed in detail in Section Nine.

See also:

- Questions: 77, 105, 106–7, 317–18.
- Feature: 26.
- A–Z entry: fasting.
- Key index entry: healthy eating.

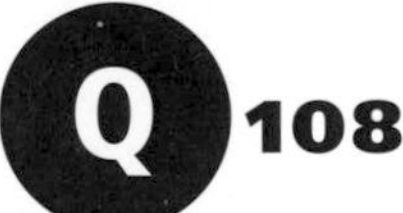

What is the lowest number of calories I can eat to slim and stay healthy long-term?

The World Health Organization says the lowest recommended dieting level (except under medical supervision) is 1,200 calories a day, but prefers 1,400–1,500. One very good rule-of-thumb is that you shouldn't diet below your own basal metabolic rate – the rate at which your body uses up (expends) calories just lying still, doing nothing. This is your basic energy output. Feature 1 shows how you can work out your own BMR. An average BMR for many women is around 1,500 calories a day.

You would then lose weight on such a diet according to how many calories you burn up in all your daily activity over and above your BMR. For very sedentary people this is as low as a few hundred; for active people it can be double the BMR – and for these people I would say dieting on the BMR would actually be too low. However, very active people rarely need to diet as they very rarely seem to get fat in the first place.

Another good rule is to increase your calorie intake if your weight loss speeds up over the sensible 1–2lb a week that dietitians recommend. You don't actually need to worry about counting your calorie intake as long as sensible weight loss is proceeding. This also holds true of weight maintenance – you don't need to count calories for life; just weigh yourself occasionally (or check your waistband for tightness!) and if nothing's changed, you're doing a good job.

See also:

- Questions: 18, 36, 87, 102–6.
- Feature: 9.

Q 109

What are the benefits and disadvantages of very-low-calorie, liquid-only diets?

VLCDs, as they are called, are most often used to get weight off severely overweight people under medical supervision, when their life is in danger or before operations. They are also sold as slimming aids to the general public.

Each meal is usually around 250 calories and, on such a regime (3 such meals a day total diet), weight loss is rapid. If only replacing one or two meals a day the results are slower. The meals are fortified with a range of vitamins, minerals and so on, and should be nutritionally balanced.

Some people find it easier to replace a meal with a formula, as all the worrying about what to eat is removed and so is the element of choice – and room for temptation and/or cheating. It's an 'eat to live' philosophy. I suppose those are the benefits if you're that sort of person.

The disadvantages could be that you have little choice, and if you enjoy real food the regime can be very dispiriting. If you want fast food to lose weight, there are plenty of quick and easy meals. Again, these formulas do nothing to re-educate you to better eating habits, lean tissue loss may be greater than on a higher-calorie regimen and, once off the system, the weight may readily return. The WHO says the use of VLCDs by individuals without medical supervision is unwise and should not be recommended. However, used to replace one meal a day, they can be useful. These diets are discussed in more detail in the A–Z.

See also:

- Questions: 105–8, 312.
- Feature: 14.
- A–Z entry: very-low-calorie diets.
- Key index entry: healthy slimming.

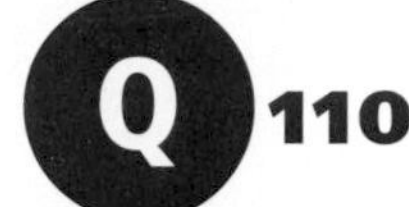

Q 110

Can you really block the calories in your food so that they are not absorbed by the system?

The prescription slimming pill Xenical works on this principle – it blocks the breakdown of dietary fat in the intestines, with the result that about 30% passes through the gut unabsorbed. The fat substitute 'food' Olestra is virtually calorie-free because of a similar principle – it passes through the gut unabsorbed. It is only used in a few food products in the USA and has not been approved in the UK. Both Olestra and Xenical may have unwanted side effects, such as diarrhoea and flatulence, if anything other than a low-fat diet is followed, and the fat-soluble vitamins are also passed through the body, which could lead to mineral deficiencies.

Over-the-counter or mail-order pills called 'starch blockers' have been on sale for years, claiming to block the starch in your food. These claims are, by and large, unproven and, in any case, within a healthy diet it wouldn't be desirable to block starch. Fat-blocking pills, often called 'fat magnets', again are of very limited, if any, use. They may block a few calories from each meal but the overall amount is too little to make any real difference to the average diet. Time and time again the UK Advertising Standards Authority condemns these products, saying their claims are unsubstantiated.

See also:

- Questions: 37, 111.
- A–Z entries: fat substitutes, slimming pills.
- Key index entries: crash diets, fats, healthy eating.

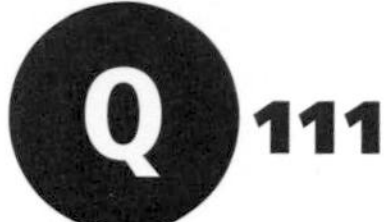

Q 111

Is it true that there are foods which contain 'negative calories'?

The idea goes that foods such as celery, cabbage, beansprouts and so on are so low in calories and high in fibre that your digestive system burns more calories digesting them than the foods actually contain, thereby creating a calorie deficit.

As with many such ideas, it does contain a grain of truth – some foods (mostly veg) are very low in calories. Also, as we've seen in Q3, when you eat, your metabolic rate speeds up via dietary induced thermogenesis. With some foods, DIT can be quite high – but the highest producers of DIT are protein foods, burning up to 25% of their calories during digestion. Sadly, all protein foods contain reasonable amounts of calories, so even allowing for this effect, you're still in a positive energy situation!

The veg mentioned above don't create a deficit, even though it'd be almost impossible to get fat on them. To eat enough celery (at 7 cals/100g) to get an average day's intake of about 2,000 calories, you would have to eat 28.5 kilos!

See also:

- Questions: 3, 18, 88, 110.
- Feature: 1.

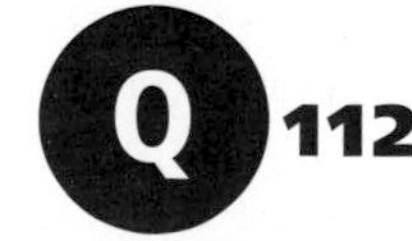

Q 112

Is it possible to lose weight without drastic diet changes or calorie counting?

If you've been eating a diet high in fat and calories that has made you overweight, the healthiest way to slim is to cut the fat right back, in which case, research shows you can eat carbs fairly freely. Such a diet would, however, sometimes entail weighing or measuring items, or at least reading the nutrition panels on packs, and the carb element should be healthy 'complex carbs', like whole grains and pasta, fruit and veg. This has been shown to be the easiest and most successful way of slimming for many people long-term.

If you've a sweet tooth or like 'junk food', then eating this way will obviously mean drastic changes to your diet. The only way to avoid this is to eat what you want, but in smaller amounts. This is calorie counting by another name – you don't look items up, weigh or measure them, but just eat two-thirds or half of what you would normally. The disadvantages of this are that you may feel hungry and it doesn't re-educate your palate to enjoy healthier foods. You would increase your chances of success by adding plenty of extra low-cal vegetables and salads to help fill you up.

The last idea you could try is to increase the exercise you do. If you burn an extra few hundred calories a day (say, an hour's cycling), then, in theory, you could lose weight without changing eating habits at all. In practice, it is best to combine exercise with a moderately reduced-calorie, reduced-fat diet. Feature 10 will help you to do that painlessly and its meal 'before' and 'afters' should cheer you up, as they show how you can still eat well.

One experiment proved most over-weight people can cut the calories in an average main course by 450 without even noticing! That would result in a weekly weight loss of nearly 1lb without doing another thing. I suggest you read Section 4 and try the retraining course in Feature 13. Also, a look through the A–Z may yield diets you like the sound of – but pick ones that score over 60%. Sadly (or gladly), weight control in the long term IS mostly about eating in a healthier way for the rest of your life – and taking more exercise.

See also:

- Questions: 35–6, 40, 79–104, 113, 118–22, 123–48.
- Features: 8, 9, 10, 11–13.
- A–Z entry: low-fat diets.
- Key index entries: fat cutting, portion control.

FAT FACT

An English professor has invented a way to make chips almost fat-free, by coating them in a secret gum solution – but a French food scientist says that is unnecessary, and that as long as you wrap ordinary chips in kitchen paper to soak up the fat within 20 seconds of them coming out of the pan, the fat doesn't get absorbed, due to water vapour inside the chip creating pressure that prevents the fat from soaking in.

FAT FACT

If you eat 200g (7oz) of boiled new potatoes instead of the same weight of most types of oven chips, you save about 184 calories.

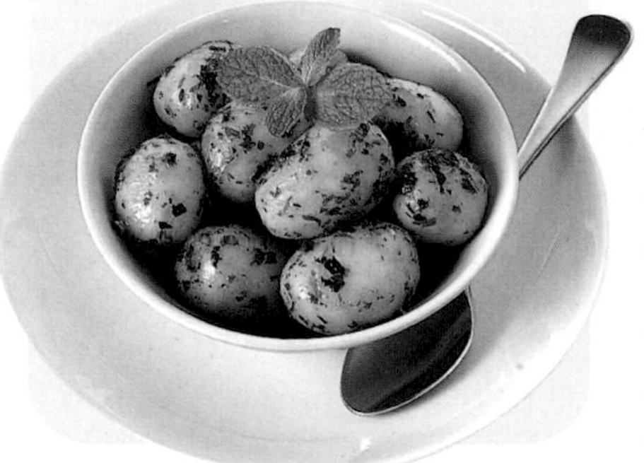

Q 113

What is the most reliable and easy way to slim and maintain weight loss?

The two things people dread, long-term, are weighing and measuring all their food and constantly having to look things up in a calorie/fat guide. This can be boring and time-consuming and, of course, everyone is looking for an easier way to keep the weight off for good. In my experience, it is good to do all these things for a week or two – actually, finding out what, say, an ounce of Cheddar cheese or a 100ml portion of ice-cream looks like is quite interesting and eye-opening. A modicum of knowledge gives your slimming and maintenance diet the greatest chance of success. Even if you follow a diet in a book, you still almost always have to weigh or measure at least some items.

The good news is that, after a while, you come to know what portion sizes look like and, broadly speaking, what foods you should be cutting back on, which to avoid and which to eat freely. This is sometimes called the 'traffic light system' and the box opposite lists foods in these three categories. Eating this way should result in fairly easy – and healthy – steady slimming and long-term weight maintenance. A few simple fat-cutting tips help make the system easier to do (see Feature 10).

Which brings me nicely to the crux of your question. A low-fat, high-carb natural diet, low on highly processed foods, is the easiest and most reliable way to get and stay slim that is also nutritionally sound and healthy. Both the World Health Organization and the US Department of Agriculture agree on this – as do most health and diet professionals.

I have to admit that I know people who have got – and stayed – slim over time via other means. A high-protein, low-carb diet is, arguably, easier than low-fat, high-carb eating and also reliable, although for long-term weight maintenance, compliance (sticking with it) may not be so good. The Hay system (food combining) is favoured by many and is probably a reliable way to stay slim, though not exactly easy to follow. The Hay system is fairly healthy, while high-protein eating generally is not. Both these methods are discussed in detail in the A–Z, where you will find all kinds of other diets and eating systems, all scored for health, palatability, ease of use, etc.

Take a look at Feature 10, which shows that it isn't hard to reduce the fat and calories in your meals while still ensuring that they look and taste good, and fill you up. In the long-term, if you think 'healthy eating' and 'fat cutting', then you shouldn't go far wrong... oh, and 'regular exercise'. All studies show that the people most successful at keeping lost weight off are those who take regular exercise. The more calories you burn up, the more you can eat without putting on weight again!

See also:

- Questions: 18, 32–5, 79–104, 112, 123–48, 333–47.
- Features: 8–13.
- A–Z entries: see individual diet entries.
- Key index entries: calories, dieting, exercise, weight maintenance.

THE TRAFFIC LIGHT GUIDE TO EATING FOR HEALTH AND WEIGHT LOSS

Eat freely:

Fresh and frozen fruit, fresh and frozen vegetables other than those listed in other sections; potatoes and other root vegetables; all salad vegetables; herbs and spices; whole grains (e.g. brown rice, bulgar wheat), whole-wheat pasta, wholemeal bread, whole-grain breakfast cereals; dried apricots, prunes; all pulses (e.g. red kidney beans, chickpeas, butter beans, lentils); all fish and shellfish; low-fat yoghurt, low-fat cheeses (e.g. cottage cheese, Quark), fromage frais, skimmed milk; poultry (skin removed) and game; Quorn, tofu.

Eat in moderation:

Refined grains (e.g. white bread); good-quality cooking oils (e.g. olive oil, walnut oil, groundnut oil); dried fruits other than those mentioned above; full-fat yoghurt, semi-skimmed milk, full-fat fromage frais; medium-fat cheeses (e.g. Brie, Edam, goats' cheese, feta); eggs; lean red meat; fresh nuts and seeds (not salted, roasted); processed and deli meats; low-fat spread; fruit juices; alcohol.

Avoid or have infrequently or in small or very small quantities:

Cakes, biscuits, chocolate, sweets, puddings, butter, lard, margarine, cream, pastry, salted snacks, full-fat cheeses, fatty meat and meat products, sugary drinks, deep-fried foods, chips.

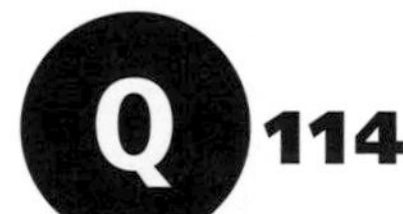

Q 114

Could a food allergy be causing my inability to lose weight?

A real allergy produces a very quick and often very obvious effect – e.g. a violent rash, vomiting, asthma. In some cases, eating a food to which you are allergic produces anaphylactic shock – a life-threatening condition. If you have no symptoms such as these then it is unlikely that you have a genuine food allergy.

Food intolerance is the term used by specialists to describe a less severe reaction to a food, which may produce symptoms such as tiredness, bowel upsets and bloating. Some people do indeed find themselves intolerant of a food or foods, but in the 'Noughties' food intolerance is to trendy people what vegetarianism was to the Nineties – with wheat, dairy and sugar being the three favourite 'bad boys'. Claims that 40% – I've even read 75% – of the population have food intolerances are wildly exaggerated, unless you count every case of flatulence after a heavy meal. Official estimates from the UK Food Standards Agency suggest that only 2% of people may have genuine cases.

Some real food allergies can actually cause weight loss (see next question). Food intolerances often show up as stomach bloating and the foods most prone to cause this seem to be wheat (particularly wheat bran) and high-fat foods. If one of these is your problem, and you eliminate it from your diet for a week, bloating should subside and you may feel better – e.g., more energetic, less tired. However, apart from the bloating effect, there is little evidence that food intolerance can actually cause weight gain. It would be scientifically impossible for a food to put more fat on you than it contains in calories – to get fat, you need to create a calorie excess (see Q18).Obviously, if you give up a range of foods, as often advised by 'allergy clinics', from dairy products and wheat to sugar, alcohol, etc., you'll undoubtedly lose weight, as you'll be cutting out a lot of calories. If you're overweight and eating such items, it also follows that they may well be causing your weight problem, but it's more likely to be due to the calories they contain than any intolerance!

Though hospital testing for allergies is reliable, currently the only reliable way to discover if you have a food intolerance is to follow an elimination diet (excluding each possible culprit food for a fortnight and noting the effect). All but the most simple elimination diets need to be done with the help of a dietitian.

Private food allergy consultancies (testing blood, hair, nails, etc.) have, by and large, been found to be unreliable when tested by undercover researchers. Not only did they advise people to give up a range of good, healthy foods to which they aren't intolerant, but they also missed genuine allergies, which may be dangerous. Some are better than others but, on balance, I wouldn't recommend them as, for one thing, it is hard for the unsuspecting punter to know which ones are good and which aren't. Interestingly, one of the top UK allergy specialists believes the igG blood test – in which raised levels are said to pinpoint 'intolerances' – simply shows higher than normal levels of exposure, i.e., these are the foods we eat the most.

Your doctor will probably be of more help than a private clinic – she/he can refer you to a dietitian and may refer you to an allergy specialist depending on your symptoms. You can also contact the British Allergy Foundation on 020 8303 8583 (helpline), 020 8303 8525 (main line).

Lastly, it is very common for people with eating disorders to seek to be diagnosed as allergic to, or intolerant of, foods like wheat and dairy as a legitimate way to avoid those foods.

See also:

- Questions: 115–6, 149.
- Key index entries: eating disorders, food allergies.

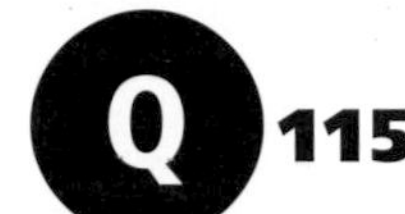

Q 115

Does avoiding wheat products help you lose weight?

Since several celebrities lost weight on a wheat-free diet, some people believe this is THE only way to lose weight. As a read through Section Three will show, there is little magic about a wheat-free diet for most of us. However, if you have been eating a lot of wheat (say, bread for breakfast, sandwiches for lunch and pasta for your evening meal) and then you cut it out, you will almost certainly lose weight, because you are reducing your total calorie intake. You will also find any problems with fluid retention minimized, because wheat and starchy carbs tend to retain more fluid in the body than a diet low in carbohydrates. Many people also report that on a wheat-free diet they feel better – more alert, less sluggish. There is, however, little scientific evidence that I can find to support this, except that high-carb foods tend to be 'comforters' (see serotonin).

Many people avoid wheat because they say they are allergic to, or intolerant of, it. Read the answer to the previous question and come back to this. It may be that our bodies aren't designed to cope with large amounts of wheat and for some people simply getting a variety of other foods and sources of starch in the diet is enough to avoid bloating and other possible symptoms of intolerance. You won't be missing many vital nutrients by giving up items high in refined white flour, which usually often contain other not-so-goodies, like sugar and fat. However, whole-grain wheat is a good source of dietary fibre, complex carbohydrates, vitamins and minerals, and shouldn't be abandoned on a whim.

You can do a one- or two-week wheat elimination and see if you lose weight and feel better afterwards. Be warned, though, wheat is contained in very many products, including lots of commercial items on the supermarket shelves, so you will need to become an avid label-reader. If you simply replace wheat with a similar amount of other starches, such as potatoes or rice, I doubt whether you will lose much weight, but you may like to try just to satisfy yourself.

Lastly, genuine gluten allergy – an allergy to the gluten in wheat, rye, barley and oats – produces the condition called coeliac disease, one of the symptoms of which may be weight loss, along with a variety of other symptoms, such as anaemia, lethargy and painful joints. This needs to be treated professionally.

See also:

- Question: 114.
- Key index entries: allergies, carbohydrates.

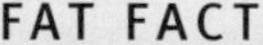

FAT FACT

The foods most often associated with intolerance and allergy are: dairy foods, wheat, wheat bran, yeast, berries, nuts, tomatoes, prawns, eggs, gluten, citrus fruits, olives, goats' milk, seeds, soya.

The foods least associated with intolerance or allergy are: rice, pears, ginger, chicken, beetroot, carrots, cauliflower, plums, garlic, avocado, celery.

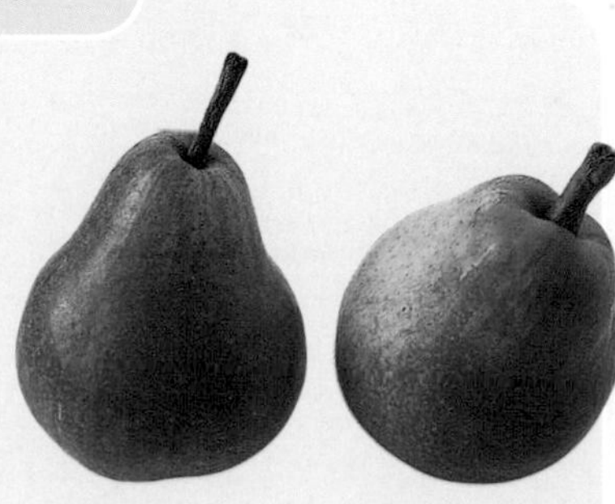

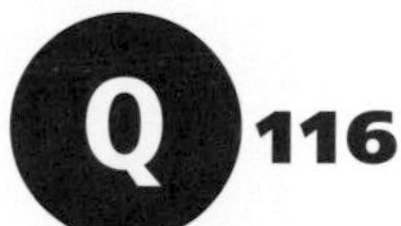

Is it a good idea to avoid dairy produce when slimming?

High-fat dairy products, like butter and full-fat cheeses, are high in calories and among the main sources of saturated fat. It is thus generally a good idea to cut right back on them, though they needn't be completely avoided as part of a varied diet, even when slimming. Medium- or low-fat dairy produce is better, as it is lower in fat and calories but still contains good amounts of calcium, protein, vitamins and minerals.

Giving up dairy produce altogether is unnecessary for slimming and, because it is our main source of calcium, may well be unwise unless you know enough about nutrition to get alternative sources in the right quantities, or take a supplement. Calcium is necessary for building and maintaining bones and teeth, and for a variety of other bodily functions. As with wheat, dairy produce is currently 'out of fashion', but there is no evidence that avoiding items like skimmed milk, cottage cheese, eggs and yoghurt will help a diet.

That said, if you are lactose-intolerant – when the body can't break down lactose (the sugar found in milk) – you will suffer from bloating and diarrhoea. You may also be intolerant of cows'-milk protein, in which case you may be fine on goats' or ewes' milk. Dairy intolerance is reasonably common – with some people mildly intolerant. If you have these symptoms, you can try a one- or two-week diet eliminating all dairy produce to see if the symptoms disappear. If they do, you should in any case see your doctor, who should also refer you to a dietitian.

The mildly intolerant may be fine on low-lactose cheeses, like Brie, Edam and Gouda.

See also:
- ▶ Question: 114.
- ▶ Key index entries: calcium, dairy produce.

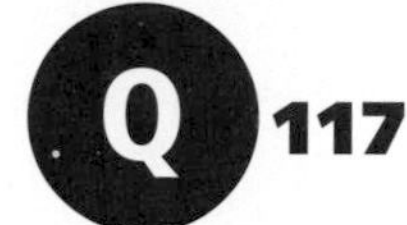

Are there disadvantages to diets which restrict me to just a few types of food?

The most obvious one is that you may suffer from nutritional deficiencies on the one hand, and a surfeit of other nutrients on the other. For example, on a diet of only carrots and apples, you'd get a surfeit of beta-carotene (which can turn your skin yellow and poison you) and a shortfall, for example, in protein, essential fats and a range of vitamins and minerals – an extreme example, but an important point.

The second disadvantage is that you will probably get extremely bored over time with the same few foods and more likely to give up your dieting efforts – though, in the short term, people seem to tolerate reduced-choice diets well (see Crash Diets in the A–Z for more on this). This is because they do take away the element of worry and indecision, and make dieting simple. However, these reasons aren't enough in themselves to recommend such a diet for most people.

The third disadvantage is that, in the long term, any weight lost on such a diet is unlikely to stay off, as you haven't learnt any new, more sensible eating habits.

A fourth, practical reason is that in slimming it is the overall calorie deficit that you create that matters, not what foods you eat or avoid. Whether you eat, say, 1,500 calories a day on a varied sensible diet or 1,500 calories of apples and carrots, your weight loss will be more or less the same. So variety restriction is fairly pointless.

There is little case, then, for following any diet that places severe restrictions upon the types of food you can eat. Much better, in the long term, to find a varied way of eating that fits in with your lifestyle and preferences rather than turning you into a faddy eater.

See also:
- ▶ Questions: 18, 79, 102–6, 112.
- ▶ Features: 10, 13.
- ▶ A–Z entry: crash diets.
- ▶ Key index entries: calories, healthy eating.

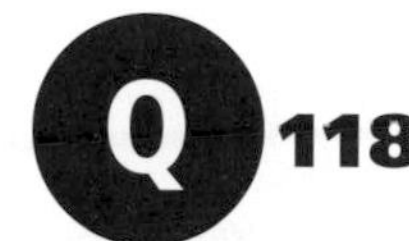

I enjoy fast food, like burgers and chips. Is it really necessary to cut these out in order to lose weight and keep it off?

The trouble with most of the food at burger bars, fried chicken bars, pizza places and Indian and Chinese takeaways is that it is surprisingly high in fat – and therefore calories. So, from both a dieting and a health viewpoint, a regular diet of takeaways isn't a great idea. Even items that you might think aren't high in fat, such as a chicken, fish or vegetarian burgers, for example, or a coleslaw side salad or salad bar main meal, usually are. For example, a McDonald's Vegetable Deluxe contains nearly 19g of fat – over double the fat in a McDonald's hamburger! The panel overleaf gives average values for basic takeaway items.

Of course, you can have the occasional treat of one of your favourite takeaways as part of even a slimming diet – nearly all food has at least some good points about it: for example, a beefburger is high in easily assimilated iron and protein, B vitamins and zinc, and is probably one of the better items described as fast food. (The bun's okay too – it's the fries and mayo that make a burger meal so high in fat.) Some takeouts ARE much lower in fat and calories than others – generally, you can get a lower-fat, all-vegetable pizza (often actually described as such on the menu) and tandoori chicken is another good option.

Another idea is to prepare 'takeaway'-type meals at home, where you can control the fat and calorie content (see the box below). In my experience, however, some takeaway addicts tend to turn up their noses at 'healthier' options, which just don't do it for them, taste-wise. In the long term I suggest that you try the retraining course in Feature 13 to help 'wean' you off your dependence on takeaways and high-fat food, while the rest of Section 4 may help get your mind in gear to do so. A read of Section 9 may give you motivation on the health score.

See also:

- ▶ Questions: 128–9, 131, 142, 165–7.
- ▶ Features: 12, 13.
- ▶ Key index entries: calories, fats in diet, healthy eating.

I love chocolate – can I eat it as part of a slimming diet?

Yes, you can, but obviously not in the kind of quantities that may have made you put on weight in the first place. As part of a calorie-counting-type diet, you could easily fit a 250-calorie bar into a 1,500 calories a day diet every day. However, on the type of slimming diet that seems to work best and be the favourite of the experts – about 25% fat content – fitting that much chocolate in every day is more of a problem.

For example, a 50g bar of dairy milk chocolate contains about 250 calories, and about 15g of fat, of which 9g is saturated fat. The 15g of fat represents over a third of your total daily fat intake – on a 1,500 calories a day diet of 42g (25%) fat – and more than the whole of your day's saturated fat intake – 8g (5%). So, on a low-fat diet only very small amounts of chocolate on a daily basis – about 100 calories' worth – really do fit in without bother. On a high-protein diet, you can eat more chocolate (see High-protein diets), but you may not then be getting a healthy diet.

I suggest you either try the retraining course in Feature 13, or find ways to get chocolatey tastes without so much fat and calories (see opposite), or designate one or two days a week as 'chocolate day(s)' and allow yourself a full bar of your favourite on those days. This latter method will only work if you aren't a 'chocoholic' as such (see Q139 if you are). It may also be worth pointing out that chocolate cravings can be due to low blood sugar, in which case see Qs 81–6 and 199, and always eat your chocolate at the end of a meal, and not as a between-meal snack.

HOMEMADE TAKEAWAYS

- Extra-lean quarterpounder in a bun with potato wedges coated in herb seasoning before baking, salad – average 400 calories.
- Chicken pieces (skinless) coated in yoghurt and Mexican herb mixture, baked and served with baked potato skins and home-made guacamole (mashed avocado, tomato, chilli and spring onion) – average 450 calories.
- Pitta pizza – top a pitta with tomato sauce, grated mozzarella cheese and slices of tomato, red onion and yellow pepper and grill until bubbling – average 350 calories.
- Greek kebabs – skewer lean leg lamb cubes, season and grill, season with lemon juice and serve with Greek yoghurt and chopped cucumber and pitta – average 450 calories.

FAST FOOD VALUES (AVERAGE PORTIONS)

Chinese	Cals	Fat (g)
Chicken chow mein	700	14
Peking duck/pancakes	750	25
Sweet-and-sour pork	500	18
Crispy pancake roll (l)	240	10
Indian/Thai		
Beef Madras	550	20
Chicken curry	700	40
Chicken korma	875	50
Chicken tikka masala	680	40
Rogan josh	700	24
Tandoori chicken	320	8
Onion bhaji (1)	190	16
Thai red beef curry	650	20
Thai green chicken curry	600	18
Pizza (per whole individual pizza)		
Four seasons	680	25
Margherita	650	23
Marinara	525	13
Pepperoni	800	40
Spicy meat	850	42
Burgers		
Quarterpounder/cheese/reg fries	750	37
Quarterpounder in bun	425	20
Chicken nuggets (6 pieces)	250	15
Chicken bar		
Chicken fillet burger/reg fries	700	32
2 drumsticks	370	22
Fish and chips		
Deep-fried cod in batter/chips	1000	55
Greek		
Large doner kebab in pitta	700	40
Tex-Mex		
Beef enchiladas	650	30
Chicken fajitas	725	30
Nachos	450	20

See also:

- ▶ Questions: 81–6, 89, 120, 139, 199.
- ▶ Features: 12, 13.
- ▶ A–Z entries: Atkins Diet, calorie counting, low-fat diets.
- ▶ Key index entries: chocolate, low blood sugar, sweet cravings.

WAYS TO GET CHOCOLATE TASTE FOR LESS

■ Low-calorie hot chocolate drinks – usually about 40 calories per cup.
■ Dip fresh fruits like strawberries into melted hot chocolate – 15 calories per strawberry.
■ Low-calorie chocolate bars – about 100 calories each.
■ Small amount of very-good-quality dark chocolate – more satisfying than a larger amount of cheaper chocolate. Two squares – about 50 calories.
■ Individual chocolate mousse, ready-made – about 80–100 calories.
■ One portion of chocolate-flavoured sugar-free 'Instant Whip'-type dessert – about 100 calories.

120

I have a sweet tooth and can't face life without desserts – any suggestions?

The solution is to base desserts around fruit, which is naturally sweet but not high in calories – and also good for you. If fresh fruit or fruit salad is not 'desserty' enough for you, try the following:
■ *Baked bananas* (bake in their skins until black and serve with a sprinkling of brown sugar and lemon juice) – about 100 calories a portion.
■ *Summer puddings* made in the usual way but with half the quantity of fructose instead of sugar – about 200 calories per 125g (5oz) slice, served with half-fat crème fraîche or Greek yoghurt (15ml, 16 cals per tbsp).
■ *Fruit kebabs*, brushed with low-fat spread and grilled or barbecued – about 50 calories per stick.
■ *Fruit fools* made by whizzing rhubarb, gooseberries or strawberries with a little fructose and 0%-fat fromage frais – about 125 calories per 150ml (1/4 pint).
■ *Fruit layers* made with puréed or whole soft fruits and Greek yoghurt, topped with no-added-sugar muesli – about 150 calories per 150ml (1/4 pint) portion.

Desserts based on fruit and calcium-rich dairy produce are not items to feel guilty about, so you win all ways.

See also:

- ▶ Question: 185.
- ▶ Feature: 13.
- ▶ Key index entries: food value charts.

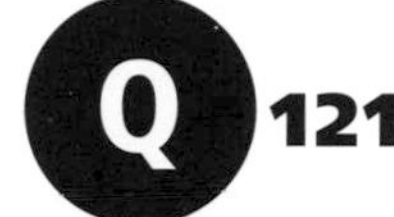

121

I adore cheese (all the full-fat kinds!) – how can my diet cope with its calories?

Like the chocolate lover in Q119, you need to find ways to get the cheese flavour and satisfaction without the calories. Here are some ideas:
■ Buy best-quality, very strong extra-mature cheeses, such as mature farmhouse Cheddar or Parmesan, and you will find that much smaller quantities tend to satisfy the taste buds.
■ Grate cheese for sandwiches; you'll use much less.
■ Mix grated cheese with grated carrot for a salad; again it goes further.
■ Make a low-cal sauce with sauce flour, skimmed milk and a little grated strong cheese and use for pasta, fish and fish pies.
■ Blue cheeses tend to be stronger and more tangy than others, so you need less. Some are lower in calories than others – e.g. Danish Blue or Irish Cashel Blue.
■ Both Greek feta cheese and most medium-mature goats' cheeses are medium-fat only, high on taste and tang, and can therefore be used in small quantities – both are good in salads.

Small amounts of most cheeses can be incorporated into any slimming diet – even a low-fat one (see the Basic Diet in Feature 9, which contains cheese). Cheese is high in calcium and protein, and makes a nutritional contribution.

One last point is that your cheese addiction may, in fact, be a salt addiction – most cheese is very high in salt. Try the retraining course in Feature 13.

See also:

- ▶ Questions: 89, 116, 185, 195.
- ▶ Features: 9, 13.
- ▶ A–Z index: Atkins Diet, calorie counting, low-fat diets.
- ▶ Key index entries: cheese, fat.

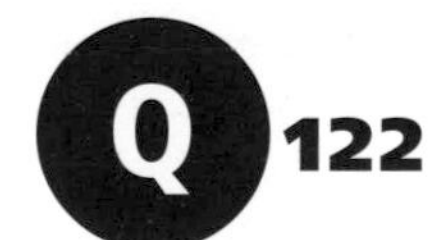

122

What are the best (quick and/or easy) cooking methods for slimmers?

Well, there's plenty of scope. The only method that is probably unwise for slimmers is deep-frying. An easy cooking method is tray-baking, perhaps with a little olive oil. This can be used for almost all vegetables, meat and fish. Stir-frying is simple and, if you eat meat, fish and poultry, marinating lean cuts and then grilling or barbecuing takes a lot of beating for flavour and ease. If I were vegetarian, I would virtually live on salads, stews and soups!

See also:

- ▶ Questions: 165–6.
- ▶ Features: 10, 11, 14, 16.

Meal makeovers

Here are three meals of the kind that may have been contributing to your weight problem, with my suggestions for alternatives that use the same main ingredient(s) but are much lower in calories and fat. In each case, the total weight of the 'after' meal is at least as much as the 'before', and often more.

SOME TIPS FOR REDUCING CALORIES PAINLESSLY

- Use cooking oil spray to coat non-stick frying pans for dry-frying.
- For creamy salad dressings, choose reduced-fat mayonnaise and mix with equal parts bio yoghurt and a little seasoning and lemon juice.
- Choose leanest cuts of meat and/or remove visible fat before cooking. Remoisten with yoghurt, herb crust or marinades.
- Choose Brie, feta or goats' cheese instead of Cheddar and Stilton.
- Add pulses to soups, stews and curries to cut down fat and add fibre.
- When stir-frying and the mix goes a bit dry, add a little water or stock to the pan, not more fat – it will do the same thing.
- Use low-fat spread or low-fat mayonnaise in sandwiches.
- Use 8%-fat fromage frais or smetana in desserts, dips and sauces instead of full-fat Greek yoghurt, cream or crème fraîche.
- Eat tea breads – such as banana bread – instead of full-fat cakes.
- Drink spritzers instead of wine (equal parts wine and soda water).
- Dress salads with balsamic vinegar instead of French dressing.
- Reduce portions by 20%, except veg and salad – increase them 50%.
- Leave casseroles and stews to go cold and remove any fat that rises to the surface, before reheating and serving.
- Make fat-free béchamel sauces by using sauce flour and skimmed milk. Season well.

MAKEOVER 1

Before – Chicken, Chips and Peas

One 200g (7oz) chicken breast fillet (skin on), baked on a tray with 200g (7oz) oven chips (large, straight-cut type) and served with 80g ($2^3/_4$oz) peas – 840 calories.

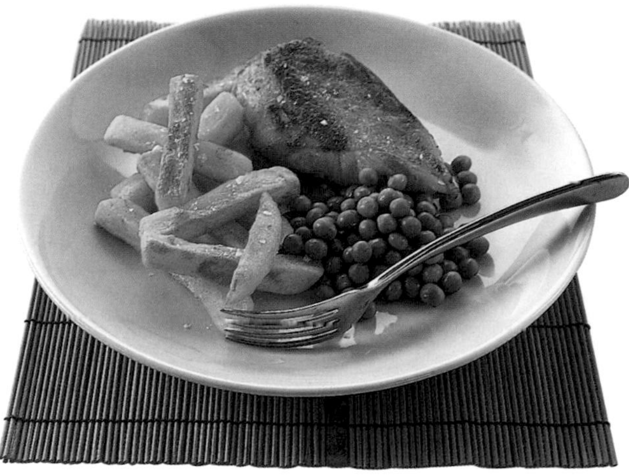

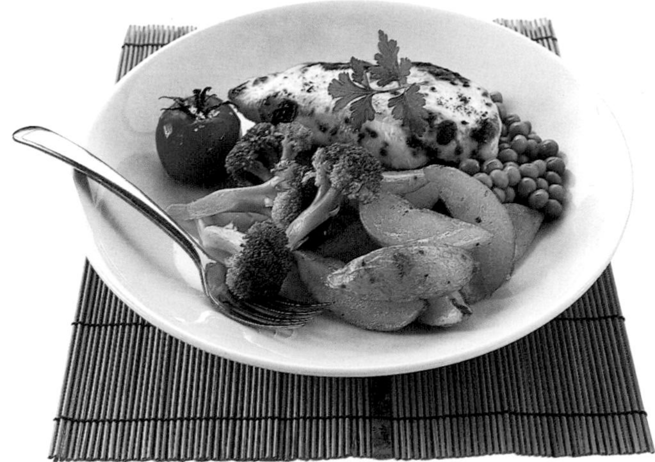

After – Baked Chicken with Potato Wedges

One 200g (7oz) chicken breast fillet (skinless), basted with whole-milk yoghurt to coat and baked on a tray, with 200g (7oz) wedges of baking potato tossed in I dsp olive oil and seasoning, and served with 80g ($2^3/_4$oz) peas and 80g ($2^3/_4$oz) broccoli and I tomato – 565 calories.

MAKEOVER 2

Before – Thai Lamb Curry
175g (6oz) stewing lamb chunks cooked in 100ml (3 1/2fl oz) Thai red curry sauce and served with half a naan bread and 150g (5oz) (cooked weight) pilau rice – 1,060 calories.

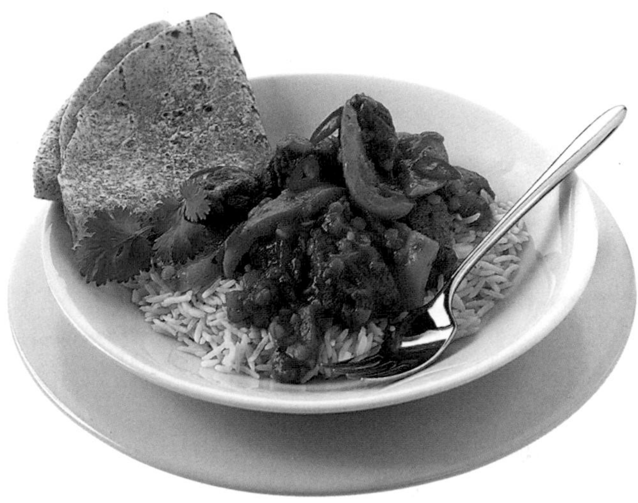

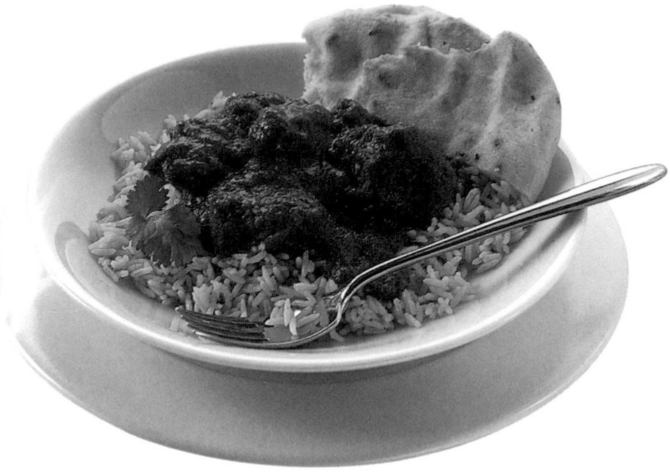

After – Lamb and Lentil Curry
110g (4oz) lamb fillet cubes and 75g (2 3/4oz) ready-cooked red lentils, one 50g (1 2/3oz) chopped onion and mixed pepper slices, fried in 1 tsp groundnut oil with l-2 tsp curry powder and 1 deseeded and chopped chilli, then simmered in 100ml (3 1/2fl oz) tomato sauce, and served with half a chapati and 100g (3 1/2oz) (cooked weight) boiled basmati rice – 560 calories.

MAKEOVER 3

Before – Pork Chop with Mash and Gravy
150g (5oz) average loin pork chop (rind on), grilled and served with 150g (5oz) potato mashed with butter and skimmed milk, 60g (2oz) green beans, l dsp plum sauce and 2 tbsp gravy – 630 calories.

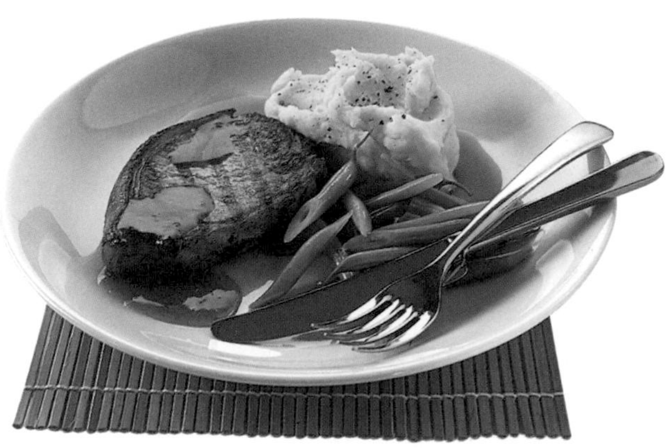

After – Pork with Pak Choi and Noodles
100g (3 1/2oz) pork fillet stir-fried in l dsp groundnut oil with 100g (3 1/2oz) pak choi, 50g (1 3/4oz) beansprouts and l dsp soya sauce, served with 200g (7oz) (cooked weight) egg thread noodles – 360 calories.

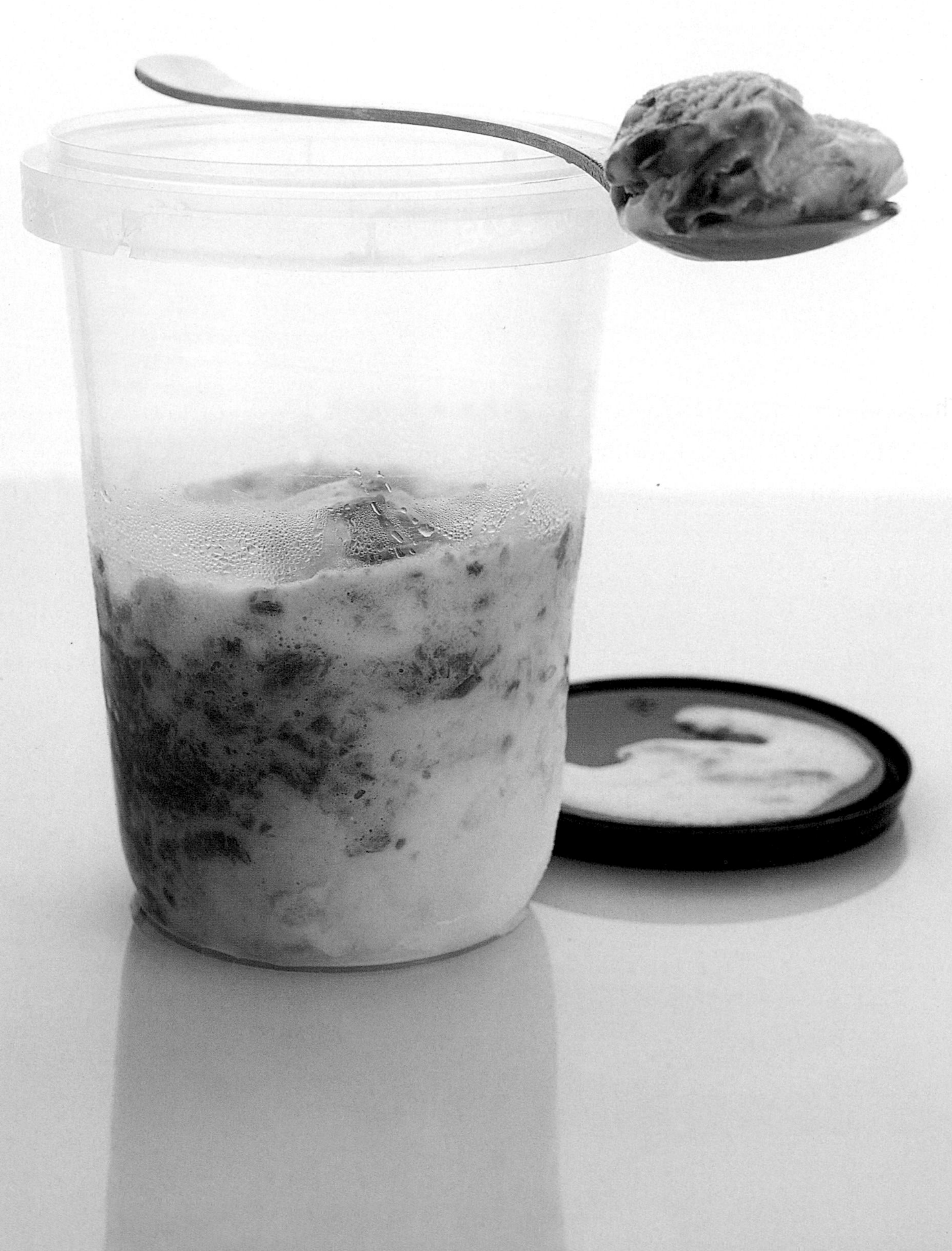

Section Four

All in the mind?

The previous section looked at the practicalities of eating a healthy, reduced-fat, reduced-calorie diet. Now we examine the difficulties many people face in turning ideas into realities. For many, the psychological, emotional and practical problems of eating to get – and stay – slim seem almost insurmountable.

Ever since gluttony was named as one of the seven deadly sins, the inhabitants of the Western world have had to contend with feelings of guilt about eating. It is this dichotomy – knowing that food is something we want, crave, need, but is also something we can so easily come to fear or even hate – that we need to resolve.

For food can be different things to different people – or different things to all of us at different times. Food is ritualistic, symbolic, mystical. The home and the family and comfort equal food. Food can be a front, a mask, a statement. It easily defines who many people are. Get the balance wrong, however, and food says for you 'I'm unhappy'... too fat, too thin, either way. Eat – or refuse – too much and food can be immoral – with the consequences of over- or under-indulgence so physically on display, the obese and anorexic alike may be stigmatized and shunned.

Here, in Section Four, we aim to unravel the mystery – and, often, misery – of our relationship with food.

123

I know I should lose weight – but how do I get motivated?

I assume you are genuinely overweight, but just can't see any bonus to be gained or incentive to be found in losing it. If you're only slightly overweight, perhaps there IS no need – in which case, see the next question – but, if you are very overweight, all I can do is tell you that when people do lose it and keep it off, they feel better in several ways – often unexpected ones.

In l997 *The American Journal of Clinical Nutrition* published a review of how people felt after they'd lost weight. The slimmers said the quality of their lives had improved in the following ways (the percentages indicate the proportion of people interviewed who agreed that their life had improved in that area): general quality of life (95%); level of energy (92%); mobility (92%), general mood (91%); self-confidence (91%); physical health (86%); interactions with strangers (69%); interactions with opposite sex (65%); interactions with spouse (56%); job performance (54%); hobbies (49%). By the way, I take the quaint expression 'interactions' to mean things like strangers smiling at you, people agreeing to come on a date with you, or your spouse allowing you back into the matrimonial bed. These findings match those from my own observations of the many people I've helped to slim over the years. People blossom after losing weight!

It might be useful for you to write a list of all the ways you think you'd feel if you were slim, and how your life would be. Also write a list of the health benefits you think you want; a check through Section 9 will help with that. You could also attempt to add up all the lost days or hours you have spent fretting or being miserable about not being more slim, or feeling guilty about eating too much. For most people that comes to a large chunk of their adult lives.

You must decide – do I accept my weight and live happily with it, or do I really want to change? The worst motivation for slimming is saying, 'I should...','I must ...', 'I'd better ...' or 'My doctor says ...'

If you aren't doing it because you want to and believe that you can, then it is not likely that you will succeed. One trick if you want to but aren't sure that you can – i.e., you're halfway there – is to think yourself into the part. This idea – called by American actor Roy Scheider 'Acting Well' – uses techniques advocated by Stanislavski's Method school of acting. You create your thin self in your mind and think about what you do, how you look, what you eat, what exercise you do, how popular you are. Over time, you become what you are imagining in a natural way. You eat better, take more exercise, lose weight, turn into your 'thin self'. Well – it worked for Roy, and he also used the same method to give up smoking.

Another tool is to join a slimming club – the comradeship and common goal works for many. While getting weighed every week may be seen as a bullying tactic, it's also a great motivator!

See also:

- ▶ Questions: 124–9.
- ▶ Feature: 11.
- ▶ A–Z entry: slimming clubs.

124

I've lost weight before and it all returns – what's the point?

Life certainly is too short to spend much of your time struggling to get thin, then getting fat again. I can hardly think of any worse way to live. If you have a Body Mass Index of no more than 25–7, you may be better off accepting the size you are and simply trying to ensure that you don't put on any more weight. Some studies show that 'yo-yo' dieting is worse for heart health than being overweight (though others dispute this). Attempting to get down to too low a weight is one important factor in the 'yo-yo syndrome', so if you do decide to 'try again', set a realistic target.

Also, don't set out this time to 'diet', but to eat in a better, different way, and to look at your whole lifestyle. How much exercise do you take? How stressed are you? What causes you to overeat? Joining a group such as Overeaters Anonymous might be a good way for you to go.

Also, weight loss for previous dieters is usually best when it happens as a side-effect of something you enjoy doing. As an example, a neighbour of mine was plump, bordering on obese, for years. A few winters ago, she and her husband developed a passion for line-dancing. What started out as one two-hour session a week ended up with them out line-dancing 5 nights a week, doing demonstrations, classes and so on. Within a year she had shed 3 stones and is now a slim size 12. She's fit, she's happy – and she eats whatever she wants.

The point is not so much getting the slimming right, but getting the maintenance right. So I quite agree – there IS no point to dieting, unless you have a strategy in place for the long term. I'd also say that, for all of us, a wise strategy is one that does include regular exercise.

See also:

- ▶ Questions: 22, 26, 32–6, 123, 125, 204–7, 313–4, 333.
- ▶ Features: 3, 4, 10, 12, 13.
- ▶ A–Z entries: Overeaters Anonymous, slimming clubs.
- ▶ Key index entries: exercise, healthy eating.

Q 125

Everyone tells me that diets don't work – so why bother?

Be very wary of the things that people tell you, because they may not be true. First read the answers to the previous two questions, which may help to resolve the 'why bother' point. Now on to the first part of your question. Diets certainly DO work. If you create an energy deficit by eating fewer calories than your body uses in energy output, you'll lose weight.

What people mean by 'diets don't work' is that 'after the diet' the weight tends to return ... and then some. This IS true – in most studies, about 95% of people have put back all their weight after a year. Other studies, however, show that certain groups of people – notably those who begin to take regular exercise – DO manage to keep the weight off.

From my own experience, it is definitely my friends who run, cycle, walk, swim, dance, enjoy the great outdoors, garden, have active jobs and so on who seem most successful in keeping their youthful figures into middle age. It doesn't take a lot. Burning up just 100 extra calories a day in, say, a half-hour walk, could mean, over a year, that you save yourself from putting on a whole stone in weight.

So diets DO work – but you need to commit yourself to a regular activity programme to keep the weight off. It would also be a help if you read all the stuff listed in the cross-references below, to find out all the background on calories and weight control.

See also:

- ▶ Questions: 3, 6, 9, 18, 24, 32–4, 74–90, 102–6.
- ▶ Features: 1, 2, 3.

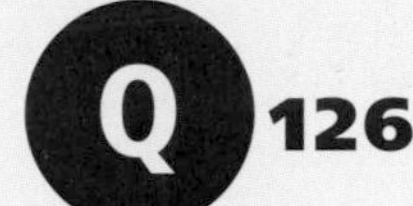

Q 126

Everyone tells me that I look just fine as I am – so why should I slim?

Perhaps you do look fine, and perhaps you shouldn't slim. Check with Feature 3 to find out. If it shows that you do need to lose weight on health grounds, then I would trust this rather than what people who know you say. Well-meaning friends will almost always say, 'Oh, you look fine!', especially in response to a heartfelt query from yourself along the lines of, 'Do you think I'm too fat?' I mean, honestly – how many people are going to look you in the eyes and say, 'Yes'? So, partly their reluctance to come clean is cowardice, and part could also be misguided kindness – they don't want you to feel bad about yourself.

However, all research shows that we live in a fat-prejudiced society. The World Health Organization reports that obesity is 'highly stigmatized in industrialized countries', even down to doctors being less interested in treating obese patients. The Association for the Study of Obesity says that very fat students are 65% less likely to get a place at college than thin ones, even if they have the same grades; that they are less likely to get a job or promotion, and that, in Britain, obese women are paid on average 5% less than others.

Unfair though all this is, it is a fact at the moment. Choose whether or not to lose weight with unbiased advice – friends are the last people to ask.

See also:

- ▶ Questions: 26–31, 127.
- ▶ Feature: 3.
- ▶ Key index entries: dieting, obesity, overweight, weight control.

Q 127

I would like to lose weight but my family don't want me to – is this a common problem and how do I deal with it?

Isn't it strange how we don't like our own fat bodies, we don't like to look at obese people on the streets, don't admire fat models or pop stars, but if our nearest and dearest are fat and want to lose weight – we panic! Your spouse and children like familiarity – old slippers, old teddy bears – and they know and love you as you are now. It is quite flattering in a way – you are loved for who you are, not what you look like.

However, there could be a less altruistic motive going on here too. It is true that some people who lose weight (usually, the larger amounts of weight) do change quite drastically – they become more outgoing, more confident, more successful, more selfish even. So the family may realize this (albeit possibly subconsciously) and, selfish themselves, want to keep you 'in line'. They see your losing weight as a threat. An under-confident spouse may wonder if you'll be swept off your feet by a newer model when you're once again slim – and indeed, this does happen now and again.

So, this not wanting you to lose weight is a more common problem than you might have thought. How to deal with it? I would quietly get on with the business of slimming and carry on in other areas of life as normal. If you do it slowly and sensibly, and try not to make a big issue of it, I dare say equilibrium will be maintained. If you do feel much better when slim (which you will) and make life changes, then let you and the family deal with them when they happen. Certainly don't stay fat because your family want you to.

See also:

- ▶ Questions: 26, 124–6, 300.
- ▶ Features: 3, 25.

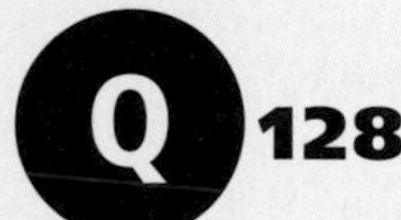

We live in a food-dominated society – how can I slim when the odds seem stacked against me?

I think this is THE big and crucial question. Indeed, it does seem as though the odds are stacked against individuals trying to lose weight, when all around is a non-stop, relentless onslaught of food promotion. Media advertising, supermarket specials, fast food, street food, dining out, eating with friends, snack food sold almost everywhere from DIY stores to newsagents. Everything is geared to try to persuade us to eat and drink more than we need or want.

The food industry is the biggest industry in the world. Never let anyone try to kid you that it is the diet industry that makes billions off our fat backs; it is the food producers and retailers who do that. We get fat – and then what happens? We are the ones who end up feeling inadequate and guilty, greedy and weak-willed.

It is NOT all your fault you are fat. However, I still do think that it IS up to the individual – having recognized that people are trying to get rich on your liking for fatty foods, sugary foods, salty foods, snacks, alcohol, or just too much of everything – to put up resistance. Try to recognize the ploys used every day to get you to eat or drink when you don't need to eat or drink, and get in the habit of tuning in to your own real hunger signals and food and nutrition needs rather than listening to these 'devils in disguise'.

It may take a while, but you can retrain your taste buds to enjoy more natural, less fattening, healthier foods, and you can train your appetite and hunger signals to let you know what they're really thinking. This way you end up eating when YOU want or need to eat, what YOU want or need to eat, and in quantities that YOU decide are right. It doesn't take willpower, but determination.

You could also read up on the way mass market food is produced – John Humphrys' book *The Great Food Gamble* (Hodder, £12.99), published in 2001, is an eye-opener. If you thought you enjoyed fast food, and all kinds of other consumer foods, you may change your mind after you read this and decide that it's organic for you from now on!

You could also become a campaigner yourself – things won't change unless enough people demand better-quality food, and stricter advertising standards, and that the food giants – and the government – don't hinder, but help, us to help ourselves in the war of the weight.

See also:

- ▶ Questions: 129–31.
- ▶ Features: 12, 13.
- ▶ Key index entries: fast food, healthy eating.

Food is my main pleasure – why should I deny myself?

Many people who live to eat do get fat, but I don't think that having food as one of your main pleasures necessarily disposes you to fatness. Food is one of my real pleasures too, but over the past few years I've come to enjoy slightly different eating patterns and types of food.

If you'd told me 10 years ago that I would positively relish bio yoghurt, fresh fruit and pumpkin seeds for breakfast, large bowlfuls of organic mixed salad greens and stoneground bread for lunch, and brown rice with wild salmon and herbs for supper, I would not have believed you. I still enjoy chocolate, wine, cheese, butter, meat, eggs, even pastry and cream, but I always buy best-quality and enjoy smaller portions of these.

Why the change? See the previous question – and I've learnt to regard my body as important, and I want to feed it well – which isn't the same as overfeeding it or overindulging it. 'Indulgence' to me now really does mean feasting on gorgeous, tasty, natural foods.

There is also, of course, a difference between having food as your 'main pleasure' and having food as 'a pleasure'. Try the following tips, which may help you to make small changes in your diet and your attitude to food that add up to a big difference.

- ■ Try the questionnaire in Feature 12 and the retraining course in Feature 13.
- ■ Substitute rich, fatty, salty or sugary foods with other strong tastes and aromatic foods that are less fattening – research shows that people who overeat prefer more intense flavours and aromas than thin people.
- ■ Listen to your body and begin reading signals. Are you really hungry? Are you full? Act on the signals you receive.
- ■ Always eat slowly and chew thoroughly, then you may naturally eat less.
- ■ Consider joining a group, such as Overeaters Anonymous, or get counselling that may help you fit food into your life in a less dominating way (see A–Z).
- ■ Don't deny yourself good food, but rethink your parameters.

See also:

- ▶ Questions: 128, 131–43.
- ▶ Features: 11, 12, 13.
- ▶ A–Z entries: diet aromas, Overeaters Anonymous, slimming clubs.

FAT FACT

Sniffing a bulb of Florence fennel is said to curb the appetite – apparently fasting Christians in the Middle Ages used this idea to help them through.

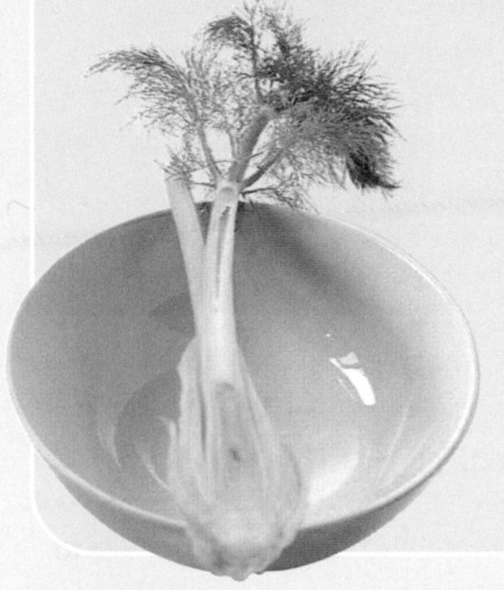

Q 130

Isn't it true that overweight people are just basically greedy and lazy?

No. The recent WHO report on obesity says that, in contrast to the widely held perception, it is clear that obesity is not simply a result of overindulgence in highly palatable foods, or a lack of physical activity. Although it is true that anyone can create for themselves an energy deficit (see Q18) and lose weight, some people do have much more of a predisposition to putting on weight than others, for reasons discussed in detail in Section One.

For most people, weight gain is something that happens gradually over a period of years (most weight gain occurring between the ages of 25 and 50), and it doesn't take a great deal of overeating to achieve gains of a few pounds – even a stone – a year. If you eat, for example, just one large slice of bread and butter a day more than you need (about 150 calories), you would put on about 15lb (7kg) in a year, on average. Moreover, the temptation to overeat is all around us – it is more a matter of food always being there so we eat it, rather than everyone being greedy.

It is also true to say that most of us don't take nearly enough exercise and that this is by far the best way to prevent weight gain in the long term – but I really don't think it would be fair to describe people who don't take enough exercise as 'lazy' across the board. Mostly people are far from lazy, but don't take enough exercise because they are very busy and have simply got out of the habit of fitting exercise into their hectic lives.

See also:

▶ Questions: 1–6, 18–27, 128.

Q 131

Is there any real answer to the fact that diet food is very, very boring?

There's no such thing as 'diet' food, really. Take a look at Feature 11 and see all the great tastes and textures, colours and aromas there are in a good slimmer's diet. The 'cottage cheese, cardboard crispbread and limp lettuce' regime has long since departed for most of us, thank goodness.

New research indicates that overweight people hate bland diets because they have a greater need than slim people for strong and intense flavours and aromas. So they don't try a slimming diet because they perceive them all to be boring and bland. However, calorie- and fat-reduced diets have become much more sophisticated, as we now know exactly how to cut calories that aren't needed while retaining loads of interest, flavour and satisfaction – as well as a decent-sized plateful of food.

I think the right way to ensure that food is kept exciting and enticing, is to go big on ethnic eating... the spices of the Middle East and India, the herbs and vegetables of the Mediterranean, the succulent fruits of the tropics, the more exotic grains and pulses. What could be better than chicken spiced with coriander, cumin and chilli,or a delicious Greek salad with feta, or a plate of pasta sprinkled with fresh basil and balsamic vinegar? I could go on. All these things are, or can be, staples of a calorie-reduced diet.

What do you want that you think you can't have? Fit in small amounts of these using the Food Value Charts at the back of the book, or go on the retraining course in Feature 13 to alter your taste buds. Read all of Section Three to familiarize yourself with cutting calories and fat without pain. Work out your own optimum slimming calorie and fat levels using Features 3 and 8. And, most of all, cheer up!

See also:

▶ Questions: 79–90, 128–9.

▶ Features: 3, 8–13.

▶ A-Z entries: calorie counting, low-fat diets.

▶ Key index entries: healthy eating, slimming.

Delicious dieting

Here is a sample day's menus for people who say that dieting is boring and tasteless. Not true! The menu here (either choice) adds up to around 1,500 calories and 25–30% fat. All dishes serve one.

The Four Most Flavoursome Meal Ideas for Slimmers

■ Mixed vegetable soups made with good-quality stock, blended to give a creamy finish without cream.
Key base ingredients: tomatoes, onion, parsley, garlic.

■ Pulse and meat casseroles – good combinations are beef and red kidney beans, lean lamb and chickpeas or cannellini beans, chicken and green lentils. Meat can be browned in a non-stick pan sprayed with low-calorie cooking oil spray.
Key base ingredients: good-quality stock, herbs, passata, onions.

■ Vegetable curries: mix some root and other vegetables or pulses and use a freshly made spice blend for maximum flavour. Use 1/2 tablespoon of vegetable oil per person for frying the onion and spices before proceeding. Good combinations include: potato and spinach, aubergine and lentils, sweet potato and broccoli. Thicken the sauce with yoghurt. Serve with boiled rice flavoured with saffron or cardamom, if you like.
Key base ingredients: chilli, ginger, turmeric, cumin, coriander seed, good-quality vegetable stock, yoghurt, coriander leaf.

■ Ethnic salads: combine robust salad leaves and herbs with fruity or spicy low-fat dressings and add a low-fat protein (e.g. chicken, turkey, lean meat, fish) plus one or two other vegetables and/or fruits and some starch (e.g. pasta, potatoes, rice). Good combinations are fresh tuna with tomatoes and courgettes, bulghar wheat with goats' cheese, pasta with chicken and peppers. Vegetables can be marinated for more flavour and to soften them a little.
Key base ingredients: fresh salad herbs, good-quality vinegar or citrus juice, small amounts of top-quality extra-virgin olive oil, garnishes (see the suggestions above).

FOODS FOR FLAVOUR

Some foods and condiments add masses of flavour to your meals for very few calories. Here are my favourites:

The Top Five vegetables: tomatoes, onions, red peppers, mushrooms, rocket.

The Top Five flavoursome fish: tuna, swordfish, salmon, monkfish, skate.

The Top Five spices: chilli, saffron, garlic, cumin, ginger.

The Top Five herbs: basil, coriander leaf, mint, flat-leaf parsley, tarragon.

The Top Five flavourings: balsamic vinegar, lime juice, soy sauce, French mustard, passata.

The Top Five garnishes: anchovies, black olives, capers, garlic croutons, truffles.

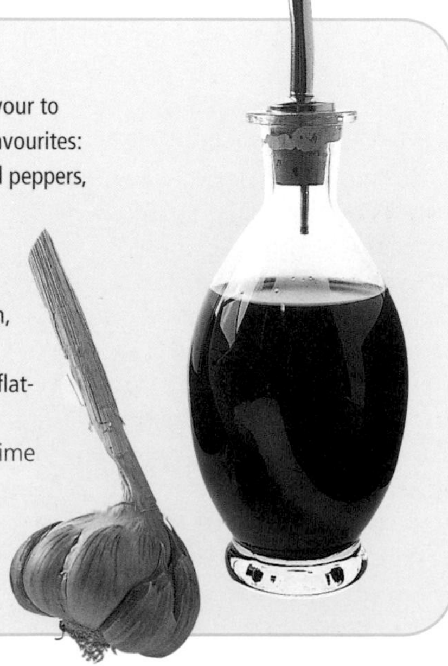

Breakfast

Menu 1

80g (2¾oz) raspberries or sliced top-flavour strawberries, topped with I level tsp golden caster sugar, 3 tbsp Greek yoghurt and finished with 1–2 tbsp no-added-sugar muesli.

Menu 2

2 large flat mushrooms, sprayed on either side with low-calorie cooking oil spray and the gills brushed with a little balsamic vinegar, seasoned and grilled or baked until tender and served on a toasted ciabatta roll and topped with I slice of extra-lean back bacon, grilled or baked and crumbled.

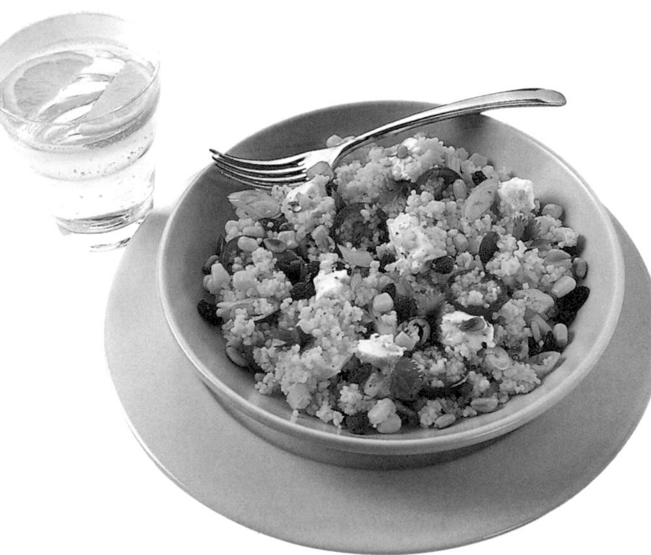

Lunch

Menu 1

Saffron couscous salad: 50g (1⅔oz) couscous soaked in vegetable stock with a pinch of saffron and tossed with 40g (1⅓oz) medium-fat goats' cheese, spring onions, sweetcorn kernels, sultanas, cherry tomatoes, a few toasted pine nuts and fresh coriander leaves with I tbsp of your favourite fat-free dressing.

Menu 2

Split pitta filled with a salad of chopped 'high-flavour' tomatoes, ready-made herb salad, 50g (1⅔oz) ready-cooked chickpeas and chopped black olives, tossed in a dressing made by beating together I level tbsp good-quality hummus with I tbsp fat-free French or Italian dressing and I level tsp fresh chopped red chilli.

Evening

Menu 1

A prawn and chicken creole made by sautéing 100g (3½oz) bite-sized chicken fillet chunks in ½ tbsp corn oil and adding chopped red onion, peppers, garlic and hot chilli, 2 chopped sun-dried tomatoes, 50g (1⅔oz) basmati rice, 100g (3½oz) chopped tomatoes, and 100ml (3½fl oz) stock. Cover and cook until rice is tender, adding more stock if necessary; add 50g (1⅔oz) prawns before serving.

Menu 2

A new potato salad made by combining 150g (5oz) new potatoes with chopped mint, parsley, spring onions and I tbsp dressing of equal parts balsamic vinegar and olive oil, with a little wholegrain mustard and seasoning; served with 1 grilled organic salmon steak and ruby chard.

Extras:

1 glass of wine and I portion of lemon sorbet.

■ To drink during day – mineral water, tea of choice, 3 cups coffee, if liked.

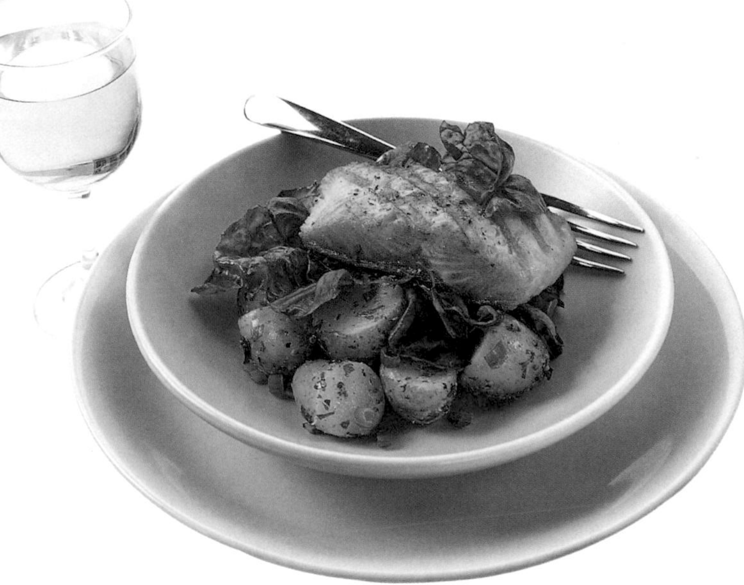

Can you define compulsive eating for me?

Compulsive eating is also called 'binge eating disorder'. It is more than an occasional mild binge on an extra chocolate bar and is more than having second portions of a particularly tasty meal. It is also more than eating half a fruit cake mindlessly once a year when you feel particularly upset. All these things many of us do on occasion. Binge eating disorder involves recurrent episodes of eating much larger quantities of food than most of us would eat in a similar time, resulting in weight gain and, often, obesity over time. Types of food eaten can be very varied, although typically foods high in fat, sugar and refined carbohydrates are favourites.

Compulsive eating differs from bulimia in that the sufferer doesn't purge (vomit or take laxatives), so all the extra food ends up as fat. According to a review published by the British Nutrition Foundation, it is thought that between 20 and 30% of all obese people suffer from binge eating disorder, and more women than men may be affected.

The American Psychiatric Association's criteria for diagnosing binge eating include:

- Eating in a short (less than 2 hours) period of time an amount of food that is definitely larger than most people would eat in similar circumstances.
- A sense of lack of control over eating during this episode.
- Binge eating episodes associated with three or more of the following – eating more rapidly than normal, eating until feeling uncomfortably full, eating large amounts while not hungry, eating alone, feeling embarrassed about how much one is eating, feeling disgusted with oneself, depressed or very guilty after overeating.

Binge eating may occur, on average, at least two days a week, and occurs in people who do not suffer from anorexia or bulimia; however, binge eating may be interspersed with periods of rigid dieting.

Binge eating is classified as a disorder and is most successfully treated with cognitive behaviour therapy. If you think you're a sufferer, it is best to talk to your doctor and get referred for further advice and help. Other questions (listed below) in this section may help you decide whether you do have BED and will offer advice.

See also:

- Questions: 133–43, 149–58.
- Feature: 12.
- A-Z entry: Overeaters Anonymous.
- Key index entries: eating disorders, food cravings, obesity.

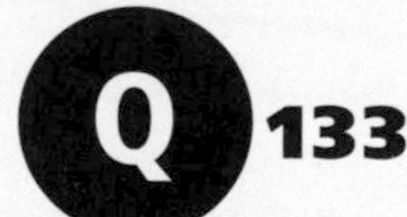

Can you recommend a strategy to beat comfort eating on carbohydrates?

Eating carbohydrate foods for comfort may have some basis in physical need and science. For example, eating foods very high in sugars and starches and low in protein may increase the activity of the neurotransmitter serotonin in the brain. This is involved in the control of our mood and behaviour (the drug Prozac works by promoting serotonin activity).

So, in effect, you may be 'dosing' yourself with carbs to try to treat depression. There is circumstantial evidence for this in that people who suffer from Seasonal Affective Disorder (SAD), who get depressed in the winter months, automatically increase their intake of carbs at that time.

Another possible cause may be that you aren't eating regularly enough and a sudden urge for carbs may be because you have low blood sugar. The British Nutrition Foundation reported in 2001 that dieters are more likely to turn to food for comfort when they are under stress than other people, and this may, I feel, be linked to blood sugar – or simply because dieters can be 'good' when not under stress, but if things go wrong, it may be 'blow the diet – I'll have a cream cake'. This is yet another reason to avoid very-low-calorie, strict diets and choose to slim slowly.

The consensus is that the likely reasons for eating carbs when you are miserable are simply that they are pleasurable to eat and temporarily help ease negative feelings. Some people turn to alcohol, shopping, gambling, etc., while others turn to food if they have life problems. If you feel that you are actually depressed, then you should visit your doctor, who may recommend medication and refer you for counselling if that would help.

If you just eat for comfort when you feel 'fed up', the following strategies may help:

- Eat small regular meals, so that when you feel below par you may be slightly less inclined to overeat. Don't ever be over-strict on yourself about food.
- Prepare alternative 'comforters' ahead of time – if you know you regularly eat bread and jam, say, in a crisis, think of alternative things that may help you to feel better, such as, soothing music. Decide in advance what you'll try instead of the food, so that you aren't 'caught out'.
- Distract yourself when you feel the urge for a carb coming on. If hungry, eat something other than carbs (e.g. a small piece of cheese). Get away from the kitchen and do something else – have a bath or go for a walk.
- Remember, just because you have a craving, it doesn't mean you have to do anything about it. Keep telling yourself you are in control and eventually you will be. You may also benefit from doing the food retraining course in Feature 13, which will help to reduce your taste for sweet, fatty, carb foods.
- Reflect on what is causing you to comfort eat and see what can be done to alter or improve the situation. This is the

most important part of the strategy in the long term. If food is filling a hole in your emotional life, or acting as support system or a mask for problems, then you may not find it easy to control until you sort out the underlying reasons. You may also like to join a group like Overeaters Anonymous.

See also:

▶ Questions: 132, 134–43, 156.
▶ Features: 12, 13.
▶ A–Z entry: Overeaters Anonymous.
▶ Key index entries: blood-sugar levels, carbohydrates, eating disorders.

I eat when I'm bored – most evenings and weekends – what's the answer?

Well, the obvious answer is to make efforts to solve your boredom problem. Sounds as if you have a busy and enjoyable job or occupation during weekdays but haven't done enough to ensure balance in your life. You need to spend time thinking about yourself, your aims, your interests.

A starting point might be to think about what you don't like about your life at the moment (apart from the overeating). The answer to loneliness is involvement with others – but how? What would you enjoy? As to lack of purpose, you need things that will make you feel useful.

Whatever the reasons for your boredom and consequent overeating, you need to tackle both long-term with lifestyle changes. Short-term, any distraction is good if food beckons – even a visit to the library or bookshop, renting a video, writing an email, sending off for a load of holiday brochures – and so on.

See also:

▶ Questions: 133, 135–43.
▶ Features: 12, 13.

FAT FACT

Hyperphagia is a medical condition in which there is an insatiable and constant appetite for food – usually caused by a deficiency of the hormone leptin in the body.

I eat when I'm angry and/or frustrated – is there a cure?

Some smoke, others drink or take drugs, you eat. Eating to suppress anger has been described as, literally, pushing the anger back down inside yourself with the food. You need to address the causes of your anger, if it's frequent, and see what you can do to minimize or rid yourself of them. If you can't do this on your own, you'd probably benefit from counselling or sessions with a group like Overeaters Anonymous, to get some of your anger out in other ways and help you overcome it.

See also:

▶ Questions: 132, 149.
▶ Features: 12, 13.
▶ A-Z entry: Overeaters Anonymous.

Q 136

I've got no willpower at all so I can never stick to a diet – have you any tips?

I don't like the word 'willpower' because, if huge efforts of will are needed non-stop during a slimming campaign, then I believe it's bound to fail. I prefer 'determination', for certainly you need to be determined and motivated in order to lose weight.

So first examine your own motivations (see Q123) and come up with the main reasons you want to slim down. Next you need to set a sensible target weight, so that you aren't trying to diet yourself too low. Now pick a suitable food intake level so that you aren't permanently hungry – Feature 1 and Q104 will help here. Then you need to make sensible food choices, ones which will also help you to feel sated and happy while you slim. Feature 9 and much of Section 3 will help you do that.

You may find the support of a slimming club helpful to you – many people find the better ones extremely motivating. You may also benefit from doing the retraining course in Feature 13, which will help you get rid of, for example, a sweet tooth or a salty tooth. You will definitely benefit from regular exercise. The more you do, the more you can eat and still lose weight.

See also:

▶ Questions: 104, 112, 123.
▶ Features: 1, 9, 12, 13.
▶ A–Z entry: slimming clubs.
▶ Key index entry: healthy eating.

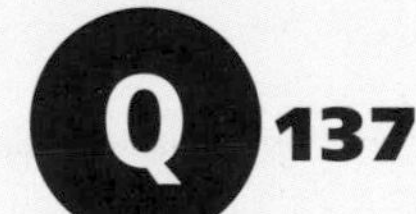

Is my need for food hunger or habit?

Many people these days have actually forgotten how it feels to be truly hungry – regular mealtimes and endless snacks on the run mean that our stomachs are rarely empty long enough to register feelings of hunger. We eat because it is time to eat. So, in a way, your need for food may well be more habit than hunger, and it is habitual eating, or eating 'because it's there' that makes us fat. If we all just ate when we were genuinely hungry, we wouldn't be fat.

How to tell the difference? It's interesting to keep a food diary for a week and record what you ate when, and why. In the 'why' column, you will find many and varied reasons, ranging from things like, 'Went for a newspaper and picked up a chocolate bar because it was a new variety and the packaging tempted me,' through, 'Dropped in on Mike and didn't like to refuse the coffee and cake'... to, 'Had a pizza while Sue and I went shopping – because we always do.' Not all your reasons will come down to habit (other reasons will be discussed later in the section) but many will.

We are creatures of habit, we love our rituals, and food and drink fit neatly into most rituals and habitual situations. The cure? A good first step is to become aware of what you are doing (keep that food diary going in your head, if you like) and then, before you eat, ask yourself, 'Is it hunger – or is it habit?' Begin saying 'no' to the food, at least some of the time. Eventually it gets easier, because you get more in tune with your real hunger signals.

See also:
▶ Questions: 134, 138, 141–2.
▶ Features: 12, 13.

What is the difference between greed and hunger?

It is said that when you eat food because you fancy it, that it is greed, and when you eat because you need to, that is hunger. However, I think this is an over-simplification. Hunger comes after a reasonable period without food – say, several hours – and may be enhanced by fresh air and exercise. If you can match one of these criteria and have hunger pangs and/or a 'grumbling' tummy, then you are probably, indeed, hungry. You'll probably enjoy your food all the more for that.

Greed is not a word I like – 'over-enthusiastic appetite' may describe the idea better. Even if you're not hungry, appetite can be triggered by the appearance, or thought, of a 'novel' food (one you haven't already just been eating) – say, a dessert after a large meal, or by a particular favourite food (say, chocolate). Habit can also make you eat more than you need – if you're always given huge portions, for instance, then that is what your eyes and your stomach (via brain signals) will come to expect.

Between-meal snacks may also be eaten because of the 'moreish' factor, rather than hunger. Snack foods such as chocolate bars, biscuits and ice-creams aren't regarded as 'staple' foods and tend to be used as treats or rewards. However, they may also be eaten when you are genuinely hungry (though this isn't actually a good idea – see Q85). 'Asking for more' isn't necessarily the province of the greedy, though, as food intake needs vary from person to person and from day to day.

One of the main differences between genuine hunger and hunger impostors is when you aren't hungry you're unlikely to choose a salad or an apple – but an item high in fat and/or sugar and/or refined starch. If you're hungry, you'll eat anything, including so-called 'healthy' foods. So if you're not sure whether you're feeling hungry or just have an 'over-enthusiastic appetite', examine what you're thinking of eating. If it's the doughnut or chocolate bar it could be you're not hungry at all!

See also:
▶ Questions: 23, 137, 141.
▶ Features: 12, 13.

I am a chocoholic. Can chocolate be addictive, like drugs?

Chocolate isn't addictive in the sense that heroin or other drugs can be, but its key ingredient, the cocoa bean, does contain some potent chemicals that have been blamed for causing chocolate addiction. It contains methylxanthines, a group of stimulant phyto (plant) chemicals including caffeine, theobromine and theophylline, which can help to keep you alert.

It also contains phenylethylamine (PEA), a substance that can cause migraine in susceptible people but which also has properties similar to amphetamine, and can enhance the body's own levels of its natural painkiller endorphins. It is also said that this substance increases libido and is the same chemical as that produced in the bodies of people in love. The seeds contain small amounts of their own endorphins and the cocoa bean is also said to contain a cannabis-like relaxant, amandanide.

However, it seems that chocolate itself usually doesn't contain enough of any of these chemicals to achieve much of an effect, let alone account for chocolate 'addiction'. (Indeed, white chocolate contains hardly any.) The British Nutrition Foundation reviewed all the evidence on chocolate recently and concluded that the levels of the methylxanthines in chocolate are so small that it is unlikely they would

FAT FACT

When students coming from Asia and the Middle East start studying at universities in America they put on an average of about 15 pounds in their first year through simply taking on board the typical US diet. This debunks the commonly held idea that some races don't get obese because they have an anti-fat gene.

have any effect, and that the phenylethylamine in chocolate cannot influence mood. One 40g piece of milk chocolate provides only 10mg caffeine – a tiny percentage of that in a cup of strong coffee – and dark chocolate has about 28mg, half that of a cup of tea.

The other, oft-cited effect of chocolate is that, as it is a high-carbohydrate food because it is high in sugar, it increases production of brain serotonin (see Q133) and therefore makes us feel happy. In fact, the BNF reports, foods that contains more than very small amounts of protein don't have this effect – and chocolate contains too much protein (because of its milk and/or cocoa content) and doesn't stimulate serotonin production at all.

The answer, then, to why chocolate is so moreish is that a) it melts at blood temperature and provides a unique pleasure experience and sensation in the mouth; b) it does release the body's natural endorphins simply because of the pleasurable experience, providing a small calming effect, and c) it provides a hedonistic buzz because it is perceived to be 'naughty' rather than virtuous. Most chocolate is also very sweet, and a 'sweet tooth' is a habit that can be hard to resist. In fact, the latest research from the Harvard Medical School and the Mount Sinai School of Medicine in the US has isolated a 'sweet tooth' gene called TIR3, meaning that a liking for sweet foods can be inherited.

Chocolate may, however, be something of a false friend. Some research by the charity MIND found that, in the long term, chocolate increases negative emotions, such as depression, because of the feelings of guilt it induces.

So is there a cure for a chocolate 'addiction'? The retraining course in Feature 13 will help to 'cure' a sweet tooth (whether or not it is inherited!). Another trick is to have chocolate as part of a more substantial item, for example, as a chocolate-coated muesli bar. This is because, normally, chocolate slips down so quickly that you can eat far too much before you think you've had enough. Eating it as part of something that needs chewing will slow down the process and help you eat less. Other researchers found that smelling vanilla blunts the need for chocolate – so vanilla perfume or essence may be on your shopping list. It is also important to keep blood-sugar levels even to prevent sweet cravings (see Q143).

There is some good news on chocolate though. Too much of it may not be good for the waistline, at 130 calories for 25g, but it is, in moderation, good for your health. Cocoa beans contain antioxidant plant chemicals called polyphenols that can help to protect against heart disease. The Department of Nutrition at the University of California reported in 2000 that a 40g bar of dark chocolate contains double the antioxidants of red wine. However, milk chocolate contains less of these antioxidants and white chocolate contains none.

Cocoa is also rich in magnesium and iron, two important minerals that may be in shortfall in our diets. Some reports also suggest that the main saturated fat in cocoa butter – stearic acid – is better for you than the type of saturated fat found in meat and cheese, however not all research agrees.

The consensus seems to be that a little bit of very good, dark chocolate as part of an overall healthy diet can fit into the scheme of things even if you are slimming, and may be good for the body – and good for the mind, as long as you never feel guilty afterwards.

See also:

- Questions: 80–81, 89, 119, 133, 138, 143.
- Features: 8, 9, 12, 13.
- A–Z entry: calorie counting.
- Key index entries; carbohydrates, chocolate, fat.

FAT FACT

Researchers in Switzerland have discovered that, by adding small amounts of calcium to chocolate, the calories and fat it contains are not absorbed so well by the body. Volunteers who ate the calcium-rich chocolate also had lower levels of the 'bad' LDL cholesterol in their blood. It seems that the calcium hinders the absorption of the cocoa butter, reducing the overall calorie value of the chocolate by 10%.

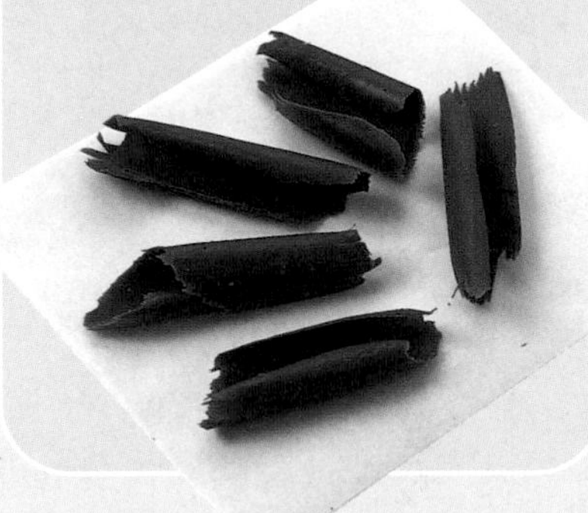

Q 140

I'm a disorganized person who hates to plan ahead – what is the best way to reduce my food intake?

You could try the 'traffic light' system in Q113. This is about as relaxed and informal as slimming can get – but it isn't as scientific as, say, calorie or fat counting, so weight loss, while probable, isn't 100% guaranteed.

You could simply try portion control – give yourself half-portions of your normal food and add extra portions of vegetables, salad and fruit; this works for many people and involves hardly any planning.

However, it's a pity that you don't want to give any time or thought to your diet. If you're overweight, which I assume you are, it is probably this 'mindless' eating that has made you fat. Why not consider putting your body first for a change and feed it more thoughtfully? Section Five is full of ideas for helping you eat better without too much fuss or change of lifestyle.

See also:

- ▶ Questions: 142, 147, 159.
- ▶ Features: 10, 13, 14.
- ▶ Key index entry: healthy eating.

141

I can't seem to turn down food that's offered, or is in my line of vision, even when I'm not hungry – any ideas on changing this inability to say 'no'?

The questionnaire in Feature 12 and the retraining course in Feature 13 could both help you in different ways. Hunger isn't your problem – false 'appetite' is. This need for food is discussed in Qs137 and 138. I believe that you can only cure this urge – which is, basically, habit – to take what's on offer by strongly motivating yourself to say 'no', until finally saying 'no' becomes more of a habit than saying 'yes'.

I devised a system for one of my earlier books (*Slim for Life*) called 'Focus – Decide – Say No'.

- ■ First you learn to focus on what's happening. You're about to grab a biscuit on the way past the biscuit barrel, so now STOP and focus. Talk your way through the moment (under your breath may be best if anyone is about). 'Now why am I heading to grab that biscuit? Am I hungry? Do I need it? Who put that biscuit tin there?' In other words, make your brain aware of the potential calorie disaster presented to you.
- ■ Now decide what to do and give yourself a valid reason. 'I don't want a biscuit. I'm not hungry and I know it contains 80 calories. If I have one, I'll have two or three. Then I'll feel bad. And it's only half an hour until lunch anyway.'
- ■ Say no. Tell yourself loudly and forcibly – 'NO. I am not going to have a biscuit now.' And move away from the situation, distract yourself with something else.

To that – which you do every time you are about to eat something you're not hungry for – I'd add a fourth element.

- ■ Look at ways to stop yourself even being in that situation. To prevent the biscuit incident, literally move the biscuit barrel into a cupboard where it is out of sight and mind or, even better, ditch the biscuit barrel altogether and stop buying biscuits.

There are always ways round 'temptation incidents'. For example, if you are going round to a friend's house for coffee, ask him/her beforehand please not to put out any cake. End of problem. Think of your most frequent tempter times and see if you can think of strategies to defuse them now, so that you don't even have to 'Focus – Decide – Say No'.

In the long term, realize that we aren't living in times of famine and that you don't have to 'stock up' calorie supplies in case you don't get anything to eat for ages. Researchers in the US say that obese Americans (a large percentage of their population) panic unless they are within sight of a food source because of this ancient urge to eat while the going's good.

See also:

- ▶ Questions: 137–8.
- ▶ Features: 12, 13.

Q 142

All my life I've existed on a diet of mostly junk food. How can I make the changes necessary to slim – and stick to them?

I think you should make changes gradually – the retraining course in Feature 13 will help you – all the while concentrating on foods and meals that you CAN have and that you DO like, rather than fretting about what you CAN'T have and DON'T like. Even the most die-hard junk-food fan can find some foods that he/she likes which are healthy and non-fattening as part of a varied diet.

Here are a few of the foods you can include on a slimming and maintenance diet without any trouble: bread, potatoes, pasta, rice, noodles, baked beans, breakfast cereals, strawberries, bananas, steak, chicken, lamb, curries, burgers and other takeaways/fast food. These are just some of the foods some people think they can't eat when slimming, but they're all good foods that contribute to a healthy slimming diet.

You'll find more help and ideas for eating all these foods elsewhere in the book – check the cross-reference list below. Hopefully you will gradually realize, as many people before you have, that there is plenty of enjoyment in food to be had even when you are losing weight, and that you don't have to abandon the familiar. Slimming isn't all lentils and crispbreads.

See also:

- ▶ Questions: 79–90, 94, 102–4, 112–3, 118–22, 129.
- ▶ Features: 10, 11, 13, 15.
- ▶ Key index entries: calorie counting, healthy eating.

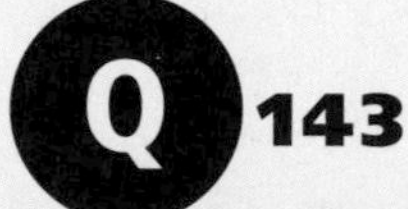

143

I can easily go all day with virtually no food, but in the evening, especially in winter, I crave food – mostly sweet snacks – and can't stop. What am I doing wrong?

You are starving your body all day, which is causing low blood sugar and very natural hunger pangs/cravings for fixes of food that will quickly raise your blood sugar – sweet foods. In winter you may also be suffering from seasonal affective disorder, which is a form of mild-to-moderate depression, and can be alleviated by starchy and sweet foods that increase the production of serotonin, the mood-enhancing chemical, in the brain.

The trouble is, if you binge on sweet food on an empty stomach, insulin is released in large amounts by the pancreas to deal with the sudden influx of sugar, which floods the system and causes the blood-sugar levels to dip too low again – so you eat more sugary foods, and so on. Here is what you must do:

- Eat regularly during the day – small, healthy meals low in sugar and including foods high on the Glycaemic Index (see Q84). Make sure to have such a snack just before you leave work (if you work).
- At home, have your evening meal fairly early and have a selection of nibbles ready-prepared by your side – try crudités or a dark rye crispbread with a little Marmite on top, for example – to keep you going while you prepare the meal.
- Try to find things to do in the evenings that you will enjoy and will keep you from feeling bored/lonely.
- When you do have something sweet to eat, eat it as part of a meal and not on its own.

There really is no point in trying to diet by avoiding food all day. It's one of the worst ways, for most people. If your cravings aren't curbed by the plan outlined above, read the answer to Q132.

See also:

- Questions: 77, 81, 84–5, 95, 97, 103, 132, 134, 139.
- Features: 12, 13.
- A-Z entries: Glycaemic Index diets, Sugar Busters.
- Key index entries: chocolate, Glycaemic Index, healthy eating, sweet tooth.

Q 144

I am overweight, but I'm also a feminist – and it's well documented that dieting is a form of female submission, isn't it?

Ever since the publication of *Fat is a Feminist Issue* there have been authors and journalists who have decried the idea that women have to be slim, and have put forward all kinds of theories as to why being slim – or trying to lose weight – is against feminist principles. Typical protests are: 'Why should we fit into an ideal that men want us to look like?'... 'If we slim down thin enough we literally almost "disappear" – it's like you're apologizing for taking up space.'... 'Thinness is weakness, not strength – so we can be dominated.'

However, I believe that most feminists would say that their mantra is that women should make their own decisions and be true to themselves; they should be able and willing to look after themselves and to put themselves first or at least equal-first. I am also quite sure that any sensible feminist would agree that the body – male or female – is a precious tool to be looked after well, because without a strong, fit, healthy body you have lost half your natural assets, and maintaining your body at a reasonable weight is, I would have thought, one of the major self-help ways to stay healthy. Therefore, I believe that sensible concern with your size concurs with the feminist beliefs, rather than conflicting with them.

A read of Feature 25 will show you all the links that overweight and obesity have with ill-health. If you are genuinely overweight (and it is easy to check using Feature 3), then any colleague, sister, friend or partner who discourages you from losing the stones on the grounds of political correctness is giving potentially dangerous advice and should, I think, be ignored.

There is no political mileage, or personal happiness, to be gained by staying fat if you'd rather be slimmer. However, any weight problem needs to be tackled in a sensible way. 'Diets' and 'dieting' have understandably developed a bad name over the past decade or two because of the number of people (mostly women) who diet to stick-thinness, who 'yo-yo diet', and who spend much of their lives ruled by food or dominated by their own need to control food. Indeed, argue feminists understandably, why replace one set of chains with another?

Your answer is to lose weight with a combination of moderate calorie reduction (perhaps a reduced-fat, high-carb diet like the blueprint in Feature 9 would suit you), coupled with an exercise regime to strengthen your muscles and get you fit, until you reach a sensible BMI, at which point you should feel psychologically and physically on top form. Such a regime can be classified as 'looking after yourself' rather than 'dieting', which is, after all, rather a passé expression nowadays. Any desire to do things in a different, more drastic way isn't a good idea and the underlying reasons and problems need to be addressed.

Women's, admittedly sometimes tricky, relationship with food and slimming is discussed in more detail in Qs149–58 and in Section Six.

See also:

- Questions: 26, 28, 35, 65, 103, 112, 127, 149–58, 198–203.
- Features: 3, 6, 7, 9.
- A–Z entry: low-fat diets.
- Key index entries: healthy eating, weight and health.

Are you a food 'addict'?

Although food isn't clinically addictive, like tobacco or alcohol, it certainly can seem that way if you want to slim down but can't stop yourself eating. This questionnaire will help you decide how much of a 'food addict' you are, and offers guidance, depending on your results.

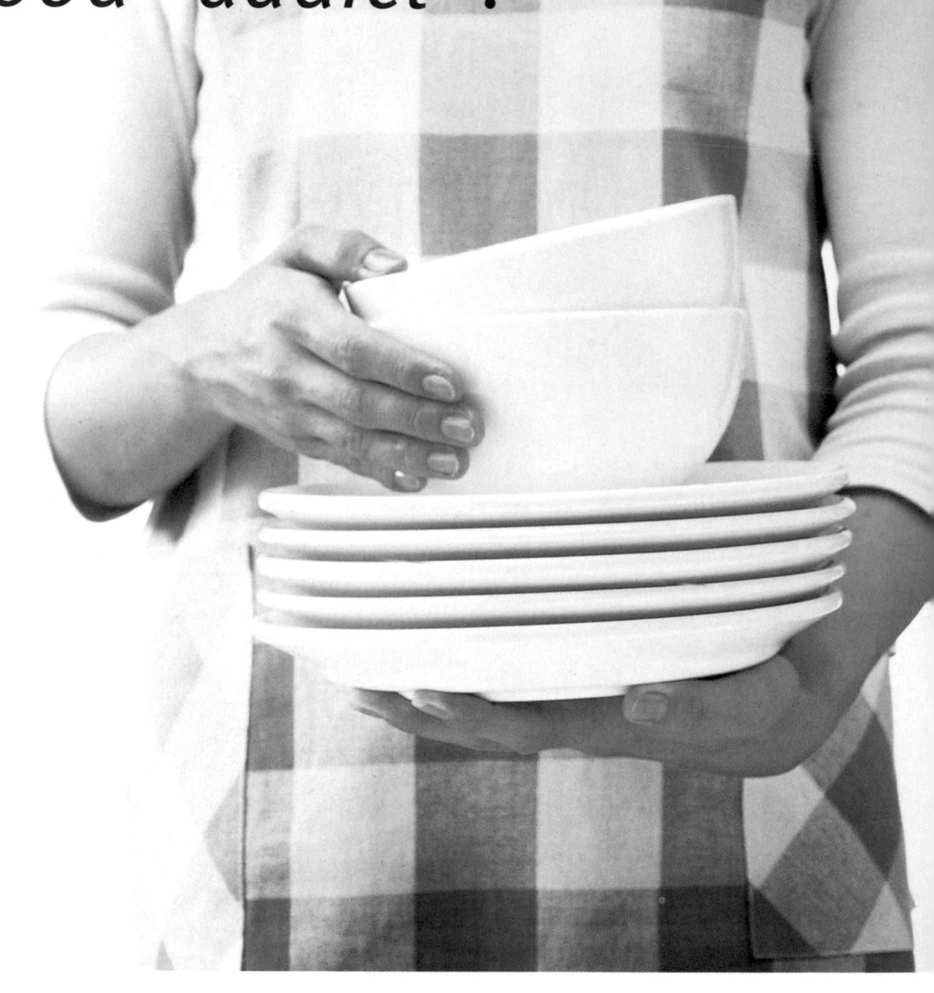

1 Which is the sort of food experience that you really enjoy most?
a A big box of assorted wrapped chocolates in front of the TV.
b A treat visit to the local steak bar.
c A luxury meal at the new trendy TV chef's restaurant.

2 How would you describe the way you eat most frequently, if left to your own choice?
a Any time, anywhere, when the mood takes me.
b A big blow-out to fill up my belly.
c Regular carefully planned meals.

3 What is your favourite type of food?
a Chocolate, sweets, bread, cake, biscuits, desserts.
b Nursery food, roasts, curries, cottage pie, puddings.
c Mediterranean, Moroccan, Californian, Thai.

4 When you have just finished an eating session, how are you most likely to feel?
a Guilty and depressed.
b Full up and comatose.
c Satisfied and happy.

5 What is your attitude to eating a prepacked convenience meal, such as a frozen lasagne?
a Fine, I eat them often.
b Not enough in them for my appetite.
c Would prefer not to eat that sort of food.

6 Which most closely describes your attitude to preparing meals?
a I tend to spend as little time as possible preparing food.
b I'd really rather someone else cooked the food.
c I really enjoy cooking.

7 If someone gave you a boxed cake from the bakery, how would you be most likely to eat it?
a Non-stop, very quickly, straight from the box the minute the giver has gone.
b Save it for teatime and have a good big slice.
c Slowly and carefully, on fine bone china, savouring every mouthful.

8 Do you ever eat walking along the street?
a Yes, often.
b Sometimes.
c Never.

9 When you go on holiday, which of these most sums up your ideal food?
a Street snacks, pub food, bar food, sweet treats.
b Places that serve food similar to what I eat at home; hotel food.
c Michelin-starred, or non-touristy places where I can eat authentic local cuisine.

10 If you shop for the weekly food, which things are you most likely to go for?
a Quick, easy, filling, low-cost.
b Repeat of last week's shop, more or less.
c Anything that looks new and interesting.

11 How often do you find yourself buying food when you hadn't planned to (e.g. at a garage or newsagent)?
a All the time.
b Sometimes.
c Hardly ever.

12 When you buy a 'treat' food, in what way will you be most likely to eat it?
a Alone – I want it all for myself.
b As a reward for a task well done.
c With spouse or friends and a decent bottle of wine.

CHECK YOUR RESULTS

MOSTLY As:
You probably are 'addicted to food', in as much as you are highly dependent upon it as a substitute for emotional fulfilment. You probably have a sweet, or 'fatty', tooth and may be a borderline compulsive eater. You have a love-hate relationship with food and are probably quite overweight.

Likely dieting problems:
Cutting down on food may leave you feeling bereft, so you need to sort out your problems in parallel with your diet.

Best advice
Seek help via counselling or an eating disorders group. The retraining programme in Feature 13 may help you. Also read Qs132–5 and 143.

MOSTLY Bs:
You are not addicted to food as such, but you are a lover of food as fuel, with a strong traditional streak. You are frightened of feeling hungry and enjoy 'a full stomach'. Your diet has probably been very high in fat – and therefore calories – and you are probably overweight.

Likely dieting problem:
you are frightened of going 'on a diet' as you think you will feel hungry and miserable.

Best advice:
Follow all the tips in this book to cut calories and fat without stinting on bulk and satiety value. See Qs23, 35, 85, 87, 112–3, and Features 8, 10, 15.

MOSTLY Cs:
You are a foodie, not a food addict. You really adore food and it probably figures a great deal in your everyday life, but you are in control. You love taste, texture, novelty. If you are overweight, you will probably just need to make some minor adjustments to your diet.

Likely dieting problem:
Getting enough flavour and excitement in a diet. Taken to extremes, your attitude may also border on obsessive. Many anorexics take obsessive interest in choosing and preparing food for others.

Best advice:
This book is full of ways to eat enjoyably and healthily. See Qs 129,131 and Features 3, 9, 11.

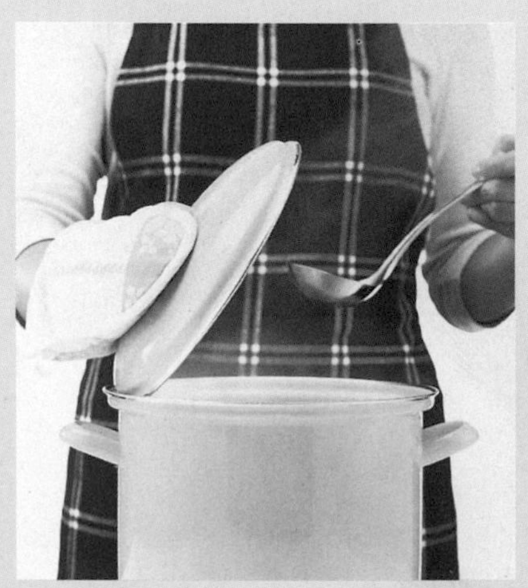

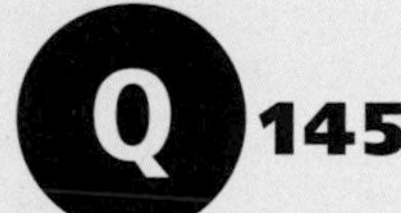

Q 145

Is there an organization like Alcoholics Anonymous for overweight people with eating problems?

The best-known one is Overeaters Anonymous, which is the ultimate self-help organization for food addicts, and has branches all over the country. They say, 'Our primary purpose is to abstain from compulsive overeating and carry the message of recovery to those who still suffer.' Telephone 07626 984674 (South-East England) or 07000 784985 (rest of UK) for more information – and check out the A–Z section for more information on what OA meetings may do for you.

Designated websites and chatrooms on the Internet also offer a similar type of service. See Internet slimming in the A–Z.

See also:

- Questions: 146–158.
- Features: 12, 13.
- A–Z entries: Overeaters Anonymous, Internet slimming.
- Key index entries: bingeing, eating disorders, psychological aspects of weight control.

Q 146

Are there any alternative remedies or natural treatments for overeating?

If by that you are asking whether you can lose weight without dieting but by taking natural herbs or going to a therapist to shed the pounds, the answer is basically no. To shed weight you need to create a calorie deficit in your body (see Q18) so that your surplus fat is burnt up for energy.

However, there are therapies and treatments which may help the process. Counselling to relieve stress, anxiety or depression may all help by getting to the root causes of why you overeat and/or your dependence on food, so counselling is probably one of the more sensible routes to take if you feel your overeating is a result of psychological problems.

There is anecdotal evidence that acupuncture and hypnosis may help strengthen a slimming campaign and other treatments that may be of peripheral help include massage and aromatherapy, by relaxing and creating a sense of self-worth. Yoga and other exercise classes may also help by improving body image and resolve. Eating under Ayurvedic principles, following a kapha-pacifying diet, may help you shed weight. A good starting point is *The Book of Ayurveda* (Gaia) by Judith Morrison.

Certain combinations of Chinese herbs may help boost the weight-loss process by speeding up the metabolism or blunting the appetite. You can also get slimming patches impregnated with scents, such as vanilla, which again seem to help blunt the appetite for some. Many of these ideas and more are discussed in the A–Z section.

See also:

- Questions: 145, 147–8.
- A–Z entries: acupuncture, counselling, diet aromas, health farms, herbal diet supplements, hypnosis, massage, yoga.

Q 147

Are there slimming equivalents of life coaches to help on a one-to-one basis?

Yes, you can take your pick from personal nutritionists who will help you to lose weight from Internet diet coaches, postal diet coaches, telephone diet coaches and so on. These are discussed in more detail in the A–Z, but the main thing to do is check out people's credentials before parting with your money, as many of these 'experts' have very little experience or expertise. Any of the top national slimming clubs may offer you more expertise and motivational help than many of these one-to-one experts.

See also:

- Questions: 123, 145.
- Features: 12, 13.
- A–Z entries: diet coaches, Internet slimming, slimming clubs.

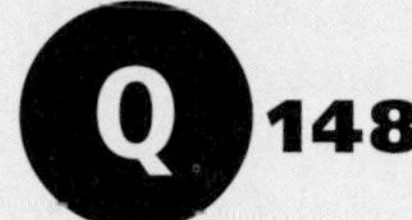

Q 148

Can you recommend any books to help me lose weight and keep it off for the rest of my life?

Hopefully, this book you are reading now will help you to do that, but if you need extra help there is a short reading list at the back of the book, divided into psychological help, practical help and low-fat healthy cooking.

See also:

- Key index entries: book list, slimming, weight loss.

Q 149

What are eating disorders, who gets them and why?

The main eating disorders are anorexia nervosa, bulimia nervosa and binge eating disorder. Anorexia is when the person restricts the amount he or she eats and drinks way below that recommended for a normal weight-loss diet, on a long-term basis. Bulimia is when the person purges – vomiting and/or taking laxatives, to keep their weight under control, often following bouts of bingeing and possibly starving. Binge eating disorder is long-term bouts of bingeing without purging (see Q132).

People who develop anorexia tend to rely on controlling food intake as a way of expressing psychological problems and/or of coping with emotional difficulties in their lives. Bulimia may develop in someone who has been anorexic and may be triggered by stress.

Anyone can get an eating disorder. There are an estimated 1.1 million sufferers in the UK. Although the most common age is between 15 and 25, and there are ten female sufferers for every man, both sexes of any age can be sufferers. It is possible that genetic make-up may influence the chances of getting eating disorders – anorexia is eight times more likely in people with a close relative who also has anorexia, and recent research has pinpointed a gene involved in appetite control which is more frequently present in anorexics. This gene may cause the brain's food-intake mechanisms to go haywire. Also, people who are under strong social, parental or academic pressures may be more at risk, when the focus may shift from such pressures to food.

Major upsets in life – e.g. a divorce in the family, exams looming, a bereavement – can trigger an eating disorder. However, anorexia can develop because of a desire to lose weight, when normal dieting habits (a sensible reduced-calorie diet) become exaggerated or distorted, and bulimia can develop as a way to eat without getting fat, therefore the pressure to be 'thin' is a risk factor.

The UK Eating Disorders Association says that eating disorders are complex illnesses in which eating or not eating is used to block out painful feelings. There is evidence that eating disorders are 'chosen' by some and the EDA says that treatment may not always be effective if the sufferer has mixed feelings about 'giving up' their illness. However, without appropriate treatment, the problems may persist throughout life. Anyone with a suspected eating disorder should see their doctor.

These days treatment concentrates as much, or more, on discovering and eliminating the psychological and other problems of anorexics as it does on aggressive re-feeding and target weights.

The following organizations can be contacted for help in the UK:

- Eating Disorders Association, telephone helpline 01603 621414 (weekdays 9am–6.30pm). Recorded information service 0906 3020012. Website www.edauk.com
- The National Centre for Eating Disorders, tel 01372 469493, www.eating-disorders.org.uk
- Overeaters Anonymous, tel 07000 784985 or 07626 984674 (South East and London), www.overeatersanonymous.org.
- National Self-harm Network tel 020 79165472.
- Samaritans Helpline 0345 909090.

See also:

- ▶ Questions: 132, 150–58.
- ▶ Feature: 12.
- ▶ A–Z entries: laxatives, Overeaters Anonymous, counselling.
- ▶ Key index entries: anorexia, bingeing, bulimia, crash dieting, starving, yo-yo dieting.

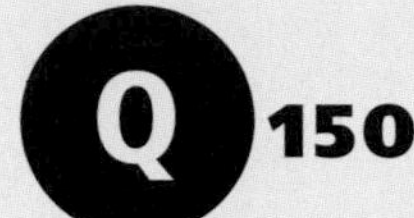

Q 150

What are the health problems associated with eating disorders?

Long-term effects of anorexia include disruption/delay of puberty in girls, disruption/cessation of menstruation, inability to conceive, chemical imbalances in the blood, loss of bone density, loss of lean tissue (leading to weakness), major nutritional deficiencies, inability to keep warm, exhaustion, tiredness and psychological problems. If treatment is successful, the body can make good recovery, but unchecked it can result in chronic heart failure and death.

The effects of bulimia may include psychological problems, major nutritional deficiencies, erosion of tooth enamel, dehydration, stomach rupture, bleeding of oesophagus, choking and irregular heart rhythms, which could cause sudden death.

People with binge eating disorder are often severely overweight with all the problems that can bring (see Feature 25).

See also:

- ▶ Questions: 132, 149, 151–58.
- ▶ Feature: 25.
- ▶ Key index entries: eating disorders, weight and health.

THE SCOFF ASSESSMENT

Eating disorder specialists use the 'SCOFF' five-point questionnaire to help diagnose people with anorexia or bulimia. The five questions are:

- Do you make yourself Sick because you feel uncomfortably full?
- Do you worry you have lost Control over how much you eat?
- Have you recently lost more than One stone in a 3-month period?
- Do you believe yourself to be Fat when others say you are too thin?
- Would you say that Food dominates your life?

If you can answer 'yes' to two or more of these questions, a likely case of anorexia or bulimia is indicated and you should seek help.

4-week retraining course

If you think you will never manage to get a taste for healthier eating or be able to control your cravings for food, this is the course to help you retrain your taste buds and your mind. In 4 weeks you can achieve a great deal.

Week 1

Days 1–3

■ Start by keeping a 3-day food diary recording all you eat and drink. Using a red pen, circle everything that you think contains high levels of either fat (e.g. fried foods, pastry, Cheddar, fatty meat, chips), sugar (e.g. confectionery, cakes, biscuits, sweet drinks) or salt (see the box below). Now, using a blue pen, circle all the following – fresh vegetables, fresh fruit, fish, game and poultry, pulses, whole grains and whole-grain products (e.g. pasta, bread). Over the weeks we will aim to decrease the red circles and increase the blue circles. (Items not circled are 'neutral'.)

Day 4

■ Go shopping and aim to shop to increase the blue and decrease the red circles by next week. Here are some swaps you might make:

Swap	For
Shoulder of lamb	Lamb fillet
Duck	Turkey
Chips	New potatoes
Cheddar	Brie
Chocolate cake	Malt loaf
Cheesecake	Fruit yoghurt
Fruit pie	Fresh fruit
Salted nuts	Fresh nuts in shell

■ Read through this book for meal and menu ideas and write down some ideas that appeal.

Days 5–7

■ Aim to eat more fruit and vegetables this week – if you've been eating little, go for 1-2 portions of fruit a day and 1 portion of fresh vegetables or salad. Eat them raw, boiled, steamed, baked, microwaved, casseroled or, if you like, made into a soup or a fruit smoothie.

Week 2

Day 1

■ Start a new food diary for the week.

Days 1–7

■ Aim to reduce the amount of sugar you have in your diet (see box opposite).

- Cut down the amount you use in hot drinks by a third on Day 1, and again, on Day 5 cut a few more grains, so by Day 7 you're having half what you were last week.
- Avoid all sweet fizzy drinks, including 'diet' drinks, and use sparkling mineral water or speciality teas.
- Try to swap very sweet foods for less sweet foods (e.g. malt loaf instead of cake, fruit yoghurt instead of tiramisu).
- Once or twice this week, have fresh fruit for dessert.
- Cut down the amount of sugar you sprinkle over foods, e.g. breakfast cereals, by a half.
- Use reduced-sugar jams and marmalades.
- You can use alternative natural sweeteners for stewed fruit (the herb sweet cicely is good and so is cinnamon).
- Try to make your breakfasts more healthy generally – swap sugary cereals for non-sugared ones and add flavour with chopped dried apricots or fresh fruit. Use whole-grain breads instead of white bread and use low-fat spread instead of butter. Use natural yoghurt instead of sweetened yoghurt.

Mindtest

Think you haven't time to pay attention to your diet or learn new cooking habits? Tick off all the things on the following list that you do regularly:

■ Vacuum your home
■ Mow the lawn
■ Clean the car
■ Ironing
■ Get your hair cut
■ Washing

Did you tick any? If you did, that means you are prioritizing your home and chores ahead of your body. Think again –

FOODS HIGH IN SALT

Salt, most stock cubes, salted and cured meats, packet soups and sauce mixes, crisps, salted nuts, pretzels, ketchups and sauces, processed cheese, hard cheese, butter and spreads.

which is REALLY most important?

■ Aim for 2 portions of fruit and 2 of vegetables each day this week.

Day 7

■ Go through your diary with your two pens and see if there is improvement from last week.

Week 3

■ Keep your diary all week.

■ Aim to reduce salt in your diet – this will give your taste buds the chance to get used to cleaner, fresher flavours (see the list of foods high in salt opposite). Two easy ways are to stop using salt at the table and to halve the salt you add to cooked dishes. A third important way is to stop buying high-salt snacks and packet foods. Look for 'low-salt' labels when buying. Add some fresh or dried herbs and spices to your food for seasoning instead of salt.

■ Aim to reduce sugar intake a bit more – down to one-quarter of your usual quantities in drinks and for sprinkling and in cooking.

Days 4–7

■ Think about reducing the fat in your diet – you will have already done this somewhat by following the plan to date, but now consider more swaps in your daily diet.

Swap	For
Pork pie	Cold cooked low-fat sausages
Meat casserole	Meat and pulse casserole
Double cream	Half-fat crème fraîche or Greek yoghurt
Cream cheese	Ricotta or fromage frais

Think of some more swaps yourself, using the Food Value Charts at the back of the book if necessary.

■ Get your portions of fresh fruit and veg up to 5 a day. Try having fruit or crudités instead of high-fat, high-salt between-meal snacks.

■ Look at your lunches. Swap high-fat items in sandwiches for lower-fat ones; swap high-fat cheese on toast for lower-fat baked beans on toast; swap high-fat baked potato toppings (e.g. cheese, butter) for lower-fat ones (e.g. baked beans, chilli, fromage frais). Swap creamed soups for vegetable and pulse soups and mayonnaise salads for salads dressed in balsamic vinegar, lemon juice, and just a dash of olive oil.

Day 7

Mindtest

Get in tune with your hunger – learn to spot real hunger from fake hunger (see Qs 137 and 138 for advice). Start underlining in your food diary any snack or meal occasion when you ate without feeling hungry. (Write down your reasons for eating in that case, and think of ways you might avoid doing the same next time.)

Do this: At lunchtime, serve yourself a healthy salad and see how long you can take to eat it – try for about 20 minutes. Take small amounts on your fork, chew them slowly and thoroughly and savour what you are eating. In future, try to eat slowly all the time – and stop eating when you are full.

■ Go through your diary as before.

Week 4

■ Keep your diary all this week.

■ Take your hot drinks without sugar and don't sprinkle sugar on foods.

■ Continue to make swaps to reduce the fat, sugar and salt content of items in your diet.

■ Aim for 6 portions of fruit and vegetables a day.

■ When you go shopping this week, aim to buy several items that are new to you – e.g. exotic vegetables, a new type of pulse, a dark rye bread instead of wheat, a pack of Quorn instead of meat, a pheasant instead of a pork joint, a new type of fish instead of haddock – and so on. Choose things you like the look of and try them.

Day 7

Mindtest

Aim to make all your meals at home look lovely, and try to go for good aromas, too. Cut things up, arrange the plate nicely, use fresh herbs and colourful vegetables.

Now prove to yourself that you can eat well and eat plenty on a reduced-calorie diet. See how much food you can put on your plate for 250 calories (about the same calories as you'd have got in a small chocolate bar). (Use the Food Value Charts at the back of the book to help you). Here is my idea:

1 x 100g (3½ oz) can of tuna in spring water, flaked (110 calories) and served with 25g (¾ oz) cannellini beans (cooked weight, 30 calories), I medium ripe tomato, sliced (15 calories), some red onion rings (10 calories) with balsamic spray dressing (2 calories), a fresh mixed herb salad (50g – 8 calories), some cucumber batons (2 calories) and 25g (¾oz) slice of dark rye bread spread with 5g (⅓oz) low-fat spread (70 calories).

Finish

■ Do the red and blue pen test with this week's food diary. Compare the results with those from Week 1.

■ Remember, your taste for food is coloured mainly by habit and can easily be altered permanently if you have the right, positive mindset.

■ Continue with the good work and look forward to a slimmer and healthier you.

FOODS HIGH IN SUGAR

Sugar, honey, confectionery, syrup, jam, sweet drinks, cakes, biscuits, many desserts, custard, sweet pastries and pies, ice-cream, sugared breakfast cereals – also baked beans and tomato ketchup!

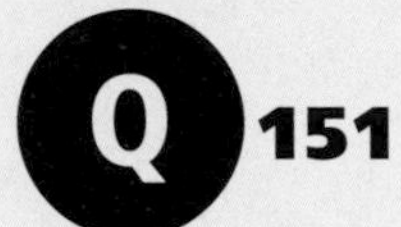

151

What are the signs of someone having anorexia and how can it be treated?

Anorexics lose weight as they reduce calorie intake, often to starvation levels. It may begin slowly – with something like a normal low-calorie diet, or they may claim food intolerances or allergies.

Eventually weight loss can be extreme, but they may try to hide this with baggy clothes and lots of layers – which also help protect them from the cold, felt because there is no fat layer. Other symptoms are constipation and stomach pains, dizzy spells, fainting, swollen stomach, face and ankles, downy hair on the body, dry or discoloured skin, loss of periods. Anorexics often enjoy long hard bouts of exercise.

Psychological symptoms may include an extreme fear of gaining weight, a feeling that they look fat not thin, mood swings and personality changes, eating rituals and enjoyment in preparing food for others, lying about what food they have eaten, reluctance to eat with others, and secrecy.

A fairly new phenomenon, a 'cousin' or 'branch' of anorexia, which has been noticed and termed 'orthorexia' by American doctor Steve Bratman, is an obsession with 'health' foods and avoiding anything that isn't pure or wholesome. An orthorexic person can become as dangerously thin as if they had anorexia.

The EDA and NCfED offer help/advice for those who think a dependant may have an eating disorder (see Q149), or the sufferer and/or the family should see a GP. The SCOFF questionnaire (page 103) may help diagnosis. It's very hard for an anorexic to self-treat (they often don't agree there is a problem) and almost equally hard for a family to help on their own.

See also:

▶ Questions: 149, 150, 152–8.

▶ A–Z entry: counselling.

152

Will rigorous dieting make me likely to suffer from anorexia?

It's possible, especially if you have any other 'risk factors' outlined in Q149. Rigorous (i.e. crash) dieting – especially with long lists of forbidden foods, or rules – makes you think constantly about your diet and can make you crave forbidden foods more, or more 'frightened' of food.

Experts tend not to think that anorexia is always, or even mostly, caused by dieting alone, because very many people lose weight without becoming anorexic, and many anorexics become so without having started off with a perceived weight problem. Certainly, some cases do begin by people simply wanting to lose weight, and taking it too far, so it is best to tackle any weight-loss programme sensibly and slowly on healthy food, as outlined in this book. The ability to know when to stop is inbuilt in most people – anorexics lose this ability.

See also:

▶ Questions: 105–6, 108, 149–51, 153–8.

▶ Features: 3, 9.

▶ Key index entries: Body Mass Index, healthy eating, slimming.

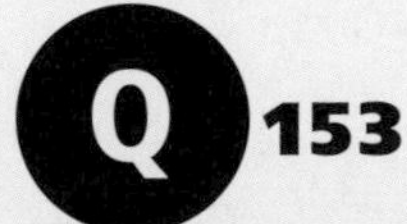

153

People tell me I'm too thin (8 stone and 5ft 7in) but I feel fat. Should I continue dieting?

You are definitely underweight because your BMI is only just over 18. A healthy BMI is between 18.5 and 25. There is no need for you to diet any more and indeed, further dieting could be dangerous. It would be a good idea if you contact the Eating Disorders Association or the National Centre for Eating Disorders (details at the end of the answer to Q149), or visit your doctor, as a feeling of 'fatness' when you are obviously not fat is one of the signs of anorexia.

See also:

▶ Questions: 149–52, 154–8.
Feature: 3.

▶ Key index entries: Body Mass Index, eating disorders, healthy eating, ideal weight.

154

I make myself sick occasionally after I've eaten, to help keep weight down, but I don't feel ill or that I have an eating disorder. Is this OK?

You are bulimic. There are different 'degrees' of bulimia and perhaps you are not as 'at risk' as someone who vomits or purges several times a day – but, without treatment, your occasional bouts of vomiting could easily get more frequent.

I suggest you contact one of the eating disorders centres listed in Q149 for help, as the earlier bulimia is treated the more chance you have of full recovery. If you are not convinced that 'mild' bulimia is a problem – read Qs 149–53 and 155–8.

See also:

▶ Questions: 149–53, 155–8.

▶ Key index entry: eating disorders.

155

How does one recognize someone who has bulimia, why do they do this to themselves, and what should I do about it?

Bulimia nervosa means 'the hunger of an ox' and the Eating Disorders Association says that the hunger is an emotional need that can't be satisfied by food alone. Bulimia is harder to recognize than anorexia, as sufferers are often of normal weight. The SCOFF questionnaire on page 103 may help a diagnosis to be made.

A typical bulimic pattern is to binge on huge quantities of food in a short space of time, and then to purge via vomiting and/or laxatives, and perhaps vigorous exercise. This means that the calories in the food aren't absorbed and the bulimic doesn't gain weight. Sometimes bulimics also alternate periods of bingeing and purging with periods of starving. Many hate themselves and fear the 'vicious circle' of bingeing and purging that they can't seem to escape. Yet other bulimics use vomiting as what they see as a reasonable habit to control weight, no more socially unacceptable than smoking.

Often bulimia goes undetected for years. Bulimics may also appear to the outside world, and even to their closest families and friends, to be well adjusted and in control, successful and confident. However, they are often chronically lacking in self-confidence, with poor body image and emotional and psychological problems.

The most likely age to develop bulimia is between 18 and 30, and some sufferers may have had, or go on to have, anorexia. Some signs of bulimia to look out for are: fluctuating weight, disappearing to the bathroom after meals; poor skin, sore throat and hoarse voice, tooth decay (especially the teeth at the front of the mouth); general lethargy and periods of exhaustion, and sometimes periods of manic exercise. If you live with a bulimic, you may also notice food disappearing, money disappearing, empty laxative and/or diuretic packs, empty food packs in the bin, secrecy and a reluctance to enjoy social meals. Another problem with spotting bulimia in someone is that bulimics often go for months without purging. Others do it only at certain times of day.

The reason why people become bulimic is not straightforward, as there may be many factors at work and there is great variation between cases – which is why it may be difficult to spot and treat.

If you know someone with bulimia, your best course of action is probably to contact one of the eating disorder centres listed in the answer to Q149 for advice or persuade the sufferer to visit their GP; however, the sufferer has to want to be treated and, of course, has to admit to the problem (many bulimics feel ashamed and won't admit to purging). As the Eating Disorders Association says, 'Recovery is not easy but is certainly possible.' In four out of five cases the frequency of the bouts of bingeing is reduced by therapy. Therapy can involve self-help groups, counselling, support groups, nutritional advice and more, including, possibly, medication.

See also:

- ▶ Questions: 149–54, 156–8.
- ▶ A–Z entry: counselling.

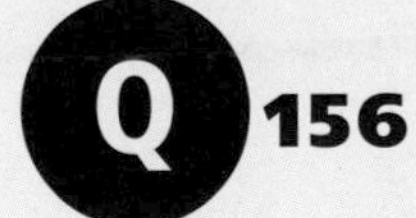

Q 156

I can normally control my food intake, but some nights I can eat huge amounts of food, like 5 packs of biscuits or 3 whole cakes. What eating disorder do I have?

If you don't purge yourself through vomiting, laxatives, etc. you seem to be a compulsive eater, with what is now called Binge Eating Disorder. This is discussed in more detail in Q132. The main symptom is weight gain, and I strongly recommend that you do seek help for your problem as soon as possible.

See also:

- ▶ Questions: 132, 149, 155.
- ▶ Features: 12, 13.
- ▶ Key index entries: eating disorders, overeating, weight control.

Q 157

At what age do anorexia and bulimia stop?

Sadly, they can begin at any age and sufferers may continue to have these illnesses throughout their lives. A considerable number of women begin to be anorexic or bulimic in their 40s, and this may coincide with 'empty nest syndrome', menopause, divorce or other mid-life problems. Chances of overcoming eating disorders are greatly increased with professional help and treatment, and with a supportive circle of friends and/or family.

See also:

- ▶ Questions: 132, 149–56, 158.
- ▶ Key index entry: eating disorders.

Q 158

Is 'night bingeing' an eating disorder?

'Night eating syndrome' is an eating/sleeping disorder recently studied in the *Journal of the American Medical Association* but first noticed by doctors in the Fifties. Its symptoms are waking with uncontrollable feelings of hunger and cravings for carbohydrates during the night, and lack of hunger in the mornings.

Estimates are that up to a quarter of obese people may suffer from night eating syndrome and 1.5% of the UK population is affected. At the moment, there is no universal cure, although sufferers may benefit from counselling. Stress and a hectic lifestyle may make the problem worse. The eating disorder associations as listed in Q 149 are a useful start point.

See also:

- ▶ Questions: 132–4, 143, 149, 160.
- ▶ Key index entries: carbohydrates, stress.

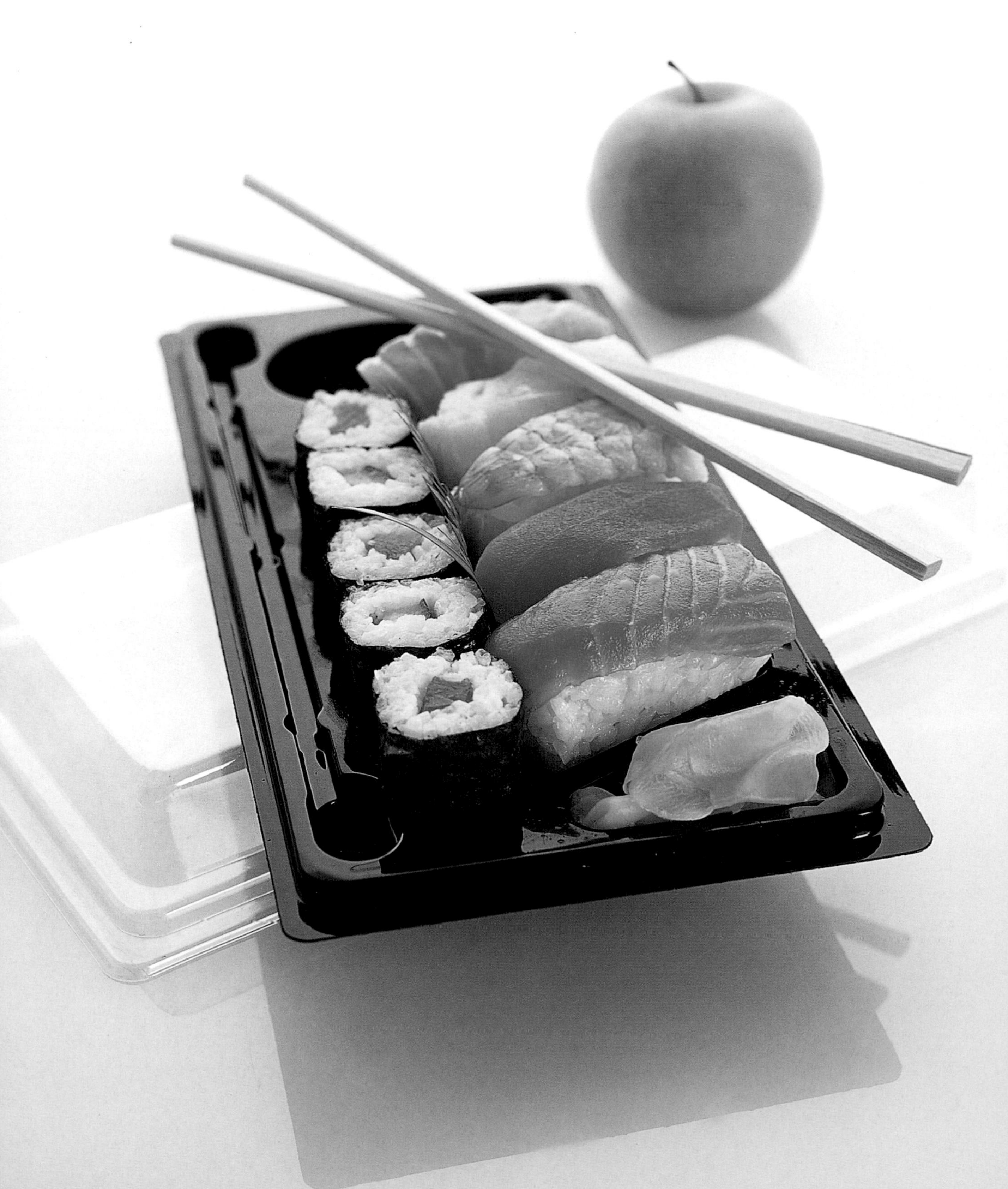

Section Five

Your diet, your lifestyle

You want to stay slim; you want to lose weight – but healthy, non-fattening food just doesn't seem to fit in with your lifestyle.

Many of us are too busy, rushed and stressed to want to pay attention to diet or cooking. Some of us are always in a car, or on a plane or train, finding little other than 'junk' food available. Business entertaining may be called for, adding yet more unwanted pounds. When we do have time to relax – on holiday, in bars and restaurants, seeing friends – the pressure's on to eat, and to drink alcohol.

Those who are responsible for cooking for children or their spouse have their own problems and temptations – and for others, finances seem to pre-empt starting that diet.

We work hard and play hard – yet when it comes to food, we are ambivalent. We like the idea of spending time on our food, but not the reality. We watch TV chefs for entertainment, not to follow the recipes. We buy cookery books to adorn our kitchens but – statistics show – rarely sit down to a proper family meal any more.

In this section I hope to help you unravel some of these strands with coherent solutions.

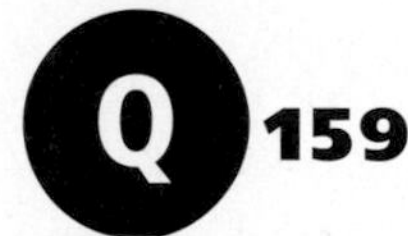

Q 159

How can I lose weight if I'm too busy to diet – I freelance from home and hardly have time to sleep?

Fact one: all eating takes a certain amount of time – whether it is 'fattening' food or 'slimming' food. If you are overweight, I expect you have been finding time to eat, even though you're very busy. Fact two: high-fat, high-sugar snacks, such as chocolate and cakes, are easier and quicker to eat than items such as fresh fruit or whole grains, even though they contain many more calories. So, I guess you have been 'filling up' on the quick-and-easy items that are the 'fattening' ones, and ignoring the healthier items.

If you want to lose weight it isn't necessary to spend a lot of time and effort on buying and eating a special or complicated diet. You just need to replace the high-fat and/or high-sugar, highly refined calorific foods with different, equally easy, ones that will fill you up for fewer calories but won't take more than an extra few minutes to eat.

You can eat ready-prepared main meal salads (which come complete with fork), ready-to-eat chilled soups, ready-in-an-instant pasta with ready-made tomato or vegetable toppings, ready-washed and -trimmed green salads, ready-cooked chilled chicken, ready-cooked prawns, decent bread... I could go on. For snacks, you can eat bananas, apples, nectarines. A read through the rest of this section will give you hundreds of ideas for reduced-calorie eating.

What you need to do is a one-off research session, to see what you can get without spending a lot of time shopping ... supermarkets on the Internet... home box schemes... local delivery services... and to make a long list of quick and easy foods that you will enjoy without having to cook. A once-weekly, 10-minute session should then be all you need to get the week's food organized. If you really do want to lose weight, you can find this time. And if you really can't, I think you should do some serious rethinking about your priorities – the health of your body should be number one.

Which brings me on to the last point – it IS worth spending a few more minutes actually eating your food, as all research shows that food eaten at a slower pace satisfies you more for less calories. And it IS worth trying to eat healthily as, again, research shows that people's bodies AND brains work better when they are getting all the nutrients they need for health. You may thus save time.

See also:

▶ Questions: 79–90, 95–104, 165–77.
▶ Features: 13, 14, 15.

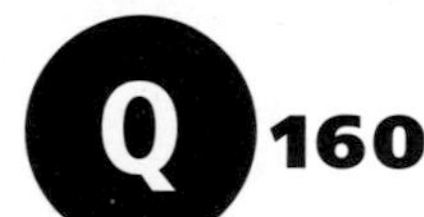

Q 160

I sleep only four hours a night – do I burn more calories than someone who sleeps a lot?

Compared with someone who sleeps, say, 8 hours a night, you have 4 extra hours of activity on top of your Basal Metabolic Rate (see Feature 1). Depending on how you spend those 4 hours, you could burn up a lot more calories, or just a few.

For example, if you sit watching TV or working at a desk, you would burn up only about an average of another 30 calories an hour, totalling 120 extra calories. If you spent the time walking or at the all-night gym, however, you could burn up very many more. Even asleep, you burn up quite a few calories (about 60 an hour for an average woman).

See also:

▶ Questions: 3–6.
▶ Features: 1, 2.
▶ Index entry: metabolism.

Q 161

Does mental activity (brainwork) burn calories?

Yes, energy is needed for your brain to function. The brain can use only glucose for energy and if it doesn't get it will begin to show signs of seizing up – sluggishness, tiredness, fuzziness, etc.

However, there is little research on how many extra calories your brain might use up in a particularly busy period of activity. It seems that the difference between reading a light novel and working flat-out all day, preparing an important report say, may not amount to many extra calories burnt.

The proof of this is that sedentary people who do a great deal of hard brain work tend to get fat because they're not physically active. The sad truth for everyone who is overworked but under-exercised is that it is the moving parts of the body that burn up most calories – if you move them, that is.

See also:

▶ Question: 162.
▶ Features: 1, 2.
▶ Key index entry: metabolism.

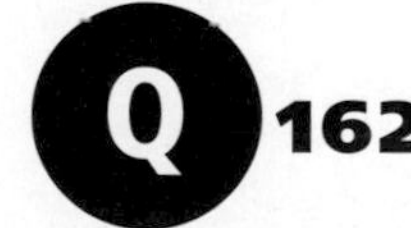

Q 162

Does stress burn calories?

It is quite common that people who are under stress do lose weight. This can be for a variety of reasons. Stress can easily diminish appetite in the short term (e.g. the looming exam, the speech to give, the divorce hearing) and it isn't unknown for people under severe stress to lose up to a stone in a fortnight. However, for some people, stress seems to increase appetite, especially for 'comfort' foods like carbohydrates.

Stress can also increase the metabolic rate – hormones released at times of stress make the heart beat faster; and stress can also make people more 'fidgety' – almost literally living off 'nervous energy'. Stress may also hasten the passage of food through the digestive system and gut, and that may then mean that less of it is actually absorbed.

However, long-term stress can also make you fat – for more on this, see the answer to Q14 – and there is some evidence that dieters under stress tend to 'comfort eat' more. In any case, I wouldn't recommend a dose of stress as a good way of losing weight – there are too many drawbacks.

See also:

- ▶ Questions: 14, 133, 161.
- ▶ Feature: 2.
- ▶ Key index entries: metabolism, stress.

163

Does smoking keep you slim?

The World Health Organization says that tobacco smoking causes a 'marked' increase in the metabolic rate in the short term and may also cause a long-term increase in the basal metabolic rate. Although not all research has come to this conclusion, the evidence is quite strong, as smoking and weight gain are inversely related and smokers almost always put on weight once they give up tobacco.

Apart from the metabolism-boosting effects, people who smoke may also be slimmer because food intake is reduced. This is partly because the physical act of smoking replaces the physical act of eating and partly because smoking can suppress the appetite. However, all health authorities agree that smoking should not be used as a means to weight control, as the adverse health implications from smoking are so great.

See also:

- ▶ Question: 164.
- ▶ Features: 1, 2.

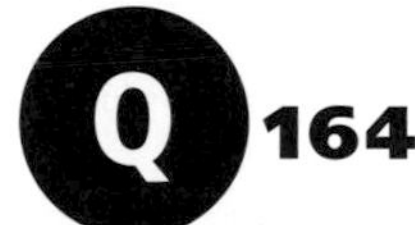

164

I've given up smoking – is weight gain inevitable?

One research paper published in the American *New England Journal of Medicine* reported that the average amount of weight gained in people who gave up smoking was 2.8kg in men and 3.8kg in women. People who smoked more than 15 cigarettes a day and then gave up tended to put on more weight and were at a higher risk of weight gain.

This weight gain is probably partly due to a slowing of the metabolic rate (see the answer to the previous question) and to an increase in appetite; because the act of eating is a substitute for the act of smoking, total calorie intake is increased.

The consensus is that the relatively small gain in weight should not be a reason to carry on smoking. I would add that I do know many people who have given up smoking and have managed to keep to within two or three pounds of their 'smoking' weight. Many people who quit smoking do so because they want to have a healthier lifestyle. Once the lungs are free from tobacco pollution, exercising becomes a much more viable option – and so ex-smokers can easily, and often do, reset their metabolism to a higher rate via regular exercise. It goes without saying that a healthy weight-maintenance diet will also help.

See also:

- ▶ Questions: 3–6, 163, 333.
- ▶ Features: 1, 2, 3, 9, 29.
- ▶ Key index entry: metabolism.

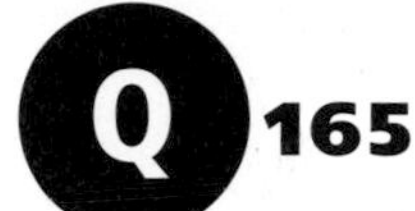

165

Can you give me some ideas for quick and/or easy, non-fattening but delicious suppers for one or two people?

It is easier than you might think, especially if you eat meat and fish, as the supermarkets have so many quick-cooking low-fat choices. Think fairly small portions, bulked out with lots of vegetables (again there are so many ready-prepared ones to choose from) and some decent-quality carbohydrate (new potatoes, rice, noodles, pasta, couscous, bulghar are all cheap, quick and easy).

The griddle or frying pan is, of course, a boon for quick after-work cooking, and I never mind cooking with a little olive oil or a small dab of butter for the main meal of the day – as long as you mostly avoid the obviously calorific foods like pastry, and save things like double cream for special occasions, you can't go far wrong. All the main-meal ideas in Feature 14 would come to no more than 500 calories or so per portion, which is fine for your supper (assuming a normal breakfast and lightish lunch plus snacks, as per suggestions in Basic Diet in Feature 9).

See also:

- ▶ Questions: 166, 191.
- ▶ Features: 9, 14–16.

Quick meals for busy people

With a well thought-out store cupboard, anyone can produce quick and easy meals in minutes. More elaborate meals can be made ahead and frozen when you're less busy.

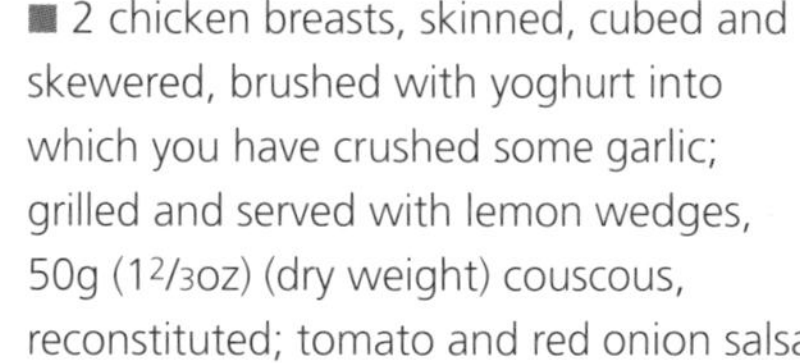

15 Quick-and-easy After-work Meals

Around 500 calories a portion; 15g (1/2oz) fat max; quantities given serve 2, but can be halved to serve 1. If no amounts given, use medium portions.

- 100g (3 1/2oz) (dry weight) wholewheat pasta topped with a seafood sauce made by simmering good-quality ready-made pasta tomato sauce with 200g (7oz) thawed mixed frozen seafood and some sliced mushrooms and fresh basil; salad.
- 100g (3 1/2oz) (dry weight) couscous or basmati rice, soaked or cooked as per instructions, or 2 medium baked potatoes, topped with plenty of ready-made ratatouille, a little crumbled feta; salad.
- 100g (3 1/2oz) (dry weight) spaghetti, cooked and topped with halved grilled filleted sardines, a few sultanas, some halved baby tomatoes, plenty of chopped parsley and a drizzle of olive oil; salad.
- 2 medium turkey escalopes, fried in a non-stick pan with low-calorie cooking oil spray, served with 100g (3 1/2oz) (dry weight) rice noodles, cooked; and stir-fry of mixed frozen vegetables with a dsp of yellow bean sauce and 2 tbsp chicken stock.
- 2 medium salmon fillets brushed with good-quality ready-made pesto sauce, grilled and served with ready-prepared baby new potatoes or wild rice; broccoli.
- Eggs Florentine: cook a 200g (7oz) bag of baby spinach in the microwave; poach 2 large eggs; make a savoury béchamel sauce using sauce flour; assemble the dish by dividing the spinach between 2 dishes, topping with the egg and then the sauce, and grate 1 tbsp each of Parmesan cheese on top; flash under grill; serve with wholemeal bread.
- 100g (3 1/2oz) (dry weight) basmati rice, cooked with a good pinch of ground curry spices; mixed with 150g (5oz) smoked haddock fillet, microwaved and flaked, and 75g (2 3/4oz) cooked petit pois; with a poached egg each on top.
- Large bowl of mixed salad leaves, tossed with 4 slices of extra-lean back bacon grilled until crisp; dressing of l tbsp olive oil and l dsp balsamic vinegar, 1 tsp wholegrain mustard, pinch of sugar, seasoning; crusty roll each.

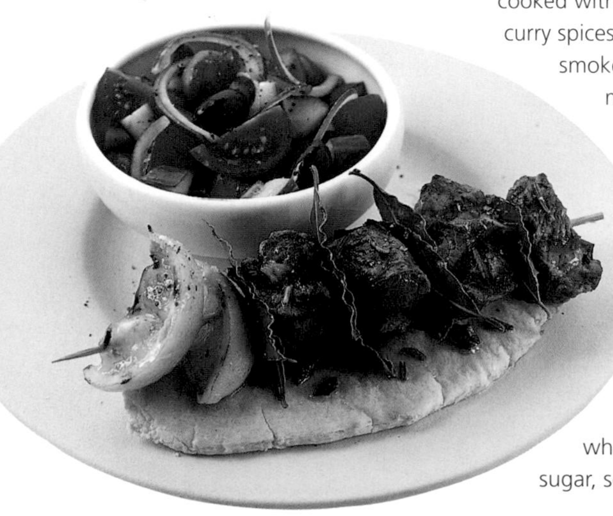

- 2 chicken breasts, skinned, cubed and skewered, brushed with yoghurt into which you have crushed some garlic; grilled and served with lemon wedges, 50g (1 2/3oz) (dry weight) couscous, reconstituted; tomato and red onion salsa.
- 2 chicken breasts, skinned, each wrapped in a foil parcel with a tsp each of chopped fresh ginger, 2 chopped spring onions, l dsp soy sauce; baked for 20 minutes and served with 100g (3 1/2oz) (dry weight) rice noodles and mangetout.
- 300g (10 1/2oz) pork fillet, sliced and stir-fried with ready-prepared carrot batons and broccoli and halved spring

DESSERTS

If you're in a hurry, there is nothing to beat fresh fruit for dessert – otherwise choose one of the many individual tubs of chilled dessert that you can buy at the supermarket or Boots. Try to pick one that is 100 calories or less and low in fat. There are also some ideas for easy puddings in the answer to Q 120.

onions, I tbsp sesame oil, soy sauce, sugar, sherry and ready-prepared ginger, plus 2 tbsp chicken stock; serve with 50g ($1\frac{2}{3}$oz) (dry weight) egg-thread noodles.

■ Two 125g ($4\frac{1}{2}$oz) venison steaks, dry-fried for 3 minutes each side and with a dash of red wine added plus I tbsp Cumberland sauce; serve with crunchy red cabbage salad and a wholemeal roll.

■ 2 medium fresh mackerel fillets, grilled and served with a sauce of Greek yoghurt mixed with horseradish sauce, baby spinach microwaved in its own pack and ready-prepared baby new potatoes.

■ Flat omelette made in a non-stick frying pan using 4 eggs, chopped spring onion, tomatoes and mushrooms (well beaten into the egg) with a knob of butter; cook over slow heat and flash under grill to brown top; serve with 50g ($1\frac{2}{3}$oz) crusty bread each and side salad.

■ 250g (9oz) cubed lamb fillet, threaded on kebabs, seasoned and grilled for a few minutes a side, with lots of lemon juice drizzled over and sprinkling of Mediterranean herbs; serve with flat bread and Greek salad (no feta).

Quick-and-easy Lunches

To serve 1. Max 450 cals, 15g ($\frac{1}{2}$oz) fat. (For takeaway lunches, see Feature 15.)

■ Broad Bean Salad: 75g ($2\frac{3}{4}$oz) cooked small broad beans tossed with 50g ($1\frac{2}{3}$oz) cubed feta cheese, 100g ($3\frac{1}{2}$oz) chopped new potatoes, some fresh mint, seasoning and oil-free French dressing.

■ Couscous Salad: selection of chopped Mediterranean vegetables, tossed in $\frac{1}{2}$ tbsp olive oil and seasoning, pre-roast and spooned over 50g ($1\frac{2}{3}$oz) (dry weight) couscous, reconstituted.

■ Open Goats' Cheese Sandwich: slice 1 thick (50g/$1\frac{2}{3}$oz) slice of rye bread, spread with a little low-fat spread and top with 50g ($1\frac{2}{3}$oz) soft goats' cheese, sliced, a few sliced cherry tomatoes, some red onion rings, fresh basil leaves and drizzle over some low-calorie balsamic vinaigrette.

■ Summer Soup: in an electric blender, mix together 225ml (8fl oz) tomato juice, 2 chopped fresh tomatoes, 2 spring onions, 3cm ($1\frac{1}{4}$inch) piece of peeled cucumber, a good clove of garlic and seasoning; adjust the seasoning and serve cold (or you could heat). Serve garnished with 20g ($\frac{2}{3}$oz) Parmesan cheese, thinly sliced, and 25g ($\frac{3}{4}$oz) wholemeal bread.

■ Miso Soup: chop a selection of vegetables (e.g. carrot, celery, onion, courgette) to make up 300g ($10\frac{1}{2}$oz) and simmer in 300ml ($\frac{1}{2}$ pint) vegetable stock with I dsp miso paste added, for 30 minutes; adjust the seasoning and serve with 25g ($\frac{3}{4}$oz) rye bread.

■ Quick Lentil Soup: in a pan, heat 200ml (7fl oz) chicken stock with a drained can of green lentils, finely chopped onion and butternut squash; season, add chopped thyme and cook for 30 minutes until vegetables are tender. Serve with 20g ($\frac{2}{3}$oz) grated tasty Cheddar and 25g ($\frac{3}{4}$oz) rye bread.

■ Mushrooms on Toast: destalk 2 flat field mushrooms and put on foil on a grill pan, gill side down; grill on high and near the heat for 3 minutes, turn over, turn heat down slightly and grill for further 4 or 5 minutes; meanwhile, make a dressing by mixing I tbsp olive oil, I crushed garlic clove, juice of $\frac{1}{2}$ lime, I dsp chopped fresh coriander or parsley, $\frac{1}{2}$ tsp chopped chilli and seasoning; when mushrooms are ready, pour over the dressing. Serve on a thick slice of wholemeal bread with a green side salad.

■ Herring Roes on Toast: simmer 200g (7oz) soft fresh herring roes in their own juice in a non-stick pan for a few minutes; serve on I thick slice of wholemeal or rye bread.

■ Vine Tomatoes on Toast: grill several tasty vine tomatoes on a foil-covered grill pan until soft, sprinkle with balsamic vinegar and oregano and serve on a 50g ($1\frac{2}{3}$oz) toasted slice of ciabatta; top with 25g ($\frac{3}{4}$oz) goats' cheese, cubed.

Quick breakfasts

To serve 1. Max 300 cals or 8g ($\frac{1}{4}$oz) fat.

■ I small banana blended with 150ml ($\frac{1}{4}$ pint) skimmed milk, juice of I small orange and I dsp honey; I small handful sunflower seeds (10g/$\frac{1}{3}$oz).

■ I small banana blended with 125g ($4\frac{1}{2}$oz) pot of natural low-fat bio yoghurt, 100g ($3\frac{1}{2}$oz) strawberries and I tsp caster sugar; I small handful (10g/$1\frac{1}{3}$oz) shelled walnuts.

■ 2 Shredded Wheat, 5 tbsp skimmed milk, 1 level tsp sugar, chopped pear or grapefruit, 1 level dsp sesame seeds.

■ 2 Weetabix; skimmed milk to cover, 50g ($1\frac{2}{3}$oz) halved black seedless grapes and 10g ($\frac{1}{3}$oz) sunflower seeds.

■ I large slice of wholemeal toast with low-fat spread; Marmite; one 125ml (4fl oz) pot of natural low-fat bio yoghurt with I tsp runny honey; satsuma.

■ 60g (2oz) muesli with 5 tbsp skimmed milk and I chopped apple.

■ 150g (5oz) baked beans in low-salt, low-sugar tomato sauce, heated in microwave and served on 40g ($1\frac{1}{3}$oz) slice of wholemeal bread with a little low-fat spread; small glass orange juice.

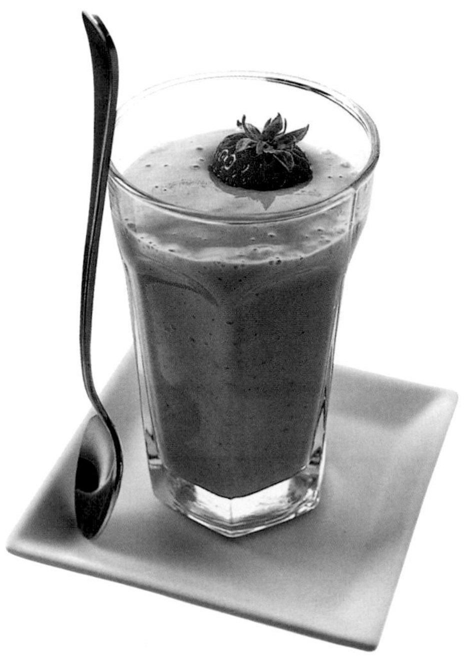

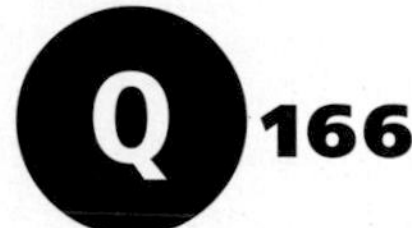

166

Is it OK to diet on nothing but convenience foods?

Everyone makes use of such things as microwave meals for one now and then, and they are a boon – but when choosing, do read the label and make sure that it doesn't contain more than about 15g of fat per serving. This will mean that you can have about 15g fat for lunch, and a little fat in your breakfast and daily snacks without going over a daily 42g total fat, which will give you a 25% fat diet for an average woman slimming on 1,500 calories a day (see Feature 8 for a full explanation).

Also, try to find ready meals that contain plenty of vegetables. Otherwise, add a pack of mixed salad leaves to your basket and eat a big side salad too. Most ready meals also contain the 'carbohydrate' element of the meal (rice, pasta, etc.). If so (for females with an average metabolic rate slimming on 1,500 calories a day), you can afford to choose a meal up to 500 calories. If yours doesn't, make sure that it is no more than around 300 calories a serving, so that you can add some carbohydrate of your own at home – the simplest would be about 50g ($1\frac{2}{3}$oz) of wholemeal bread or roll.

Meals like beans on toast are also fine sometimes – the pulses are very healthy and the tomato sauce is a good source of lycopene; make the bread wholemeal and it's a very good meal, low in fat unless you add lots of butter to your toast. I'd add an orange afterwards, otherwise you won't get any vitamin C. This will also help the body absorb the iron in the beans and bread.

If you choose very carefully, varying your choices, you may well be fine nutritionally on a diet of convenience foods and things on toast, especially if you add fresh fruit and salad. However, one of the main disadvantages of many of the ready meals is that you don't get very much on your plate – many slimmers could each TWO portions easily! So without high satiety value, you may feel hungry and increase the amount of food you eat in snacks between meals. Some are not all that tasty or exciting, either, although some brands are quite good.

Feature 14 gives some more ideas for 'things on bread'. Convenience meals in a pack are saving you time and trouble – but check out the other ideas in this section of the book and you'll see that there are many simple main meals and lunches that you can prepare almost as quickly, from scratch. If you have a wide variety of foods and tastes on your slimming plan you are more likely to stick with it and succeed.

See also:

- ▶ Questions: 159, 165, 167, 176–7, 183.
- ▶ Features: 8, 9, 14, 15.

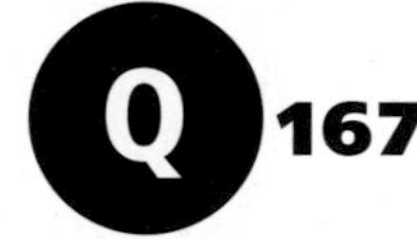

167

Is there such a thing as a non-fattening takeaway or fast-food meal, for my main meal of the day several nights a week?

Assuming you are one of the many people who work late, then call into a takeaway on the way home – there are some items you could choose which would be better for your waistline, but the trouble is that, in my experience, you will be so hungry that caution goes out the window and you choose the most calorific thing you can see on the menu – plus, of course, there are all the food aromas as you order, to get your taste buds going!

This is one of the trickiest problems to solve. It would be best if you could adjust your schedule or, failing that, have something nice but not so calorific in your briefcase or bag that you can eat during your last hour at work – say, a small ham sandwich or even a bag of low-fat crisps. This will take the edge off your appetite and then you could wait until you get home, where you can heat up a (decent-quality) ready meal or cook a quick steak or bowl of pasta – or re-heat something you made earlier, perhaps.

The thing about losing weight is that you have to be committed, and you have to plan. If what you eat is last on your list of priorities, of course you are going to have problems. You have to decide what is most important to you. Hopefully you'll decide that you do want to lose weight and feel good about your diet, in which case you may like to invest an hour or so at weekends in making a few simple things for the freezer (assuming you're very busy all week). If you're not short of cash and live in a city, you can probably even find companies via the Internet who will bike you round a healthy meal to order.

That said, Feature 15 does include a (fairly short) list of takeaway meals that can be fitted into most slimming plans. Sushi is great, so is tandoori chicken, for example. Sadly, however, very many takeout foods – including most of the menu in Indian, Chinese, Thai, Mexican, pizza houses, burger bars, chicken bars, fish and chip shops – ARE full of fat and therefore high in calories and best saved for occasional use. A list of common takeaways with their calorie and fat value appears on page 82.

TIP: One of the most important things to remember for very busy people is to eat 'little and often' throughout the day, to keep blood-sugar levels even and stop you from wanting to 'pig out' the minute you stop work and realize you're ravenous. See 'Small Snacks' in Feature 14.

See also:

- ▶ Questions: 36, 84, 95–7, 100, 104, 118, 122, 142, 159, 166, 168.
- ▶ Features: 8, 9, 13, 14, 15.
- ▶ A–Z entry: Internet slimming.

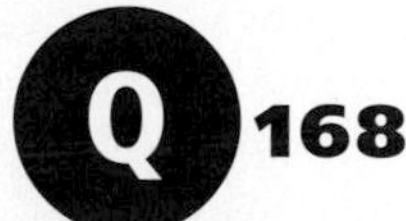

168

I work shifts, and often work nights – I have yet to find a diet I can follow, have you any ideas?

Shiftworkers sometimes get in a muddle with set diets because some days – particularly when shift hours change – they may have an extra meal, or two main meals, instead of a breakfast and main meal – that kind of thing. Shiftworkers also tend to snack on high-fat items, like chocolate and biscuits, more than the national average.

If that is what is bothering you, the best way to cope is first to understand that losing weight doesn't necessarily mean sticking to three set meals a day in strict order and, second, that to avoid getting very hungry and snacking on chocolate, etc., you need to plan ahead a little.

If you can lose weight on 1,500 calories a day (which most people can), in theory you could divide these calories up any way you want over any 24-hour period. As 'little and often' is best for health and will also suit your lifestyle best, you could divide it into, say, four mini-meals a day of 300 calories each (and have the extra for milk, drinks, treats).

It is best to stick with mini-meals that are easy to eat and quick to prepare – and another tip is to choose things that can serve as breakfast, lunch, supper, whatever. It is also best to take your food along to work with you, if the only alternative will be a badly stocked cafeteria – when working nights, buying decent food is always a problem.

You could keep a weekly food diary, each day divided into four spaces into which you write what you've eaten as soon after eating it as is practical. That way, at the end of the week you can see how many of your mini-meals you've had. Even if one or two extra show, you should still lose weight slowly. On days when you want to sleep all day to 'catch up', perhaps there will be fewer meals to record, anyway.

Mini-meal ideas – each about 300 calories:

- Calorie-counted ready-to-eat sandwich of 250 or less; piece of fruit.
- Big bowl of ready-to-eat, chilled-counter vegetable soup with 1 small slice of bread.
- Bowl of wholegrain cereal with skimmed milk and fresh and dried chopped fruit.
- 150g (5oz) baked beans on 40g ($1\frac{1}{3}$oz) toast with low-fat spread.
- Banana sandwich using two 25g ($\frac{3}{4}$oz) slices wholemeal bread and low-fat spread.
- Ready-cooked chicken breast portion with side salad and small roll.
- 2 small eggs, poached, on wholemeal toast with low-fat spread; I satsuma.
- Breakfast bowl of cooked pasta, topped with ready-made Italian tomato sauce and a little grated Parmesan.
- Ham sandwich: two 25g ($\frac{3}{4}$oz) slices of wholemeal bread OR medium bap with low-fat spread filled with 50g ($1\frac{2}{3}$oz) low-fat ham and plenty of salad.
- 200g (7oz) baked potato topped with 50g ($1\frac{2}{3}$oz) baked beans and 20g ($\frac{2}{3}$oz) grated Parmesan.
- 200g (7oz) cooked basmati rice mixed with chopped chicken, salad vegetables and pine nuts, tossed with oil-free French dressing.

The Food Value charts at the back of the book will give you other ideas. If this 'four meals a day' idea doesn't appeal to you, just do your own thing. If your weekly calorie total gives you an energy deficit, how you ate those calories doesn't really matter.

See also:
- ▶ Questions: 85, 95–6, 102–4, 143, 173, 177.
- ▶ Features: 13, 14, 15.
- ▶ A–Z entry: calorie counting.
- ▶ Key index entries: healthy snacks, hunger.

FAT FACT

Nurses have one of the highest levels of overweight of any professional group in the UK – with gifts of chocolate and other food, and shiftwork being the main reasons cited.

169

I haven't time for breakfast and I prefer to have my main meal late in the evening. Is it true this causes weight gain?

As Q100 explains, it is how many calories you eat over the course of the day (or week) that matters, not when you eat them. As long as you aren't creating a positive energy situation (taking in more calories than you're burning off), then you shouldn't put on weight eating this way. That said, I don't think your pattern of eating is by any means ideal – but if it works for you, you like it and you're healthy, then why worry?

See also:
- ▶ Questions: 95–100.
- ▶ Key index entry: healthy eating.

170

I'm always ravenous when I get home from work, even though I eat lunch. We don't have an evening meal until 8pm, when my partner gets home, so how do I stop myself from snacking?

'I get too hungry for dinner at eight' applies to lots of people, and no wonder. Most working people have their lunch around 1pm – and seven hours is too long to try to go without eating anything and not expecting to feel hungry. Matters are compounded if you have to spend an hour in the kitchen after work preparing a meal – of course you will pick, it's only natural.

What you need to do is give yourself an 'allowed' snack when you get home from work – something around 100–200 calories. If this contains foods low on the Glycaemic Index (see Q84), then it should keep hunger well at bay until 8. Some suggestions are: 2 dark rye crispbreads topped with Marmite and slices of tomato (80 calories); I individual tub of diet fruit yoghurt and an apple (130 calories); 10g (1/3oz) walnuts and a satsuma (100 calories); I heaped tbsp reduced-fat hummus on I mini pitta (130 calories).

To make amends for this extra snack, give yourself slightly smaller portions of the rest of your meals throughout the day – to reduce any meal by 50 calories you would only have to serve yourself, say, 30g (1oz) less meat or half a slice of bread less. Check out the Food Value Charts at the back of the book for more help.

One other solution you could incorporate is to have half your lunch at 1pm and the remainder at 2 or 3, if that's possible (or simply have lunch later).

See also:

- Questions: 18, 84–6, 172
- A–Z entry: calorie counting.
- Key index entries: Glycaemic Index, hunger.

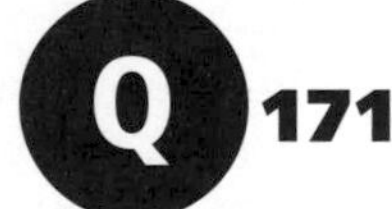

Q 171

How do I resist the coffee and snacks trolley that comes around twice a day when I am at work?

If you know when it comes, the best bet is to make sure you have had a small healthy snack just before it arrives – as you will see in the Basic Diet (Feature 9), you can easily fit two snacks a day into you diet. Snack suggestions appear in that feature and in the answer to the previous question.

See also:

- Questions: 84–5, 95, 101.
- Feature: 9.
- Key index entries: appetite, healthy eating, hunger, snacking.

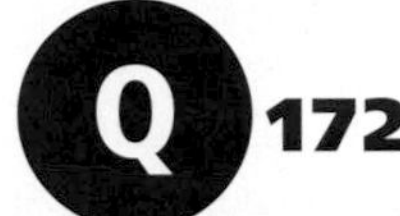

Q 172

Is skipping lunch a good way to save calories, as it is always a very busy time at work for me anyway?

Skipping lunch isn't ideal for most people, as blood-sugar levels will begin to dip without anything to eat since breakfast. As a compromise, you could have a reasonably large breakfast, including items low on the Glycaemic Index (see Q84) and take to work a couple of portable snacks to eat at quiet moments during your working day – ideally, one at around 12 noon and the other around 3.30pm. Two 150-calorie snacks would be ideal, again, with a low GI, which will help keep your blood-sugar levels stable until you have your meal. See the Food Value Charts at the back of the book.

As I have said before, how much you eat is what counts in maintaining, or losing, weight. HOW and when you eat are more important for other reasons – perhaps health, convenience and helping you stick to any diet regime. What works best for you is what matters most – but for most people, skipping lunch inevitably means the (sometimes uncontrollable) urge to eat something high in calories and/or fat and/or sugar or starch in the late afternoon or early evening.

See also:

- Questions: 18, 84–6, 95–9.
- Key index entries: Glycaemic Index, hunger, snacking.

Q 173

My company cafeteria majors on pies, chips, sausage, curry and so on – otherwise there is quiche and salad, cheese and biscuits or things on toast. What is the best bet, calorie-wise?

Take your own lunch to work! Seriously, most of the things you mention are high in fat and best avoided on anything except an occasional basis. A quiche salad is much higher in fat and calories than you would think, because of the pastry, egg and salad dressing, and is probably no better than sausage and chips. Cheese and biscuits are also high in fat and high density, meaning that you don't get much on your plate, and there are no vegetables or salad with this, either, which isn't good.

If taking your own lunch to work and eating it in the cafeteria isn't feasible, is there anywhere else locally you could go for a more slimmer-friendly lunch? Otherwise, I'd find out who is responsible for the menu at your works cafeteria and see if you can get them to put at least one 'healthy option' on the menu each day. If the cafe franchisee isn't helpful, go to your company boss and ask him or her instead. The list of fast foods shown on page 82 may help you make the best choices from what is currently on offer.

I think all places of work large enough to have a cafeteria should be responsible enough to make sure that the food on offer is varied, with something suitable for all needs. With so high a proportion of people overweight, and many more trying to follow reduced-fat diets for their health's sake, it hardly makes sense to provide only high-fat, high-calorie food. All employers, please take note!

See also:

- Questions: 118, 167, 172, 176.
- Feature: 15.

Q 174

I travel most days of the week and have put on over a stone through eating at take-outs, pubs and roadside cafés. How can I do better, without inconvenience?

The best idea would be to take an insulated lunchbox with you, filled with tempting lower-fat foods and snacks (Q 176 will help here). You can pull off the road for half an hour – and probably save yourself time as well.

If this isn't possible, stock up in the supermarket with ready-made, calorie-counted sandwiches, wraps, sushi or other 'healthy options' lunch foods.

If eating at the occasional roadside café is inevitable, Feature 15 will give you more ideas on what to pick that will do least damage. Also bear in mind that when you are at home and in control of what you eat is the time to major on low-calorie, very healthy meals, plenty of veg and so on – all outlined in the Basic Diet in Feature 9.

See also:

- Questions: 118, 166, 167, 175–9.
- Features: 9, 14–15.
- Key index entries: healthy eating, junk food, takeaway food.

Q 175

I travel abroad on business much of the year and am often entertained in homes and restaurants, with little choice. Otherwise it's hotel and airline food. How do I avoid putting on weight?

There's no simple solution, but several tactics may help you to cut down on surplus calories wherever you happen to be eating.

If being entertained, first, avoid pre-meal nibbles, or take just one, or at most two, if offered. During the meal, say no to extras like bread, butter, spring rolls, chapatis, or whatever. Stick to the main items. If self-service is called for, give yourself small portions. If offered seconds, refuse politely. Most hostesses the world over don't mind too much if you refuse dessert. And say no also to any chocolates or other titbits that arrive with coffee.

Alcohol is easy – just say you're not drinking at the moment. This may be a horrifying thought, but drinking alcohol honestly isn't a prerequisite of being the perfect guest. If you can't bear the thought of avoiding all alcohol, just take the first drink and have it slowly. For more tips on alcohol avoidance see the answer to Q 187.

If on your own in the hotel, simply order the plainest things you can find: grilled steak, fish or chicken, salad, new potatoes. On a plane there are usually fewer calories in airline meals than you might think, as portions are quite small. Just leave the roll, butter and dessert.

In general, keep a wary eye on your mouth and what goes in it; avoiding unnecessary calories when travelling becomes easier with practice.

See also:

- Questions: 178–88.
- Feature 15.
- A–Z entry: Dine out and Lose Weight.

Q 176

Can you give me some ideas for healthy low-fat lunch-box meals for adults?

Very many sandwiches, filled rolls, wraps, etc. are quite low in fat and calories. If making up your own lunchbox, simply choose decent-quality bread, a low-fat protein filling (e.g. lean ham, chicken, turkey, tuna, prawns) or occasionally a medium-fat filling (egg, Brie), add plenty of salad items, dress with a little low-fat mayonnaise (or nothing) and there you are. Pittas are great – easily stuffed with feta and salad or tuna and salad, or buy your own wraps and roll them up with more exotic fillings – chicken and pesto, seafood and chilli. If buying in your sandwiches, simply look for the words 'low-fat' and/or 'low-calorie'.

You will want to add other items to the pack: always choose a piece of fresh fruit and then pick one (or possibly two, depending upon your metabolic rate and dieting level – see Section One) more item from: individual tubs of yoghurt or fromage frais, a small bag filled with some ready-to-eat dried fruit and fresh nuts or pumpkin seeds, malt loaf, teabread, plain scone, good-quality fruit cake.

If you get bored with all bready-things, think about sushi, or various lunch salads which you can pack in a little box and eat with plastic fork! You can buy several ready-made, but if you want some ideas for salads to make at home there are several in Feature 15.

Add a bottle of mineral water or a flask of tea – most drinks add too many calories to your lunch for little benefit and low-cal fizzy drinks just encourage a sweet tooth. In warm weather, or warm offices, take your lunch in an insulated lunchbox or bag – these are now widely available.

See also:

- Questions: 101, 104, 121.
- Features: 1, 15.

Food to go

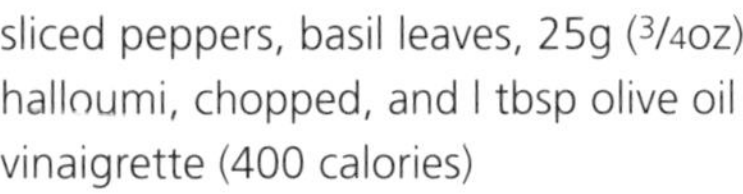

If you're always on the move, here are some ideas for healthy (or at least reasonably healthy, now and then), reduced-fat, reduced-calorie meals, all of which can be included in an average 1,500 cals/day slimming diet.

Sandwich meals

- Any wrapped sandwich labelled as containing less than 300 calories per portion with less than 10g fat.
- Subway branches – any 'Less than 6g fat' range, e.g. 6" subs – 300–465 cals and 2–6g fat.
- Bistro Express – Hot and Crispy Baguettes, Spicy Chicken – 310 calories, fat n/k.
- Any of the following from an independent outlet (e.g. sandwich bar) – a wholemeal bread sandwich filled with salad (no mayonnaise) plus one of the following: chicken, turkey, smoked ham, tuna, prawns, low-fat soft cheese, chicken tikka, egg.

Café and pub food

All calorie and fat values approximate – order side salad or plainly cooked vegetables as accompaniment.

- Chilli con carne and rice – 350–500 calories; 10–20g fat.
- Shepherd's or cottage pie and vegetables – 500 calories, 15g fat.
- Vegetarian lasagne – 500 calories; 16g fat.
- Jacket potato with beans – 300 calories; 1g fat; portion (12g/$^{1}/_{3}$oz) of butter – 92 calories, 10g fat.
- Jacket potato with tuna and sweetcorn topping – 450 calories; 10g fat.
- Ham salad and roll (no coleslaw or mayo) – 450 calories, 6g fat; 75g/2$^{3}/_{4}$oz coleslaw – 150 calories, 12g fat.
- Ham tuna, chicken or prawn and salad sandwich – 400–500 calories, 5–12g fat.
- Ham, tuna, chicken or prawn baguette and salad – 500–600 calories, 7–15g fat.
- Little Chef Gammon Platter with Salad – 550 calories, 14g fat.

Fast Food

- Hamburger, standard – 250–280 calories, 8–12g fat.
- Cheeseburger, standard – 300–330 calories, 11–16g fat.
- 6 chicken nuggets – 210–250 calories, 9–15g fat.
- McChicken Sandwich – 375 calories, 17g fat.
- KFC Chicken Drumstick with BBQ beans and corn on the cob – 345 calories, 14g fat.
- Lamb kofta skewer with salad and small pitta – 470 calories, 15g fat.
- Tandoori chicken, average portion – 320 calories, 8g fat.
- Plain rice, average portion – 200 calories, 2g fat.
- Pizza Express individual Pizza Marinara – 525 calories, 13g fat.
- Chicken Burritos, average portion – 580 calories, 14g fat.
- Chicken enchiladas, average portion – 600 calories, 10g fat.

Packed Lunch Salads

- Any supermarket or Boots 'main meal' salad containing 400 calories or less (check label), with 15g fat maximum.
- Couscous and Red Pepper: 50g (1$^{2}/_{3}$oz) (dry weight) couscous, reconstituted in vegetable stock and mixed with grilled, sliced peppers, basil leaves, 25g ($^{3}/_{4}$oz) halloumi, chopped, and I tbsp olive oil vinaigrette (400 calories)
- New Potato and Egg Salad: 175g (6oz) cold cooked new potatoes, roughly chopped and mixed with I medium hard-boiled egg, chopped, I slice of lean back bacon, grilled and crumbled, 50g (1$^{2}/_{3}$oz) small cooked broad beans, wedges of Little Gem lettuce and I tbsp dijonnaise dressing mixed with I tbsp low-fat natural bio yoghurt and seasoning (375 calories).
- Rice and Bean Salad: 150g (5oz) (cooked weight) basmati rice mixed with 100g (3$^{1}/_{2}$oz) cooked mixed pulses (well drained) OR chickpeas, 3 pieces ready-to-eat dried apricot, chopped, I tbsp pine nuts, chopped celery and cucumber and oil-free French dressing to taste (375 calories).
- Pasta and Tuna Salad: 150g (5oz) (cooked weight) wholewheat pasta shapes mixed with 100g (3$^{1}/_{2}$oz) flaked bluefin tuna in water, well drained, 25g ($^{3}/_{4}$oz) cooked sweetcorn kernels, chopped tomato, parsley, cucumber and oil-free French dressing to taste (300 calories).
- Pasta and Prawn Salad: 150g (5oz) cooked weight wholewheat pasta mixed with 100g (3$^{1}/_{2}$oz) cooked peeled prawns, a few chopped mushrooms, a few lightly cooked small broccoli florets, and I tbsp dijonnaise dressing mixed with I tbsp low-fat yoghurt and seasoning (325 calories)

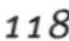

177

Are there any snacks, like peanuts and crisps, which are just as tempting but not so fattening?

You can buy several brands of reduced-fat, reduced-calorie crisps and savoury snacks – in the UK, Boots do a good 'Shapers' range, with every pack under 100 calories. Other brands include WeightWatchers Weavers, KP Skips, Golden Wonder Lites. Popcorn is another good idea – it is filling and reasonably healthy, and a small bag will satisfy you at around 115 calories. Pretzels and Twiglets are both fairly low in calories, too, but make sure to buy small packs, and remember lots of savoury snacks are high in salt.

Another good idea for home use is to buy fresh nuts in their shells, and crack them open yourself. Not only are the nuts healthy, tasty, salt-free and good for you, but if you have to crack them it will slow down your rate of eating to a quarter your usual rate. Yes, nuts are high in calories, but only if you eat too many of them!

See also:
- ▶ Questions: 86, 95, 171.

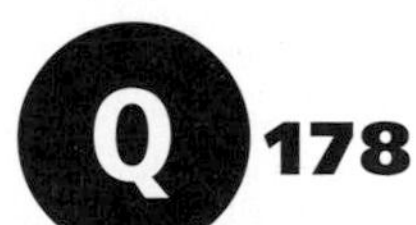

178

I have to stay in hotels a lot – can you advise me on wise choices from the typical hotel menu?

Of course, hotel menus will vary depending on where you are in the world but, assuming 'international' standard hotels, choices can be remarkably similar. If dining alone, just have a main course – this will immediately bring your calorie total down to a reasonable level. Choose anything grilled or roast – fish and chicken being a good bet. Tenderloin of pork is a very lean hotel favourite. Lamb often comes with a fair amount of fat still attached, so perhaps is best avoided.

Sauces can add a lot of fat and calories to your meal, so choose wisely. 'Mediterranean'-style sauces based on tomato are fine, though they may be high in olive oil. 'Meunière' means butter – these and rich cream sauces are ones to pass on, or have in very small amounts, as are béchamel, au gratin, and hollandaise. Ask the waiter for your meal without the sauce, or for the sauce served separately so you can put just a dab on, if necessary. Also ask if you aren't sure what a dish contains in the way of butter, oil, cream.

Definitely ask for your side vegetables to come without butter garnish, skip the bread (or at least the butter with the bread). You can also save lots of calories by asking for rice cooked plain and for new or baked potato rather than roast or chips. You may prefer to stick with the protein and vegetable element of the meal and skip the starch (potatoes, pasta, bread, rice). This isn't a particularly healthy way to eat, but it is a fairly simple way of keeping the calories down (but not the fat).

Some ethnic main courses will be fine, but there isn't room here to second-guess all that you may be offered. The answer to Q182 comes with advice on ethnic eating – when in doubt, avoid. Hotel 'help yourself' buffets are useful but, for the unwary, some of the salads on offer are very high in fat. If they are 'glistening', they are probably thick with mayonnaise or oil.

For dessert, if you're being wise you'll stick with fruit salad or fresh fruit platter.

See also:
- ▶ Questions: 88, 175, 179–88.
- ▶ Feature: 15.
- ▶ A–Z entries: Atkins Diet, Dine Out and Lose Weight.
- ▶ Key index entries: carbohydrates, protein.

179

I eat in restaurants a great deal – what kind of food should I choose to fit in best with a reduced-calorie regime?

Follow the guidelines for hotel eating in the previous question. Q182 provides more detailed advice on ethnic eating.

At least in restaurants, a varied menu should always give you plenty of choice – it is unlikely that everything on the menu will be laden with too many calories. Of course, this can work against you if, by nature, you find yourself drawn to the most fattening things! The temptation factor is the main problem when dining outside the home, be it other people's homes or restaurants.

If you are being entertained in restaurants, you may want to read the answer to the next question.

FOOD FACT

Researchers at Yale University in the USA have found that if women eat a high-protein, low-carbohydrate lunch, they then tend to eat fewer calories in the evening. The reason, the researchers say, is that the protein triggers a greater secretion of hormones that act to blunt the appetite.

See also:
- ▶ Questions: 174–5, 178, 180–88.
- ▶ Feature: 15.
- ▶ A-Z entries: Atkins Diet, Dine Out and Lose Weight.
- ▶ Key index entries: calories, carbohydrates.

Q 180

I am entertained in restaurants at least three lunches and two evenings a week, which has made me gain weight. How do I cope with this? I often have no choice but to eat the full three courses with wine.

Assuming that you can pick your own menu from what is on offer, Q178 offers plenty of tips on reducing the total calorie content of your meal without seeming to be a spoilsport. For ethnic menus the box on page 121 may be of some help.

Other tips for not offending your host appear in the next question. Much of the etiquette when being entertained in restaurants is exactly the same as that expected when being entertained in private homes.

I should also point out that if you have three lunches and two evenings out each week, that also leaves four lunches and five evenings when you can control your diet. Going on the swings-and-roundabouts principle, perhaps at these times you could be a bit harder on yourself. It is the overall number of calories you consume that counts, not the total in any one particular meal. Also, try to take some extra exercise if you know you've had a particularly calorific week.

See also:
- ▶ Questions: 18, 175, 178–9, 181–8.
- ▶ Feature: 15.
- ▶ A–Z entry: Dine Out and Lose Weight.

Q 181

I am invited to dinner in people's homes once, and sometimes twice, at weekends, where there is no choice but to eat what I am offered. How do I eat fewer calories while I'm dieting without causing offence?

There is nothing worse than turning up for a carefully prepared dinner and announcing that you are on a diet. Perhaps there is – bringing your own food. I know people do it but, unless there is medical reason, it seems obsessive. If you know the host well, have a word beforehand and say that you're trying to lose a few pounds (on doctor's orders, if you like) and so he/she isn't to feel offended if you have smaller than usual portions and may refuse the dessert. If you don't know the host well, follow the tips below. However, for anyone who dines out rarely, an occasional evening's overindulgence isn't going to make a great deal of difference to your total calorie input in the long term, so perhaps the best policy is to sit back and enjoy it!

- Avoid more than one pre-dinner canapé. No one will really notice.
- Avoid like the plague nuts, crisps and other high-fat savoury nibbles left out in bowls – they ruin your appetite for the meal, anyway. Again, no one will notice whether you eat these or not.
- Sip drinks very slowly, putting your glass down between sips. If you're driving, you have the excuse not to drink.
- Don't take bread or butter with your meal – this won't offend the host.
- If food arrives on a 'self-service' basis, take only small portions of the high-calorie items. If there are several people present, no one is likely to notice. You could even pass on the sautéed potatoes or the like without causing comment.
- If your host dishes food out herself/himself at the table, when she/he is dishing yours out, smile and say, 'That's lovely, thank you,' before she/he gets a chance to dish too much out.
- If seconds are offered, smile ruefully and decline gracefully.
- Many hosts don't feel offended if you skip dessert – if yours insists, it is fine to ask for a small portion. If there is a choice, avoid the rich, creamy dessert and go for the fruit dessert.
- Avoid the cheeseboard and after-dinner chocolates, etc.

Also bear in mind that going out once or even twice at weekends, and eating a bit more than you would have done at home, aren't the end of the world for your diet – it leaves all week to be more restrained. A supper or dinner party is to be enjoyed – not something that makes you feel guilty. A long walk the next day helps, too.

See also:
- ▶ Questions: 175, 178–80, 182–88.
- ▶ Feature 15.
- ▶ A–Z entry: low-fat diets.
- ▶ Key index entries: calories, carbohydrates.

PARTY NIBBLE CALORIES

Piece of salmon sushi – 50
Breadstick – 20
Mini chicken kiev – 50
One carrot crudité and cheese dip – 25
Mini pizza (2 mouthfuls) – 100
Breaded prawn – 40
Baked potato wedge with dip – 45
Won ton – 35
Individual quiche (2 bites) – 100
Red pepper slice and salsa dip – 10
Cocktail sausage – 40
Hummus/roast veg crostini – 50
Mini samosa – 80
New potato with sour cream topping – 60
Chicken vol au vent (2 mouthfuls) – 80
Marinated olive – 5

182

We take three holidays a year, often to all-inclusive resorts. Overeating seems inevitable – how can we avoid this?

Most all-inclusive holiday resorts offer plenty of activities and opportunities to exercise and work off those surplus calories, so take advantage of that and then you don't have to feel guilty. One report published in *Men's Health* magazine found that a high percentage of people came back from their holidays having lost weight, rather than put it on.

If you want to be able to eat plenty without guilt, you could swap one or two of your laid-back inclusive resort holidays for an all-in 'activity' holiday, such as sailing, skiing, walking, cycling or some such. There is nothing to beat the satisfaction of eating a huge Provençal meal in the evening having tramped through the lavender fields and hills all day long! Nice food is always much nicer when you have a ravenous appetite – too much food on all-inclusives, including cruises, is eaten just because it is there and not because you need, or even want, it. Otherwise you could consider forgoing your inclusives and swapping for a 'pay-as-you-go' swish hotel – that'll certainly make you watch how much you eat.

The box on the right gives 'bests' and 'worsts' for a variety of meals in the most popular holiday destination countries. In hot weather, salads, fish, vegetables and fruit are all appealing and can save the day, calorie-wise. The main things to watch out for at help-yourself buffets, in which all-inclusives seem to specialize, are the mega-oily dressings on a lot of the side dishes. Take only very small portions of any salad that is glistening – it will be dripping in oil or mayonnaise.

See also:
▶ Questions: 175, 17–81, 183–88.

A WEIGHT-WATCHERS' GUIDE TO HOLIDAY FOOD

Calorie and fat values aren't given, as portion size and recipes can vary enormously.

Italy
Best: spaghetti napoletana, liver and bacon, seafood risotto/pizza, melon and Parma ham, grilled vegetable platter, chicken cacciatore, tuna and bean salad, chicken with rosemary.
Worst: cannelloni, meat lasagne, pasta carbonara, most risottos, meat pizzas.

America
Best: grilled steak and salad, Cajun steak or chicken, plain beefburger.
Worst: french fries, cheeseburger, chicken Maryland and other deep-fried foods.

Spain
Best: grilled fish with Catalan sauce, seafood paella, grilled tuna and salad, chicken casserole with tomatoes and olives, gazpacho soup, marinated mushrooms, tortilla.
Worst: deep-fried foods, pastries, Catalan custard, chorizo.

France
Best: Provençal dishes such as tuna niçoise, ratatouille, grilled fish, moules marinière.
Worst: rich sauces including meunière, béchamel, hollandaise; fatty cassoulets and stews.

Greece/Turkey/Cyprus
Best: chicken and pork kebabs with tzatziki and salad, Greek salad, doner kebab, lamb kofta, grilled fish, rabbit stifado, dolmades , keftethes (meatballs), tabbouleh.
Worst: moussaka, pasticcio, deep-fried calamari, taramasalata, lamb stews.

North Africa
Best: couscous, grilled vegetables, chicken and vegetable tagine, chicken with lemon.
Worst: brik, lamb tagine.

Thailand/Far East
Best: prawn or chicken sizzles, dry or vegetable curries, vegetable, fish or chicken stir-fries.
Worst: curries made with coconut milk, fried rice, fried desserts such as banana fritters.

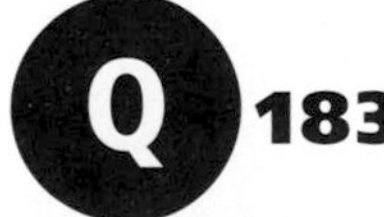

183

Surely the best way to eat out and stay slim is to say 'no' to all the carbohydrates?

Certainly this is one way to cut calories when eating out, and for people who are unsure which choices are high-calorie or high-fat and which aren't, it is a fairly simple and foolproof way of doing so. If you just avoid the potatoes, rice, pasta, bread, couscous and so on, you will save on average about 300–400 calories on the total meal. If you love meat, for example, you may like to do this.

You could probably, however, save more if instead you deliberately go for items very low in fat, and take the plainly cooked carbohydrate items such as new potatoes or plain boiled rice. This is also, long-term, a healthier way of eating – though going the low-carb route now and then won't do you any harm.

See also:

- ▶ Questions: 175, 178–82, 184–88.
- ▶ Feature: 15.
- ▶ A–Z index: Dine out and Lose Weight.
- ▶ Key index entries: calories, carbohydrate, high-protein diets, protein.

When eating out, on balance is it best to have a starter and main course or a main course and dessert?

You can choose starters that are quite low in calories and you can also choose desserts which are quite low in calories, so it's a matter of personal preference. The other questions in this section will point you towards good choices and steer you away from the less good.

There may be something to be said for having a starter, as it will take the edge off your appetite and you may be less inclined to overeat on your main course. It is also the thing to go for if you are following a high-protein, low-carbohydrate diet.

Also, in some restaurants it is quite hard to find a dessert that is on the 'good' rather than the 'less good' list. So my inclination would be to go for the starter. On the other hand, if you love desserts, when the dessert menu is handed round you will need an iron will to refuse, even if you have had a starter!

See also:

- ▶ Questions: 175, 178–83, 185–8.
- ▶ Feature: 15.
- ▶ A-Z entries: Dine out and Lose Weight.
- ▶ Key index entries: desserts, sweet tooth.

Which desserts are least calorific – or should I choose cheese?

Fresh fruit, fruit salads and sorbets are the absolutely blameless desserts, while several others come 'in the balance', for example ice-cream, meringue and zabaglione. Anything with a lot of pastry, cream and/or chocolate and anything laden with mascarpone cheese are all very high in calories, fat and sugar. If you only eat out once in a blue moon, however, I don't see why you shouldn't have what you feel like, and perhaps cut back a bit on your calorie and fat intake the following day.

I would say that a 'good' or a 'reasonable' dessert would definitely be a better bet, with respect to calories and fat, than the cheeseboard. If you choose cheese (much of which will be high in fat, calories and saturated fat), you will also be offered butter and fat-rich crackers, oatcakes, etc. After a starter and a main course, you don't need the protein, fat, etc., that a cheeseboard has to offer.

If you are a 'cheeseaholic' and really do want to try the cheeses on offer, I suggest you plan for this, skip the starter and have a very low-fat main course – perhaps pasta with tomato sauce, or some grilled white fish with plenty of vegetables. Then you can eat your cheese without feeling guilty.

See also:

- ▶ Questions: 175, 178–84.
- ▶ Feature: 15.
- ▶ A–Z entries: Dine out and Lose Weight.
- ▶ Key index entries: calories, cheese, desserts, fat.

I eat sensibly but drink a bottle of wine every evening. Is alcohol consumption the cause of my steady weight gain?

It could be – a bottle of wine has about 500–600 calories in it and, if you are drinking that on top of a normal day's food intake – meaning that the wine is all 'excess' calories – then you could put on about a pound a week (as excess intake of 3,500 calories roughly equals a pound in weight gain for many of us).

If your weight gain has been much slower than this, you are probably eating a little less to 'allow' for the wine. However, the fact remains that it is quite hard to stay slim when drinking anything more than a glass or two a night.

As an example, if you are female with a fairly average metabolic rate, you may need about 2,000 calories a day to maintain your weight. A bottle of wine equals at least a quarter of your day's calorie requirement, so in order not to gain weight you can only have maximum 1,500 calories a day of food. Unless you are careful, it is easy to go over this amount. You would also need to be extra diligent in getting all your nutrients, vitamins, minerals and so on in your food, as the wine contains no major nutrients except alcohol, sugar and some trace elements.

Of course, a bottle of wine a day is double the recommended maximum for a female – you could be setting yourself up for health problems other than your weight gain. The answer to the next question will hopefully help you to cut down your intake by at least half. The Basic Diet in Feature 9 will also help you to shed the excess weight. You don't have to give up wine completely to do so, but more than a glass or two a day is hard to fit into an average slimming diet without the nutritional balance suffering.

See also:
- ▶ Questions: 180–81, 187.
- ▶ Feature: 9.
- ▶ Key index entries: alcohol, calories, healthy eating.

187

What tips do you have for cutting down on alcohol? I have to attend a lot of drinks parties and I drink most days.

First you have to get into the right 'mindset' – you need to want to reduce your alcohol intake. If you really do, the following tips should all help you:

* Drive to parties, so that you can say you are driving. If you like the company present, you honestly don't need alcohol to enjoy the evening.
* Have a pint of water before you begin drinking – thirst can make you drink more than you need.
* Alternate one alcoholic drink with a soft drink, or mix wine with equal parts soda water for a spritzer.
* Sip your drinks slowly and put your glass down whenever you can. If you see a waiter approaching you with a bottle, be strong and turn your back, avoiding his/her eye.
* Single measures of spirits mixed with low-cal mixers are a better bet than wine for many people. A single measure contains only 50 calories and one alcohol unit, while an average glass (150ml/1/4pint) of 12.5% strength wine contains 2 units and about 100 calories.
* Fill your spirits or wine glass with water – nobody will notice that you're not drinking if you don't want to tell them.
* Remember, it's your life – drink (sensibly) if you want to, but not if you don't.
* As a substitute for wine at home, 'adult' cordials, like elderflower, nettle and citrus, mixed with ice cold water, are excellent.

See also:
- ▶ Questions: 178–9, 186.
- ▶ Key index entries: alcohol, calories, entertaining.

188

Because I eat out a lot, I don't want the restriction of a 'set diet'. Are there simple guidelines to make sure I do lose weight?

I think your best bet is to follow the 'traffic light' system outlined in Q113. If you are sensible and don't cheat, this should produce steady weight loss without any calorie or fat counting, or any other fiddly methods of weight loss. You might also consider trying a high-protein/low-carbohydrate diet as outlined in the A–Z. It's not as healthily balanced as a good healthy eating diet should be, but it does achieve results.

See also:
- ▶ Questions: 79, 112–13, 159, 174–87.
- ▶ Features: 8, 10, 13, 14, 15.
- ▶ A-Z entry: Atkins Diet.
- ▶ Key index entries: calories, carbohydrates, high-protein diets, protein, socializing.

189

I have a family of ravenous children and obviously cook a lot, but find I'm always tempted to nibble while cooking; have you any tips for breaking this habit?

The main thing to do is make sure that you are not ravenous while you are in the kitchen and preparing food. What you need to do is eat 'little and often' during the day so that you never reach the 'ravenous' stage, choosing foods and snacks low on the Glycaemic Index as outlined in Q84. Even if you are trying to lose weight, you shouldn't ever need to reach the point where you feel starving.

Also, keep a lidded container on your work-top, filled with things to eat while you're preparing food – crudités with fat-free dip, or dark rye crispbread spread with Marmite, for example. These will add very little to your day's calorie or fat tally and will keep your mouth busy while you cook. Prepare these before you do anything else.

Of course, it is difficult to avoid ever tasting anything while you cook and not how cooks operate – you have to taste to make sure all is as it should be. If you frequently cook your family something that you love and feel won't fit in with

FAT FACT

One in 25 adults in the UK is dependent upon alcohol, and over 30,000 people die each year from alcohol-related incidents or health problems.

Alcohol is implicated in 26% of drownings, 15% of car crashes and 36% of deaths in fires.

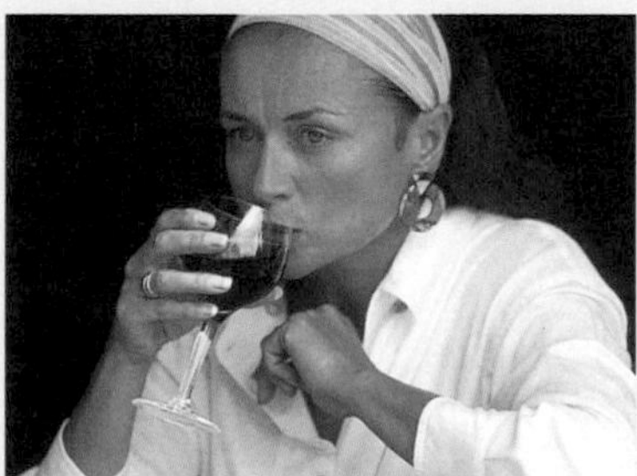

your diet, however, you make life even harder for yourself. If that happens often, perhaps you could do some rethinking on what you're feeding the family. Should they need many more calories than you do, perhaps you could cook 'healthy' for them and simply increase their portion sizes and add extra starch items, such as bread and potatoes. It's always a good idea to get your children keen on lean meats, fish, vegetables and grains, and not relying too heavily on pies, fries, etc.

See also:

▶ Questions: 84, 95–6, 170, 190.

▶ Key index entries: Glycaemic Index, healthy cooking.

190

How can I stop myself from eating the food I bring back from the supermarket for the children's lunch boxes – cakes and so on?

Your wanting to eat the children's cakes suggests to me that you are suffering from fluctuating blood-sugar levels, probably because you're trying to diet and not eating often enough, and/or of foods low on the GI (see the previous question).

You will be tempted to eat sugary items if you get back from the shops, unpack the food and notice cake when your blood-sugar levels are low. Eat a low-GI food before you go shopping and have a ready-prepared snack waiting in the fridge for you when you get in.

Don't try to diet on too few calories – check your metabolic rate and your proper dieting calorie intake using the cross-references below. Also consider giving your children more items in their lunch boxes which perhaps you won't feel too guilty about 'pinching' – fruit, dried fruit, fresh nuts, seeds, good-quality fruit cake rather than sugary sponges, lower-fat crisps and so on. It's good to help them grow up with less of a sweet (and salty) tooth than you have yourself. Take a look at the retraining programme in Feature 13.

See also:

▶ Questions: 84–5, 95–6, 104, 176–7, 189.

▶ Features: 1, 13, 15.

▶ Key index entries: Glycaemic Index, healthy eating, snacking.

191

I have a tight budget and need a main meal of the day of about £1 a head for four. Can you advise on healthy non-fattening meals that would fit the bill?

In general, you can keep costs down by:

■ Buying fruits and vegetables in season and/or locally produced and/or sharing bulk-buys with neighbours.

■ Basing several meals a week around pulses – dried pulses are cheaper than canned ones and only need soaking overnight, and sometimes pre-boiling. If you are organized, it needn't take much time. Add small bits of meat to your pulses for flavour and 'complete protein'.

■ Eating less protein and more grains and potatoes – many of us eat more protein than we actually need for health. Dishes of pasta, brown rice and other low-cost grains or baked potatoes, topped with vegetables sauces and a little grated cheese, are ideal low-cost meals.

■ Eggs are low in cost and you can eat up to 7 eggs a week. Combine them with in-season peppers or spring greens.

■ Some oily fish are low-cost and very healthy – try mackerel or herring fillets grilled with seasonal vegetables, or buy them in cans for quick lunches.

■ Concentrate on slow-cooking methods, like stews and casseroles, when using meat, as slow-cook cuts are cheaper and often tastier. Let them cool and skim fat off the top before reheating (cheaper cuts are usually fattier). If you buy standard mince, pre-cook it to remove the fat.

■ Root vegetable and pulse soups make excellent winter suppers.

See also:

▶ Questions: 192–5.

▶ Key index entries: budget eating, healthy eating.

192

I can't afford to diet – how are people on low incomes expected to buy five fruits and veg a day, for example? I have only £15 a week to spend on my food.

One of the best ways to save money on fruits and vegetables is by buying in bulk, but that is probably not an option for you unless you can organize a co-op with like-minded neighbours. Even then, if you live alone you may not be able to store the food, especially if you don't have a freezer or a cool place. However, this doesn't mean death to your diet – let's look at ways you can eat to slim (and get your fruit and vegetables) without spending over your limit.

First of all, although it is a good idea for your health's sake to eat five portions of fruit and veg a day, it isn't a prerequisite of successful slimming (see Q94).

FAT FACT

Research from University College, London, found, in a study of 2,700 households, that poor women are almost three times as likely to be obese as better-off women.

Even if you manage 2–4 portions a day, you will still be doing better than a great many other people. However, because eating more fruit and veg does help a slimming diet along by 'bulking up' your plates for few calories, let's look at ways to work some into your low-cost diet.

■ Pulses – baked beans, butter beans, red kidney beans, lentils, etc. – all count towards your daily veg intake and are some of the lowest-cost foods you can buy. See the answer to the previous question for tips. They are also low in fat and calories, high in fibre and low on the Glycaemic Index, to keep you feeling full, and have an almost perfect balance of protein and carbohydrate. Completely versatile and indispensable, in other words!

■ Although it doesn't taste as good as fresh, long-life orange juice is a good and inexpensive source of vitamin C and will keep well for several days, even when opened (in the fridge).

■ Fresh fruits that tend to be cheapest are apples, bananas, kiwi fruits and satsumas. Buy whichever is the least expensive at the time and buy enough for the week – one a day. Kiwi and satsumas are highest in vitamin C, but apples are good for the blood and bananas are a great source of energy. You should be able to afford seven pieces of fruit a week at an average of 15p a piece.

■ Basic vegetables in season – such as cabbage, greens, carrots, onions, swede – should be fairly inexpensive and you should be able to buy one portion a day for about 20p. Other veg may also be cheap at times and/or may be on special offer. If you have a garden and are able to, consider buying easy vegetable and herb seeds to grow your own (gardening also burns calories and will help with the diet).

■ If you do have a freezer, or a freezer compartment to your fridge, large packs of peas or sweetcorn kernels can be a good buy. A portion is about 3 tablespoons (80g/3oz) and a I kilo (2lb) pack will last you for about 12 meals. This works out at about 16p a portion. Both are high in fibre and vitamin C and fairly low in calories.

■ For other cost-saving ideas, see Qs191 and 193.

So, following these tips you could have 1 glass of orange juice, 1 piece of fresh fruit, I fresh vegetable, I pulse and I frozen vegetable a day for a total cost of around 90p. As I said, you don't have to have all that – a varied choice of 3 or 4 of these would be acceptable, and the remainder of your cash can be spent on bread, potatoes, cereal, tea and all the other healthy items that can make up a low-cost slimming diet.

See also:

▶ Questions: 94, 191, 193.

▶ Key index entries: budget eating, dieting, healthy eating.

LOW-COST AND EASY – FOODS TO EAT ON A STUDENT BUDGET

■ **Carbohydrates:** bread, dried pasta, rice, couscous, bulghar wheat, egg thread noodles, baking potatoes, breakfast cereals.

■ **Proteins:** medium or low-fat cheeses*, such as Brie, Edam, Camembert, feta, halloumi, mozzarella, goats' cheese; extra-lean ham*, cooked turkey*, eggs, canned tuna, mackerel; baked beans and all cooked canned pulses; fresh chicken thigh portions*, skimmed milk* or buy long-life, natural yoghurt*, Greek yoghurt*.

■ **Fruits:** fresh apples, bananas, kiwis, satsumas and other fruits in season; dried apricots and peaches, prunes, figs, raisins; canned fruits in natural juice; lemons (keep well and ideal for dressings/flavouring).

■ **Vegetables:** fresh tomatoes, lettuce, onion and cucumber (price varies on salads, but low-cost for several months of the year); canned tomatoes, canned peppers, white cabbage and carrot (these roots both store well, good for salads and in soups).

■ **Miscellaneous:** dried herbs and spices, seasoning, ketchup, Worcestershire sauce, soy sauce, vinegar, olive oil, stock cubes, low-fat spread*, ready-made tomato sauce for pasta, low-fat cook-in sauce for chicken, pasta or fish, Marmite, low-sugar jam, runny honey, hummus, curry powder.

(* need to be stored in a fridge. If possible also store fresh fruit and veg in a fridge.)

193

I am a student living in a bedsit with minimal cooking facilities – what can I eat that can be cooked on two rings or in a microwave, that is cheap and filling but non-fattening?

The previous two questions will give you a general idea of which foods are low-cost and healthy, and here I can give you a few more specific guidelines for your own situation. Look at the box above for a list of the low-cost, quick-and-easy foods from each food group that can form part of your healthy slimming diet. Then look back here for ideas on how to prepare these in your bedsit to make them into decent meals that will fill you up without piling on pounds.

Take a little time to plan out what you may need for a few days ahead (but if you don't have a fridge you'll have to buy any starred items that you want just before you eat them) which will save time and money in the long run.

Here are some ideas for meals:
Breakfast: cereal with skimmed milk or yoghurt and fresh or dried fruit OR bread, low-fat spread and low-sugar jam, yoghurt and fruit.
Lunch: egg on toast OR lean ham and tomatoes OR cheese and salad sandwich OR leftover cooked rice salad with chopped apple, ham and apricot OR leftover couscous salad with raisins, chopped onion, carrot and cooked chicken.
Evening: one-pan soup with chopped carrot, white cabbage, onion, canned tomato, canned lentils, stock from cube, soy sauce and seasoning to taste (add some spice if you like); simmer together for 30 minutes.
OR baked (microwaved) potato with ready-to-eat tomato sauce and grated medium-fat cheese, e.g. Edam or mozzarella.
OR stir-fry of sliced chicken thigh portions (ready-skinned and boned) stir-fried in a little oil with sliced carrot, white cabbage and onion, soy sauce and seasoning to taste. Serve with egg thread noodles.
OR pasta shapes, boiled and served topped with ready-to-eat tomato sauce (with basil or herbs flavour), stirred with canned tuna.
OR omelette served with tomato and onion side salad and crusty bread.
Dessert: Greek yoghurt with honey or fresh fruit; low-fat bio yoghurt topped with muesli

See also:

▶ Questions: 191–2, 194–5.
▶ Key index entries: budget eating, healthy eating, teenagers.

Q 194

Can a vegetarian slimming diet give me all the nutrients I need for health?

Yes it can – but even with a normal maintenance vegetarian diet, because you are living off a more restricted diet than omnivores, you may need to try a little harder to get all your requirements. On a vegetarian slimming plan, you have to be even more vigilant about getting a healthy range and variety of foods, because you are eating less and there is thus potentially more chance for shortfalls of nutrients.

If you are following a reduced-calorie diet without meat, poultry or fish, the nutrients that you are most likely to fall short on without care are iron and B vitamins (rich in red meat), selenium (fish and offal) and zinc (offal and meat).

Many vegetarian slimmers also cut down on, or out, dairy products such as cheese, and eggs – partly because they can be high in calories and fat and sometimes because not all vegetarians eat dairy or eggs anyway. This may mean a possible shortfall in calcium and/or protein. (Eggs are also a good source of iron.)

What you need to do to replace the nutrients from meat, poultry and fish is to eat plenty of dark leafy green vegetables and salads, pulses, whole grains, nuts and seeds, dried peaches and apricots (for iron, selenium and B vitamins). If you don't eat dairy, good sources of vegan calcium are poppy seeds, sesame seeds, tofu, fortified soya milk, almonds, soya beans, figs, haricot beans, spinach, brazil nuts, chickpeas, kale, white bread, broccoli, spring greens and white cabbage.

Good sources of vegan protein are tofu, Quorn, pulses, textured vegetable protein (TVP), nuts, soya milk, pasta and whole grains.

If you do eat dairy produce, go for low-fat types such as skimmed milk, yoghurt and cottage cheese most of the time, which will still provide you with calcium and protein, and save medium- or higher-fat varieties, such as Cheddar cheese, for less frequent use (or in much smaller quantities). In fact, by avoiding fish you may be low on the essential fatty acids in the omega-6 group. Replace these in the diet with flaxseeds, walnuts, rapeseed oil and groundnut oil, or take an omega-3 supplement (1,000mg a day).

If you follow these guidelines and try to get as varied a diet as possible, you shouldn't fall short of any nutrients. The Vegetarian Diet in Feature 16 gives a blueprint for healthy reduced-calorie vegetarian eating.

See also:

▶ Questions: 195–7, 299.
▶ Feature: 16
▶ A–Z entries: raw food diets, vegetarian diets.
▶ Key index entries: essential fatty acids, healthy eating, minerals, protein, vitamins.

FOOD FACT

Compared with meat eaters, vegetarians have 30% less heart disease, up to 40% less cancer, and are slimmer and with lower blood pressure.

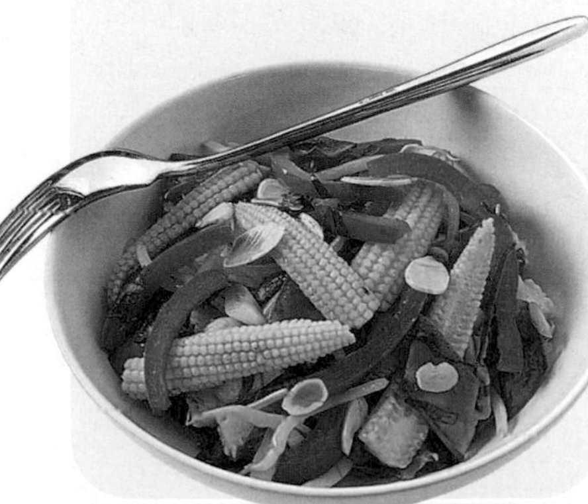

Is it OK to cut out meat and dairy produce from my diet and save calories that way?

If you cut these items out without replacing them with anything else, you will certainly save calories (assuming you had been eating a reasonable amount of them on a regular basis) and will probably reduce the total fat and saturated fat content of your diet. Thus far, good. However, a read of the answer to the previous question will show you that you may fall short of a variety of nutrients if you don't make an effort to replace them. So just cutting out large chunks of your diet isn't as good an idea as you may think.

If you like meat and dairy, why not simply eat less of them (and choose leaner, or less-fat varieties) and follow a varied healthy diet such as the one in Feature 9.

If you don't like meat and dairy, the blueprint Vegetarian Diet in Feature 16 will show the kind of varied diet you should be eating to replace key nutrients such as iron, calcium and protein.

Remember, any kind of fad/restricted diet is not often the best way to reduce calories. As a group, the statistics show that vegetarians are generally slimmer and healthier than meat-eaters, but other factors may be involved. For example, there are many more non-smokers amongst vegetarians, and veggies tend to take more exercise and live generally 'healthier' lives than the rest of us.

If there IS a food connection, it is more likely to be because vegetarians eat more fruit, vegetables, nuts, seeds and whole grains than meat-eaters. They have a similar health profile to people who eat a traditional Mediterranean diet, which does contain fish and small amounts of meat and dairy – but, again, is high in plant foods.

So, on balance, I would say that, unless you have any objection to eating fish and small amounts of lean meat and low-fat dairy, including these foods in your diet is probably the easiest way to get a healthy slimming diet.

See also:

- ▶ Questions: 103, 112, 116–7, 121, 194, 196–7.
- ▶ Features: 9, 16.
- ▶ A–Z entry: vegetarian diets.
- ▶ Key index entry: healthy eating.

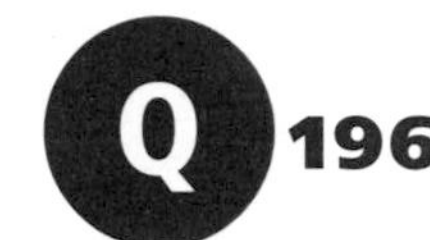

Is it easier to lose weight if I give up meat?

If you have been eating a great deal of fatty meat, I suppose if you gave it all up you would lose weight without making any other changes – but see the previous two questions. Nutritionally, cutting out one large and important food group isn't a good idea. You may also find that you feel bored with your new regime, or feel deprived, unless you replace meat with other foods. There is also evidence that protein foods, when eaten, speed up the metabolic rate more than carbohydrate foods or fat (see the answer to Q88) and may also keep hunger at bay for longer.

If you really want to give up meat, do so – but replace it with fish and high-quality plant foods, like pulses, whole grains, nuts, seeds and so on. Remember – you need a way of eating that you can follow for the rest of your life if you want to stay slim, which is actually more important than getting slim.

See also:

- ▶ Questions: 88, 103, 112, 117, 194–5, 197.
- ▶ Features: 9, 16.
- ▶ A–Z entry: vegetarian diets.
- ▶ Key index entries: faddy eating, healthy eating.

FOOD FACT

A study from the University of York in 2000 found that 'going vegetarian' may be linked with eating disorders in young women. Avoiding meat is a common way for such women to be able to eat fewer calories legitimately. A quarter of the females questioned said that they avoided meat as a way to lose weight.

By changing to a vegetarian diet, will I definitely lose weight?

There are good and bad vegetarian diets, and high-calorie and low-calorie vegetarian diets. Although, statistically, vegetarians are, on average, slimmer than non-vegetarians, there is no cast-iron guarantee that you will, indeed, lose weight by giving up animal foods. I have known vegetarians become overweight on a diet of pastries, cheese pies, oily pasta, sugary desserts and chocolate. It is surprising how many vegetarians do have a sweet tooth.

So if you plan to go vegetarian to lose weight, read the answers to the previous three questions and look at the basic blueprint Vegetarian Diet in Feature 16 – do lots of the foods in it appeal to you? Would you be able to eat like that on a long-term basis? If the answer is 'yes', a veggie diet may be for you. If not, I'd go for a more mainstream healthy diet such as the one in Feature 9.

See also:

- ▶ Questions: 79, 85, 93, 102–3, 112–3, 116–7, 194–6.
- ▶ Features: 9, 16.
- ▶ A–Z entry: vegetarian diets.
- ▶ Key index entries: healthy eating, slimming.

The blueprint vegetarian diet

This plan contains around 1,500 calories a day and is generally within the total fat guidelines for such a diet (explained in Feature 8). There is a little dairy produce in the diet but suggestions for vegans are given.

Instructions:

Every day have 250ml (9fl oz) skimmed milk or soya milk for use in drinks or as a drink on its own. Also have 2 small daily snacks of a small palmful of shelled pumpkin, sesame, sunflower seeds or walnuts, cashews, almonds (unsalted), plus a daily piece of fresh fruit of choice OR a few dried peaches or apricots. Vary these snack choices as much as possible. Unlimited on the plan are leafy greens, salad greens, tomatoes, onions, fresh and dried herbs and spices, vinegars, lemon juice, oil-free/calorie-free dressings. Breakfasts serve 1; lunches and main meals serve either 1 or 2 (explained in the text).

Vegans can substitute soya milk and yoghurt for dairy versions throughout.

Day 1

Breakfast: 150ml (1/4 pint) low-fat bio yoghurt with I small sliced banana and I segmented orange, I tsp runny honey and I level dsp flaxseeds.
Lunch: 400ml (14fl oz) portion of ready-made, chilled-counter mushroom and garlic soup (or homemade using field mushrooms, vegetable stock, garlic, onions and seasoning to taste – simmer for 30 minutes and blend in blender), served with 50g (12/3oz) wholemeal bread.
Evening Meal: Baked Aubergines (to serve 2): slice 1 large aubergine, brush slices with 1/2 tbsp olive oil, season and bake at 190°C/375°F/Gas 5 until soft and golden (about 20 minutes). Arrange the slices in gratin dish and top with 75g (23/4oz) sliced mozzarella cheese (or marinated tofu slices). Pour over 250ml (9fl oz) ready-made tomato sauce (or home-made using own recipe), top with wholemeal breadcrumbs and I dsp grated Parmesan (or chopped nuts) and bake for 30 minutes. Serve with 25g (3/4oz) crusty bread each and a dark green side salad.

Day 2

Breakfast: 1/2 grapefruit, I medium slice of wholemeal bread with low-fat spread and I medium boiled egg (or have 150ml/1/4 pint low-fat bio yoghurt, if not having the egg).
Lunch: Baked Potato with Peanut Butter (to serve 1): bake or microwave one 225g (8oz) baking potato until cooked through, then serve with I tbsp crunchy organic peanut butter (unsweetened variety) warmed slightly in a pan or the microwave and beaten with I tbsp natural bio yoghurt and seasoning. Serve garnished with beansprouts or fresh herbs; mixed salad.
Evening Meal: Chilli Beans and Tortilla (to serve 2): heat 1/2 tbsp corn oil in a non-stick frying pan and sauté 1 chopped onion and I chopped green pepper until turning golden; add a crushed garlic clove, I level dsp paprika, I tsp ground cumin and I red chilli, chopped; stir and add one 400g (14oz) can of mixed cooked pulses, well drained, and one 400g (14oz) can of chopped tomatoes with chilli (or plain), and seasoning to taste. Simmer for 20–30 minutes, stirring occasionally, then crush 40g (11/3oz) tortilla crisps and sprinkle over the beans; top with 25g (3/4oz) grated mozzarella and flash under the grill. Serve with a large green salad.

Day 3

Breakfast: Medium bowlful of good-quality muesli with skimmed milk to cover, I portion of chopped fruit or berries and I level dsp flaxseeds.
Lunch: Homemade Pizza (to serve 2): spread a ready-made good-quality 2-portion pizza base with ready-made tomato sauce (or homemade using own recipe), and plenty of chopped or sliced vegetables of choice (e.g. red peppers, mushrooms, artichoke, red onion, olives) and some chopped fresh herbs of choice (e.g. basil, parsley). Finish with 50g (12/3oz) grated Mozzarella or marinated tofu slices and bake at 200°C/400°F/Gas 6 for 15–20 minutes until bubbling. Serve with a dark-green side salad.
Evening Meal: Vegetable Pasta Gratin (to serve 2): parboil, steam or microwave a selection of 450g (1lb) mixed vegetables

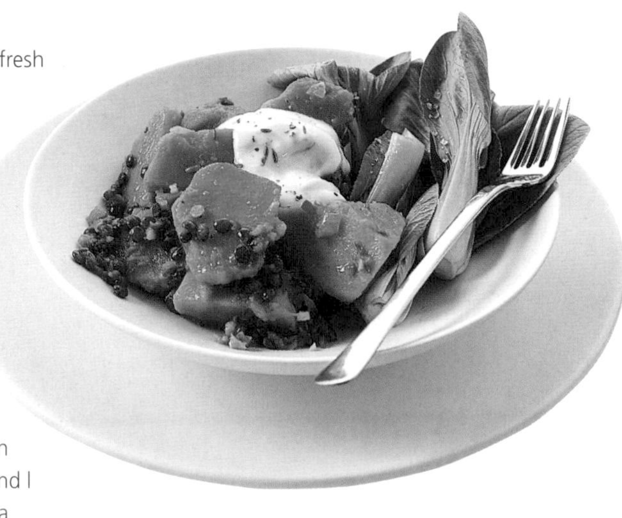

(e.g. broccoli, carrots, peas, mangetout, green beans, sweetcorn), cut or sliced as necessary, until just tender; drain and tip into a gratin dish. Meanwhile, cook 75g (2¾oz) wholewheat pasta shapes in salted water, drain and mix with the vegetables. Make a white sauce by mixing 20g (⅓oz) olive oil margarine with 25g (¾oz) sauce flour in a saucepan over medium heat until you have a roux, add 350ml (12fl oz) skimmed milk and I tsp mustard powder, and stir until you have a sauce. Add 40g (1⅓oz) grated Mozzarella cheese and seasoning to taste, and pour over the pasta and vegetables. Top with I dsp grated Parmesan cheese and brown under the grill for a few minutes to heat through until the top is bubbling and golden. Serve with a dark-green side salad. If vegan, use 30g (1oz) chopped nuts in the sauce instead of the cheese.

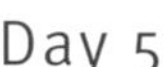

Day 4

Breakfast: As Day I.
Lunch: To serve 1: make a sandwich of 2 medium slices of wholewheat or dark rye bread, spread lightly with low-fat spread and fill with 50g (1⅔oz) Brie and plenty of slices of tomato.
Vegan alternative: fill with 50g (1⅔oz) marinated grilled tofu and I field mushroom brushed with olive oil, grilled and seasoned to taste. I portion of fresh fruit.
Evening Meal: Spiced Lentils and Sweet Potatoes (to serve 2): heat I tbsp groundnut oil in a non-stick frying pan and sauté 400g (14oz) peeled sweet potato chunks for a minute; add I chopped onion and sauté for a few more minutes, then add I crushed garlic clove, I deseeded and chopped fresh chilli, I tsp cumin seeds, I tsp chopped fresh ginger and I tsp ground coriander seed. Stir for a minute or two, then add 200g (7oz) cooked (or canned) brown or Puy lentils and 150ml (¼ pint) vegetable stock; bring to a simmer and cook uncovered for 30 minutes, adding extra stock if the mixture gets too dry. Season to taste and stir in 2 tbsp natural yoghurt before serving. Serve with broccoli or pak choi.

Day 5

Breakfast: I large slice of wholemeal bread with a little low-fat spread topped with 150g (5oz) baked beans in tomato sauce; ½ grapefruit.
Lunch: Fruit and Nut Rice (to serve 2): cook 100g (3½oz) brown basmati rice until tender and leave to cool a little before combining it with 50g (1⅔oz) fresh beansprouts, 25g (¾oz) chopped pecan or cashew nuts, I dsp sunflower seeds, 4 chopped dried apricot halves, 1 small chopped banana and a dressing made of 2 tbsp low-fat bio yoghurt mixed with I tbsp hummus, a little lemon juice, and seasoning to taste. Follow with I portion fruit of choice.
Evening Meal: Vegetable and Quorn Hotpot (to serve 2): heat 1 tbsp olive oil in a flameproof casserole and sauté I thinly sliced onion for 5–10 minutes until soft and just turning golden. Meanwhile, cut 200g (7oz) new potatoes into bite-sized chunks. Add I crushed garlic clove and I tsp each ground paprika, cumin and coriander to the pan with a pinch of saffron strands and stir well. Add the potato chunks with 175g (6oz) Quorn chunks, 75g (2¾oz) spring greens, 200g (5oz) canned chopped tomatoes, 5 tbsp vegetable stock and seasoning to taste. Stir again, cover and cook in the oven preheated to 180°C/350°F/Gas 4, or on the hob, for about 45 minutes or until all is tender. Serve with 25g (¾oz) crusty bread each.

Day 6

Breakfast: One medium bowlful of good-quality muesli with skimmed milk to cover, I piece of chopped fruit or berries and I dsp flaxseeds.
Lunch: One 400ml (14fl oz) bowlful of ready-made chilled lentil soup (or homemade using own recipe) served with 1 large slice of wholemeal or dark rye bread; I orange.
Evening Meal: Wholewheat tagliatelle (or other pasta) cooked in boiling salted water until barely tender. Toss with olive oil, rocket or baby spinach leaves and 10g (2tsp) freshly grated Parmesan or 50g (12/3 oz) diced firm tofu.

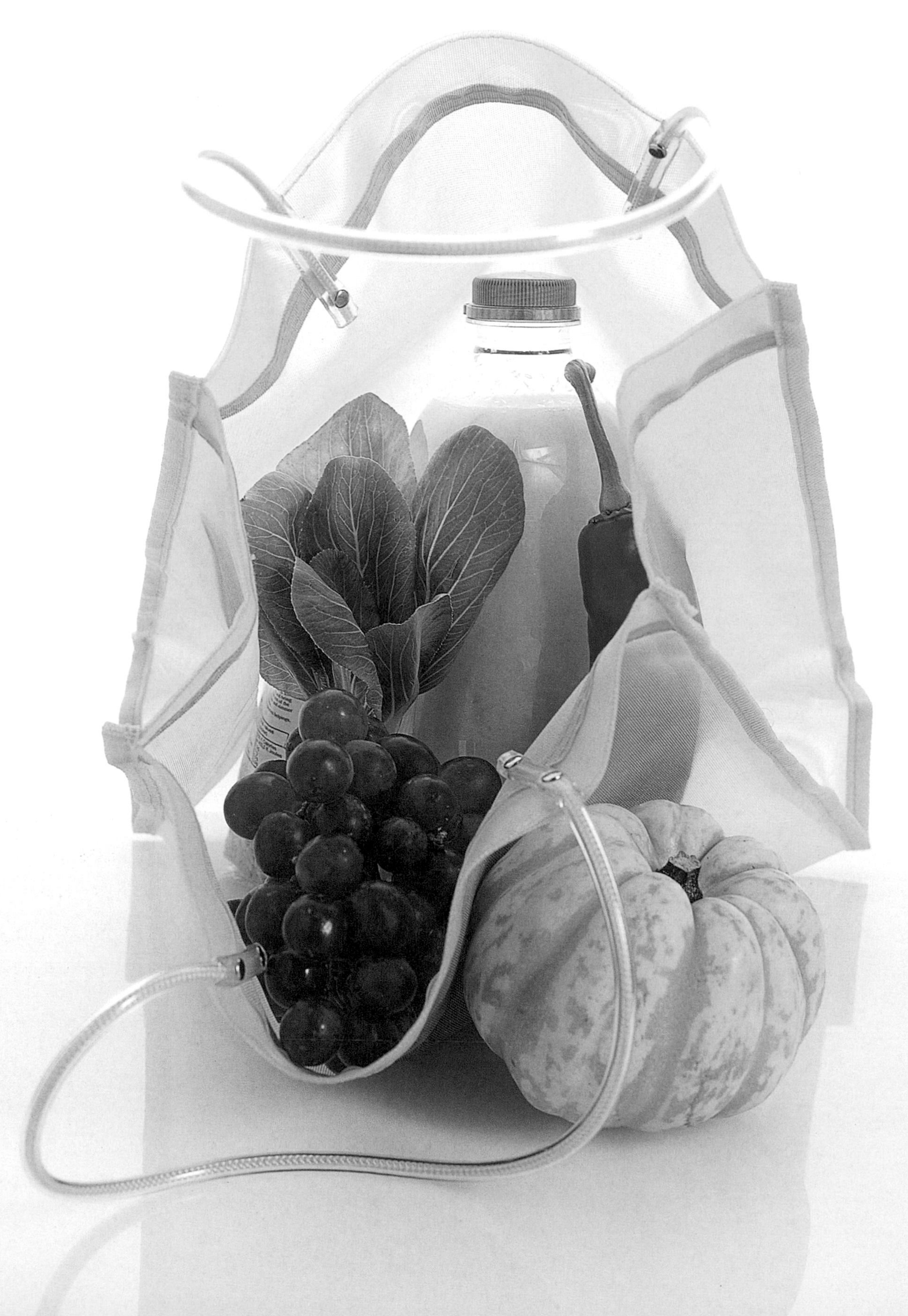

Section Six

For women only

In the Western world, more women than men are obese, and it isn't hard to see why. Although men have their own problems, it does sometimes seem as though women have more odds stacked against them in their efforts to stay slim.

From adolescence through to late mid-life, they need to cope with the physiological fluctuations of monthly periods, most will experience pregnancy and lactation, and all will go through the menopause. All these life events can affect women's ability to stabilize their weight. Hormonal changes mean that mood, too, may be affected and this can, in turn, bring problems in coping with food. All this can have a cumulative effect on weight over the years.

It is also true that, in the majority of households, it is the female who organizes the menus, shops for food, prepares and cooks most of the meals. Also, the relationship with food seems to be more complicated – perhaps more compelling – in women than it is for men.

This section looks at all the problems specific to women attempting to control their weight.

However hard I try to lose my stone, every month before my period I put on around 5 pounds. How can I avoid this?

Much of this weight gain is fluid, not fat, which accumulates as a result of changes in the levels of the hormones oestrogen and progesterone at this time. You will notice that in the few days before your period you don't 'go to the loo' as often as usual. Some of the weight gain may also be due to constipation – a common problem at the same time of the month and again because the hormones tend to relax the muscles of the colon and so elimination isn't so efficient. You may also suffer from bloating through extra production of gas in the intestines, once more because of the hormonal influence.

Once the period gets under way, the fluid is excreted in the urine, the constipation and bloating disappear and, hopefully, everything is back to normal – along with your weight. More help with minimizing fluid retention appears in the answer to Q 203 and in Feature 17.

However, if you eat more than your body needs for fuel (you create a positive calorie balance – see Q 18) in the few days before your period as well, over time, you may put on weight. If you think you are eating a lot more than normal at this time, see Qs 199-202. You do burn up extra calories in the pre-menstrual period, so a little extra food won't put body fat on you, however.

Women trying to slim should not weigh themselves in the week before a period as this weight gain can make you depressed, even if you know it's not fat. An ideal solution is to weigh yourself no more than once a month, say, on the last day of your period. Then you get a real idea of how the slimming campaign is going.

See also:

- Questions: 199–203.
- Feature: 17
- A–Z entry: diuretic diets.
- Key index entries: constipation , fluid retention, hormones, metabolism, PMS.

Before my period, and now and then at other times of the month, I crave sweet foods, particularly chocolate. Why is this and what can I do about it?

As background, first read Qs133 and 139, which give you general information on carbohydrate and chocolate cravings.

The reason that so many women do have cravings for sweet foods before a period is, it seems, usually because of the lack of circulating hormone oestrogen. Oestrogen is a 'stimulating' hormone for women, increasing production of serotonin (nature's Prozac), norepinephrine (noradrenaline) and endorphins (natural painkillers and pleasure-stimulators). Oestrogen is at its peak in your body at ovulation (mid-cycle) and at this time women often describe feeling particularly well and happy.

After ovulation, oestrogen levels decline quite rapidly and by the time the period is due they are at their lowest, and PMS is in full onslaught in many women. This may trigger the cravings for sweet foods – it could be the body's way of replacing the chemicals like serotonin, which will make you feel better. See also Q200, which explains about the other female hormone, progesterone, and cravings.

This is one explanation, but there could be others, and causes may vary from woman to woman. Production of insulin – the hormone regulating blood-sugar levels – may also be affected by female hormonal fluctuations, adding to the 'chaos'.

One thing does seem to be certain – once you start giving in to the sweet food cravings, they are very difficult to control or stop. This is because the blood-sugar levels may fluctuate (see Qs85 and 86). Experts in PMS and diet advise eating 'little and often', using foods low on the Glycaemic Index (see Q84) and high in fibre in the week or so before a period, as a good way to control sweet cravings at this time. Some examples of such snacks are: an apple and a dark rye crispbread; a pot of natural bio yoghurt and a few dried apricots; a pear and a few spoonfuls of baked beans. These snacks also have the benefit of offering a little natural sugar – fructose. Your main meals should be as near to the types suggested in Feature 9 as you can make them and following the programme in Feature 13 should also help.

Some experts recommend chromium supplements, which some women find help ease the cravings, but there is no hard scientific evidence that these work, only anecdotal evidence. Never allow yourself to get too hungry at this time – and see Q201 for an explanation of increased hunger pre-periods.

See also:

- Questions: 84–6, 133, 139, 198–202.
- Features: 9, 13, 17.
- A–Z entries: chromium, Glycaemic Index diets, Sugar Busters.
- Key index entries: blood-sugar levels, cravings, Glycaemic Index, healthy eating, hormones, PMS, serotonin.

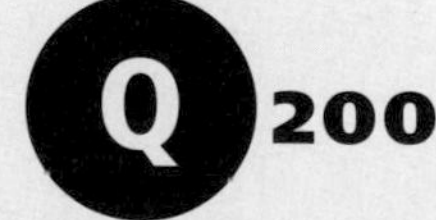

At period time I crave carbohydrates, particularly bread. Why is this?

In premenstrual cravings, some women go for very sweet foods, others prefer very high 'doses' of bread, potatoes, pasta and other starchy carbohydrates – and, indeed, some women crave both. You should read the previous question, but it is also likely that fluctuating levels of progesterone may be at play here.

After ovulation, progesterone levels increase for a few days until the body is sure that it isn't pregnant, then levels of this hormone drop rapidly until, just before the onset of the period, levels of both progesterone and oestrogen are low. (If you become pregnant, progesterone levels will remain high throughout the pregnancy and, interestingly, it seems that post-pregnancy, it is the sudden drop in progesterone that may cause postnatal depression.)

Progesterone is the 'calming' hormone, as opposed to oestrogen's 'stimulating' properties, and just before your period your body may signal to your brain that it needs an alternative source of 'calming'. Starches are the best of all foods at producing this effect.

Your doctor should be able to advise you on possible therapy which will help to ease premenstrual hormonal upheaval and therefore food cravings. However, a good, healthy diet, such as that in Feature 9, can go a long way towards easing these problems, and the plan in Feature 17 may be of extra help.

It is important to try to avoid alcohol and coffee in the premenstrual phase, as these tend to make all the symptoms worse, and to get your carbohydrates from 'whole' sources, such as whole grains, pulses and root vegetables, rather than from refined foods.

See also:

▶ Questions: 84–6, 133, 198–9, 201–3.
▶ Features: 9, 13, 17.
▶ A–Z entries: Glycaemic Index diets, low-fat diets.
▶ Key index entries: carbohydrates, comfort eating, cravings, Glycaemic Index.

Q 201

I definitely feel hungrier and eat more in the few days before my period is due. Do you have a cause and cure?

A read of the answers to the previous two questions may help you to understand why you may get cravings for carbohydrate foods. However, many women, whether or not they get cravings, simply feel hungrier and eat much bigger portions of normal meals before their periods, and then worry that this will either cause weight gain or prevent weight loss if they are trying to slim.

There is a physiological reason for this – aided by the increase in progesterone, women's metabolic rates speed up after ovulation and before their period. This means that you burn more calories and your body 'tells' you that you need more calories to cover this extra energy burst. You can tell your metabolic rate is increased because after ovulation you will tend to feel hotter (you tend to wear fewer layers or want the heat turned down lower). Average increased energy expenditure is thought to be around 250 calories a day, but it could be more for many women.

So don't feel too bad about yourself when you find you're eating more before your period; unless you actually go completely overboard, it shouldn't hinder your diet or make you fat and therefore there is no need for a 'cure' as such. Follow the tips in the answers to the previous few questions on what and when to eat.

See also:

▶ Questions: 198–200, 202–3.
▶ Features: 9, 13, 17.
▶ Key index entries: appetite, healthy eating, hormones, hunger.

FAT FACT

98% of women – and 68% of men – get food cravings from time to time. However, for women, the most common time for these to occur is in the week preceding their period.

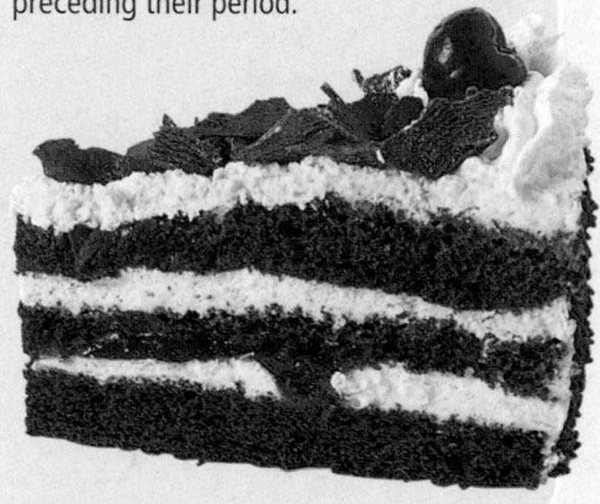

Q 202

I tend to suffer from depression before my period is due and this makes me 'comfort' eat. What can I do about it?

A healthy diet (all the time, not just in the days before your period) can help to alleviate PMS symptoms, including depression. Such a diet will include plenty of complex carbs, vitamin B-complex rich foods such as whole grains, lean meat, fish, nuts, seeds, lentils and vegetables. Vitamin B6 is particularly linked with easing of PMS symptoms and is found in good amounts in fish, poultry, fortified breakfast cereals and nuts. There is also some evidence that a diet rich in essential fatty acids (plant oils, oily fish), calcium (low-fat dairy produce, dark leafy greens, white fish) and magnesium (found in many of the foods listed already) can help minimize PMS symptoms, including depression.

The diet will also help regulate blood sugar levels and reduce the physical need to comfort eat. For more information on comfort eating and food cravings, see the cross-references below. It may also be an idea to see your doctor, who may be able to help in other ways – for example, going on the contraceptive pill can minimize PMS and depression by altering hormone balance.

See also:

- Questions: 133, 156, 198-201, 203.
- Features: 9, 13, 17.
- Key index entries: comfort eating, cravings, depression, healthy eating, hormones, PMS.

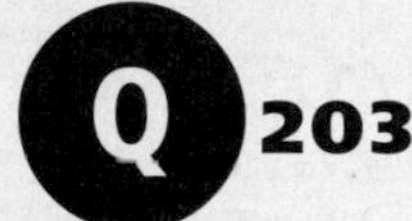

203

Before every period I swell up due to fluid retention, which makes me feel fat and miserable. What can I do about it?

Again, it's those female hormones at work here – according to some experts, oestrogen tends to make the body retain salt, which in turn means water retention. (At any time of the month, if you eat a lot of salt your body will retain extra water because it is literally trying to dilute the extra salt to safe levels.) Other experts believe that lack of vitamin B6 and/or magnesium, both of which are important in retaining fluid balance, may cause pre-menstrual fluid retention.

The truth is that we still don't know exactly what causes PMS fluid retention in women (and why most don't suffer from it). The fluid will probably become most apparent in your breasts and abdomen and can cause not only bloating and weight increase but also pain, especially in the breasts (although not all premenstrual breast pain is due to fluid retention)

You can help to minimize this fluid retention by eating a low-salt diet and by avoiding foods containing highly refined starches and sugars, such as cakes and biscuits, which also contribute to fluid retention (the 'blotting paper' syndrome). It is also wise to avoid all the salty, sugary, refined foods and drinks in any case, as they add little to your diet in terms of nutrition and, as we've seen in previous answers, such snacks can add to your premenstrual misery by making cravings and other symptoms worse. High insulin levels, stimulated by sugar, can cause more sodium retention, creating a vicious circle.

A diet rich in potassium will also help eliminate fluid – most fruits and vegetables contain good amounts of potassium. Foods rich in vitamin B6, magnesium, calcium, vitamin E and essential fatty acids may also help. You should also drink plenty of water, as this helps to dilute the salt – paradoxically, this won't increase the fluid retention. Although coffee is a diuretic, it's wise to avoid it at this time of the month as it can aggravate PMS symptoms, especially breast pain.

You will find more information on foods and drinks that can help both with PMS symptoms and can act as 'diuretics' (ridding your body of surplus water) in Feature 17. If you find it hard to cut right back on sugary and salty foods, try the retraining programme in Feature 13. Don't take diuretic pills – long-term, they can actually increase the fluid retention problem and have other adverse effects.

Lastly, don't forget that a day or so after your period begins your body fluid level should return to normal. A healthy diet all month long will help the symptoms to be less severe next month.

See also:

- Questions: 198–202.
- Features: 13, 17.
- A–Z entries: diuretic diets, diuretics.
- Key index entries: fluid retention, hormones, PMS, salt, water.

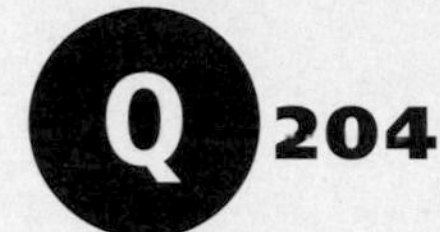

204

Why do women naturally have much more body fat than men?

Women's extra body fat is there for a purpose. A certain amount of fat is essential for women to ovulate and menstruate and, therefore, in order for them to have children. If a woman's body fat percentage drops below about 17% – and, indeed, if her Body Mass Index drops below about 18 – then she is at risk of losing her periods. Women tend to store fat on hips and thighs, which in past eras would supply long-term energy, if necessary, for pregnancy and breast-feeding when food supplies were uncertain.

Another reason why women have fat is to attract the male. Fat on the hips and thighs and breasts gives women the classic curvy 'hour-glass' figure that men are said to prefer. It is only in fairly recent times that thinness has been so sought after – and, even today, surveys show that a majority of men still prefer women not to be too slim. So, well-distributed fat has been nature's way of ensuring attraction and survival of the species.

FAT FACT

A major Internet survey of young women found that 85% dieted not to please men but because they felt pressurized by other women to do so. Only about 15% of them said that men had criticized their size or shape in any way.

Women's fat percentage and distribution seems to be governed by the hormone oestrogen – interestingly, when men take oestrogen as part of a sex-change process they develop extra fat on their hips and thighs.

See also:

- Questions: 1–2, 29–30, 34, 41, 45.
- Features: 3, 4
- Key index entries: body fat, body mass index, hormones.

FAT FACT

According to the World Health Organization, after puberty both males and females develop a greater taste for fat in their diets – but the rise in fat appetite starts earlier and is much greater in females. This may be due to females being genetically programmed to lay down fat stores in preparation for pregnancy.

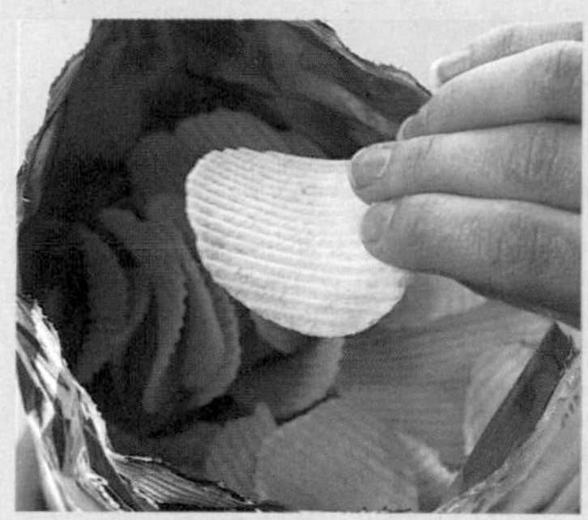

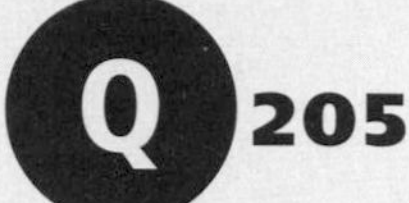

Q 205

I have been dieting and regaining weight for 20 years now. Is my metabolism shot to pieces?

The idea that yo-yo dieting permanently lowers your metabolism has almost gone into folklore now – but it isn't altogether true. Go back and read the answers to Q6, Feature 1 and Qs 32–34 first to get the background on your metabolic rate, weight loss and weight cycling (yo-yoing).

As you will have seen now, if you lose weight and then regain it, there is a tendency for your body to contain less lean tissue (muscle) after you have dieted and then regained the weight than it did before you began dieting. This is because when you lose weight you lose lean tissue and fat, but when most people put weight back on, they gain mostly fat. Fat is less metabolically active than lean and so repeated dieting and weight regaining will predispose the yo-yo dieter to having a lowered metabolic rate, making it slightly harder to lose weight next time.

However, most studies indicate that the change in lean tissue isn't great – particularly if you haven't crash-dieted – and that the reduced metabolic rate because of this isn't great either. For example, one famous scientific trial at what was then the government-sponsored Dunn Clinical Nutrition Centre in Cambridge found that the metabolic rates of people after repeated bouts of dieting were not significantly lowered.

(What you will also have found out from reading the earlier questions is that when you lose weight, your basal metabolic rate naturally lowers, whether you diet just once, or whether you yo-yo diet.) The fact is that however many years you have yo-yo'd, your metabolism can 'improve'. As we've seen, an individual's metabolic rate isn't a static, unchanging thing. So even if, at the moment, you have a lower proportion of lean tissue in your body than you would have had had you never dieted, it is possible to increase your lean tissue percentage once again and raise your metabolic rate once more.

The way you can do this is through exercise. When I wrote above that 'when most people put weight back on, they gain mostly fat', I was not implying that this is inevitable. It isn't. If people were to do adequate regular exercise, a fair proportion of the new weight gain would be lean tissue.

Resistance exercise to build muscle, as outlined in Sections Two and Ten, will raise your metabolic rate, as will regular aerobic exercise. Obviously, you are 20 years older now and, even without dieting, as we have seen in Q72, the body naturally tends to lose lean tissue as you age, so you may never be able to bring your muscle percentage up to the level it was in your 20s. However, you can definitely make significant improvements – and I suggest that you follow the programmes outlined in other parts of the book (see cross-references below) and embark on a gentle calorie-reduced diet at the same time, creating no more than a 500-calorie-a-day deficit (see Q104). If you don't aim for too low a body weight and follow all this advice, your previous years of yo-yo dieting should not impede your progress to a slimmer body.

Once at a sensible weight, though, you will need to continue with the exercise programme and understand that, at a lower weight, your metabolic rate will naturally be lower – therefore you need to make a permanent adjustment in your calorie intake to account for this, or weight will return. I stress this is NOT because you are an ex-yo-yo-dieter – it happens to all slimmers. And the more exercise you do, the less likelihood there is of lost weight returning and the more you can eat without gaining weight.

See also:

- Questions: 3–6, 32–4, 206–7.
- Features: 1, 3, 9, 6, 7, 28–30.
- A–Z entries: crash diets, gyms, weighted workouts.
- Key index entries: crash dieting, exercise, metabolism, yo-yo dieting.

The PMS and diuretic diet

The following diet may help to minimize symptoms of PMS such as bloating, breast pain and headaches, and may help beat fluid retention at any time.

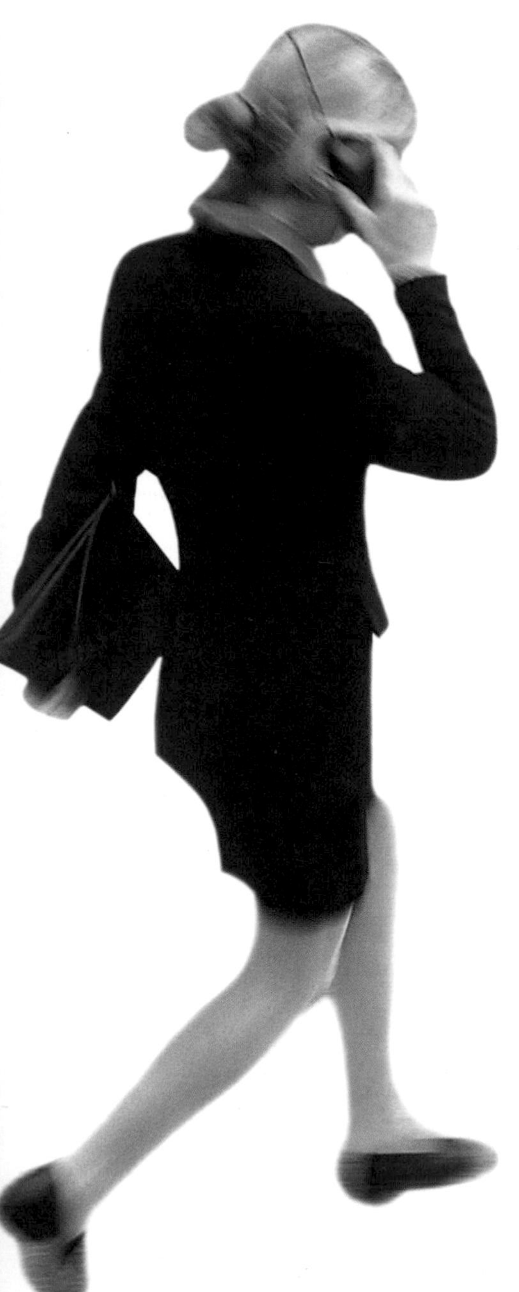

Foods to go for:

Fruits: all fruits are beneficial – almost all are rich in potassium, which balances sodium and helps to eliminate fluid. Particularly diuretic fruits are melon and citrus fruits.

Vegetables: all vegetables are beneficial; again, most are rich in potassium. Particularly diuretic vegetables include asparagus, celery, cucumber, watercress, lettuce, tomatoes, sweet peppers, carrots and onions.

Herbs: several herbs have a diuretic action – one of the best is parsley. Dandelion leaves are good, too, and young leaves can be used in salad; nettles are excellent but best used as a tea (don't eat the raw leaves!).

Fish: oily fish are rich in essential omega-3 fats, which may help PMS symptoms caused by inflammation. Try salmon, tuna, trout, mackerel, herring, sardines.

Instructions:

■ Drink plenty of fluid – water, redbush tea, herbal teas (particularly nettle and dandelion), and vegetable juices are all good.

■ Apart from the meals listed below, have 2 small snacks a day, each of I small handful nuts and/or seeds (unsalted, fresh – walnuts, brazils, almonds, sesame seeds, pumpkin seeds, sunflower seeds and pine nuts are all good) plus 1 slice of melon or 1 piece of citrus fruit.

■ Eat small, not large, amounts of complex starches – whole-grain breads, brown rice, etc. Some people may find they do better on rice and potatoes rather than wheat.

■ Avoid added salt and very salty foods (see page 104 for a list of foods with a high salt content).

■ Avoid alcohol, coffee, cola, sugar (see page 105 for a list of sugary foods), and refined starch (e.g. white flour).

■ You may like to find a source of the sugar substitute stevia, which is diuretic and may not interfere with blood-sugar levels. You are unlikely to find it in the UK except on the Internet. It should be harmless, but it has not been tested in the UK, so I can't vouch for its total safety. For more information, try www.stevia.net.

■ You may like to try supplements of vitamin B6, evening primrose oil, or flaxseed (especially if you don't regularly eat fish).

■ Or try sweet cicely, a herb which you may have to grow yourself as it isn't easy to find at the garden centre or in supplement form.

WHERE TO FIND IT

Good sources of vitamin B6: wheatgerm, pulses, whole grains, oily fish, bananas, poultry.
Good sources of magnesium: nuts, seeds, lentils, bulgar wheat, brown rice.
Good sources of calcium: low-fat dairy, dark leafy greens, canned fish, seeds, nuts.
Good sources of vitamin E: vegetable oils, nuts and seeds, avocados, oily fish, brown rice, asparagus.

The Plan

Breakfast every day:
Have a good bowlful of low-fat bio yoghurt with plenty of fresh fruit (e.g. citrus, berries, melon) and some seeds sprinkled on.

Alternatively, have a fresh fruit and yoghurt smoothie: blend 2 portions of soft fruit (no hard skins) with 200ml (7fl oz) of yoghurt and chill (have a little runny honey in it too if you like).

Day 1

Lunch: A salad of brown rice, segmented orange, sliced avocado, sliced cooked chicken and some walnuts, pine nuts and parsley. Dress with walnut oil vinaigrette made without added salt, and serve on bed of mixed salad leaves.
Evening: I mackerel fillet, baked or grilled and served with a tomato and onion side salad, with a little olive oil and balsamic vinegar vinaigrette (no salt) and a portion of broccoli.

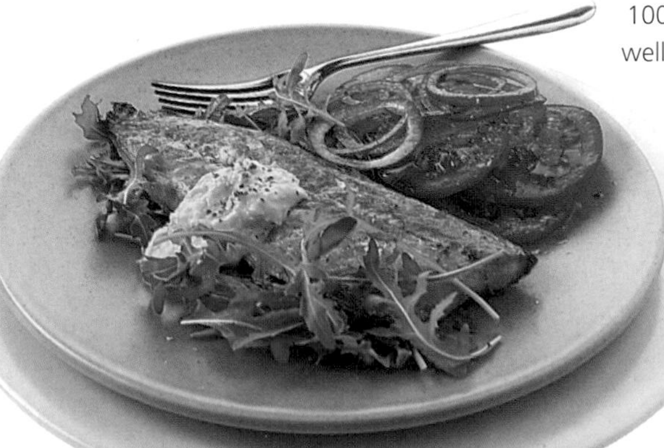

Day 2

Lunch: A salad of asparagus tips, tomato, cooked salmon, sunflower seeds and plenty of lettuce (e.g. Cos or little gem) dressed with a little olive oil and balsamic vinegar. 1 small slice of wholemeal bread.
Evening: I tuna steak, grilled, with I portion cooked brown lentils and a salad of celery, cucumber, lettuce and watercress.

Day 3

Lunch: A bowlful of watercress soup (made with a bunch of good watercress simmered with a little potato, salt-free vegetable stock and a dash of skimmed milk, pepper to taste).
1 small slice of dark rye bread.
1 orange.
Evening: Portion of chicken, marinated in pesto, baked or grilled and served with chard or spinach and cooked green lentils.

Day 4

Lunch: Salad of carrot and hazelnuts in olive oil vinaigrette served with 100g (3½oz) tuna in water, well drained.
1 banana.
Evening: Cooked, drained chickpeas mixed with char-grilled red peppers and served in a mix of chilli oil and balsamic vinegar.
Large salad of mixed leaves and herbs including parsley.

Day 5

Lunch: Asparagus soup (ready-made from chilled counter if liked); I small slice of whole-grain bread; I orange.
Evening: I whole trout, grilled or baked and served with lightly toasted almonds. Stir-fried spring greens or chard; grilled or baked tomatoes; 2 tbsp brown rice.

Day 6

Lunch: Grilled herring fillet served with a mixed leaf and cucumber salad, dressed with a little French dressing.
Evening: Pork brochettes made by cubing pork tenderloin and threading the pieces on skewers alternately with button onions; brush with olive oil, season with black pepper and grill for 10 minutes, turning occasionally. Serve with a stir-fry of mixed yellow, red and orange peppers, sliced, stirred in groundnut oil and with some passata added at the end; 2 tbsp brown rice.

Day 7

Lunch: A medium portion of ready-made tabbouleh with 2 tbsp ready-cooked (canned is fine) green lentils stirred in, plus some freshly chopped mint. Watercress and tomato salad dressed in French dressing.
Evening: A portion of chicken baked with garlic and lemon juice, served with steamed broccoli and carrot; a slice of cantaloupe melon; 1 small banana.

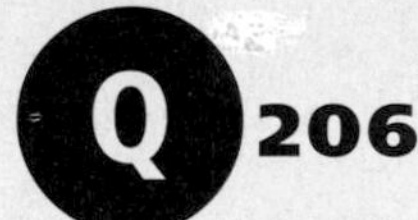

Q206

Have years of yo-yo dieting damaged my health?

Yo-yo dieting (sometimes called 'weight cycling') involves periods of very low calorie intake resulting in weight loss, followed by periods of non-dieting or overeating that result in the initial weight loss being regained, and perhaps further weight being gained. This pattern of dieting is more common in women than in men. It seems that women whose weight fluctuates constantly are more at risk of heart problems than are women who maintain a permanently raised weight.

One recent study published in the *Journal of the American College of Cardiology* found that yo-yo dieting raised the risk of heart disease and heart attacks in women. Worryingly, they found that a mere three yo-yo cycles of losing as little as 10lb (4.5kg) and then regaining it increase the risk by 12%. The main connection seems to be that yo-yoing reduces levels of the 'good' HDL cholesterol in the blood. HDL is one of the main protective factors against coronary heart disease. Other studies have found a similar connection between yo-yoing and heart disease, and there are also possible links with high blood pressure, diabetes and gallstones.

Years of yo-yo dieting may also result in deficiencies of nutrients such as calcium (which may predispose you to osteoporosis over time) or essential omega fats (which influence health in many ways).

However, these adverse effects of yo-yoing may also be true of women – and men – who maintain artificially low weights over a period of time (without yo-yoing). Yo yo dieting may also be bad psychologically, as it can produce long-term feelings of frustration, guilt, depression, anger and low self-esteem.

FAT FACT

According to a leading underwear manufacturer, British women's average statistics have changed quite considerably since the 1950s. The average shape in 1960 was only 34-24-35, now it is nearly two sizes larger at 36-28-38.

The good news is that it is never too late to repair at least some of the damage. If you maintain a reasonable body weight, eat a healthy balanced diet not too low in calories, and take regular muscle-building and weight-bearing exercise, you can improve blood cholesterol profiles, total nutrient profiles and – depending on your age and other factors – you may even improve your bone density.

See also:

- ▶ Questions: 104–12, 205, 207, 300–19.
- ▶ Features: 3, 30.
- ▶ A–Z entries: gyms, weighted workouts.
- ▶ Key index entries: cholesterol, omega fats, osteoporosis, weight-bearing exercise.

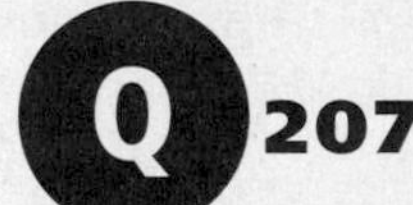

Q207

After years of yo-yo dieting, will I ever be able to lose the weight and keep it off?

As Q205 explained, the consensus of opinion from obesity specialists throughout the world is that the metabolic rate of an overweight person who has yo-yo dieted for years is not significantly lower than that of someone who hasn't, all other factors being equal.

As we've seen, you may have a slightly lower lean tissue mass after years of weight cycling than you might otherwise have had. With correct management of your diet, your exercise levels and what is termed by professionals 'behaviour modification', however, you can alter this state of affairs, lose weight and keep all, or most, of it off.

The main guidelines are as follows:

- Be happy with a final weight that isn't too low (see Section One). For previous yo-yo dieters, a Body Mass Index of around 25 is a better goal than one of less than 23. Aiming too low is a typical cause of the beginning of the yo-yo cycle.
- Aim for slow, steady weight loss of about 2lb (1kg) a month at first, for example, by eating a healthy balanced diet that reduces calorie intake by not more than 500 a day. Recognize that, as you get near your chosen weight, weight loss will slow down considerably, all other factors being equal. Don't worry about this. More detailed help on creating an energy deficit appears in Section Three.
- Take regular weight-bearing and aerobic exercise to help burn off calories and to increase lean tissue. This is perhaps the single most important part of the strategy and, again, Section One will explain this in detail.
- Use Section Four to help motivate you to do all this.
- Once you are at, or near, a sensible maintenance weight, recognize that regular exercise and modified eating habits will need to be part of your life from now on.

Lastly, you may have noticed that I said you can keep all or most of your weight off with these measures. The consensus of opinion is that there are, as yet not quite understood, physiological changes – having nothing to do with all the known factors that influence metabolism (see Section One) – that facilitate weight gain as we age, particularly in 'middle age'. This means that, in all probability, for most people a small gradual weight gain is normal and on the cards at this time, however closely you stick to the recommendations above. In old age, the reverse normally occurs, and a small gradual weight loss is normal.

See also:

- ▶ Questions: 1–40, 74–158, 205–6, 333–65.
- ▶ Features: 1, 2, 3, 9, 12, 13, 29, 30.
- ▶ A–Z entries: crash diets, gyms, Overeaters Anonymous, slimming clubs, very low-calorie diets, weighted workouts.
- ▶ Key index entries: energy equation, lean tissue.

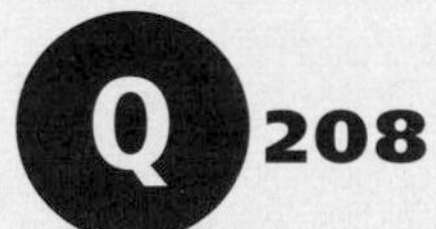

Q 208

Is it true that people are allergic to foods they crave the most?

There doesn't seem to be any hard scientific evidence to back up this theory, which seems to be based more on circumstantial evidence than on proper trials. It's a theory that has had wide coverage in recent years, the idea being that if you crave a particular food – often refined carbohydrates and sugary foods are cited – then that means you are, in fact, intolerant of that food and, by giving up the culprit food(s), you will feel healthier – and lose weight.

Certainly, if you avoid a range of foods such as simple carbohydrates, which provide a great deal of calories in most people's diets, then you will probably lose weight – but simply because you're cutting down on calories.

In truth, most food cravings can be explained by low blood-sugar levels or other hormonal disturbances – e.g. pregnancy or premenstrual syndrome. The 'allergy' theory has proponents but until it's proved scientifically I'd take it with a large pinch of salt (unless you're allergic to it).

See also:

- ▶ Questions: 199–201, 203, 222.
- ▶ A–Z entry: The False Fat Diet.
- ▶ Key index entries: allergies, bingeing, cravings.

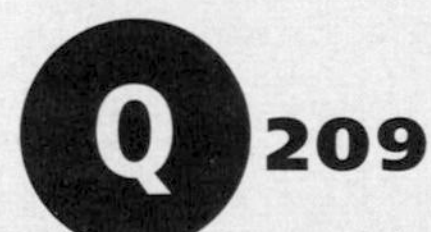

Q 209

Does having sex burn off lots of calories?

Not really. If you just lie there and let your partner do all the hard work, you probably won't burn up more than an extra one or two calories a minute for the duration – hardly any more, in fact, than if you were just lying in bed asleep. The actual orgasm only uses up a handful of calories.

If, however, you are taking a very active role (a good gauge of this is how exhausted you feel at the end), you may well be burning up an extra 6 or 7 calories a minute. Of course, the total amount burnt will depend upon how long the sex actually lasts. The average length of sexual intercourse is a rather meagre 4 minutes. I think we can safely say in that case that, active or not, sex isn't going to help you lose a great deal of weight. One four-minute sex session, including orgasm, would burn only enough calories to cancel out half an apple or one rye crispbread. A brisk walk is a much better idea in that respect, because it's bound to last longer.

However, in the long term, regular (say, at least 3 times a week) sex may bring some other small benefits. During sex, your body manufactures chemicals similar to those released when you eat chocolate and carbohydrates. Therefore, if you are the kind of person who tends to binge, regular satisfying sex may reduce this need and thus reduce calorie intake. Sex and orgasms also help to flatten the stomach, by working the abdominal muscles.

See also:

- ▶ Features: 29, 30.

DIET MYTH

'A session of sex will burn up 500 calories.'

Sadly, not true: the average sex session will burn up just 28 calories.

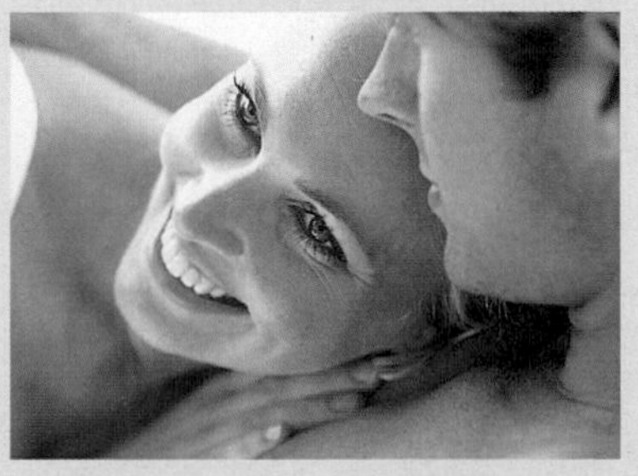

Q 210

What is cellulite?

Cellulite is a term used to denote the sometimes dimpled appearance of fat on the bottom, hips or thighs of women. 'Cellulite' fat is scientifically similar to 'normal' body fat. The dimpled appearance is, however, not a figment of women's imaginations and, although there is still furious debate about this, the explanation seems to be that women's fat cells are grouped in sacs and held in place between the layers of tissue that make up the skin by vertical fibrous strands of connective tissue. These strands cannot expand, so, especially when weight is gained or the skin is squeezed, the fat globules distort and push through, producing the classic orange-peel look.

The female sex hormone oestrogen causes most women to lay down most fat on their bottom, hips and thighs – where 'cellulite' is most obvious. Poor skin tone/elasticity, and lack of exercise don't help.

See also:

▶ Questions: 211–14.

Q 211

Isn't cellulite caused by toxins?

No – there is no scientific evidence for this, although many cellulite 'therapists' would disagree and will provide a 'detoxing' diet as a cellulite cure. If a detoxing diet helps cellulite to look better, it is usually because detox regimes are low in calories and therefore result in weight loss, including some fat and fluid loss from the offending areas. The subject is also usually required to follow other cellulite-busting strategies at the same time, including exercise and massage, which may help.

See also:

▶ Questions: 210, 212, 213–4.

Q 212

Why don't men get cellulite?

Men's connective tissue is, apparently, formed differently from women's (see Q210), with the result that the fat cells don't bulge through in the same way. Also, male hormones dictate that, in men, fat usually tends to be laid down in the abdominal area and trunk rather than on the hips and thighs. Lastly, men's outer skin is much thicker and provides a firmer layer so that subcutaneous fat is less noticeable.

See also:

▶ Questions: 210–11, 213–14.

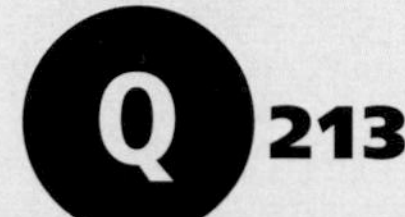

Q 213

Why do even slim women get cellulite?

Even a slim woman has a body fat composition of around 20% fat and, as we have discussed, women's natural oestrogens mean that fat is often deposited on the bottom, hips and thighs, where the cellulite (explained in the answer to Q 210) appears. Skin tone, strength and elasticity may also be poor, and this may increase with age, hence older slim women are more likely to suffer from cellulite than young ones. However, slim women who take a lot of regular lower-body exercise (e.g. runners, dancers, ice-skaters) very rarely have any signs of cellulite.

See also:

▶ Questions: 210–11, 212, 214.

FAT FACT

There are no magic potions to rub in, or pills to take, that you can buy to shift the fat we call 'cellulite'. None have proved effective in properly conducted scientific trials.

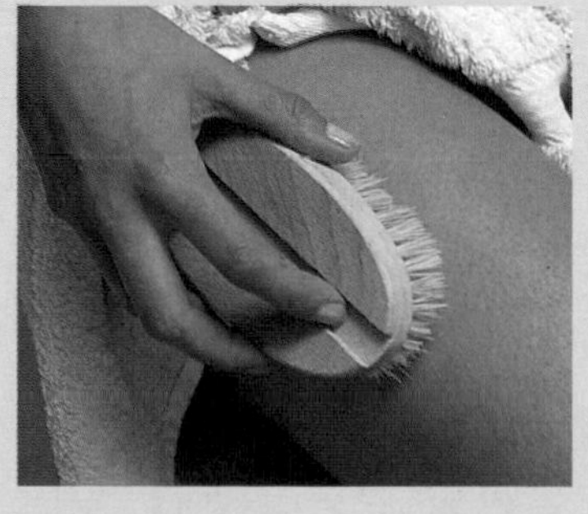

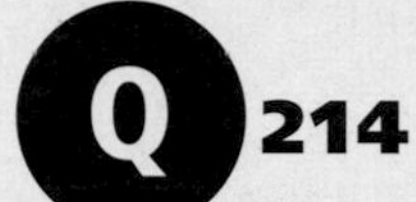

Q 214

How can I get rid of cellulite?

Diet, exercise and massage. A reduced-calorie diet of the sort on pages 92–3 will help to create a calorie deficit and shift the fat forming the cellulite appearance. However, no diet can make the fat disappear from your lower body only – you will lose fat from elsewhere too. Exercise will also help burn off the calories and shift the fat; and lower body exercise, such as cycling, walking, and toning exercises, will improve the appearance of the cellulite. Lastly, field trials show that regular vigorous massaging of the skin above the cellulite (using, for example, a loofah and a low-cost moisturizing cream) may also improve its appearance.

This combined effort will show results if kept up long enough, but don't expect fast results. When the body loses fat, it is first lost from the abdomen and upper body, and last from the lower body area. In this respect women are at a disadvantage to men as the female body may try even harder to 'hang on' to its lower-body fat for reasons already discussed. Think in terms of six months and plenty of effort and you won't be disappointed.

See also:

▶ Questions: 210–13.

▶ Features: 9, 29, 30.

▶ A–Z entries: cellulite treatments, Hip and Thigh Diet.

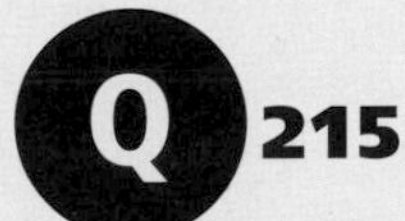

215

I'd like to become pregnant soon, but I'm very overweight. How important is this?

To some extent it depends on exactly how overweight you are. If very obese, you may be advised to slim down to a BMI under 30. Overweight women are more likely to suffer from diabetes or high blood pressure during pregnancy and there may also be other problems, like increased risk of back pain, varicose veins and haemorrhoids.

It is also in your interest not to be obese if you want to conceive soon, as there is evidence, according to the British Nutrition Foundation, that 'excessive stores of body fat can impair fertility', and women with a BMI over 30 have a lower pregnancy rate than those with a BMI under 20.

Go back to Feature 3 and work out your BMI. If it is over 30, see your doctor and discuss your weight with him/her.

See also:

- ▶ Questions: 26, 28–9.
- ▶ Feature: 3.
- ▶ Key index entries: healthy eating, healthy weight, slimming.

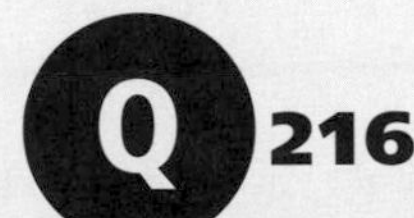

216

I want a baby but I am quite underweight, with irregular periods. Will my weight affect the baby's health?

Women who weigh less than 105lb (47.5kg) are more likely to have a small baby and, according to some studies, small babies may have a higher risk of some diseases in later life – for example, heart disease, high blood pressure and insulin-dependent diabetes. Also, your own health may be at risk if you don't take in enough nutrients during pregnancy – e.g., if you don't eat sufficient calcium, the foetus will take it from your body and this could predispose you to osteoporosis.

Restricting food intake in the pre-conceptual period and during pregnancy can also adversely affect the foetus. It may fail to grow sufficiently in the womb and this can sometimes lead to delayed physical and intellectual development.

In general, the healthiest babies seem to be born to women with a BMI of 20 to 25. Even if you gain a normal amount of weight during the pregnancy, you still run a high risk of having a low-birth-weight baby – in other words, waiting until you are pregnant to increase BMI is too late.

Having a reasonable amount of body fat is important to fertility (see Q204). If periods are infrequent, you aren't ovulating properly; so, if you want to become pregnant, you need to see if, by following a diet increased in calories and nutrients, you can regain regular menstruation. First check whether you really are underweight by finding your BMI (Feature 3). If you are, the Basic Diet in Feature 9 can be used as a weight-gain diet if you increase portion sizes; or supplement it with a meal replacement drink (e.g. Complan) twice a day.

If an eating disorder is causing underweight, read Qs 149–57, and get professional help both for your eating problems and for advice on pregnancy. Indeed, if periods remain irregular despite improved diet, see your doctor anyway.

See also:

- ▶ Questions: 28–9, 204, 319.
- ▶ Features: 3, 9.
- ▶ Key index entries: eating disorders, weight.

FIT FACT

At a BMI of 18, only 10% of women are fertile. Body fat is linked with oestrogen levels, necessary for egg development.

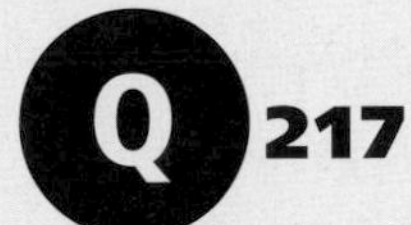

217

What is the best way to lose weight during pregnancy?

Why do you want to lose weight during your pregnancy? If you are seriously overweight before conception, you could lose weight to get your BMI down to a reasonable level (see Feature 3) before conceiving – which is the most sensible way of tackling a weight problem, for both you and the baby.

If you find yourself pregnant and are seriously overweight, you should see your doctor or prenatal clinic dietician for advice. Although there are several possible health problems associated with what is described as 'maternal obesity' during pregnancy, it is uncommon for women to be prescribed a strict reduced-calorie diet during pregnancy. A 13lb (6kg) gain is the minimum recommended for obese women.

If you're slightly overweight when you first become pregnant – say, with a conceptual BMI of around 26–9, you will probably be advised simply to monitor your weight and try to put on no more than the recommended lower amount of gain – about 15–25lb (7–11.5kg) – during the pregnancy. A moderate weight problem is best treated after the birth. If not overweight, welcome your pregnancy weight gain as a sign that your growing baby is well and healthy.

Don't try to follow any kind of calorie-restricted diet during pregnancy without professional and personal advice from those who have your case notes and who can monitor you in person.

See also:

- ▶ Questions: 215, 218–24.
- ▶ Features: 3, 18.
- ▶ Key index entries: Body Mass Index, healthy eating, nutrients, pregnancy.

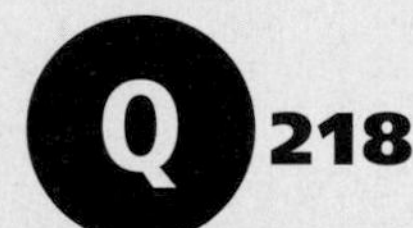

Q 218

Should I eat for two now I'm pregnant?

The UK Dietary Reference values for pregnancy suggest that, on average, women need only an extra 200 cals/day during the last 3 months of pregnancy. Other expert guidelines suggest up to an extra 300 cals/day during the last 4–5 months. Almost every woman is different and these can be but guidelines. The best approach is to 'follow your appetite' (using common sense – I use the word 'appetite' in its real meaning) and if you're gaining weight roughly according to advice you've received (read Q220), you're doing fine.

This means you don't need to 'eat for two' – if you mean doubling calorie intake! Certainly, in the first few months of pregnancy you hardly need eat any extra at all. This is even more pertinent if you start overweight – these early months are an ideal time to ensure you don't put on more, over the whole pregnancy, than absolutely necessary for a healthy baby.

Research shows that in pregnancy the body adapts to conserve energy, especially if you don't eat enough, by slowing down thyroid gland activity. And at this time the foetus is so small it doesn't need many calories – rather, it needs nutrients for growth and health. Also, towards the end of pregnancy the mother is naturally less active and calories are conserved that way, too. Lastly, when you're pregnant the gastrointestinal system becomes more efficient at absorbing nutrients.

When you do begin to eat more in the last half of the pregnancy, as a guide, 250–300 extra calories a day can be covered by one of the following:

- An average chicken salad sandwich.
- Increasing portion sizes of breakfast, lunch and main meal by 15% (one sixth).
- A large (90g/3¼oz) slice of fruit cake.
- A medium (225g/8oz) baked potato with baked bean topping.
- 250ml (9fl oz) semi-skimmed milk and 1 large slice of bread with low-fat spread and Marmite. As you can see, the extra doesn't amount to a great deal.

There is also evidence to indicate that the last thing you should do is to increase intake of saturated fats – found in greatest quantities in full-fat dairy produce, fatty meat and many processed sweet and savoury snacks. Research at St Thomas's Hospital, London, in 2000 found that a diet high in saturated fat increased the blood cholesterol levels in the foetus, creating an increased risk of the baby later developing heart disease and diabetes.

So what is most important during your pregnancy is that you get a healthy, varied, balanced diet rich in all the nutrients needed by your growing baby, as advised by your prenatal dietician (see Feature 18).

See also:

- ▶ Questions: 215, 219–22.
- ▶ Features: 8, 18.
- ▶ key index entries: healthy eating, metabolism, pregnancy, saturated fats.

FAT FACT

Some experts believe that the stretch marks common during pregnancy can be prevented with a diet rich in Vitamin E, lean protein and pantothenic acid (vitamin B5, found in wheatgerm, whole grains, pulses and nuts).

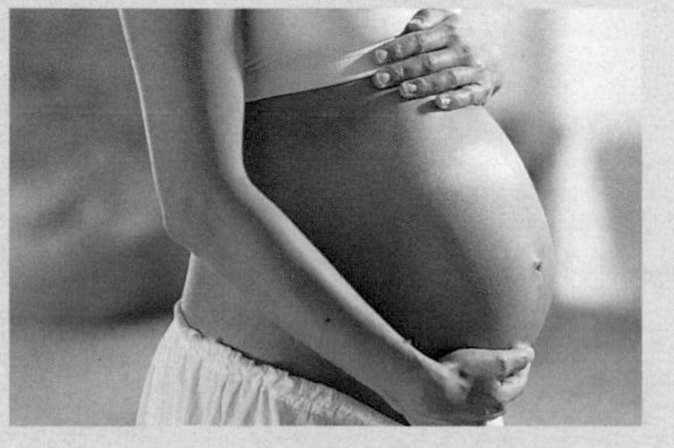

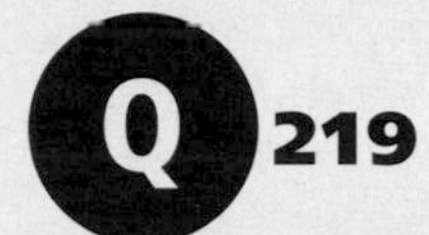

Q 219

I'm putting on weight too fast during this pregnancy; what advice can you give me?

The average total weight it's wise to gain is described in the next question. If you were an average weight (BMI 20–25) at the start of pregnancy, after the first 3 months you should gain, on average, no more than about 1lb (0.5kg) a week until the last 4 weeks, when weight often stabilizes. If you are gaining much more, it's wise to go for a check-up straight away. The weight gain may be fluid, which needs medical advice.

If you know you're eating a lot more than usual (and definitely more than the extra 300 cals/day outlined), this could be the reason for weight gain. Cut down on fatty, sugary foods and substitute complex carbs, like wholemeal bread and potatoes, fruit and, to a lesser extent, nuts, seeds and lean fish or chicken. If ravenous between meals, snack on fruit, rye crispbreads, or similar. Feature 18 provides more guidelines.

If underweight at the start of pregnancy, gaining more weight than average may not be a disadvantage. Talk to your specialist about your fears – they should weigh you regularly anyway and advise you even without your asking. Above average weight gain shouldn't negatively affect baby's health.

See also:

- ▶ Questions: 215–18, 220–24.
- ▶ Features: 3, 18.
- ▶ Key index entries: healthy eating, pregnancy, weight control.

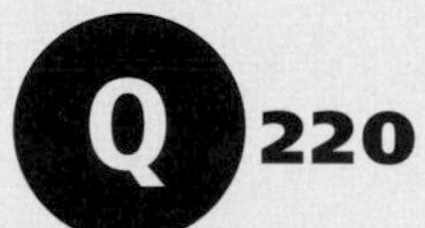

220

What is the right amount of weight to gain during pregnancy?

The trick is to gain enough weight to ensure optimum weight, health and nutrition for the baby, but not so much that you have an uncomfortable pregnancy and/or complications, and are not left with masses of fat to lose after the birth.

The recommendations for weight gain are usually based on those produced by the USA National Academy of Sciences Food and Nutrition Board in the l990s. These recommend weight gain of anything from 13–40lb (6–18kg), depending on pre-pregnant weight. See Table 1 above.

Based on these, ideal average weight gain for the ideal female Body Mass Index of 22.5 is 30lb (13.75kg). This is higher than the ideal gain recommended in the '70s and '80s of 20–28lb (9–12.5kg), which was based on women's average weights in the 1950s – which were considerably less than they are now.

The weight of the foetus, placenta and other essentials is usually about 20–22lb (9–10kg); the rest of the gain is maternal fat. At an average weight gain of 30lb (13.75kg), up to 10lb (9.5kg) would be fat. Research shows that although high weight gain in pregnancy may be associated with more complications, prolonged labour and retained maternal weight after the birth, the extra weight appears not to affect the baby adversely – rather, it may be born with a higher-than-average birth-weight, which may not be a disadvantage. The weight gains shown above represent ideals for optimum health of the baby, and least risk to it.

On average, most gain will take place from the fourth to eight month. A gain of 3lb (1.35kg) or so is adequate in the first three months; after that about 1lb (0.5kg) a week until week 36 is about right.

TABLE 1

Mother's Body Mass Index at conception	Recommended weight gain during pregnancy
Less than 20	26–40lb (12.5–18kg)
20–25.9	24–36lb (11.5–16kg)
26–29	15–25lb (7–11.5kg)
30 or over	13lb (6kg) minimum

See also:

- ▶ Questions: 215–19, 221–24.
- ▶ Features: 3, 18.
- ▶ Key index entries: Body Mass Index, healthy eating, hormones, pregnancy, weight control.

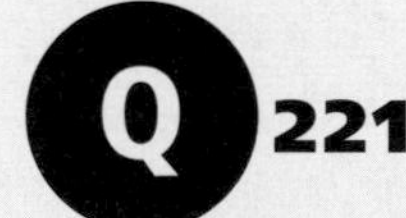

221

If an average baby weighs about 8lb, can't I just put on 8lb so when the baby is born I will be my correct weight again?

The weight that you gain is not just the baby's birth weight but includes weight due to several other factors. The list on the right shows that about 20–22lb (9–10kg) of your weight gain is in items over and above any fat that you may put on, and this is what is called 'essential' weight.

After the birth, you will lose about 10–13lb (4.5–6kg) from the weight of the baby, amniotic fluid and placenta. In the next few days you'll lose a few more pounds as the extra fluids and blood return to normal. The uterus (womb) gradually shrinks, too, so that about 2 weeks afterwards you should have lost most of this extra 'essential' weight of pregnancy. (Breast size may actually increase.)

In addition to the gain described above, most women put on several pounds of fat. Although, as research shows, laying down fat in pregnancy is not absolutely essential to ensure a healthy baby (as it takes what it needs from the mother's tissue), maternal fat deposition is encouraged by the huge rise in the production of the female hormone progesterone. This is thought to be the body's way of ensuring there will be enough food for the baby after its birth. (In times of famine, the mother will make breast milk from her fat stores.) Our bodies still behave as they used to, although famine is much less likely.

At an average gain of 30lb (13.75kg) (see Q220), maternal fat deposits would be about 10lb (4.5kg). Interestingly, this is almost exactly enough to breast-feed baby for the first 10 weeks of its life! (10lb/4.5kg equals 35,000 calories and a new-born baby will need about 500 calories a day or 35,000 calories over 10 weeks.)

By eating very, very carefully during pregnancy you could limit your extra body-fat gain to less than 10lb but you certainly should not consider low-calorie dieting as a way to avoid gaining fat during this time. Breast-feeding after pregnancy is a much better way to get your figure back quickly.

See also:

- ▶ Questions: 215–20, 222–29.
- ▶ Features: 3, 18.
- ▶ Key index entries: healthy eating, postnatal weight, pregnancy, weight control.

TABLE 2

Total weight gain excluding maternal fat during an average pregnancy	
Foetus	7–9lb (3–4kg)
Amniotic fluid ('waters')	2lb (1kg)
Placenta ('afterbirth')	1½lb (700g)
Enlarged uterus	2lb (1kg)
Mammary glands (breasts)	1½lb (700g)
Extra blood	4lb (2kg)
Extra tissue fluid	2lb (1kg)
Total	20–22lb (9–10kg)

Healthy eating for pregnancy

The menus and advice on these pages will be appropriate for the average woman during pregnancy, but you should seek personal advice on diet from your own antenatal clinic dietician, especially if you are under- or overweight.

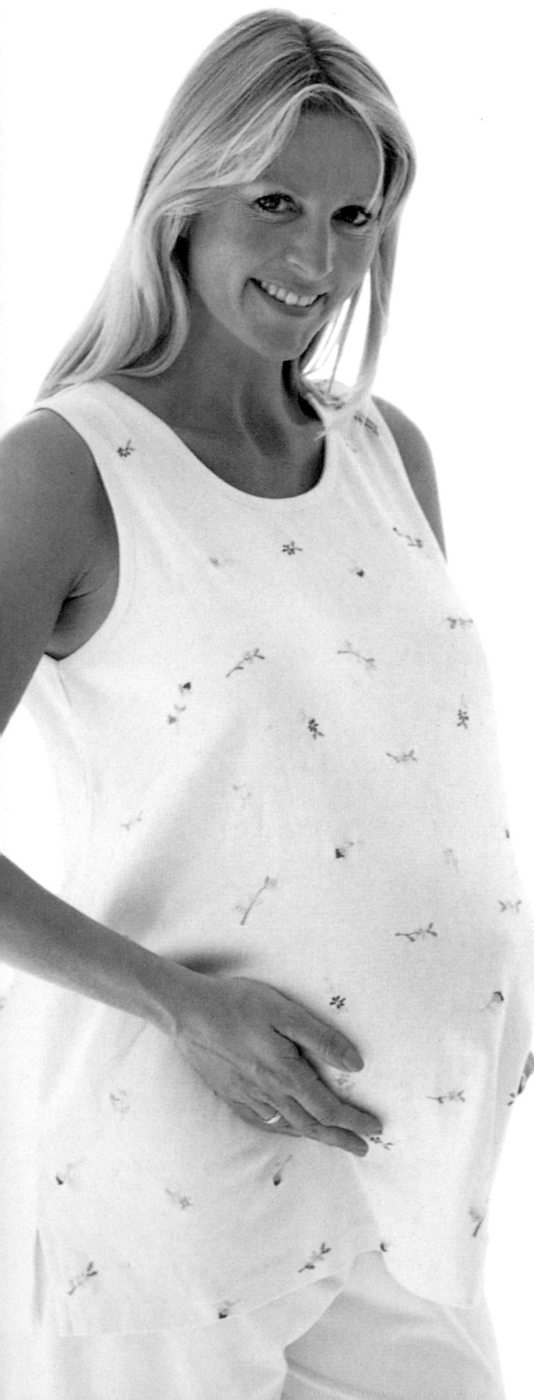

Throughout the Pregnancy

You should follow a basic healthy diet similar to the Diet Bible Basic Diet which appears in Feature 9 on pages 74–5, maintenance version. In particular, however, you need a few nutrients in slightly larger quantities than average (see the box below) and the list that follows shows where to find those nutrients:

Extra protein: low-fat dairy produce, such as skimmed milk, low-fat cheese, yoghurt, lean meat, poultry, game, pulses, Quorn, tofu, fish, seafood.

Extra vitamin A: hard cheese, eggs, orange, dark green and red vegetables and fruits.

Extra vitamin B2: yeast extract, fortified breakfast cereals, seaweed, game, hard cheese.

Extra folate: yeast extract, pulses, fortified breakfast cereals, asparagus, sweetcorn, purple sprouting broccoli, Brussels sprouts and other leafy greens.

Extra vitamin C: fresh fruit and vegetables, particularly citrus fruits, berry fruits, kiwi fruit, mangoes, peppers and leafy greens.

Extra vitamin D: sunlight on the skin, oily fish, eggs, many breakfast cereals.

During the first three months of pregnancy and before conception

At this time you need extra folate – your specialist will prescribe you folate supplements but you can find extra folate within your diet.

During the last 3–5 months of pregnancy or as advised by your specialist

Extra calories: 200–300 a day, to produce a weight gain of about 1lb (0.5kg) a week to week 36. The Food Value Charts at the back of the book will help you choose suitable foods.

Extra vitamin B1 (thiamin): Quorn chunks, yeast extract, vegeburger, sunflower seeds, fortified breakfast cereals, bacon, peanuts, pork, whole grains.

ADDITIONAL DAILY NUTRIENT REQUIREMENTS FOR PREGNANCY

- Extra calories – 200–300 (last few months of pregnancy only)
- Extra 6g protein
- Extra 100ug vitamin A
- Extra 0.1mg vitamin B1 (last 3 months of pregnancy only)
- Extra 0.3mg vitamin B2
- Extra 400ug folate (preconception and for first 12 weeks of pregnancy)
- Extra 10mg vitamin C
- Extra 10ug vitamin D

Other nutrients to look out for

You may be surprised to see that there is no mention of additional iron or calcium during pregnancy. This is because absorption of both rises during pregnancy, and loss of iron in menstruation ceases, so there is therefore no official recommendation for extra amounts of either for adult women. However, you should, of course, make sure you do get adequate amounts of both in your diet.

■ Find iron in dark leafy green vegetables, red and other meats, pulses, whole grains, nuts, seeds, curry powder.

■ Find calcium in dairy produce, fish, leafy greens, soya, nuts, seeds, white bread, muesli.

Also make sure you get enough fibre in your diet – many women in the later stages of pregnancy become constipated, and a high intake of fibre, together with fluids, can help to avoid this.

■ Find fibre in fresh and dried fruits, veg, pulses, whole grains, nuts, seeds.

GOOD SNACKS FOR MORNING SICKNESS AND FOOD CRAVINGS

A small amount of a fairly bland, low-fat food can help to alleviate sickness during the early months of pregnancy. There is no need to go for something high in fat and sugar, such as sweet biscuits or cake. Instead try:

■ Traditional oatcake spread with low-sugar jam.

■ Small slice of white bread spread with low-fat spread and a little organic peanut butter.

■ Dark rye crispbreads spread with Marmite.

■ Small slice of wholemeal bread spread with mashed banana and a little honey.

■ Slice of malt loaf.

All these ideas will also stem off cravings for other less healthy food items which you may find occur later in pregnancy.

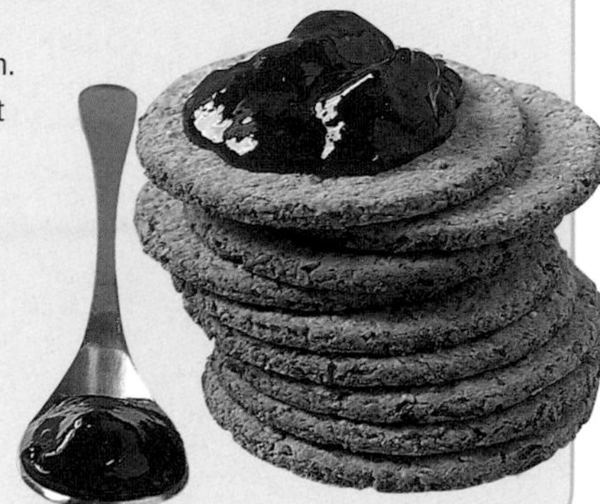

Foods to avoid

■ Liver and liver pâtés and products – because the high amounts of vitamin A they contain are toxic in pregnancy and can cause birth defects.

■ Cod liver oil and supplements – again, contain high amounts of vitamin A.

■ Mackerel, shark and swordfish may contain harmful levels of mercury.

■ Coffee – total caffeine consumption should be no more than 300mg a day (up to 4 cups of coffee).

■ Alcohol – very small amounts may be okay, but it is better to be safe and give up completely.

■ Soft cheeses, such as Brie and Camembert, soft mould-ripened cheese and unpasteurized cheeses, and blue-veined cheeses such as Stilton should all be avoided as they can contain the listeria bug, which can cause poisoning. Cheddar cheese and cottage cheese are fine, and should be substituted in any meal or recipe.

■ Prepacked/deli salads and deli meats – again, may harbour food poisoning bugs.

■ Raw or lightly cooked eggs – may contain the salmonella bug.

■ Underdone or raw meat and poultry – can contain food poisoning bugs.

■ Unpasteurized milk, soil-dirty fruits, veg and eggs – can give you toxoplasmosis.

Sample meal ideas

Breakfasts

■ Orange juice or fresh orange, Weetabix, wheatgerm, skimmed milk, I slice of toast, low-fat spread, low-sugar jam.

■ I hard-boiled egg, 2 slices of toast with low-fat spread, 1/2 grapefruit.

■ Baked beans on wholewheat toast with kiwi fruit to follow.

■ Natural low-fat yoghurt, muesli, chopped orange and added sunflower seeds and wheatgerm.

■ Strawberries with half-fat Greek yoghurt and muesli on top.

Lunches

■ Tuna, hard-boiled egg, tomatoes, Cos lettuce, French bread and French dressing.

■ Lean ham, new potatoes, broad beans, mint, red onion rings and sliced tomato.

■ Cheddar, carrot, hazelnuts, sunflower seeds, brown rice, French dressing.

■ Hummus with pitta bread, onion rings, herb and green salad, tomato.

■ Lentil soup, wholemeal roll, kiwi fruit.

■ Well-cooked chicken slices and chickpeas marinated in pesto dressing, served with mixed salad and white bread.

Evening Meals

■ Roast beef dinner using lean beef, new potatoes, selection of fresh vegetables.

■ Macaroni cheese with added broccoli florets and halved baby tomatoes.

■ Salmon portion with new potatoes or brown rice and two green vegetables.

■ 2-egg omelette with oven-baked potato wedges and a large mixed salad.

■ Vegeburger with crispy potato skins, tomato salsa, and herb salad.

■ Quorn stir-fry with a selection of thinly sliced brightly coloured vegetables, yellow bean sauce and chopped chillies.

Desserts if you feel like one sometimes

■ Low-fat ice-cream with fresh fruit coulis.

■ Greek yoghurt with strawberries.

■ Rice pudding with fresh fruit.

■ Banana with low-fat custard.

■ 8%-fat fromage frais with berries, muesli.

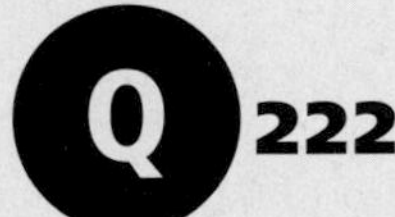

Q 222

If I crave particular foods when pregnant, does my body need their nutrients?

Most pregnant women 'go off' certain foods and develop a strong taste for others – this is normally called having 'cravings' and may be for basic ordinary foods such as oranges, or may be for more unusual items like caviar or dill pickles! Cravings for non-food items, such as coal – which do happen – are called pica.

If you crave fatty, salty or sugary foods a lot during pregnancy, it is best to try to control these cravings, using techniques described in Qs 132–43 and 199–202 for non-pregnant women. These types of foods don't supply good quantities of the essential nutrients you and the baby need, and also tend to be high in calories and perhaps saturated fat (see Q218).

It isn't true that all cravings are a result of your body needing the nutrients they contain – as we've seen, a lot of craved foods contain hardly any nutrients at all except calories. Although some believe that cravings are linked to nutritional need, there is little if any scientific evidence that any craving is based on a physical requirement for a particular nutrient. If you crave 'pica' non-foods, talk to your doctor.

See also:

- ▶ Questions: 132–43, 199–202, 218.
- ▶ Features: 18.
- ▶ A–Z entry: Glycaemic Index diets.
- ▶ Key index entries: carbohydrates, cravings, Glycaemic Index.

Q 223

Is plenty of exercise the best way to keep my weight down during pregnancy?

You don't really want to keep your weight down, as such, during pregnancy – you want to gain approximately the amount recommended for your pre-pregnancy Body Mass Index (see Q 220). If, however, you mean that you see exercise as a way to ensure that you don't put on too much weight during pregnancy, then you are partly right. Regular exercise, suitable for pregnancy, can help to keep you fit and a reasonable weight. It does depend, though, upon your definition of 'plenty' of exercise.

A lot of the more vigorous types of exercise – such as jogging or gym work – become increasingly difficult to perform in the later stages of pregnancy, and may actually be detrimental to the bone composition of the foetus. It may be preferable to cut exercise down to small easy sessions rather than long, calorie-burning bouts. Many women find they're very tired in pregnancy and prefer rest to a lot of exercise.

If you've been a regular exerciser, you'll probably find you can do a lot more than someone who hasn't. If you've only done mild or moderate exercise, though, you shouldn't suddenly begin to do a lot more when pregnant. Walking and swimming are probably the most ideal forms of aerobic (calorie-burning) exercise for pregnancy.

A pregnant women is – or should be – a perfectly healthy woman, and there is no reason in that case why you shouldn't exercise whenever you feel you want to, but you should take advice from your own prenatal clinic on the best forms of exercise for your state of health and pregnancy. NOTE: If you have a history of miscarriage and/or any problems in early pregnancy, seek professional advice before exercising.

See also:

- ▶ Questions: 224–7.
- ▶ Feature: 28.
- ▶ Key index entry: exercise.

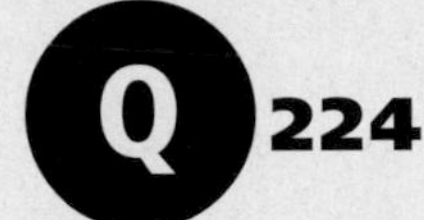

Q 224

Should I put my feet up and avoid exercise now I am pregnant?

If you have been a regular exerciser, there shouldn't be any need – if you and the foetus are healthy – to avoid exercise for the next 9 months. You will probably benefit from continuing to exercise in a moderated way, as you will find you get tired and, later, your bump will make some exercise hard, if not dangerous. There is new evidence that vigorous weight-bearing exercise later in pregnancy significantly reduces bone density in the baby.

Some women do use pregnancy as a great excuse to do little and eat plenty – but live to regret it after the birth, when they are overweight and unfit.

As with many things in life, common sense and moderation are the keys. Check with your prenatal clinic that it's okay to do what exercise you want to do. NOTE: Women with a history of miscarriage and/or with any problems in early pregnancy should seek professional advice before doing any exercise.

See also:

- ▶ Questions: 223–7.
- ▶ Key index entries: exercise, pregnancy.

FAT FACT

Vitamin company Sanatogen did a survey of pregnant women's cravings in 2000 and amongst the top ten most weird were garlic bread dipped in fruit yoghurt, ice lollies dipped in mustard, custard-covered beetroot and stuffed olives with lemon curd.

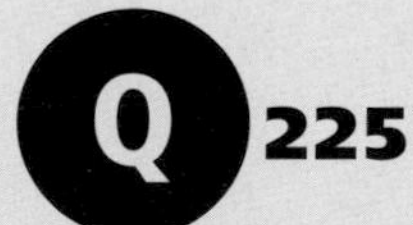

225

When my baby is born what is the best way to get my figure back to normal?

Breast-feeding, healthy diet and progressive exercise. Because breast-feeding uses up around 500 calories a day, it is an ideal way to create a small calorie deficit so that you gradually lose any surplus pounds you gained during the pregnancy. See the answer to Q229 for more information on that. Breast-feeding also contracts the uterus quickly, so that it shrinks back to normal size, has many health benefits for the baby, and is convenient, so I strongly recommend breast-feeding rather than bottle-feeding.

You do need extra nutrients while breast-feeding, and the answer to Q229 will also explain how to ensure those in your diet. Whether or not you are breast-feeding, you don't need high-fat, high-sugar and/or high-salt snacks, such as cakes, biscuits, crisps, creamy desserts and so on. So if you were eating a few too many items like that in your pregnancy, now is the time to make a big effort and cut right back on them.

You also need to begin to exercise your body back into shape. Qs 226 and 227 deal with that. There is no great rush, though – many women do feel very tired and some feel stressed postnatally and you shouldn't feel guilty if you don't exercise every spare minute of the day. Just do what you can to make yourself look and feel better – anything is better than nothing, and making a little time for yourself each day is an important part of getting your 'self' back together in the months after your baby is born.

See also:

- Questions: 226–9.
- Key index entries: exercise, healthy eating.

THE POSTNATAL 'T' FACTOR

A gene – called 825T – has been discovered which explains why some women get their figures back quickly after the birth and others don't, however hard they try. Reported in The Lancet in 2000, the gene causes women who have it to remain overweight in the year after giving birth, while women without 825T regain their figures without trouble and, seemingly, without doing anything special. About a third of white Western women may be carriers of 825T – but, even if you do have the 'fat gene', regular exercise of at least two hours a week can overcome the disadvantage, the researchers found.

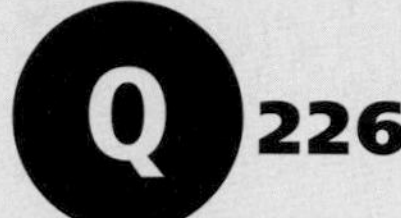

226

How soon after the birth can I begin exercising?

If you had a non-Caesarean delivery, you should get out of bed and walk around a little within hours of giving birth, to improve circulation. In the first day or two, you can do very gentle exercise to help get your stomach muscles working again (see the box overleaf) and gradually increase the amount of walking that you do.

Once home you can carry on walking – taking the baby out in its buggy, for example – twice a day for short periods. You can begin the exercise programme in Feature 6 a week after the birth, taking it gently at first and stopping immediately if anything hurts. It is better to do two or three moves correctly and slowly. Also pay attention to posture as this will quickly help you get your figure back.

If you have had a bikini-incision Caesarean, delay all the above until after three weeks, while those who have had an 'up and down' Caesarean should wait until after the six-week check-up before beginning a full exercise programme. After the six-week check-up you can do whatever exercise you want, within reason, bearing in mind that with a small baby to cope with most mothers do find extra rest and sleep just as important as exercise.

See also:

- Questions: 225, 227.
- Features: 5–7.
- Key index entries: exercise, posture.

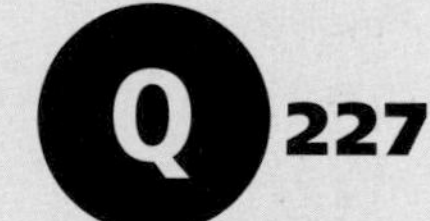

227

What is the best exercise to get my stomach back into shape after the birth?

Unless you've had a Caesarean, begin gently reminding your stomach muscles they exist in the first day by doing the exercises overleaf. Carry on with this for the first week and then, if you feel up to it, begin the 10-minute tone routine in Feature 6 (or just its stomach exercises). Make the curl-up as easy as you like – as long as you do it regularly, your muscles will gradually strengthen and you can come up further as you progress. There's no rush.

After your six-week check-up, if you still have a 'tummy' (most do), the scales may tell you if some of it is fat, in which case see Qs 228/9, and you can also incorporate other stomach-strengthening exercise, including hill-walking and swimming. Don't forget – breast-feeding is great for helping to shrink your stomach back to size.

See also:

- Questions: 225–6.
- Feature: 6.
- Key index entry: exercise.

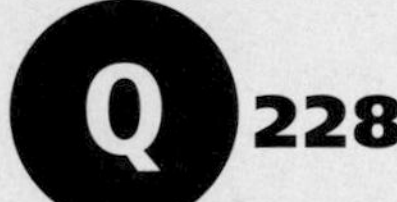

Q 228

How many cals/day should I eat to lose weight after the birth if not breast-feeding?

Follow the Basic Diet in Feature 9 for gradual weight loss, or work out your Basal Metabolic Rate (Feature 1) and, using Q104, work out how many cals/day you need to lose weight steadily and follow whichever plan suits you best, using Qs 102–3 and 112–3 or in the A–Z.

When busy with a new baby, you need a simple diet, so low-fat might be best, or the traffic light plan (page 79). Don't try to lose weight too quickly; you need good nutrition when stressed (new mothers are).

See also:

- Questions: 102–4, 112–13.
- Feature: 9.
- A–Z entries: calorie counting, low-fat diets.
- Key index entries: healthy eating, high-carbohydrate diets, high-protein diets, metabolism, slimming.

FAT FACT

The average weight gain after each successive birth for women in the Western world is 2¼lb (lkg), over and above any increases that may happen not associated with pregnancy.

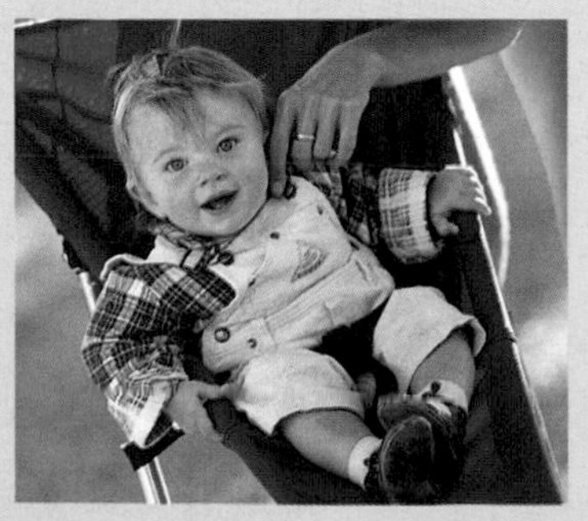

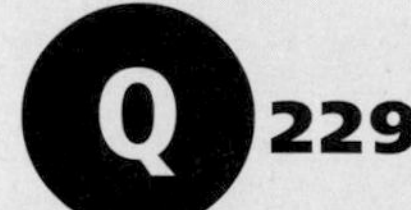

Q 229

I need to lose weight but I'm breast-feeding. How can I slim safely?

As breast-feeding uses up around 500 cals/day for the first 4 months of sole feeding (after which most babies also take weaning foods), you'll lose weight gradually if you eat the same number of cals/day as you would to maintain weight if not breast-feeding. For most this is around 2,000 cals/day. On a gentle diet like this, breast milk won't dry up and is quite safe.

The main thing to ensure is that when you are, in effect, reducing your breast-feeding diet by 500 calories a day, it is not at the expense of the nutrients your baby's needs. One good way to ensure this is first to cut out all the high-fat, high-sugar and/or high-salt items from your diet, such as cakes, biscuits, sweets, crisps, etc. Get a healthy diet with plenty of fruit and veg, complex carbs, lean protein (red meat is good especially if you lost a lot of blood at the birth), fish, and plenty of essential fats, so vital for the baby's brain development. Also drink plenty of water.

The Basic Diet in Feature 9 (maintenance) is a good all-round healthy diet, but you could double the daily milk allowance to provide extra calcium and protein and you may also like to take a calcium supplement. See how you get on with this for 2 weeks – if you're losing weight gradually, the baby is thriving, and you don't feel hungry, you can probably continue down to a suitable weight.

Talk your diet through with your doctor or postnatal dietician if you have worries.

See also:

- Questions: 79–90, 96, 101–4, 112–3 225–7.
- Features: 8, 9, 10, 11, 12, 14.
- A–Z entry: low-fat diets.
- Key index entries: healthy eating, slimming.

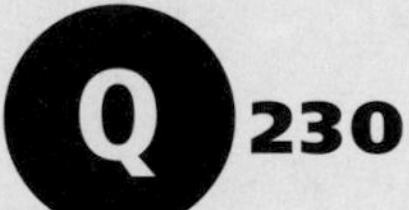

Q 230

Is weight gain inevitable for a woman during and after the menopause?

Despite the fact that so many women say they gain weight during the menopausal years, recent studies – particularly two important ones in the USA, reported in the *International Journal of Obesity* in mid-2001, have concluded that neither the perimenopause (the years immediately before the menses cease), menopause nor HRT is the cause of weight gain.

The conclusions drawn, by studying hundreds of women from 17 years before to 22 years after menopause, were that from about the age of 35 to 65, women, on average, gain total body weight gradually and steadily, and neither loss of ovarian hormones nor their replacement with HRT makes a detectable difference.

The World Health Organization broadly seems to agree – its major report on obesity in 2001 said most weight gain associated with menopause has been attributed to reduced activity. The US studies concluded that although many women gain several pounds during menopause this is simply part of the 'bigger picture' of a gain of around 0.43% per year during mid-life. For a woman weighing 10 stone (64kg) this would represent under 1lb (0.5kg) a year.

In fact, in one of the trials, about 3 years after onset of menopause there was an average 3% weight loss in the women studied – a blip which researchers couldn't explain. It does, therefore, seem that you don't have to gain weight over the menopause, but that most women do slowly gain weight throughout middle age, due to the slowing down of the metabolic rate and a typical lack of physical activity.

So, if weight gain in mid-life is probably not associated with menopause, is it still inevitable during the 'mid' decades of life?

FIRST WEEK POSTNATAL STOMACH EXERCISES

1. On the first day, lie on your bed (or on a mat on the floor) on your back with a pillow under your head and your knees bent, feet flat on the bed (or floor). Now slowly extend your legs until they are straight out in front of you. Draw one leg back in slowly, trying to feel your stomach muscles working, then draw in the other one. Repeat once or twice at first, twice a day, gradually building up to 10 reps in each twice-daily session over a week.

2. Lie on your bed (or on a mat on the floor) on your back with a pillow under your head and your legs out straight but relaxed, arms at your sides. Now lift your left leg up and over your right leg to try to touch your left heel on to the bed or floor next to your right leg. Try to feel your stomach muscles working. Slowly move the left leg back into place and repeat with the right leg. Repeat once or twice at first, gradually building up to 10 reps over a week.

Even in fit people, a small change in body shape in mid-life does seem to happen (see Q27), but large gains can be kept at bay with a sensible diet, resistance exercise to maintain muscle (or blunt muscle loss) and aerobic exercise to burn calories.

As one of the US studies says, a powerful predictor of elevated BMI (increased weight) was physical inactivity – suggesting the most useful intervention for preventing weight gain in mid-life women is increasing physical activity.

So why then do so many women say they've piled on weight over the menopause? Experts say lowered levels of oestrogen in the body tend to redistribute body fat, increasing deposits around the waist, while legs and arms may get thinner. Therefore dress size will increase, and women taking synthetic progesterone as part of HRT may suffer fluid retention. Others become very tired during the menopausal years or have other adverse symptoms, which undoubtedly makes it harder to motivate themselves to exercise, and comfort eating may also be a factor.

Although there seems to be no evidence to prove it, I don't doubt that some women do gain weight over the menopausal period, over and above the 'normal' slow mid-life increase. After all, the figures quoted in the research are based on averages not individuals. Plumper women tend to produce more oestrogen after menopause and some experts believe this may encourage weight gain. Perhaps a 'menopausal weight gene' will be found in some women, just as the postnatal 'fat' gene has been found in some mothers (see Q225).

See also:

- ▶ Questions: 10, 27, 41, 333–65.
- ▶ Features: 1, 3, 17.
- ▶ A–Z entry: weighted workouts.
- ▶ Key index entries: aerobics, exercise, hormones, menopause, weight training.

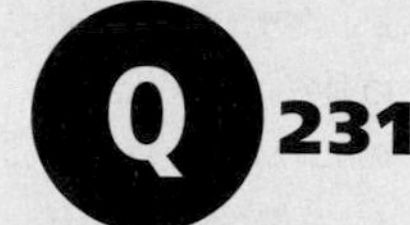

Does HRT cause weight gain?

First read the previous question. As you'll see, recent studies have found no link between weight gain and HRT. In fact, one of the large US studies actually found that the women on HRT during and after the menopause maintained a slightly lower weight than those not taking it, and other studies have come to the same conclusion. In some women, HRT does cause fluid retention, which can make the body look larger. However, this is fluid, not fat.

A low-salt diet, high in fruits and veg, can help minimize fluid retention – see Feature 17. If you find you're putting on weight with HRT – fluid or fat – you may find a change to a different formulation helps. You may also find that natural progesterone cream (prescription only in the UK) may help hot flushes and other symptoms without causing fluid retention.

See also:

- ▶ Questions: 10, 27, 41, 230, 333–65.
- ▶ Features: 1, 3, 17, 28-30.
- ▶ A–Z entry: diuretic diets.
- ▶ Key index entries: healthy eating, hormones, menopause, weight control.

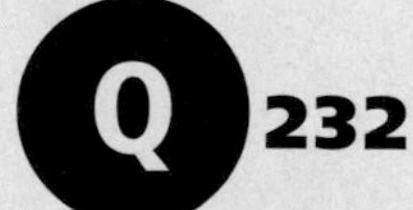

Is it possible to lose weight while going through the menopause and on HRT?

Yes, many women have successfully lost or stabilized weight during this time. In recent research scientists have not found any actual physiological reason why weight gain (or difficulty in losing it) should be associated with menopause, (see Qs 230 and 231). The best strategy is to increase regular exercise output by following the advice in Section Ten, while choosing a healthy slimming diet like the Basic Diet in Feature 9 or menopause diet in Feature 19.

As you age, metabolic rate generally decreases slowly and you need to work a bit harder to keep it 'stoked up' through exercise. A combination of resistance and aerobic exercise works best. As weight tends to increase around abdomen and waist during menopause, and arms and legs get thinner, it'll also improve overall shape.

See also:

- ▶ Questions: 230–31, 233–36.
- ▶ Features: 1, 9, 19, 28–30.
- ▶ Key index entries: exercise, healthy eating, menopause

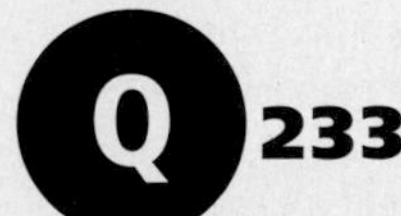

Q 233

Is it true that mid-life weight gain for women is healthy?

This is partially true. If you try to maintain too low a body weight during mid-life you may predispose yourself to reduced bone mass and higher risk of osteoporosis. This is partly because body fat helps retain stores of oestrogen, loss of which is a major factor in post-menopausal bone loss. Low body weight also generally means lower bone density – thin people have less bone mass on average than heavier ones. It's also been said that plump women tend to have fewer menopausal problems, though I can't find research to back this up.

Those are two good reasons not to aim to maintain too low a body weight in mid-life. A BMI in the upper range of 'healthy' (i.e., nearer 25) may be prudent. A good rule-of-thumb is that if you were very slim in your youth and 20s, you shouldn't worry if you put on a stone or so by around 50 – it is probably doing you more good than harm, especially if you exercise regularly.

However, it isn't healthy to gain too much weight. Feature 25 shows the long list of health risks associated with overweight. A recent study found 'middle-aged' women were much more likely to suffer from 'Syndrome X', including insulin resistance and the pre-diabetic state if overweight, and the conclusion was that women should avoid mid-life weight gain. Obesity in post-menopausal women is also linked with increased risk of breast cancer, high blood pressure, heart disease and arthritis of the weight-bearing joints.

The message seems to be that weight gain in mid-life should be kept small, BMI should be kept within reasonable bounds (if yours is over 28 you may have cause for concern) and a programme of healthy eating and exercise should be undertaken to facilitate all this. The plan outlined in Feature 19 is ideal for health protection and gradual weight loss, if necessary, during menopause and after – the Basic Diet in Feature 9 is also suitable, though additional calcium may be necessary.

See also:
- Questions: 27, 230–32, 234–7.
- Features: 6, 9, 19, 27–30.
- A–Z entries: gym, weighted workouts.
- Key index entries: exercise, healthy eating, hormones, menopause.

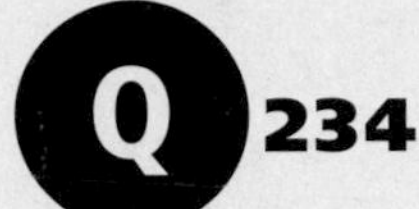

Q 234

My body seems to have slowed down since menopause (e.g., I find myself dawdling instead of hurrying, as I used to). Is this possible and what can I do about it?

There is a natural and fairly inevitable 'slowing down' as one ages. You wouldn't expect a 75-year-old to be as lively as a 5-year-old, for example. Although this 'slowing down' can be blunted with dedication, determination, regular exercise to improve strength, suppleness and aerobic capacity, and a happy and inquisitive outlook on life, it is asking a bit too much of your body and yourself that you keep everything in 100% condition.

This may account partly for your feeling that you are slowing down. However, in your 50s or 60s you shouldn't be feeling 'old'. A fit 60-year-old can be as fit as the average 35-year-old, so don't give up.

Some menopausal symptoms themselves – for example, generalized aches and pains and tiredness – can make you feel under par and therefore less likely to stride out as you used to. If this is the case, after menopause things should get back to normal, although it can take a long time. 3–4 years is the average, but it can be up to 10 years.

If you recognize a problem and don't want it to be there, you're halfway to a solution. You have the motivation to change things – so make an effort to hurry up when you find yourself dawdling; make a written plan for a regular exercise schedule which will improve your circulation and may rejuvenate you; think about your breathing – breathe deeply to oxygenate body and brain. Find interesting things to do – people walk slowly when not interested in what they are walking towards, but hurry when there is something of interest. Get a check-up in case there are any medical problems. HRT may help, as may a healthy diet.

See also:
- Questions: 27, 230–33, 235–7.
- Features: 1, 2, 6, 9, 19, 28–30.
- A–Z entries: exercise classes, cycling, gyms, swimming, weighted workouts.
- Key index entries: exercise, fitness and age, metabolism, weight and health.

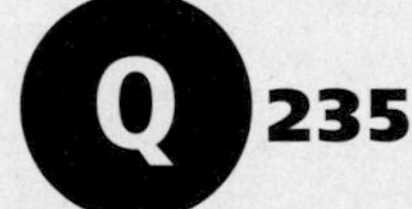

Q 235

I'm in my mid-50s and on a strict calorie-controlled regime, but I can only maintain my weight, not lose any. Is this normal?

A small weight gain of around 1lb a year (one study puts the exact figure at 0.43% of body weight per year) is average for people aged 35 to 65. The reason for this is that there is a natural physiological slowing down of the metabolism, mostly accounted for by loss of lean tissue (muscle) over the age of 35, coupled with a strong tendency for people to take less physical activity as they age. These factors can lower the metabolic rate considerably.

So as you get older, unless you increase activity levels a little year on year, including resistance work to retain lean tissue, you will find it slightly more difficult to lose weight. However, you shouldn't find it impossible. I have helped many people in their middle and late years to lose weight when they said they couldn't – with a combination of low-fat eating, behaviour modification and an hour a day of regular gentle or moderate intensity exercise.

Research shows that almost anyone can lose weight on a diet of about 1,500 cals/day – certainly, even if your metabolic rate is very low, you shouldn't need to eat fewer than 1,200 cals/day to produce a weekly weight loss of a pound.

I am wondering, therefore, two things. One – are you already quite slim and aiming for too low a body weight? If you are, that would explain the difficulty. Work out your Body Mass Index with Feature 3. If it is within the healthy range of 20–25, I think you should forget about trying to diet, take more exercise and simply be happy to maintain your current weight.

Two – DO you take any exercise? After the age of 35, your lean tissue may decrease at a rate of about 1% a year (equalling about half a pound of muscle lost per year for a 10-stone woman) and this can significantly reduce metabolic rate over time. So start a progressive routine of light resistance exercise coupled with three-times-a-week walking, cycling or aerobic work at the gym to get your metabolism ticking over at a better rate. Build as much activity as you can into your daily life and you should see improvements.

You could also check out Section Three, as a matter of interest, to see if you really do 'know your calories' – often, people who think they are hardly eating a thing are taking in a lot more calories than they think they are. If you really are overweight, you could try the Basic Diet in Feature 9 for two weeks exactly as laid out, coupled with 3 hours of exercise a week.

See also:

- Questions: 4, 10, 21, 27, 29, 79, 104, 230–34, 236.
- Features: 1–3, 9, 19, 27–30.
- A–Z entries: exercise classes, gyms, weighted workouts.
- Key index entries: exercise, fitness and age, metabolism.

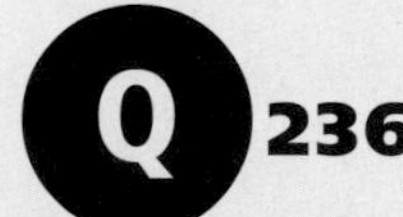

Q 236

Should one eat less as one gets older?

Over 35, our metabolic rate gradually slows, and this is progressive, so at, say, 70 you will burn up about 350 cals/day less than you did at 35 (the equation is an average of 50 cals/day less for every 5 years of your life). So, if you don't want to put on weight, you either have to eat a little less or exercise more. The advice for people in their 50s and 60s is, roughly, the advice to anyone – cut down on 'junk'-type foods like high-fat, high-sugar, high-salt processed snacks, etc., eat as healthy and varied a diet as you can, and with your doctor's permission increase exercise as much as you're able, depending on health and circumstances. Maintaining a reasonable weight in mid- and later life is one of the best ways to stay healthy.

As you get older – into the 70s or 80s – many find the appetite diminishes and the digestive system becomes slightly more difficult to please, which will alter your eating patterns. If you have any nutrition, eating or digestive worries, or want to begin exercising, see your doctor.

See also:

- Questions: 27, 233, 235, 237, 300–306, 319.
- Features: 3, 9, 19.
- Key index entries: ageing and weight, exercise, healthy eating.

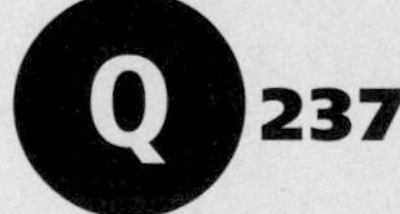

Q 237

Is it ever too late to start a diet? My mother is 75 and very overweight.

In theory, there is no reason why a person of 75 (or older) shouldn't reduce calorie intake and lose weight, but it would be best if it were done with the help of a doctor and/or dietician who knows them.

It is often hard to persuade older people to diet – many resist changing the eating habits of a lifetime, especially if all else around them is changing. Familiar food is a comfort. Their digestive system also may not take kindly to new foods.

So dietary changes need to be carefully monitored, even if psychologically acceptable to the person. The advice to 'take more exercise' often can't apply to obese elderly people because they simply can't. If weight is lost, mobility should increase and the 'vicious circle' reversed.

If your mother is obese, she should already be being monitored by her doctor or outpatients clinic and they should make the correct decisions about her diet. Obviously obesity is a leading cause of health problems and can result in early death, and it's been found even losing 5% weight for an obese person can make a big difference to health. So it would be good if she can make a few changes and lose some weight – but she has to be happy with them.

If you are responsible for shopping for and/or feeding your mother and her doctor knows of her weight but hasn't given you any particular instructions for her diet, read Section Three for more information on healthy eating. Average requirements for nutrients in old people are the same, apart from the reduction in calories and perhaps a requirement for dietary vitamin D (cod liver oil is the easiest way to get this) if she doesn't get outdoors much. Even if you only take on board some of the ideas in the Basic Diet (Feature 9), it may help both her weight and nutritional status. You could also look at the calorie content of foods in the food value charts at the end of the book, and perhaps try first to cut down on high-fat, high-sugar snacks.

See also:

- Questions: 27, 236–7, 300–306.
- Features: 3, 9.
- Key index entries: ageing and diet, ageing and weight, healthy eating.

The menopause diet

This diet is suitable for gradual weight loss for all peri-menopausal, menopausal and post-menopausal women. By following the instructions it can also be used as a weight maintenance plan.

The menopause plan here may not only help you to lose weight but is also healthy for this time in your life. It is rich in calcium to help prevent osteoporosis and also contains adequate amounts of all the other nutrients that may help alleviate the symptoms of menopause, including hot flushes, bloating, irritability and tiredness.

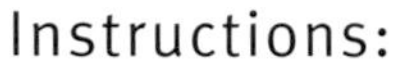

Instructions:

- Have 450ml (3/4 pint) skimmed milk or calcium-enriched soya milk a day, preferably as a drink on its own.
- Avoid coffee, alcohol and highly spiced foods, which may make hot flushes worse. Weak tea is fine, and so are herbal teas, redbush tea, green tea and water. Drink 2 litres (3 1/2 pints) of fluid each day. Caffeine hinders calcium absorption.
- Avoid added salt in foods, which can make bloating worse. Use fresh and dried herbs instead, or use salt substitute (Losalt).
- Eat plenty of vegetables and salad – those listed in the menus are suggestions, but you can add more or vary the choices.

GOOD FOODS FOR THE MENOPAUSE

- Oily fish, nuts and seeds for essential omega oils; good for general body and brain condition.
- Whole grains, lean red meat, pulses – rich in B vitamins.
- Nuts, seeds, white fish, leafy greens, white cabbage, low-fat dairy produce – rich in calcium.
- Pulses, including soy beans, lentils, chickpeas – contain natural hormones (isoflavones) which may help menopausal symptoms and are also rich in nutrients. Linseeds contain lignans, which may also help menopausal symptoms.
- Vegetables, including yams, beansprouts, seaweed, dark leafy greens – contain natural hormones, plant chemicals, vitamin C and minerals which help menopausal health.
- Fruits – most are rich in potassium which can help alleviate fluid retention.

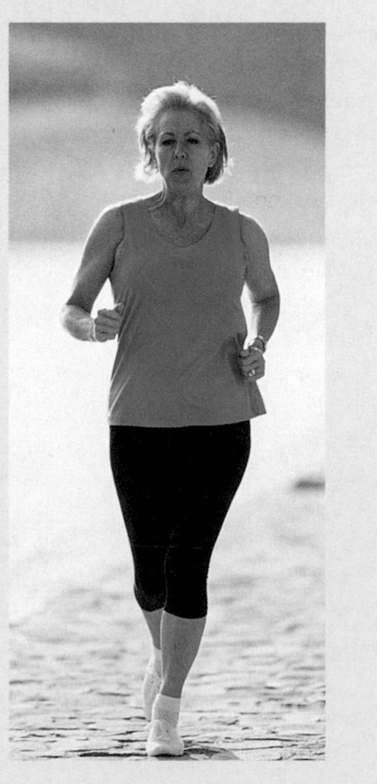

Every Day

- Have 2 small daily snacks between meals – one of a small handful of dried apricots, peaches or figs, the other a small handful of almonds, walnuts or brazils.

Breakfast: Every day for breakfast have 1 bowlful of low-fat natural bio yoghurt topped with 2 tablespoons muesli plus some flaxseeds and/or sesame seeds and a few pieces of almond, walnut or brazil nut, plus 1 piece of fresh fruit
OR
I average bowl of whole-grain cereal (e.g. Weetabix, Shredded Wheat) with skimmed milk to cover (from allowance), plus I piece of fresh fruit and nuts and seeds as for Breakfast I.
(If you don't need to lose weight, add a slice of wholemeal bread with low-fat spread and a little low-sugar jam or marmalade or honey.)

Now follow the plan as laid out – for weight maintenance just increase portion sizes by about 20%.

Day 1

Lunch: Medium slice of white bread, toasted, with 50g ($1\frac{2}{3}$ oz) portion of smoked mackerel pâté and a large mixed side salad tossed with oil-free French dressing; 1 kiwi fruit or plum.
Evening: Sliced silken or semi-firm tofu, stir-fried with a selection of thinly sliced carrot, white cabbage, broccoli, greens, yellow bean sauce, stock and some chopped herbs of choice, in a little groundnut oil.

Day 2

Lunch: Selection of ready-made sushi; I orange
OR
Salmon pâté on 3 dark rye crispbreads; I orange.
Evening: Breast of chicken portion, skinned, brushed with chilli oil and baked on a tray with I sliced yellow pepper and I sliced courgette, chopped garlic, sage leaves and rosemary until all is cooked, served with 4 tbsp cooked green lentils, all with a dash of balsamic vinegar sprinkled over.

Day 3

Lunch: Salad of baby spinach leaves tossed with cooked baby new potatoes, I hard-boiled egg, sliced, alfalfa sprouts, all tossed in a dressing made from I tbsp French dressing thoroughly mixed with I dsp organic peanut butter.
Evening: I average sweet potato, baked in the oven and served with 3 tbsp ready-made cheese sauce topped with I tsp grated Parmesan; 2 green vegetables (e.g. kale and peas).

Day 4

Lunch: 50g ($1\frac{2}{3}$oz) slice of white bread or roll served with I large bowlful ready-made (chilled counter) broccoli soup topped with I tbsp grated Parmesan or Cheddar; I orange.
Evening: I average whole trout, dry-fried in a pan and served with I heaped tbsp flaked toasted almonds, green beans, pak choi.

Day 5

Lunch: 50g ($1\frac{2}{3}$oz) slice of wholemeal bread served with 40g ($1\frac{1}{3}$oz) Brie or Camembert and a large salad with oil-free French dressing.
Evening: 300g ($10\frac{1}{2}$oz) slices of peeled butternut squash, sliced, brushed lightly with olive oil, seasoned and baked in the oven for 40 minutes or until tender, with 4 tbsp cooked Puy lentils dressed in balsamic vinegar and a large leaf side salad.

Day 6

Lunch: I portion of tabbouleh made from 50g ($1\frac{2}{3}$oz) (dry weight) bulgar wheat, soaked according to package instructions and mixed with I chopped fresh tomato, a handful of chopped mint and parsley, I large chopped spring onion and I tbsp olive oil and lemon juice dressing, with either 40g ($1\frac{1}{3}$oz) feta cheese crumbled on top or I hard-boiled egg.
Evening: 2 small lamb loin chops, extra-trimmed, baked in a tray with 2 sliced red peppers and I sliced red onion tossed in 2 tsp olive oil and some seasoning, for about 40 minutes or until cooked. Serve the chops with half the red pepper mixture and 2 tbsp brown rice – reserve the remaining pepper/onion for the next day's lunch, store in fridge.

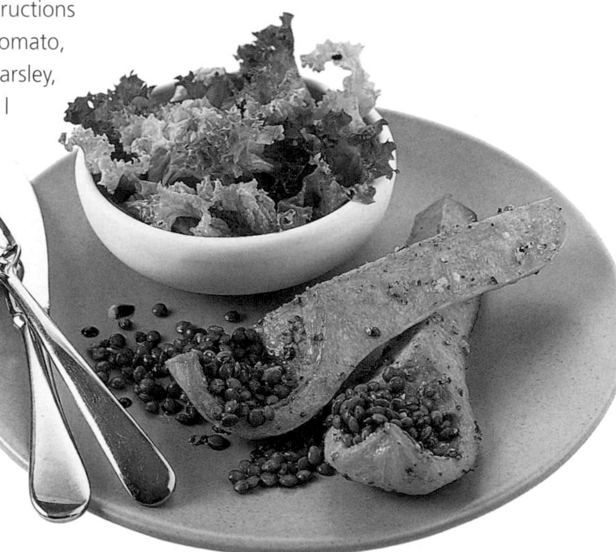

Day 7

Lunch: 50g ($1\frac{2}{3}$oz) slice of white bread, toasted and served with 50g ($1\frac{2}{3}$oz) hummus and the remaining red pepper and onion, served cold and mixed with I tsp balsamic vinegar, basil leaves and seasoning.
Evening: 100g ($3\frac{1}{2}$oz) fillet of salmon, grilled, dry-fried or baked and served with I tbsp pesto sauce (made to usual recipe with olive oil, basil, garlic, pine nuts – or use good-quality ready-made), 2 new potatoes and 2 green vegetables (e.g. broccoli and broad beans or carrots and some dark leafy greens).

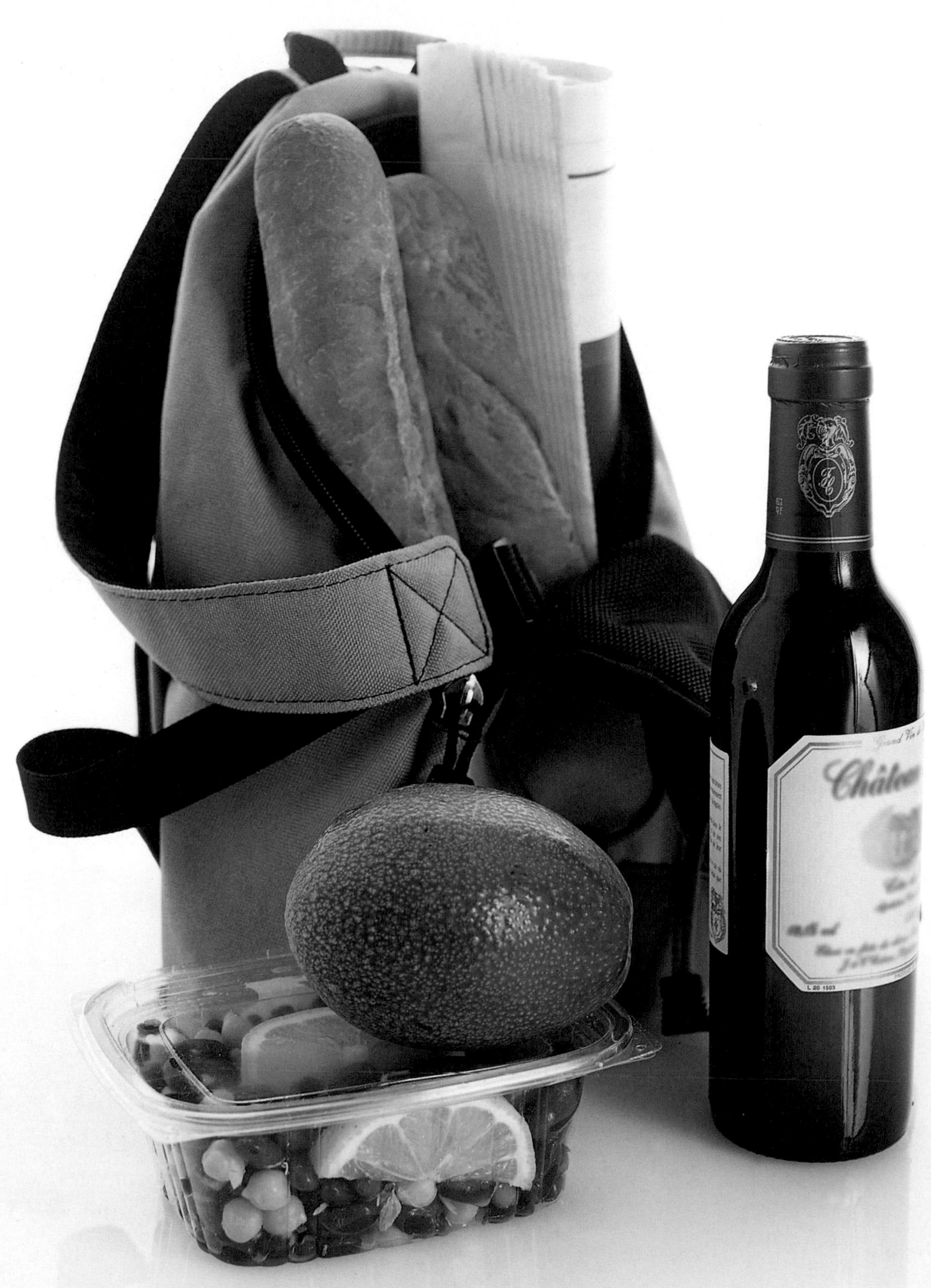

Section Seven

For men only

While men don't have periods, pregnancy or the female menopause, nevertheless they do have plenty of stresses and problems of their own which can, and often do, influence their food and drink intake and therefore their weight and health.

Despite the advent of the third millennium and so-called equality, it is still men in the Western world who are more likely to do certain types of job that are more likely to predispose to unwise diet – for example, the higher percentage of travelling sales reps, delivery men, long-distance drivers and international business travellers are male, and professionals such as lawyers and accountants, and company directors are predominantly male. It is most often males who have literally to 'wine and dine' clients.

And how about the typical 'lad' – not just a myth. We all know the pub- and club-going, male-bonding, takeaway-loving male who enjoys food and drink as much as he enjoys sex.

And how about the legion of males with their stay-home wives who believe they do him proud with a cholesterol-laden three-course evening meal; the lone career guy with an empty fridge living on late-night takeouts and TV dinners? Then, finally, the mid-life crisis... no exercise since leaving full-time education, an ever-expanding girth and the first warning from the doctor – 'You need to lose weight'.

Every scenario a cliché – but all still so often true. And men hate to diet even more than women hate to diet. This section offers some solutions.

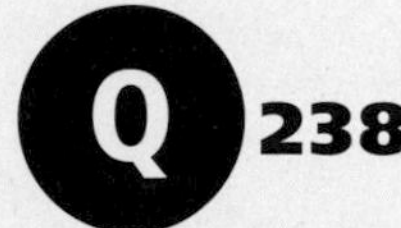

238

Is there any difference between the type of a diet a man should follow for weight loss and that for a woman?

The main difference is that the average man has a higher metabolic rate than the average women – because he is heavier, taller and with a higher percentage of lean tissue (muscle). Therefore he will need to eat more calories (food) on his reduced-calorie diet than she does, otherwise he will feel too hungry and he may lose weight too quickly.

Section One, in particular Feature 1, will help you sort out what your own personal metabolic rate is and Q104 will help you decide what kind of calorie intake you should be going for.

Apart from that, men and women can follow the same 'healthy eating' type of diet outlined in my Basic Diet in Feature 9. People with a higher metabolic rate will simply increase portion sizes, which will give them more nutrients across the board – carbohydrate, protein, fat, vitamins and minerals.

Some men may need a little more protein than this – for example, men who do hard physical work all day, or men who are professional sportsmen. If that sounds like you, you could follow the Basic Diet but, instead of increasing portion sizes of all types of food to increase your total calorie intake, you could first increase the protein element of the meal (fish, chicken, lean meat, pulses, low-fat dairy produce, etc.) and then, if you are losing weight too quickly, also add on extra carbohydrate (bread, potatoes, pasta, rice, etc.).

However, I have a feeling that most men reading this question, who need to lose weight, will NOT be professional sportsmen or highly active. Most men (like most women) who need to diet have been taking too little physical activity long-term, and such men starting a moderate activity programme (for example, a combination of the programmes in Features 6 and 29) are unlikely to create a need for much extra protein, at least in the early months.

Should you turn into a bicep-bulging, marathon-running person, you may need to take professional advice on your diet as it'll be outside the scope of this book.

See also:

- Questions: 1–6, 102–4.
- Feature: 9.
- Key index entries: calories, healthy eating, metabolism.

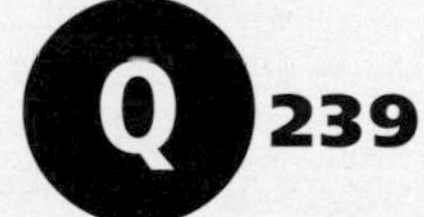

239

I'm not overweight on the scales and yet I look flabby. I'm 40. Do you think I am carrying too much fat?

If you look flabby, particularly around the midriff and upper arms and you have little muscle definition anywhere on your body – perhaps with slim arms and legs – it sounds to me as though you are a classic apple-shaped male. The scales won't register overweight, as your slim arms and legs cancel out your fat abdomen and waist, but as various other questions in this book explain, an apple shape is something to avoid, or work to get rid of. Read the items cross-referenced below, which will help you decide if this is indeed your problem.

Otherwise, if you are reasonably well proportioned but just look a bit 'soft', you may not be overweight but just need to do some all-body resistance work to tone up your muscles. Feature 6 will help at first and then you can progress to harder resistance work – a gym would be ideal, or buy simple home equipment.

Double-check your Body Mass Index using Feature 3 to make sure that you aren't actually overweight – if by chance you are, the Basic Diet in Feature 9 will help you shed a few pounds. Forty is a fairly crucial time for many men – you either decide to keep yourself trim and fit, or tend to begin to 'go to seed'. And you don't want to do that, do you?!

See also:

- Questions: 28–9, 56, 66–7, 247–50, 252.
- Features: 3, 6, 9, 21, 28–30.
- A–Z entries: exercise equipment, gyms, weighted workouts.
- Key index entries: apple shape, body mass index, exercise, weight and ageing, weight and health.

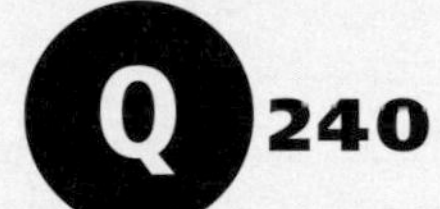

240

What is 'body fat percentage' and how can I work out what my ideal is?

The answer to Q30 will tell you most of what you want to know about body fat percentage and what is a reasonable amount of body fat for a man. Men carry less body fat than women, on average, and more muscle. Weighing on the scales won't tell you how much of your weight is fat unless you buy the new (and expensive) type of scales which do attempt to give you your BFP – but how accurately, I'm not sure.

You can go to a gym or health club and most will be able to read off your body fat percentage with specialized equipment that is quite accurate. Otherwise, you can buy small body fat monitors for home use; they are, however, quite expensive.

I do think that for most people, worrying too much about your exact body fat percentage is a bit of a red herring. In truth, you can tell fairly accurately, just by looking at yourself in the mirror, whether or not you are carrying a lot of fat over and above your ideal percentage – you will look flabby and soft, rather than firm and trim.

As I said at the beginning, scales won't measure body fat. However, people who are overweight according to the scales (with a Body Mass Index several notches higher than it ought to be) will, in 99 cases out of 100, also have a higher body fat percentage than average.

There are, however, some exceptions. For example, if you are a bodybuilder, you might weigh heavy on the scales and have quite a high BMI, but have a body fat percentage much lower than average. That is when knowing your body fat percentage would reassure you that you don't need to start the slimming campaign. But you'd know that anyway. For most of us ordinary mortals, if the scales say we're fat, we're fat.

See also:

- ▶ Questions: 29–31, 239, 248–51.
- ▶ Feature: 3.
- ▶ A–Z entry: body fat monitors.
- ▶ Key index entries: apple shape, body fat percentage, body mass index, exercise, weight and health.

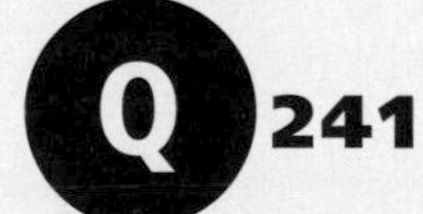

Q 241

I used to play football twice a week – but I've given up. How much less do I need to eat so that I don't put on weight?

Assuming three hours a week of fairly vigorous exercise (though, with football and other team sports, it is hard to be precise about calories burnt because your physical involvement is so variable), this would work out at around 7 calories used a minute, which comes to 1,260 calories burnt in total for your training and match. That equals 180 calories a day, which in turn equals a pint of mild beer, or two slices of bread, or a 9oz (250g) potato that you would have to decline every day in order not to put on weight. The food value charts at the end of the book give you more values for everyday foods.

I think the real issue here though is that, having given up three hours' worth of exercise a week in the form of football, it would be sensible for you to replace it with something else perhaps not quite so energetic. If you've given up football because you are 'too old' or incapacitated, is there any form of exercise you could now take instead – a half-hour walk or cycle session a day, or similar?

So many men as young as their late 20s, and certainly by their 30s and 40s, give up almost all exercise and then wonder why they get fat and start having health problems. So don't eat less – just get out and keep active. Even if you're still slim and fit at the moment, it only takes a small amount of regular overeating (like 180 calories a day) and a few months of inactivity for all kinds of negatives to begin happening to your body.

See also:

- ▶ Questions: 239, 257–8, 340.
- ▶ Features: 28–29.
- ▶ A–Z entries: cycling, gyms, walking.
- ▶ Key index entries: calories, exercise, exercise and health, weight and health.

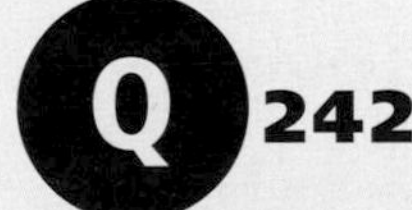

Q 242

I'm a typical male – I love takeaway curries and Chinese food, fish and chips, and so on. Are there any wise choices or is everything bad news, health- and calorie-wise?

Refer back to the answers to Qs 118, 167, 174 and 176, and to Feature 15, which will answer all your queries on the subject of takeaways. You will have now seen that there are some better choices amongst a host of not-so-good ones, and these better choices should fit in reasonably well with a varied diet, without putting weight on or risking your cholesterol levels.

Even so, I would still advise you to try to limit your forays to the takeouts to once or twice a week. Unlike some people, it doesn't sound as if your circumstances virtually force you to eat fast food, but that you simply prefer it. In that case you might try the retraining course in Feature 13, and Feature 14 and Q165 provide ideas for quick and easy meals. Q188 may also give you ideas for balancing your overall diet. If lack of time is your problem, you can even incorporate a few 'ready meals' into your diet and some advice on that is given in Q166.

See also:

- ▶ Questions: 118, 165–7, 174, 176, 188.
- ▶ Features: 13, 14, 15.
- ▶ A–Z entry: ready meals.
- ▶ Key index entries: fast food, healthy eating.

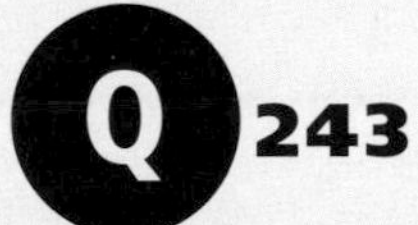

Q 243

Which is more fattening – beer, spirits or wine?

Each of these has roughly the same calorie content (about 90–100 calories): half a pint of ordinary beer or lager, a double of spirits, or a small glass (about a fifth of a bottle) of wine.

You will see then that whichever tipple you prefer doesn't make a lot of difference, calorie-wise, unless you are likely to down significantly more of one than the other in the same length of time.

For example, I would find it much easier to down a glass of wine than a half-pint of beer for the same calorie content – but you may, of course, be different.

If you enjoy spirits, and could get by on a single with a low-calorie mixer (e.g. a Scotch and low-cal ginger ale), you could have two of those for roughly the same calorie value as the single glass of wine.

When thinking about alcohol you also need to consider how many 'units' you're drinking (for your health's sake) and how many milligrams of alcohol you are putting into your bloodstream (for your driving's sake – and perhaps even your driving licence's sake). These things are considered in more detail in Feature 20.

See also:

- ▶ Questions: 101, 180, 186–7, 244–6.
- ▶ Feature: 20.
- ▶ Key index entries: alcohol, calories, healthy eating.

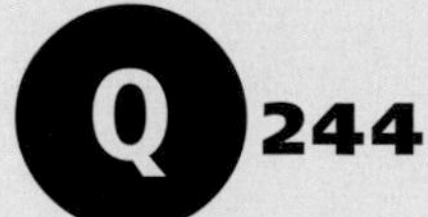

Q 244

Do you have any tips for cutting down alcohol consumed in the name of business?

The answer to Q187 gives tips for cutting down alcohol consumption when you have to attend a lot of parties, cocktail parties and so on. Q180 addresses the problems of cutting down on wine at the meal table. I think you'll find plenty of ideas there to help you and they will all work without causing offence to any business client.

However, the main item on the agenda is to get your head into the right attitude to carry out these ideas. If you have spent years of heavy regular drinking it isn't so easy to cut right back, or give up, even if you think you want to. You may find at first that you crave a drink when you usually have one – and because it may be the sugar content of the drink that you crave, rather than the alcohol (even dry drinks contain a lot or sugar), the tip that I have found works best is to have a quite sugary soft drink, such as an elderflower or citrus cordial (not kid's squashes – the grown-up sort). They are sweet but not sickly, and they also look kind of 'alcohol-coloured' in the glass. Of course, this depends upon the bar, club, restaurant, etc. being able to provide you with this. Alternatively you might try the low-alcohol versions of beer, cider or wine, but often they don't taste very authentic.

Otherwise your best plan is to cut down by watering (or soda-ing) down your drink a little at first, and gradually more and more. This won't work with beer or red wine but will work with white wine and spirits.

The moment you realize that you can function on less alcohol (and you will actually function better), the whole thing of drinking less becomes easier and easier. However, if, having given all the ideas a fair trial for a few weeks, you still aren't managing to cut down it might be an idea to contact AA and also see your doctor.

AA helpline: 020 7833 0022; online www.alcoholics-anonymous.org.uk.

See also:

- ▶ Questions: 180, 187, 243, 245–6.
- ▶ Feature: 20.
- ▶ Key index entries: alcohol, weight and health.

ALCOHOL FACT

Research at Illinois University found that going for a run after drinking can reduce the risk of alcohol-induced cancers, because the running mops up the levels of free radicals that are produced in the body after alcohol consumption. (Presumably, however, the risk of alcohol-induced jogging accidents is increased.)

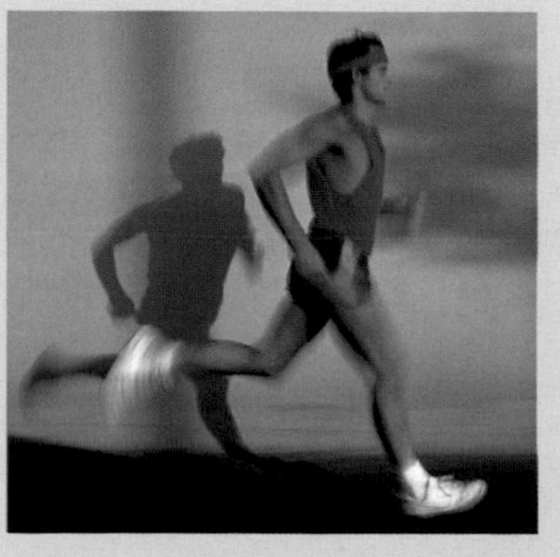

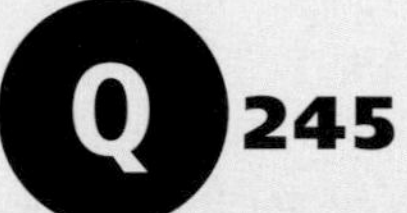

Q 245

I am overweight, but as alcohol helps to prevent heart disease in men, shouldn't I carry on drinking and cut down calories elsewhere?

Drinking just one glass of red wine or dark beer a day is enough to help prevent heart disease and provide other health protection, so you can cut all the rest of your drinking out as an obvious and easy way to save calories without having to worry that your health will suffer.

ALCOHOL FACT

According to UK government statistics, I in 25 adults are dependent on alcohol and 33,000 people a year die from alcohol-associated incidents or health problems.

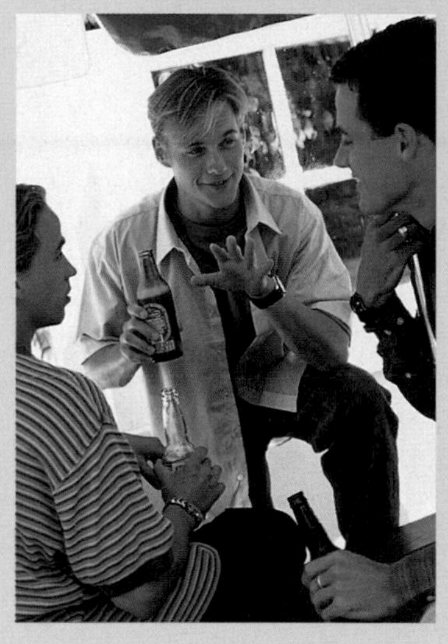

More than four units a day is likely to cause you more health problems than benefits. Although alcohol has a few trace nutrients in it, by and large it is 'empty calories' and you would be much, much better off cutting back on that than on healthy nutritious foods if you want to save calories. In fact, if you don't want to drink alcohol at all, a glass of red grape juice will have a similar protective effect to the red wine; it contains the beneficial polyphenols found in the grapes.

You will find more information about alcohol in Feature 20 and more information on a healthy diet in Section Three.

See also:

- ▶ Questions: 243–6.
- ▶ Feature: 20.
- ▶ Key index entries: alcohol, healthy eating, healthy slimming.

Q 246

Does beer drinking really cause a 'beer belly'?

A beer belly is a fat stomach by another name. Whether you take in too many calories via pints of beer or via too many takeaways or too much food on your plate too many times a day, and thus create a 'positive calorie balance (see Q18) – you will eventually put on weight. It is just that a lot of men do get fat through too many 'beer' calories (e.g. five pints in an evening are around 1,000 calories, so if this is in addition to a normal adequate diet, the beer will put weight on).

The reason that, in many men, the extra pounds of fat seem to end up on your stomach rather than elsewhere is twofold. One, men are more prone to put weight on their midriffs than women (men tend to be 'apples', women, 'pears'). Two, when anyone puts on weight, it tends to go first to the upper body (face, chest, belly) and lastly to the lower body. So, when you are gaining weight around your middle you are in fact also gaining it on your face and perhaps your chest – but it is always the belly that you and other people notice. If you carry on gaining weight, you will also gain it in other areas of your body, but, being male, it is the belly that will stand out!

See also:

- ▶ Questions: 18, 48, 56, 247–51.
- ▶ Features: 20, 21.
- ▶ Key index entries: alcohol, apple shape, healthy eating.

DRINK FACTS

- ■ Men can hold their drink better than women, it has recently been discovered, because women have less of a key enzyme in their stomachs (alcohol dehydrogenase) which breaks down alcohol so it can be absorbed into the bloodstream.
- ■ Scientists in Israel have found a way of increasing the flavonoids in white wine so that it is as good for you as red wine, without altering the wine's flavour.
- ■ Researchers in Australia have come up with a way of reducing incidence of alcohol-abuse-related brain damage – by adding some vitamin B1 to the drink.
- ■ Just three units of alcohol are enough to diminish sexual performance; six may be enough to prevent orgasm, and more than that is increasingly likely to prevent achievement of erection.
- ■ Studies on a 1,000 men in Tokyo found those who regularly drank 1–3 glasses of wine or sake a day had IQs about 4 points higher than those who didn't.
- ■ Binge drinking is much more dangerous than regular drinking.
- ■ Heavy drinkers who don't drink wine have a higher death rate than those who do.
- ■ A 10-year study of Australian beer drinkers found those who had 1–2 beers a day had a 20% lower risk of dying from heart disease than teetotallers.
- ■ Matured malt whisky contains more phenolic compounds than unaged whisky.
- ■ A man drinking one pint of beer a day over and above his normal calorie needs would put on around 19 pounds in weight over a year.

Diet and alcohol

The majority of people in the UK and the rest of the Western world drink alcohol regularly. Although small amounts may be good for health, more than one or two drinks a day can impair health and contribute to weight problems. Here we look at the facts.

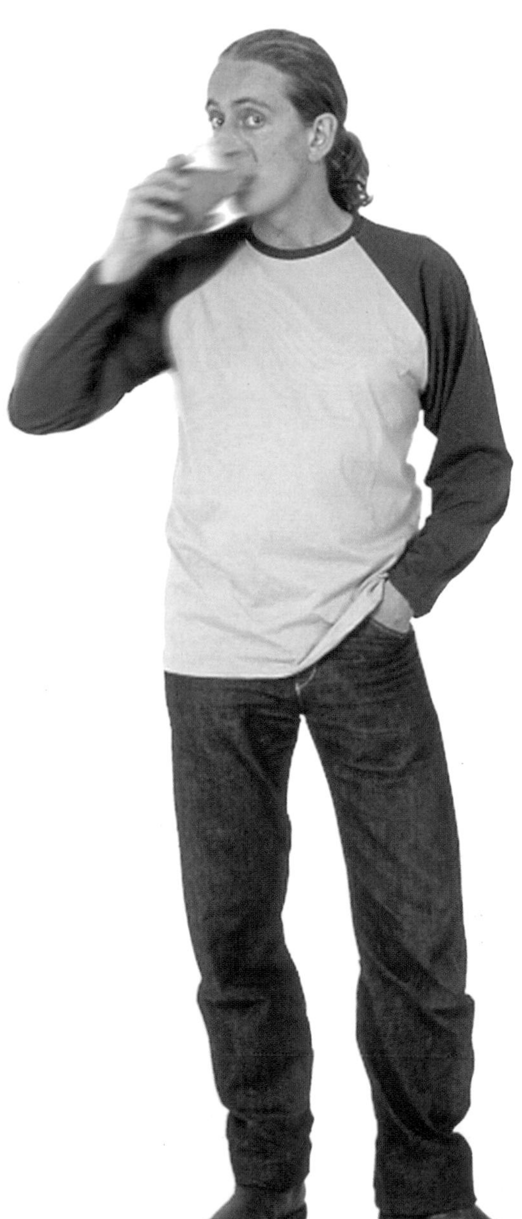

What are safe limits for drinking?

In the UK, the Department of Health issued some guidelines for safe drinking in 1995, the main points of which are as follows:

- Consuming 1–2 units of alcohol a day gives a significant health benefit in reducing coronary heart disease for men over 40 and for post-menopausal women.
- It is better to drink the units regularly rather than save them up and binge. Occasional binge drinking is not linked with any health benefits.
- Men who drink 3–4 units a day and women who drink 2–3 units a day don't face any significant health risks (except in pregnancy). Women's lower level reflects their smaller livers (which process the alcohol), body fat percentage, enzyme amounts and body size.
- Women who are pregnant should not drink more than 1 or 2 units a week and should avoid getting drunk (however, other recommendations suggest that pregnant women should drink no alcohol at all and I feel this is the safest option).

TABLE OF ALCOHOL UNITS AND CALORIES

Drink	Units	Calories
Beer, lager, 3.4%, half-pint	1	90
Beer, lager, strong (7%), half-pint	2	140–220
Cider, standard dry or medium, half-pint	1	100
Cider, strong, half-pint	1.5–2	120–180
Port, single 25ml measure*	1	40
Sherry, single 25ml measure*	1	40
Spirits, all kinds, single 25ml measure	1	50
Wine, red or white, dry, 9% or less by volume, 125ml glass	1	90
Wine, red or white, dry, 12% by volume, 125ml glass	1.5	90
Wine, red or white, dry, 14% by volume, 125ml glass	2 (approx)	100
Wine, champagne, average 125ml glass	1.5	100
Wine, sweet dessert, 15% volume, average 80ml glass	1.5	120

*Average pub measures of sherry and port are 50ml, or 2 units.

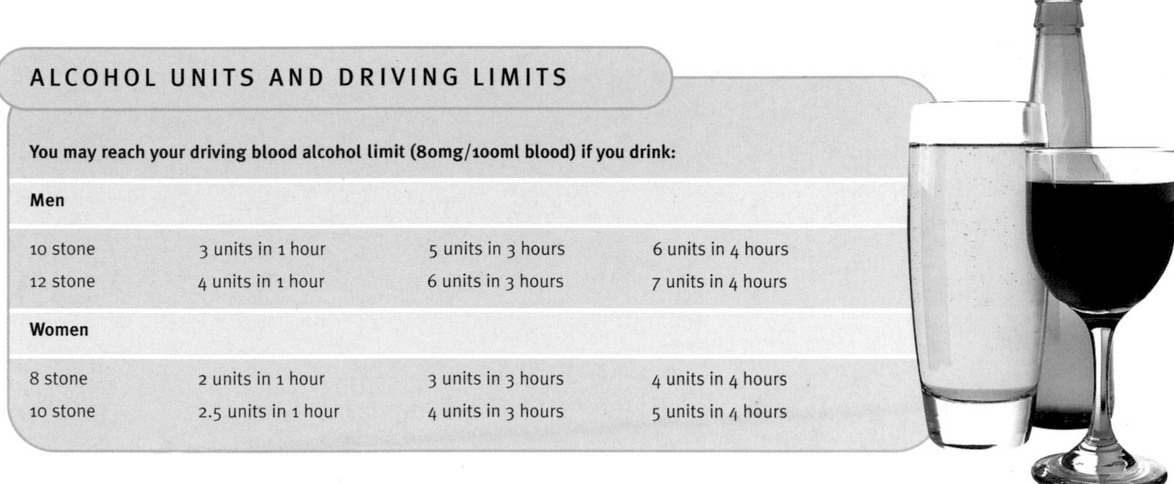

ALCOHOL UNITS AND DRIVING LIMITS

You may reach your driving blood alcohol limit (80mg/100ml blood) if you drink:

Men			
10 stone	3 units in 1 hour	5 units in 3 hours	6 units in 4 hours
12 stone	4 units in 1 hour	6 units in 3 hours	7 units in 4 hours
Women			
8 stone	2 units in 1 hour	3 units in 3 hours	4 units in 4 hours
10 stone	2.5 units in 1 hour	4 units in 3 hours	5 units in 4 hours

- Consistently drinking 4 or more units a day for men or 3 or more for women is not advisable due to increasing health risks.
- Individual reactions to alcohol vary.

Units and calories in alcoholic drinks

The table opposite gives average units in various alcoholic drinks plus the calorie content of the drinks. However, when checking the table, bear in mind, particularly with wine, that the amount of alcohol in a similar type of drink can vary enormously. For example, wine can contain from about 9% up to 14% alcohol by volume, and this will alter how much wine you can drink for one unit. Beers and lagers also vary from around 3.4% up to 8% or even more, and this needs to be considered.

The other variable is the size of your glass, and wine glasses vary tremendously. Though the average pub glass is 125ml, those in people's homes or restaurants can easily hold double that. So a large glass of 14% strength wine could contain 4 or so units, rather than one.

Drinking and driving

Alcohol is one of the few things you can eat or drink which is absorbed straight into the bloodstream, beginning when it reaches your gullet. It is also the only 'nutrient' that can't be stored by the body, so when you drink, the liver has to process the alcohol and get rid of it via the urine, breath, skin and so on.
The liver can process around one unit of alcohol an hour, though this varies from person to person depending on the state of your liver, your sex, weight, whether or not you have just eaten, and so on.

The chart above shows roughly how many units you can drink in what period of time before becoming 'over the limit' for driving – and in effect this also means that if you go over these recommendations you will be intoxicated. 'Over the limit' in the UK means a blood alcohol concentration of over 80mg per 100ml blood.

The chart is only a guide; people vary considerably. The safest is to not drink at all if you are driving.

Health benefits of alcohol

Most alcoholic drinks contain plant chemicals (phytochemicals) that can help to protect against heart disease if drunk in moderate amounts. Dark beers and stouts and red wine seem to contain more of these types of phytochemical (flavonoids) than do paler beers, white wine and spirits. The flavonoids act as antioxidants, helping to keep the arteries from clogging up with cholesterol. Red wine also helps to prevent blood clotting, increases 'good' HDL cholesterol in the blood and can protect against stroke.

Alcohol may also protect against Alzheimer's disease and peptic ulcers and can improve brain alertness and IQ in middle-aged men. Alcohol also aids digestion by encouraging the secretion of digestive juices in the stomach and is thus useful when taken with food, and can reduce stress levels.

Research at the Harvard School of Public Health found that drinking 2 glasses of wine a day lowers LDL cholesterol levels enough to account for a reduction of nearly 25% in risk of coronary heart disease.

Health drawbacks of alcohol

All the benefits of alcohol are found when it is taken in small or moderate amounts – between 1 and 4 units a day for men. When people drink much more than this, all the drawbacks of alcohol abuse begin to kick in.
They are:

- Increased risk of CHD and stroke.
- Increased risk of cancers of the digestive system.
- Increased risk of liver disease, malnutrition, osteoporosis (even in men) and mental health problems, including depression and confusion.

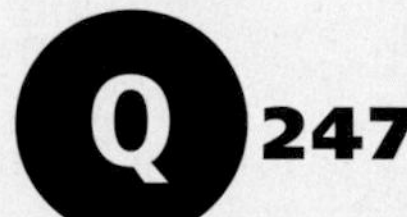

I'm not overweight but I've put 4 inches on my waist in the last 10 years. I am 50. Is this normal, and is it reversible?

This is the typical male pattern of weight gain – the 'apple' effect, discussed elsewhere. Without regular, fairly dedicated exercise, the waist size of both men and women does naturally increase over the years – for women this is more marked past menopause, when their diminished female hormones mean they become, in effect, more 'male' in their physical characteristics. For men, any small gain in adulthood tends to gather around the abdomen and waist, at any age.

The thickening waist for men is also compounded by poor posture with age (the middle may literally 'sag', as the area between hips and ribcage is supported only by muscle) and by lack of specific exercise for the midriff. Studies show that even very fit men increase girth by around 2 inches (5cm) as they get older, so there is some inevitability about it – but it can be minimized if you are determined enough.

For most men, however, 4 inches (10cm) is quite a lot to gain in 10 years and I would guess that you have put on some weight, even if you aren't actually overweight. I expect you've also given up most forms of exercise that may keep your midriff well toned. You need to set aside regular time, several times each week, to exercise all your stomach muscles, and consider losing a few pounds, which will almost certainly go from your stomach and waist first, through watching what you eat and taking more aerobic exercise.

If you were very slim as a young man, however, a 4-inch waist gain may not be as bad as it sounds. If your BMI is well within limits (see Feature 3), your waist circumference within recommended guidelines (Feature 3 again) and you feel fit, a 30-inch waist at age 30 that turns into a 34-inch waist at 50 isn't too disastrous.

See also:

- Questions: 28, 31, 56, 248–51.
- Features: 3, 6, 21, 28–30.
- A–Z entries: gyms, weighted workouts.
- Key index entries: apple shape, exercise, weight and health.

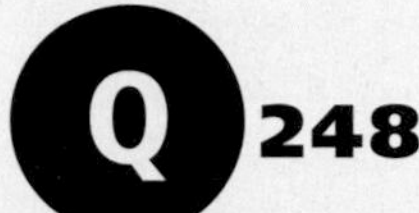

When I gain weight, why does it always go to my belly first?

Men tend to be 'apple-shaped', women 'pear-shaped', due to the differing patterns of fat laying-down because of different hormone levels. So, if you put on weight, in most men it naturally gravitates towards the stomach. There is also evidence that stress can increase abdominal fat (see Q324), so try to de-stress.

In both sexes, weight tends to go first on to the upper body, and this upper body weight is also the first to disappear if you slim. The typical 'pot belly' seems to contain a type of fat much easier to disperse than fat elsewhere, so at least that is good news.

See also:

- Questions: 48, 56–7, 246–7, 249–51.
- Features: 3, 6, 9, 21, 28–30.
- Key index entries: apple shape, exercise, weight and health.

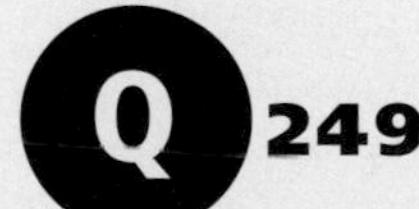

How do I slim my pot belly but keep the rest of my shape the same?

If you're a little overweight and follow a calorie-reduced diet for a few weeks you should find that the fat goes from your stomach more noticeably than elsewhere. For the explanation for this, see the previous question. You should also do exercises for the midriff to tone you up and make the stomach look slimmer.

See also:

- Questions: 48, 247–8, 250–51.
- Features: 5–6, 9, 21, 28–30.
- Key index entries: apple shape, exercise, weight and health.

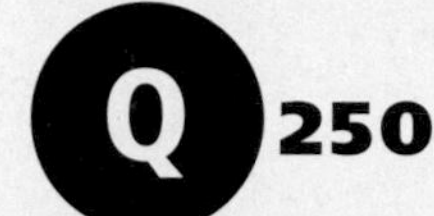

Is a pot belly a cause for concern, healthwise?

A large 'pot' is worrying because it is more closely linked with health problems than is fat elsewhere. Indeed, some experts believe that waist circumference (and 'pot') is more important than your actual weight in predicting future health risks. Other parts of the book explain this in more detail.

See also:

- Questions: 56, 324.
- Features: 3, 25.
- Key index entries: apple shape, weight and health.

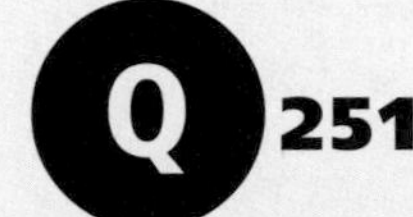

Can any man have a 'six pack'?

In theory, most men can, but in practice, not really. What is known as a 'six pack' is the outline of the divisions of the rectus abdominis muscle that runs down either side of the centre of the stomach from ribcage to 'belly button' (in fact there are four 'divisions' on each side, so really it should be called an eight-pack). All men have this muscle – but it can be seen in so few men because it is usually covered by a layer of fat, and is rarely exercised enough to be well defined.

Those young men who work very hard and very regularly on their stomach muscles, have a low body fat percentage and who do achieve a 'six pack', can feel justifiably proud of themselves. For most males, the effort required to get that sought-after physique is just too much and there are more important things in life. Men don't actually need to be that honed and toned in order to be healthy – you just need a reasonable waist circumference and an absence of obvious 'pot'.

See Feature 21 to rate your chances of achieving a six pack. If you want to go for it, don't wait. The older and flabbier your stomach gets, the harder it will be!

See also:

- Questions: 41, 45, 56, 62, 246–50, 252.
- Features: 3, 5, 6, 21, 28–30.
- A–Z entries: gyms, weighted workouts.
- Key index entries: exercise, muscles, stomach.

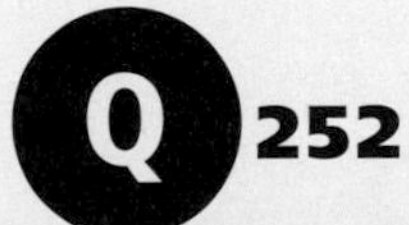

252

The scales don't tell me I weigh too much, but the weight is distributed all wrong – I want to get it off my middle and on to my chest and arms. Is this possible?

You can't actually shift your weight from your middle to your chest and arms as such, but by following a good programme of diet and exercise this is what you could probably achieve:

1 Reduction in the amount of fat in your stomach area (reduced-calorie diet).
2 Increased muscle tone in your stomach (mid-body exercise and other exercise, such as hill-walking) to produce a slimmer look.
3 Flatter appearance to your stomach (posture work).
4 Increased definition and muscle bulk to your arms somewhat (resistance training).
5 Bigger-looking chest (resistance work and posture).

When you diet to lose fat on your stomach you will lose a small amount of fat also from your arms but, as answers to other questions in this section explain, fat goes most readily from the midriff in males and so your arms shouldn't go stick-thin in the process.

What you absolutely cannot do is lose fat off your stomach and put fat on your arms at the same time, because if you are reducing your calorie intake to get rid of your belly, you can't put fat on your arms while doing so. The only way you can achieve a bigger look to your arms is by training the muscles there and bulking them up.

The amount of bulking you can achieve is determined genetically by your natural body shape (see Feature 4). I would guess that you are predominantly ectomorph with some endomorph tendencies – large middle and slim legs and arms is typical – which means that you may find it hard ever to get anything more than a small amount of extra muscle mass on your limbs. When your stomach has shrunk, though, you will look much more in proportion anyway.

See also:

- Questions: 41, 48, 56–8, 60, 66, 248–9.
- Features: 3–6, 21, 30.
- A–Z entries: gyms, weighted workouts.
- Key index entries: body shape, exercise, muscle.

FAT FACT

Just one extra pound (0.5 kilo) of muscle on your body means that you will burn up an extra 50–100 calories a day, depending on your own metabolism.

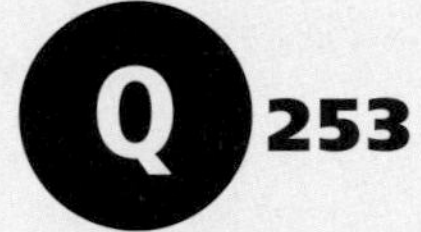

253

Is there a way of losing weight that doesn't involve starving, operations, slimming pills or aerobic classes?

Oh dear, do I detect a touch of cynicism? You need to know that weight loss needn't involve any of these tortures and, in fact, preferably doesn't – with the exception of the aerobics classes, which appeal to some people and can be a good idea. (However, you should know that the proportion of men going to aerobics classes is a mere 5%, so you may feel out on a limb.)

All you need to do is a) alter your eating habits somewhat – making sure that your new regime still fits in with your lifestyle so that you'll stick to it, and b) take up some form of regular exercise both to burn calories and to increase your muscle mass – this has to be something you don't dislike.

You absolutely mustn't go headlong into a crash diet – especially one that has been designed for a woman's appetite and metabolism – which is almost bound to end in failure. You need enough calories and 'meal appeal' to keep you satisfied.

Operations and pills are only for a small minority of people (generally very obese people) with their doctor's approval.

It sounds as though you've been watching women attempting to regulate their weight over the years and think you have to do the same. Sadly, much of what women feel they need to do to lose weight is far from wise. The cross-references below will point you in the right direction.

See also:

- Questions: 37–8, 79, 102–4, 106.
- Features: 8, 9, 11, 13, 14–15, 28–30.
- A–Z entries: gyms, low-fat diets, weighted workouts.
- Key index entries: aerobic exercise, calories, healthy eating, men and slimming, metabolism, muscle mass.

The central issue

Men worry more about it than almost any other body part, and few men are truly pleased with the shape theirs is in. Yes – it's the stomach, of course. Here's what you need to know.

Fat equals fat

All food or drink 'surplus to requirements' converts to fat on your body – but fat is particularly good at doing so. Fat is the most efficient nutrient at turning into body fat, using only around 3% energy in the conversion. At 9 calories a gram (about 50 calories per teaspoon), fats and oils are the highest-calorie food or drink you can get.

Protein for lean

Lean protein is a particularly good food for men. It converts readily into bodily lean tissue (muscle), is only 4 calories per gram and up to a third of the protein that you eat is burnt off in 'dietary-induced thermogenesis' (see Q3) before it has a chance to turn into fat. Lean red meat, poultry (no skin), game, white fish, pulses and low-fat dairy produce are all excellent sources and can form the basis of many meals.

Caution with the carbs

Carbohydrates, such as bread, pasta and rice, are good for you (especially if they are the whole-grain variety and so are starchy root vegetables. These 'complex carbohydrates' can form part of your diet – but go easy on any fat you have with them (dairy sauces, butter, cheese for example). Carbohydrates that come ready-loaded with fat, e.g. pastry, or sugar, which is a carbohydrate in itself and often comes packaged in high-fat foods (e.g. cakes, biscuits) are less 'good for you' and are also likely to end up on your belly as fat, so are best avoided.

Go for greens

If you want to get rid of that paunch of yours fast, choose plenty of green leafy vegetables and salads with your quota of lean protein and small portions of complex carbohydrates. In fact, vegetables of any colour are good (especially the brightly coloured ones as they're so full of protective phytochemicals). Jazz them up with lots of fresh herbs and spices.

Alcohol alert

Happily, small amounts of your favourite alcoholic beverage can be fitted into a flab-busting routine, but do go easy – see the answer to Q244. Just that one pint of beer a day over what your body really needs in terms of calories can put over a stone in weight on you in the course of a year – much of which, because you are male, will go straight to your belly.

The insulin factor

If you drink a lot of alcoholic drinks (which contain not only alcohol but also simple carbohydrates) over a long period of time these may eventually cause your insulin-producing mechanism to get 'worn out'.

Insulin is released in the body in response to high intakes of sugar (simple carbohydrates). When the insulin mechanism is overloaded you may get what is known as insulin resistance, a syndrome that is linked with a fat belly and increased risk of diseases such as diabetes and heart disease. (See the box on 'Syndrome X' that appears in Feature 25.)

Avoid this possibility by having alcohol and simple carbohydrates in small doses and concentrating mainly on getting lean protein, vegetables and complex carbohydrates. Also eat meals that are generally smaller, but more frequent.

FAT FACT

There is evidence that a high-stress life can increase abdominal fat by raising levels of the hormone cortisol in the body, which tends to encourage central fat accumulation.

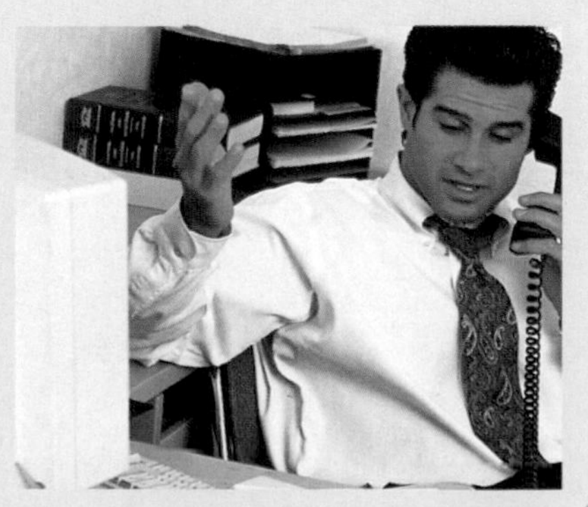

FAT FACT

The male hormone testosterone predisposes overweight men to gain weight on the abdomen rather than on the hips and thighs. In one study, men given supplements of oestrogen found themselves developing the classic female 'pear shape'.

The blueprint eating plan

The Diet Bible Basic Diet in Feature 9 on pages 74–5 is a perfect starting place where you can see what foods you should be eating to shrink your gut, and help yourself to health at the same time. Check out Features 14-15 and 25 for many more ideas to fit in with your lifestyle.

Burning the fat

No amount of abs exercises will work to give you a great stomach if the muscles are hidden underneath a layer of fat. In that case, you need not only to reduce your total calorie intake with our tips but also take more fat-burning exercise to help burn off the surplus fat. Power walking, cycling and swimming are ideal. Check out Feature 29.

Force be with you

To get a six pack (or something approximating one) you need to work your abdominal muscles every day, starting with the routine in Feature 6 and moving to the abs exercises in the panel over the page. A mere ten minutes a day will do.

Never too late

Research shows that the older you get, the harder you will have to work to maintain your stomach in good condition. Even élite athletes, doing regular vigorous training, monitored over a 20-year period in middle age, gained 2 inches (5cm) around their waists and their body fat percentage increased by 5%.

However, older men who begin eating well and taking regular exercise can expect to see impressive improvement in their body shape. In one trial, men aged from 60 to 72 doubled their muscle strength over a 12-week period of monitored exercise, while other research shows that very fit men of 70 can have a similar body profile and aerobic capacity to men of average fitness aged about 45.

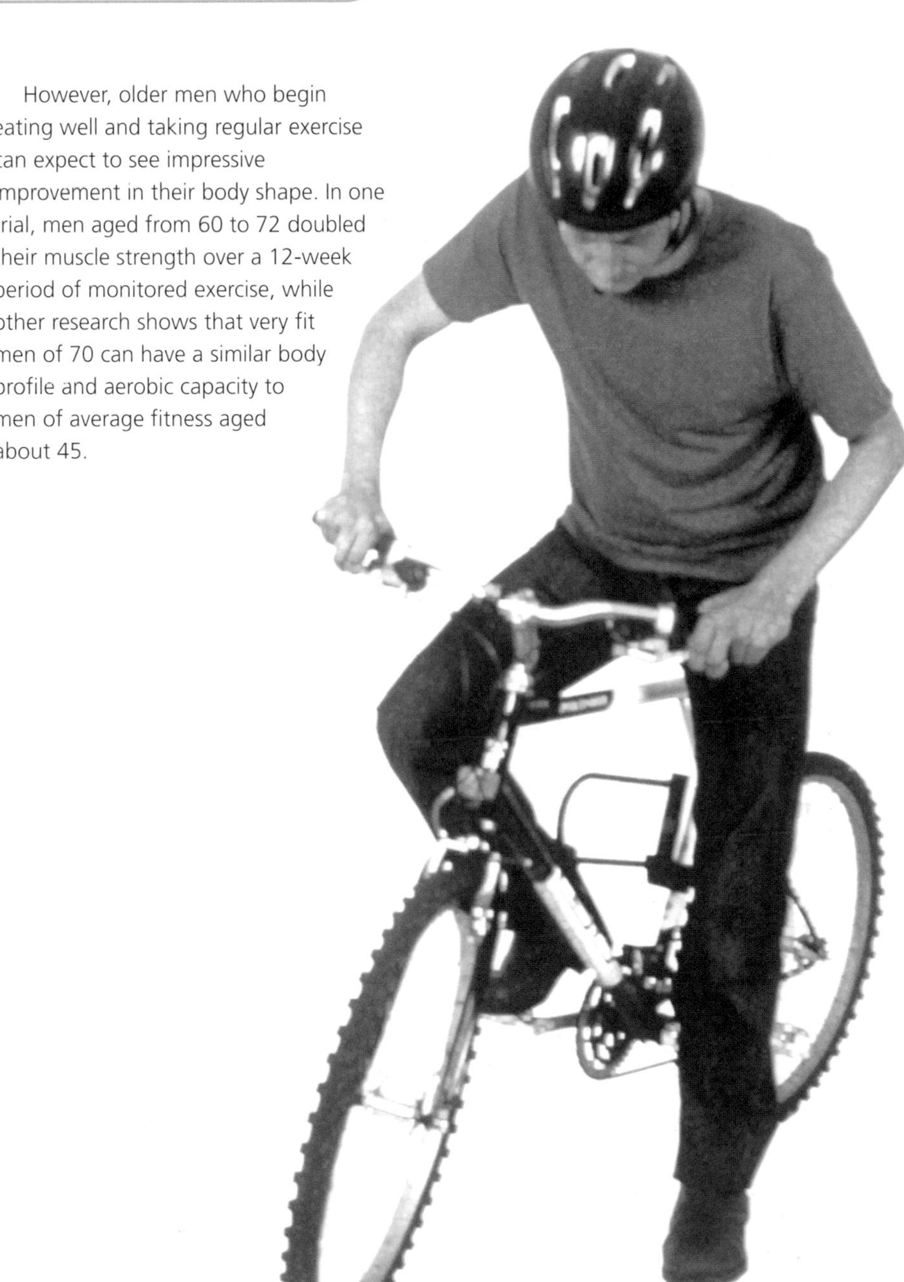

The six-pack exercises

If you are unfit, begin by doing the abs and other exercises in Feature 6 first, then progress to these, warming up, cooling down, and following instructions as explained in Feature 6. Do these exercises at least 5 times a week. NOTE: If you have a weak back, strengthen the back first before attempting these exercises (see Feature 6).

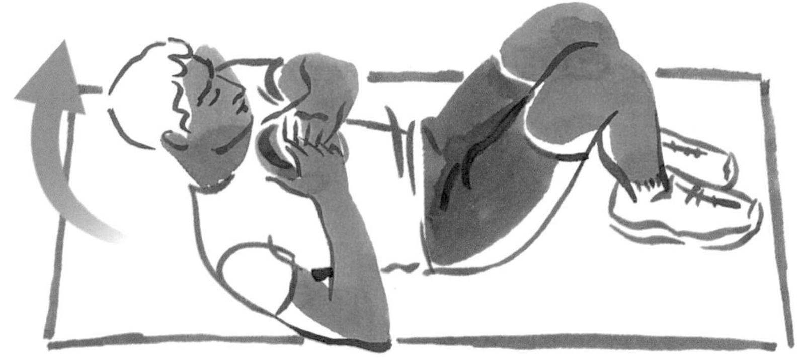

Weighted crunches (for rectus abdominis – 'six pack')

Lie in a similar position as for the standard crunches in Feature 6 but have a 2.5kg weight plate clutched to your chest. With your chin close to your chest, curl up until your shoulder blades are about 6 inches (15cm) from the floor, holding firmly on to the weight plate. Pause for a moment then slowly return to floor. When you can do 12 reps easily (after about two weeks, probably), you can increase the weight if you like.

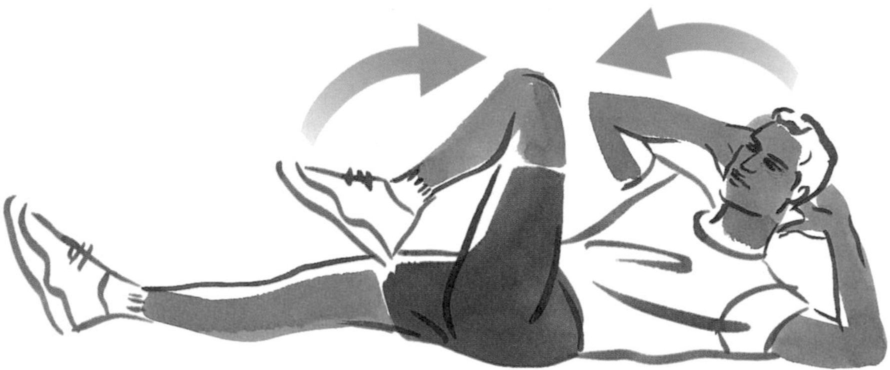

Push and pull (for all ab muscles especially obliques, i.e. waist)

Lie flat on your back with your hands loosely placed on the sides of the head and knees bent, feet on the floor. Raise your right shoulder from the floor and, at the same time, bring the left knee in to meet the right elbow while the right leg raises off the floor an inch or two (but stays straight). In a flowing movement, now lower your right elbow and raise your left shoulder, at the same time moving the left leg out and down (until it is an inch or two off the floor) and your right leg in so that the right knee meets the left elbow. This back-and-forward, flowing movement works the abs constantly, with alternating work on your obliques.
Repeat (without the straight leg touching the floor until you've finished a set).

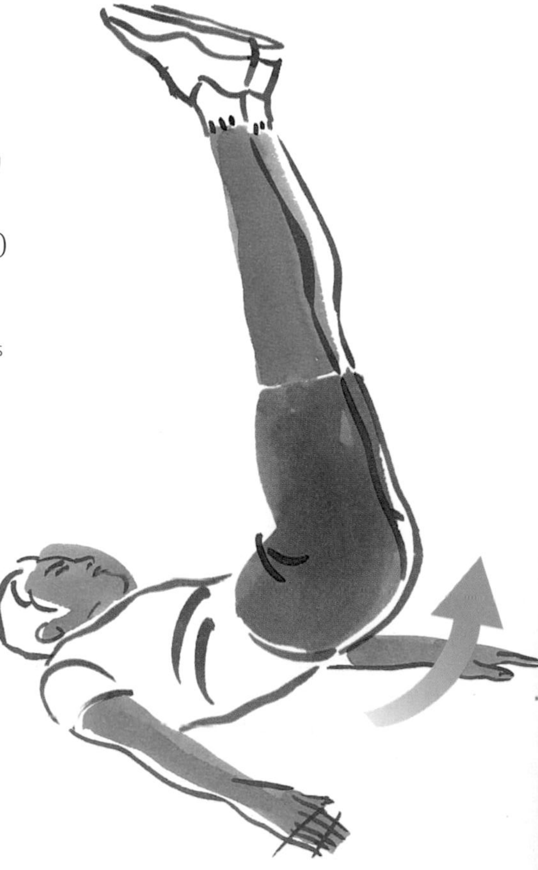

Reverse crunch (for transversus abdominis – lower stomach)

Lie on your back with your legs together, arms out at 45 degrees to your sides for support. Slowly raise your legs to vertical. Breathe out, contract your abdominals and lift your bottom and lower back off the floor, pushing the base of the feet towards the ceiling. Repeat.

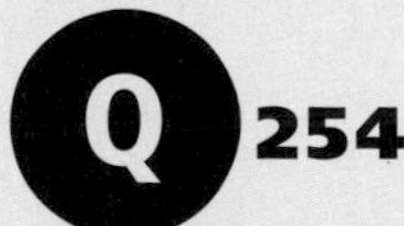

Can I do anything about my embarrassing flabby 'breasts'? I'm not very fat, but I get teased about them and would love firm pecs.

The name for this is gynaecomastia – meaning the over-development of breast tissue in males. Being overweight is normally the cause of this – you don't have to be obese to notice the syndrome, but I would guess that you are probably at least 1 or 2 stone(s) overweight, with a typical male 'apple shape'. (Check out your Body Mass Index as explained in Feature 3.)

What happens is that the fatty body tissue produces the female hormone oestrogen, which stimulates the development of fat in the breast area. If you lose weight (all over) you will reduce oestrogen levels and the 'breasts' will reduce in size.

You should also cut right back on alcohol if you have been a heavy drinker. Alcohol abuse reduces the ability of the liver to break down complex steroid hormones and can make gynaecomastia worse. Low levels of testosterone in the body may also contribute to breast development – you should see your doctor and, if a test shows this is the case, he may offer testosterone supplements.

Lastly, regular exercises to strengthen the pectoral muscles (see the cross-references) should help to improve your chest profile, too.

See also:
- ▶ Questions: 28, 56, 252.
- ▶ Features: 3, 9.
- ▶ A–Z entries: gyms, walking, weighted workouts.
- ▶ Key index entries: apple shape, food value charts, hormones, weight distribution.

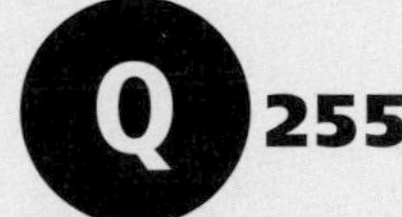

Is it true that if I wear a sweatsuit to exercise, I will burn off twice the calories?

No. What wearing a sweatsuit will do for you is to make you hotter and increase your perspiration loss, so that after the exercise you will have lost a pound or two of fluid from your body. This should be immediately replaced – by you drinking water or similar – otherwise you could be dehydrated. In other words, sweatsuits are not only a waste of time but also potentially dangerous. I am afraid there is no real shortcut to burning off calories through exercise – you have to put in the work!

See also:
- ▶ Questions: 333–7.
- ▶ Features: 28, 29.
- ▶ A–Z entries: cycling, gyms, walking.
- ▶ Key index entries: calorie burning, drinking, fat burning, metabolism.

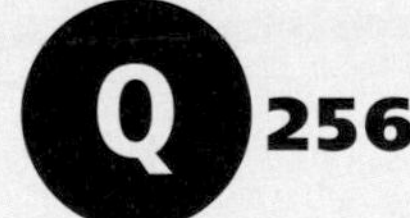

Does regular sex keep you slim?

First turn to Q209 and read the answer to the women's question on sex and calories. Should you definitely NOT be a 'four-minute man', and should you enjoy sex on a very regular basis, you could burn up a fair amount of calories in the process. Men tend to use up more calories having sex than women do, as women are often a lazy lot (or too exhausted after a day running the world and then doing the cooking, cleaning and child-minding) and tend to prefer the 'lie here and enjoy it' position most of the time, while men do all the hard work.

So let us assume that you have sex four times a week at 30 minutes a time (let's be generous!). Two hours of sex at 7 calories a minute (on average) comes to 840 calories burnt per week. That is about equivalent to a hungry male's evening meal, or four pints of beer, or a takeaway pizza. So, as long as you don't send out for the pizza after the sex, I suppose you could lose about 1lb a month (or not put ON 1lb a month) in weight with two hours' sex a week.

See also:
- ▶ Questions: 6, 18, 209, 333–8.
- ▶ Feature: 2, 28.
- ▶ Key index entries: calorie burning, energy equation, metabolism,

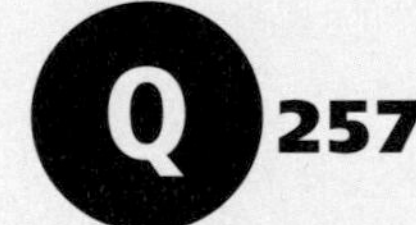

Is there any fat-burning exercise class that isn't aimed primarily at women?

A recent survey of exercise classes found that you are most likely to meet fellow males at boxercise classes or Ashtanga yoga classes. Boxercise is no surprise, although apparently 40% of devotees are female. You may be amazed to learn that you can burn fat through yoga, but Ashtanga is fast and furious and quite hard. The A–Z section at the end of the book contains information on both of these pursuits.

See also:
- ▶ Questions: 253, 258, 334–7.
- ▶ Features: 28, 29.
- ▶ A–Z entries: exercise classes, yoga.
- ▶ Key index entries: aerobics, calorie burning, exercise, fat burning, yoga.

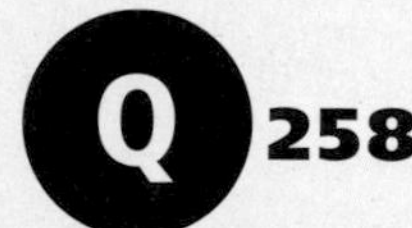

I dislike both the gym and outdoor exercise, so what exercise can I do to burn calories?

There are various things you can do at home – for example, skipping (an excellent, quick way to burn calories and get fit), or using a mini-trampoline, exercise bike, treadmill or rowing machine. For all the pros and cons of these, see the A–Z section. You could also pursue indoor sports such as badminton, tennis, squash, or swimming. I suppose you are including walking in your list of outdoor activities that you dislike, but if you hadn't thought of walking as an outdoor exercise, it really is an excellent calorie-burning activity, especially if you're not very fit to begin with. To make it more purposeful, you could do what many have done before and get a dog.

See also:

- Questions: 257, 333–47.
- Features: 27–9.
- A–Z entries: dancing, exercise classes, exercise equipment, sports, walking.
- Key index entry: exercise.

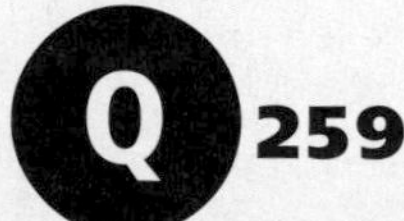

Is there a male menopause and if so is it the cause of my weight gain? I am 55.

Yes, it seems that there is a male menopause, which could indeed have various side-effects, including weight gain. Although the major symptom of the female menopause – loss of periods – is obviously not a factor for men, there is, according to studies presented at the British Endocrine Society's conference in 2001, an average decrease in levels of the male hormone testosterone in mid-life males.

Levels start to decline at a similar age to the female menopause – around 50 – and reduced testosterone can cause not only weight gain, loss of muscle mass and loss of energy, but also depression, mood swings, lowered sex drive, memory loss and irritability.

The explanation from one of the partner universities conducting the latest research is that low levels of testosterone seem to reduce the blood supply to the brain, which means, basically, a general shutdown or slowing of the metabolism – in other words, the factory that is the male brain is on go-slow and the menopausal symptoms described are a natural result of that.

As with women, menopausal symptoms vary from man to man and may be slight or severe. If you feel this may be your problem, do see your doctor. Work is under way in developing a male testosterone-replacement HRT. Such HRT for males may also include the female hormone oestrogen, which has been found to protect men against osteoporosis and may also protect them against mental decline and memory loss.

In the meantime, a programme of sensible eating and increasing the amount of both aerobic and resistance exercise will help minimize symptoms. For, although declining hormones can promote weight gain, that doesn't mean the situation isn't containable with a healthy lifestyle – as many post-menopausal women will confirm.

Staying in shape as you get older becomes harder, but is by no means impossible. The bonus is that with healthy diet and by taking more exercise you are also giving yourself natural protection against the diseases and infirmities of old age.

See also:

- Questions: 27, 72–3, 236, 247.
- Features: 1, 3, 9, 25, 27–30.
- A–Z entries: calorie counting, metabolism-boosting diets, weighted workouts.
- Key index entries: aerobic exercise, ageing, hormones, metabolism, mid-life, resistance exercise, weight and health.

Do men get eating disorders?

The number of men contacting the Eating Disorders Association for help is increasing. It is now thought that about 10% of anorexics and bulimics are male, but as people still think of these as 'female' problems it apparently takes twice as long to diagnose a male sufferer.

Although many of the 'triggers' that can cause eating disorders in females (see Qs 149, 151 and 155) may also be present in males, there are also male-specific triggers. One is being bullied, another is being teased for being overweight. Men are also more prone to over-exercising and bodybuilding, which may accompany or predate an eating disorder. Such men are often described as having 'machismo nervosa', although this isn't an official term.

If you think you may have an eating disorder, or you know someone who has, you can contact the Eating Disorders Association on 01603 621414 or the National Centre for Eating Disorders on 01372 469493. Cognitive behaviour therapy works well for many men.

See also:

- Questions: 29, 132–3, 149–58.
- Feature: 3.
- Key index entries: bingeing, comfort eating, eating disorders, healthy eating, weight assessment.

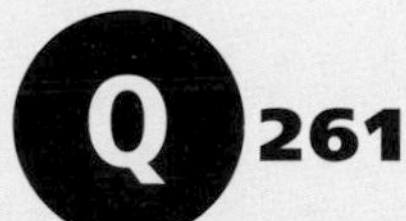

261

I'm single and like cooking, but how can I make meals enjoyable without the butter/pastry/oil/cream and so on that are the backbone of my menus?

You just need to learn a few new tricks. The meals in the diet features throughout this book will help you on the way (some are listed in the cross-references below). You'll soon see that there is a list of ingredients that crop up regularly, all of which are high on taste and low – or fairly low – in calories and/or fat.

For example, passata, balsamic vinegar and all vinegars, all spices, all herbs, lemon juice, lime juice, fresh garlic, onions, verjuice, wine, soy sauce, sea salt, chilli essence, capers, olives, anchovies, French whole-grain mustard. From these you can make a wide range of sauces, marinades, flavourings and garnishes. Oil, butter and even cream can still be used, but in small quantities, and there is no need to rely on them every time you grab a saucepan and get cooking.

For example, instead of pan-frying a steak and then adding cream to make an easy sauce, you could add chopped garlic and a dash of red wine, reduce it for a few minutes and there you have a delicious healthy sauce. To liven up a chicken breast, marinate it in lime juice and a dash of olive oil with garlic and chilli essence before baking it with olive-oil-tossed and seasoned sliced red peppers.

There are so many things to try. If you enjoy cooking you should feel excited, rather than bored or daunted, by what's available to buy and what's possible to cook. A browse amongst the cookery books in your local store will prove my point – not all are sold as low-fat or low-calorie cookbooks, but quite a lot of the 'new wave' chefs and ethnic cookbooks contain very many healthy non-fattening recipes. Quite a few also have nutritional panels with each recipe which is another boon.

One thing is absolutely certain – there is no need at all to feel that healthy eating is diametrically opposed to cooking and enjoying your food. And neither is it more time-consuming or more difficult, once you get the hang of the new easy methods. Enjoy!

See also:

- ▶ Questions: 79, 89, 112, 122, 129, 131.
- ▶ Features: 8–11, 13–15.
- ▶ A–Z entries: calorie counting, low-fat diets.
- ▶ Key index entries: calories, cooking, fat, slimming.

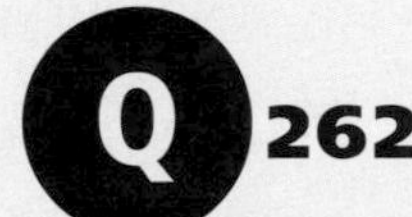

262

What are the best cooking methods for a single male who is a fairly hopeless cook and wants to lose weight?

At least you are prepared to cook for yourself, rather than relying too much on takeaways and convenience meals – so good for you. You could start by getting a novice's cookbook to bone up on a few easy methods. I hate to mention it, but Delia's *How To Cook* Parts 1 and 2 are ideal, and although people always think her food is 'fattening', in fact there is a lot of low-fat and low-cal stuff there, explained clearly – and she is always a 'tasty' cook, with plenty of male appeal in her dishes.

So, on to your question. Well, grilling and dry-frying in a pan are simple methods for lean and tender cuts of meat such as steak, pork tenderloin, lamb cutlets, and for most fish. All you need to do is get the element and pan hot enough so that you sear the outside of the meat or fish, turn once after a couple of minutes, and do the other side. Beware, though – overcooked lean meat goes tough and becomes dry, and overcooked fish breaks up and becomes dry.

Stir-frying is every man's favourite stand-by and none the worse for that. You just chop everything up small, throw it in your wok according to how long it takes to cook (hard veggies first, meat usually second, soft veggies and seasonings last). To save pouring in too much high-calorie oil, you can keep the pan moist by adding a very little water or stock towards the end of cooking time.

In winter, stews (on the hob) or casseroles (in the oven) are both ideal – there is much room for manoeuvre and they both tend to be perfectly edible even if slightly under- or overcooked. You can throw in lots of veg, and need use hardly any fat. You can fling in spices and call it a curry, or chop the veg up smaller and call it a soup. You can purée some of the finished dish if you have an electric blender, to thicken without adding fat, flour, etc. Leftovers keep well in the fridge.

In summer, you need think no further than main-meal salads – ready-cut and washed leaves, herbs, etc. make the job easy – just add your protein (cooked marinated chicken, for example, thinly sliced) and some carbohydrate (bread, chopped cooked new potatoes, cooked pasta or rice) and there you are. There are plenty of ideas throughout this book for lower-fat salad dressings and, indeed, for all the types of meal suggested here.

Keep your portions reasonably small and fill up on extra veg, side salads and fruit, and you should be successful.

See also:

- ▶ Questions: 79–90, 96, 104, 121–2, 131, 261.
- ▶ Features: 8, 9, 10, 14.
- ▶ A–Z entries: calorie counting, low-fat diets.
- ▶ Key index entries: calories, cooking, fat, healthy eating.

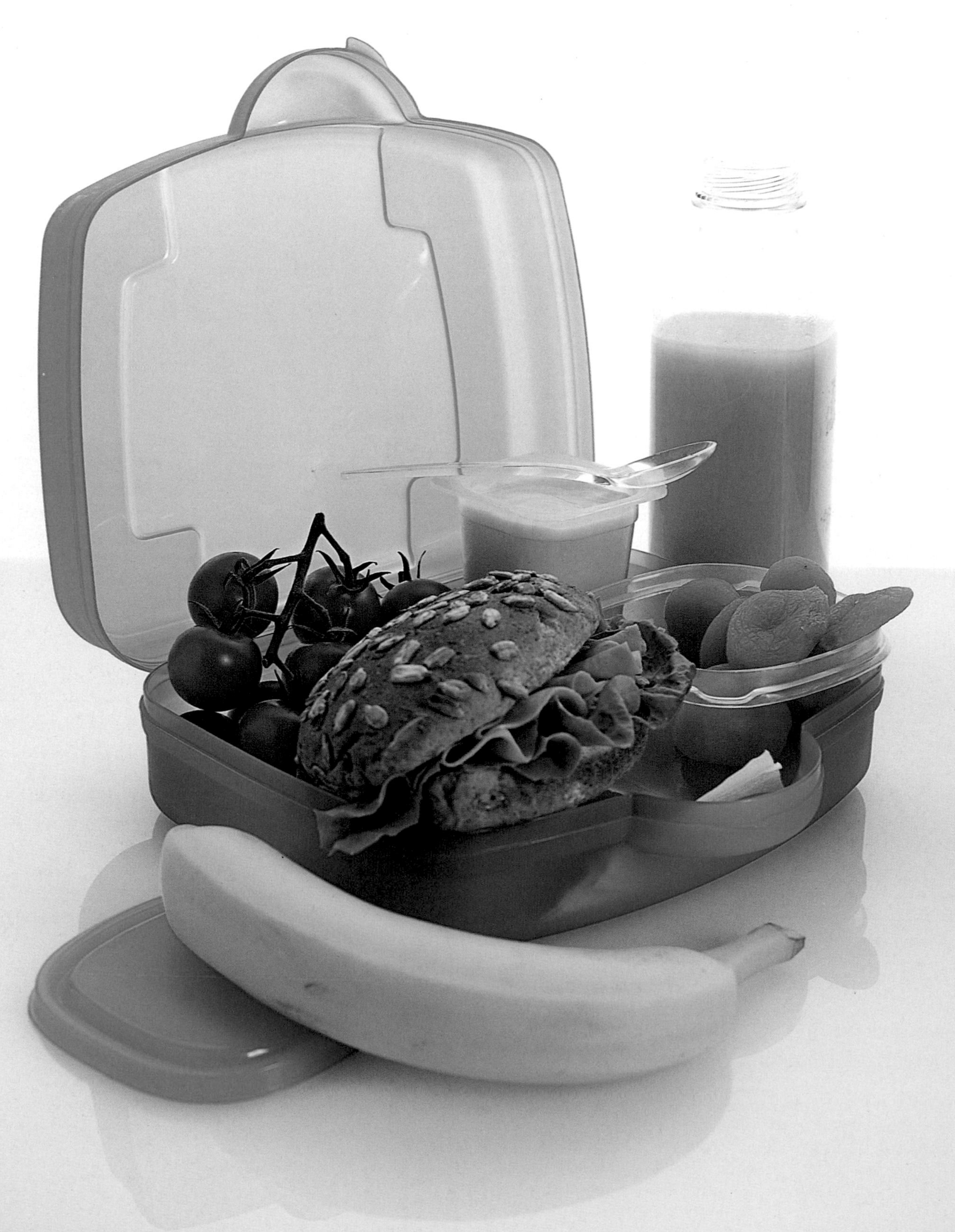

Section Eight

For kids (and parents) **only**

It is a fact today that children of the Western world (and across much of the rest of the world) are fatter than they have ever been. Look at the statistics – among children in the UK from birth to age 4 from 1989 to 1998 the proportion overweight has increased from 14.7% to 23.6%, the proportion obese has risen from 5.4% to 9.2%. Among children in the UK aged from 4 to 11, the proportion of overweight or obese boys increased from 6% in 1984 to 10.7% in 1994 and girls from 10.3% to 16.1%. By age 15, according to figures from the Obesity Resource Information Centre, 17.3% of girls and 16.4% of boys are obese, with many more overweight.

Child health experts agree that the cause is eating too many calories for their needs – encouraged by the huge fast- and snack-food industry – and taking little exercise. Our children's health is already suffering as a result. The numbers of young people aged 15–24 dying of heart disease in the West is rising year on year; and children as young as 8 have been found to have early signs of heart disease. It is known that obesity in adolescence frequently translates into obesity in adulthood – and shortened lifespan. No wonder that a report on childhood obesity published in the British Medical Journal in 2001 concluded that 'overweight in UK children is a serious public health problem'. In America, the Surgeon General recently said, 'This is the most obese generation of children in our history. The message is about saving lives.'

In this section we look at ways of helping our children to a slimmer, healthier – and longer – future.

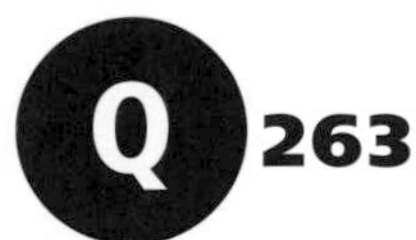

263

How do I tell if my child is overweight?

Believe it or not, there is no national or international consensus on the precise definition of overweight and obesity in children. For several years, doctors have been inclined to use 'percentile' weight for age charts (shown in Feature 22), which need to be interpreted on an individual basis, taking into account the child's height – obviously if your child is much heavier than average but also much taller than average, then he or she may not be overweight at all.

However, in 2000 a British team from the Institute of Child Health with the International Obesity Task Force produced a set of international cut-off points for overweight and obesity in children based on the Body Mass Index (see Feature 3). This produces guidelines for children based on their weight and height from age 2 to 18, after which the standard Body Mass Index charts are used. These cut-off points correspond to an adult BMI of 25+ for overweight and 30+ for obese. Although these cut-off points for children have not yet been taken on board internationally, many experts believe that they offer the best assessment of overweight or obesity in children.

An adapted chart appears in Feature 22 – so if you want an initial assessment of your child's weight you can use the percentile chart or the BMI chart – or both – and get a good idea.

Some experts also suggest simply looking at your child with the rest of his/her class at school and seeing if he/she seems much bigger than most of the others as a reasonable way to tell if there is a weight problem. It is also advisable to see your doctor, who will no doubt be able to add a professional opinion and further advice.

See also:

- Questions: 264–8.
- Feature: 22.
- A–Z entries: fat camps, Fitkids.
- Key index entries: children, exercise, weight.

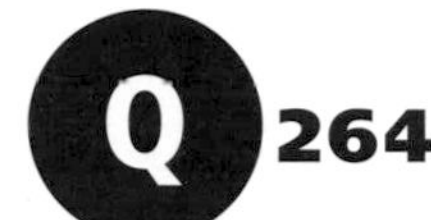

264

How important IS overweight in children?

The introduction to this section will give you a potted overview of the problem. We are facing an obesity epidemic that looks set to get even worse unless we can find solutions quickly. The main problem is that studies show that a high percentage of children and adolescents become fat adults, with all the health implications that brings, as outlined in Feature 25.

There are not many truly fat children who manage to lose the weight and go on to be slim adults, so it is obviously much better to prevent overweight in your child as a way to combat adult obesity. And, if your child has become overweight, the sooner you do something about it, the easier it should be to resolve.

See also:

- Questions: 263, 265–8.
- Features: 22, 25.
- A–Z entries: fat camps, Fitkids.
- Key index entries: children, overweight and health, weight and health.

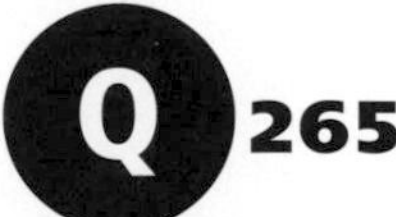

265

What is the best way to prevent a child from becoming overweight?

When children are small, many parents encourage their children to 'eat up' and equate a healthy appetite with a healthy child. This is understandable, as many very small children are faddy about food, have poor appetites and are consequently underweight. Any parent who has dealt with such a child may feel nothing but relief if that child later begins to eat like a horse, or if she/he has another child who relishes all food.

Getting your kids to eat well is perceived as a sign of being a 'good parent'. For many children, though, a healthy appetite for decent food is but a short trip to a big appetite for all kinds of food, followed by the first signs of overweight. So that is one pitfall to look out for. Encourage your child to eat well – but that doesn't mean overeating.

It is also important to look after yourself as a parent, and eat sensibly yourself. Research shows that overweight tends to run in families, as does the amount of exercise taken. The overweight factor may be partially due to a genetic predisposition (see Q7) but, even so, children tend to take their eating habits from parents and older siblings, and if what is offered, and what everyone else eats, is healthy and balanced, reasonably low in fat and sugar, then the child is unlikely to get fat, especially if the

FAT FACT

A study from Toronto University concludes that too much fat in the diet in childhood and adolescence can impair memory and concentration – brains function on glucose and the researchers believe that saturated fat may impede glucose metabolism in the brain.

parents encourage lots of physical activity. Take your child out hiking, swimming, cycling – help him/her to join sports clubs.

Sadly, PE and sports at school are tending to be sidelined by curriculum demands and so even school sports may not offer as much exercise as it once did. By the time children – particularly girls – are into their teens, their exercise habits (or lack of them) are pretty much entrenched, so it is important to develop your child's awareness of physical activity by encouraging her/him at every opportunity. Lead by example – and keep slim and fit yourself!

Lastly, you need to take an active interest in what your child is eating. Research shows that modern children tend to eat a great deal of 'snack' foods both outside the home (from the school café or tuckshop, from shops on the way home, at other children's houses) and in the home. Many kids have access to a 'snacks' cupboard and a fridge stocked full with crisps, cakes, fizzy drinks and so on. Peak times for 'raiding the larder' are when they get home from school (especially if no one is there) and over the weekend. Hundreds of surplus calories can be eaten this way, and they are likely to contain little in the way of good nutrition. Self-choice school lunches for children are also, in my opinion, a bad idea, as a high proportion of kids will pick the fattiest, most calorific thing on the menu. A lunch packed by yourself is a safer alternative and the only way to know what is being eaten.

One good way to monitor your child's calorie intake is to revive family meal times – sadly a minority of families now regularly sit down to a main meal or breakfast together. 'Proper' meals have been replaced with eating on the hoof or in front of the TV. One recent report found that increasing numbers of children can't even use a knife and fork when they start school because their meals consist of hand-held pizzas, burgers and nuggets.

FAT FACT

There is research to show that children who were breast-fed are less likely to become obese than bottle-fed infants. Three to five months of exclusive breast-feeding is associated with a 35% reduction in obesity at age 5–6.

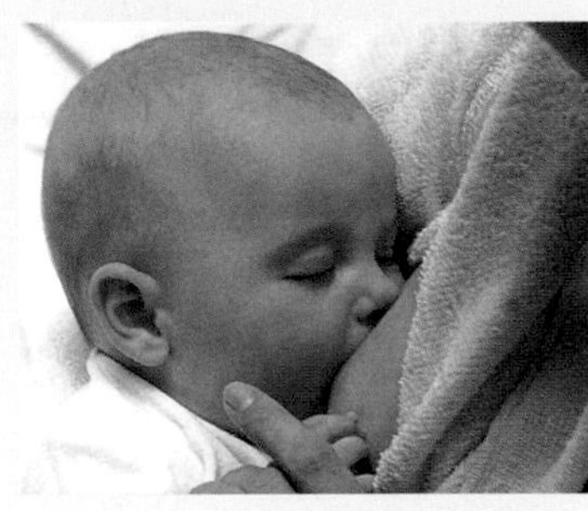

If you don't want your child to be overweight, you need to take back control of what he/she eats and drinks and how much exercise he/she does. Maybe letting the kids go down the 'fast food and TV' route gives you, the parent, more time for the rest of your life, but children are too young to know what is best for them, or care about their health. Other parts of this section will help you to give them a good diet that they will enjoy eating.

Given the choice, most children will pick high-fat, high-salt or high-sugar snack foods rather than fresh fruits, salads and fish. And, if allowed to get into the habit, they will also prefer to sit and be entertained than get out and be active. Too much freedom to choose their own diet and too many hours spent in front of the TV/computer will, in the end, make a very high percentage of them fat.

See also:

- Questions: 263–4, 266–74, 277–90.
- Features: 22, 23, 24.
- A–Z entries: fat camp, Fitkids.
- Key index entries: children, exercise, healthy eating, overweight.

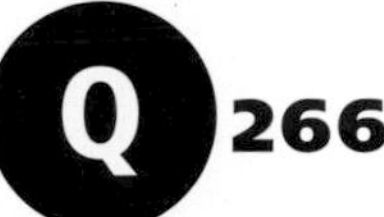

Q 266

Is it true that you should never put a child on a low-calorie diet?

This is one of those trick questions with no simple answer. Every time a child loses weight he/she has probably reduced his/her calorie intake significantly to do so – or taken a great deal of exercise to burn the calories off. Although many experts say you shouldn't put overweight children 'on a diet', as we've seen, very many children DO need to lose weight – so it's catch-22 – if you can't put your child on a diet, how is he/she ever going to lose weight? Calorie restriction seems to me to be an almost essential part of the equation.

Here we have the dilemma of what a 'low-calorie diet' actually means. If you give your overweight child a healthy diet with restricted fat and restricted sugar but with extra fruit and vegetables and bread, for example, so that the total calorie content is reduced but he/she still has plenty to eat, that is a reduced-calorie diet, I would say. But perhaps a low-calorie diet conjures up a picture of a poor child existing on meagre rations of lettuce, cottage cheese and water. So if 'low-calorie' in your book equates with 'crash dieting' then, of course, the answer is no, don't put your child on one of those.

This is not only because it will be demoralizing and miserable for the child, but also because even overweight children need all the nutrients that other children need, to grow and build bone, muscle, organs and so on. They also need enough of all the vitamins and minerals to help this along and guide them to health. A poorly thought-out calorie-reduced diet, especially one too low in calories overall, may easily not supply all these needs.

It is fair to say that any parent who feels their child is overweight should first see a doctor (who may refer you to a dietician) for advice and secondly follow the diet guidelines they are given. This will then be an officially approved, well-balanced, calorie-reduced diet, which is fine.

Having said that, obviously if your child has been eating a great deal of sweet snacks, crisps, greasy chips and so on, no dietician is going to tell you that you can't make an effort to cut these out, or down, to help reduce calorie intake. Often such methods will be enough in themselves to help a child slim down over time and this is, let's face it, dieting by any other name.

I suppose the key is that children should be helped to lose weight, if they need to, in a gradual, non-obtrusive way that won't have them feeling hungry or rebellious, or which will make them feel 'at fault' or depressed with their weight. Some experts therefore believe that the best way to slim down a fat child is simply to try to maintain his/her weight at its current level and wait until he/she literally 'grows into' it.

For example, a 10-year-old boy who weighs 10 stone now may not be overweight at all if he still weighs 10 stone at age 14. (This is just an example, children vary and height is a factor.) To ensure that your 10-stone 10-year-old doesn't put on any more weight, you do still need to watch the calories, but looking at this long-term picture of his weight may be better for the child psychologically and physically. You never once need say to the child 'you have to lose weight' and he can follow a 'calorie-containing' diet rather than a 'calorie-restricted' diet, so it may make him feel better all round. All you do is check his weight from time to time, and if he hasn't put on any more, all is well.

Again, the doctor or dietician who knows you and the child may offer the best advice on which method to follow. All the advice on feeding overweight children in the rest of this section is general, given in the best of faith, but it is always wise to treat your child as an individual.

See also:

▶ Questions: 263–5, 267–99.
▶ Features: 22–24.
▶ A–Z entries: fat camps, Fitkids.
▶ Key index entries: calories, healthy slimming for children, weight.

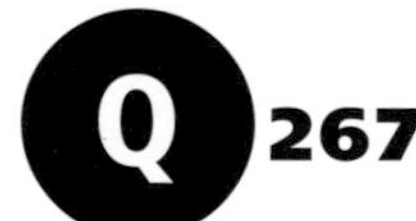

267

What is the best way to slim a child down?

The previous question will tell you, in broad terms, the lines along which you should be thinking if you have an overweight child. Here are some more detailed guidelines you can follow:

- Aim at a weekly weight loss of a maximum of ½–1lb (225–450g). This will mean reducing his/her daily calorie intake by about 250–500, which isn't drastic and should ensure adequate nutrition.
- If your child has been eating regular snacks of sweets, cakes, biscuits, pastries, crisps, and drinking a lot of high-sugar drinks, such as cola and lemonade, these are the first things to cut right back on, replacing them with less energy-dense foods such as those suggested in Qs 281–4. For some children, this alone is enough to produce 1lb a week loss.
- Increase his/her energy output by encouraging cycle rides, kicking a ball around, walk with your child to school, and so on. More ideas appear in Q282.
- Limit takeaway meals and meals eaten outside your control – prepare food yourself where possible.
- Don't reward good behaviour with snacks or chocolates and aim gradually to alter his/her mindset into accepting that food isn't always associated with 'leisure and pleasure' time: for example, that a visit to the cinema need not mean a huge box of popcorn and a litre of cola.
- Reduce portion sizes of high-density, high-fat foods, such as pies, pastries, Cheddar cheese, fatty meats, and increase portion sizes of fruits, vegetables. Portions of bread, potatoes, pasta, etc. can remain about the same.
- An easy method for both parent and child to follow is the 'Traffic Light' system described in Q113. This divides food into 3 categories – Green for go, Amber for proceed with caution, and Red for stop.

Other ideas for helping children control calorie intake appear throughout this section. It isn't easy persuading an overweight child to change eating habits, but with the right approach from you it can be done.

See also:

▶ Questions: 263–6, 268–92.
▶ Features: 22–24.
▶ A–Z entries: fat camps, Fitkids.
▶ Key index entries: healthy slimming for children.

FAT FACT

The amount of time allocated to physical education in primary schools has fallen by 50% in 5 years, according to the British Heart Foundation, and by the time girls are 15 two-thirds of them do so little exercise as to be officially classed as 'inactive'.

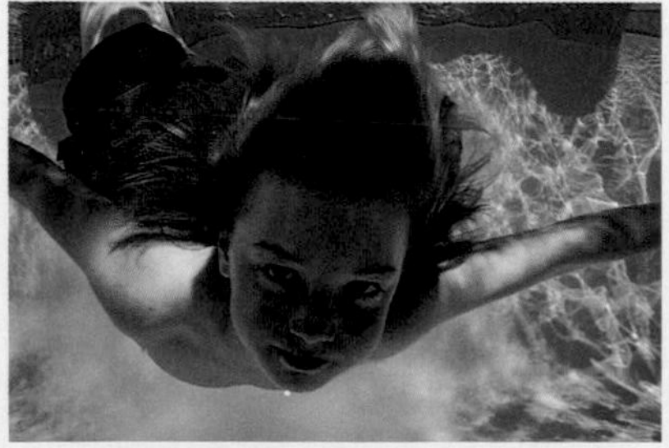

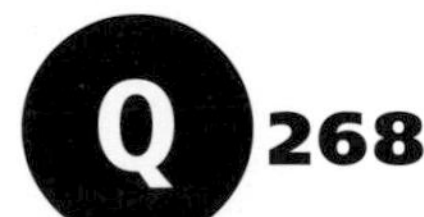

268

Should I take my overweight child to the doctor or try to do something about it myself?

In theory, it is always best to visit the doctor and let him or her weigh the child, assess the problem and help you with a strategy if needs be. He/she may refer you to a dietician, which is very useful, and you may get diet sheets and other advice.

In practice, things don't always go that smoothly, particularly if the child has very low self-esteem. Sitting in a surgery having her/his size discussed by her/his parent and a doctor is quite demoralizing, and it can backfire, with the child refusing to co-operate, or becoming depressed. The situation needs handling with tact.

I think it is best to help a child to slim without him/her quite realizing what is going on – this really is possible if you are happy (as you should be) with a very slow weight loss. Yet I feel the doctor visit is the right way to go. Perhaps you could telephone the doctor beforehand to explain the problem and perhaps he/she would be willing to invent another reason for the visit for the child – e.g., a general check-up. During this there is, quite naturally, a weigh-in, and at that point the subject of weight control can be gently worked in. Some doctors are excellent at this tactful handling of a problem.

Otherwise, if the weight problem seems minor (check in Feature 22) and you think you can beat it simply by altering snacking habits as per the previous questions, then perhaps you can get away without a visit. What you don't want to do is give any child a complex about his/her weight and the perceived problem. Encourage, or even slightly cajole, but never bully them about their weight/diet. Q296 discusses the psychology of slimming for children and young teens in more detail.

See also:

- Questions: 263–7, 296–9.
- Features: 22–4.
- Key index entry: healthy slimming for children.

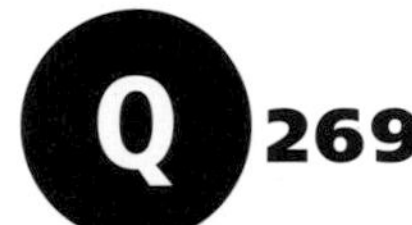

269

How can I stop my child aged 7 from liking junk food such as burgers, which will no doubt make him fat eventually?

The occasional lean burger won't make your child fat as part of a healthy balanced diet and nutritionally they aren't all bad, containing good amounts of iron, B vitamins and protein in the burger and calcium in the bun. For more on 'junk' food and takeaways, see Qs 118, 142 and 167 and Feature 15. You will see that there are a few reasonable fast-food choices, along with plenty of high-cal, high-fat ones. Most junk food is also high in salt and some is made from low-quality meat – two other factors to consider.

If your child is pre-teen, you will see from the chart in Feature 23 that he/she doesn't need as many calories as an adult or a teenager, and neither should he/she be eating so much fat. So if regularly having adult-sized portions of these meals then he/she is probably getting more of both than needed and may put on weight that way. For example, your seven-year-old needs a maximum of about 76g of fat a day, and about 1,970 calories. As you will see from the list of kid's favourites overleaf, an average (small) cheeseburger in a bun with French fries and a regular milkshake contains about 1,150 calories and 44g of fat. So one meal has provided over 58% of daily calorie needs and 58% of fat allowance. The rest of the day's meals need to be lower in fat and calories and contain fruit and veg to give a balanced diet that won't put weight on.

Worried about encouraging eating disorders?

I should point out that because of the rise in the number of cases of teenage eating disorders (and in even younger children) there is an understandable fear from some parents about encouraging their children to diet. If the child is genuinely overweight, this fear should not prevent you from reducing her/his weight by the means outlined here and in the answer to the next question.

The incidence of health problems associated with overweight and obesity is so much greater than the risks of an eating disorder developing in an overweight child who slims that I feel the sensible course of action is to help prevent the child from becoming an obese adult. Research indicates that it is very unlikely that your overweight child will turn into an anorexic one if you responsibly and sensitively help her/him to slim down. The problems of teenage eating disorders are discussed in detail in Qs 296–9.

So the first thing to do, if serving your child burgers, pizzas, nuggets, chips and so on at home, is to reduce portion sizes and offer veg, salad and fruit with them. The second thing to do is restrict these meals to a maximum of a few times a week – perhaps reducing frequency gradually over a period of weeks to soften the blow. I realize this is not easy – I personally know several children who literally live on nothing but burgers, pizza and chips for main meals – and I'm talking about children with well-off, well-educated parents who should perhaps know better.

The third thing to do is to drum up a repertoire of alternative meals to which he/she doesn't object. There are several ideas throughout this section, and also in

Sections Three and Five. If any child has a normal appetite and you continue to present them with meals other than the one or two favourites (without making a big issue out of it), they usually capitulate through hunger and wind up enjoying the food in question. You need to be quietly determined. One compromise might be to cook home-made 'junk'! For example, burgers made from lean steak mince (preferably organic), pizzas with more tomato and less fatty topping than supermarket ones and so on. Check out Feature 24 for more suggestions. Also encourage him/her to exercise to burn off surplus calories before they turn into fat.

As I said at the start, there is nothing really wrong with the occasional fast-food meal, but the best way to help your child to long-term health and weight control is to introduce a wide variety of foods, including fresh fruits, veg and salads, from toddlerhood onwards and to rely on convenience foods as little as possible. The taste for salty, sugary and fatty foods is learnt early, and it is a lot easier to prevent them from getting the junk-food habit than it is to cure once it has taken hold!

See also:

▶ Questions: 265, 270–72, 274, 286, 289.
▶ Features: 15, 23, 24.
▶ Key index entries: children and weight, food value charts, healthy eating, junk food, takeaways.

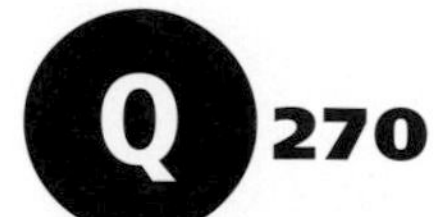

Q 270

My son has a huge appetite and is putting on weight, yet if I cut his portions he gets very hungry and I feel guilty. What can I do?

First check with the growth charts that he really is overweight – if prepubescent, his increased appetite and weight may be natural. If really overweight, you need to cut his calorie intake a little, but rather than cut the portion in total, make sure the parts you reduce are those that are densest – highest in calories weight for weight. In general, these will be foods highest in fat.

For example, if you usually offer 2 large lamb chops, but substitute 2 small well trimmed ones instead, you might save many calories.

■ 2 large untrimmed lamb chops, total weight 300g (10½oz), grilled: 830 calories and 68g fat.

■ 2 small trimmed lamb chops, total weight 200g (7oz), grilled: 250 calories and 14g fat.

So that you still have a plate of food that looks plenty, what you do then is add extra of the lower-density, lower-fat, lower-calorie foods. For example:

■ Double the portion of peas: adding an extra 75g (2¾oz) peas will add 50 calories.

■ Increase the portion of mashed potatoes by one-third: adding an extra 100g (3½oz) potato (mashed with a little butter) will add 104 calories.

So you've taken away 100g (3½oz) of food via the chops, losing 580 calories in the process. But you've added 175g (6oz) of food for a total value of only 154 calories. So,you have more food on the plate by 75g (2¾oz) but have saved a total of 426 calories!

Feature 10 gives other examples of how easy it is to offer a large plateful of food while reducing the calories on the plate considerably. The Food Value Charts at the back of the book give calorie and fat values for common foods, while the Traffic Light system explained in Q113 is also good to follow, as you don't even have to worry too much about portion sizes – he/she can 'eat all they want' of the 'Green for go' foods. You can apply the same calorie-reducing principles to puddings, too, and in fact any meal at all. There are plenty more ideas throughout the book. The final thing to do is bulk up the plate even more with low-calorie salads and veg.

Other points to note about appetite appear in Q23. It is especially important with hungry children who may be getting overweight to try to slow down their rate of eating and get them to concentrate more on the taste, texture and enjoyment of food. It is better for children to eat at a table with the family and chat during the meal – the rate of eating will naturally slow down then. Food gulped down mindlessly while watching TV gets eaten at twice the rate and the child is likely to ask for seconds as his/her appetite mechanism won't have time to register being full.

It is also a good idea to ensure a child doesn't go for too long without anything to eat. I am all for between-meal snacks if healthy – a 100-calorie snack of a slice of bread with low-fat spread and Marmite will take the edge off appetite at hungry times (say, on getting in from school) so at mealtime he/she won't be so ravenous.

CHILDREN'S FAVOURITE FAST FOODS

Their approximate calorie and fat content per portion

	Cals	Fat
Small portion of deep-fried cod in batter with small portion of chips	700	36
Jumbo fried sausage and small portion of chips	650	40
Individual small pizza margherita	650	23
Six chicken nuggets with regular fries	475	26
Cheeseburger (small) with regular fries	750	34
Strawberry milkshake, regular	400	10
Burger-bar hot chicken sandwich	400	18

See also:

- ▶ Questions: 23, 85, 87, 272, 290.
- ▶ Features: 23, 24.
- ▶ Key index entries: appetite, calories, fat, weight control for children.

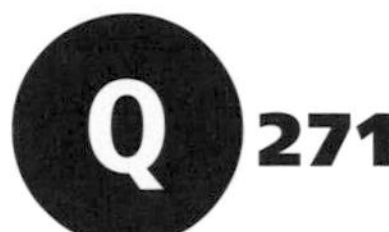

271

Is it OK to reduce the fat in my children's diets or do they need more than adults?

After weaning and until about the age of five, children do need a little more fat than adults and older children. Breast milk is about 50% fat, and 'follow-on' milks (usually given from six months of age to one) are about 42% fat. The fat amounts recommended in the charts in Feature 22 for young children reflect a gradual cutting down of percentage fat intake from 42% at age 1 down to 35% at 5. From 1 to 2, whole milk should be given, and from 3 to 5, semi-skimmed can be given, but fully skimmed milk should be reserved until after 5. Bear in mind that, although these young children need a higher percentage of fat in their diets, it is still preferable if the fat comes packaged as part of decent-quality food rather than 'junk'. Whole-milk yoghurt and full-fat cheeses are ideal.

Once at school age, children don't really need more fat than adults – so consider 35% of the calories in their diet as fat to be plenty. It is a good idea to get children to accept a diet high in carbs, adequate in protein and lowish in fat as they get older, so that by the time they are adult they don't find they have to make any massive changes to their eating habits. What often happens is that teenagers – particularly boys – have their growth spurt and the accompanying higher need for calories, so they feel justified in 'stoking up' on high-fat meals as this is the easiest way to fill up, fat being higher than other nutrients in calories, gram for gram. For those few years, many teenage boys can, almost, eat what they like without putting on weight (though some still manage to get fat).

Then the growth spurt stops, adulthood begins – and if the eating habits don't change, weight gain results. So even though they do need fat, it is best if you can make sure that the fat they eat is mostly unsaturated, and that their diet includes plenty of the healthy-fat foods, such as oily fish, nuts, seeds and good-quality plant oils. These fats will also help them to health in so many ways – essential fats can help brain development, memory, skin and much more.

The fats to cut right back on without compunction are the saturated fats found in items such as cream, cream cheese, fatty cuts of meat, pastry, batters, deep-fried foods, cakes, biscuits and puddings, takeaways and fast food. There is no need to cut out all of the medium-fat saturated fat foods such as most cheeses, eggs, milk and lean meats, which provide a range of minerals and vitamins important for growth and health. Low-fat foods such as semi-skimmed milk, low-fat cheeses, low-fat yoghurt and skinless poultry are all useful in a child's diet especially if prone to gaining weight easily or already overweight. For more advice on healthy fats, see Feature 8.

See also:

- ▶ Questions: 272, 277, 281, 283, 287–90.
- ▶ Features: 8, 23, 24.
- ▶ Key index entries: calories, fat, weight control for children.

FAT FACT

When the Food Commission looked at 385 products targeted at children, only one in ten could be regarded as healthy, while over 75% contained excessively high levels of saturated fat, sugar and salt.

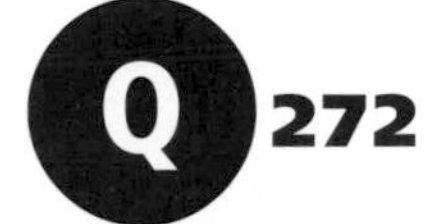

272

If my child is overweight, is fat the first thing in her diet that I should restrict?

Most doctors and nutritionists will probably tell you the first things you should restrict – or even cut out altogether – are low-nutrient 'junk' foods and drinks which offer little nutrition but are high in calories. Some, but not all, of these will be high in fat, others high in sugar, some in both.

Some parents find that by just cutting out all sugary drinks, for example, they can save hundreds of calories a day. For example, a can of cola is about 130 cals, a sparkling orangeade about 140, a half-pint (300ml) glass of squash is about 50 cals, enough powder to add to half a pint (300ml) of milk to make an instant 'fruit shake' is about 80 cals, and a 9fl oz (250ml) blackcurrant drink about 150.

Few children drink tea, coffee or water, instead sticking to sugary beverages, and the calories mount up. Better alternatives are water or plain semi-skimmed milk, or diluted fresh fruit juice. (Fruit juices and smoothies may contain vitamin C and other trace elements, but can be high in cals and their fructose promote tooth decay.) Milk has calories but is a good source of calcium; water is calorie- and cost-free.

Next think about cutting out sweets and chocs, then snacks like crisps. Also consider cutting out high-fat, sugary puddings. Along with these, cut out or down savoury pastry items like sausage rolls and pasties. These are generally the first things to restrict and for many children will be enough in themselves to instigate weight loss. There is more information in other parts of this section.

See also:

- ▶ Questions: 79–81, 89–90, 265, 267, 271, 281, 283.
- ▶ Features: 8, 23, 24.
- ▶ Key index entries: fat, calories, sugar.

Is your child overweight?

Check out your child's weight using either of these methods; Q263 gives more information.

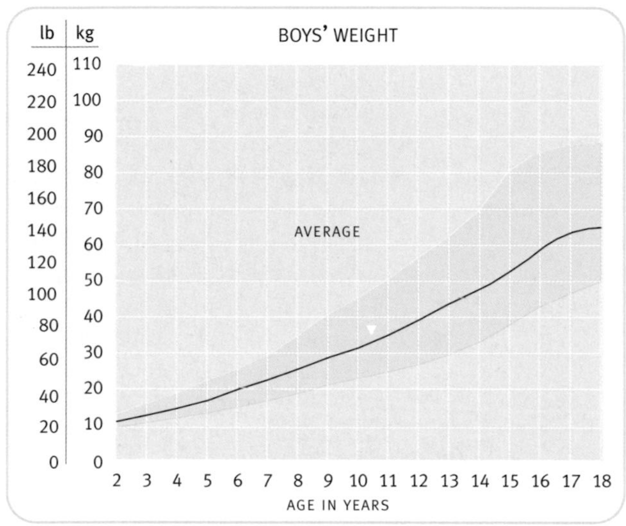

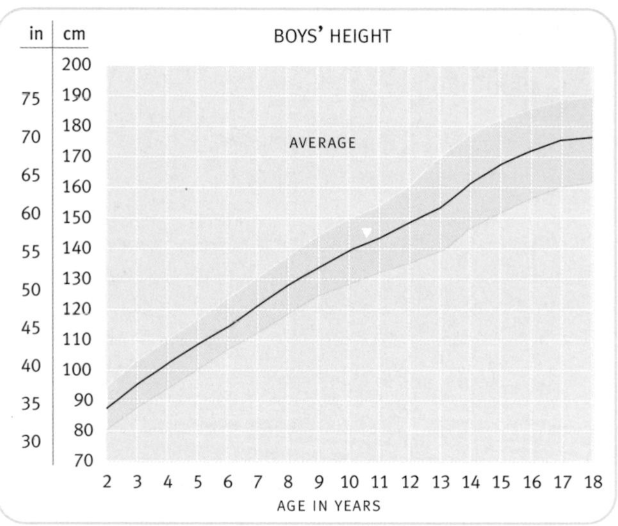

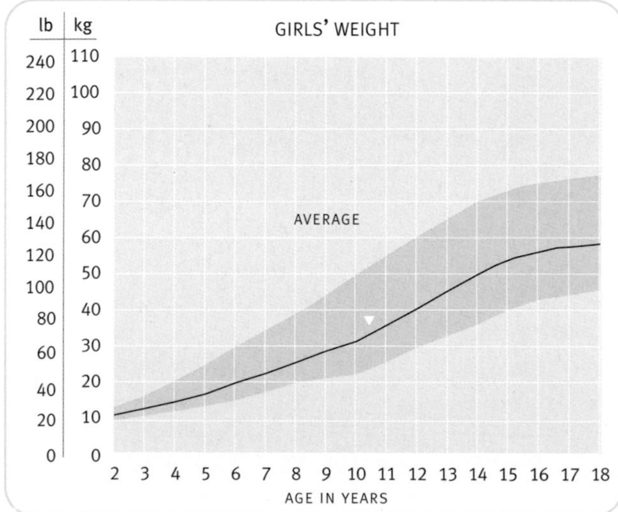

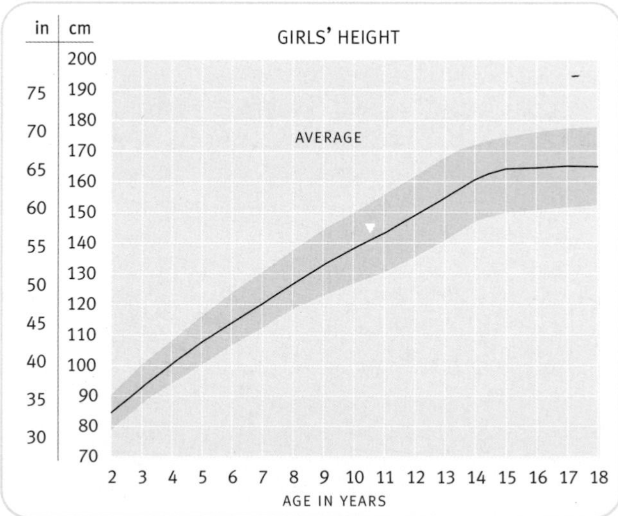

The growth charts

The charts above show average weights for age and heights for age, for children aged 2–18. The upper and lower lines represent the limits within which most children fall, while the centre line represents the average.

International cut-off points

The charts opposite represent the cut-off points for every age from 2 to 18, over which you child is either overweight (BMI Chart 1) or obese (BMI chart 2). These charts have been adapted from those produced by T. J. Cole for the Institute of Child Health and the International Obesity Task Force.

■ To find out your child's body mass index, divide his or her weight in kg by his or her height in metres squared. (For more information on doing this see Feature 3.)

BMI CHART 1

Your child is overweight if he/she is...

Age	With a BMI of more than Boys	Girls
2	18.4	18
3	17.9	17.6
4	17.6	17.3
5	17.4	17.1
6	17.6	17.3
7	17.9	17.8
8	18.4	18.3
9	19.1	19.1
10	19.8	19.9
11	20.6	20.7
12	21.2	21.7
13	21.9	22.6
14	22.6	23.3
15	23.3	23.9
16	23.9	24.4
17	24.5	24.7
18	25	25

BMI CHART 2

Your child is obese if he/she is...

Age	With a BMI of more than Boys	Girls
2	20.1	20.1
3	19.6	19.4
4	19.3	19.1
5	19.3	19.2
6	19.8	19.7
7	20.6	20.5
8	21.6	21.6
9	22.8	22.8
10	24	24.1
11	25.1	25.4
12	26	26.7
13	26.8	27.8
14	27.6	28.6
15	28.3	29.1
16	28.9	29.4
17	29.4	29.7
18	30	30

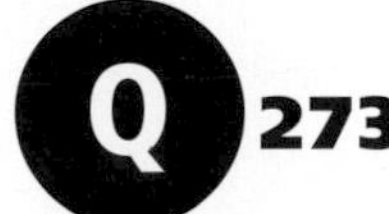

273

Is a high-fibre diet suitable for all children?

Very small children shouldn't be given a lot of very-high-fibre foods as their digestive systems aren't equipped to cope; and such foods may hinder absorption of minerals like iron and calcium. Young slim children with a small appetite may find high-fibre foods particularly daunting as they take a lot of chewing and may make them feel full up before getting many calories.

These are exactly the properties which make fibre-rich foods a good addition to the diets of overweight older children. Foods such as whole-wheat pasta, pulses, dried fruits and vegetables help to fill hungry children up and should form part of their healthy calorie-controlled diet unless there is any medical reason not to do so (check with your child's dietician).

See also:

- Questions: 83–5, 277.
- Features: 23–4.
- A–Z entry: high-fibre diets.
- Key index entries: digestive system, fibre, minerals (absorption of).

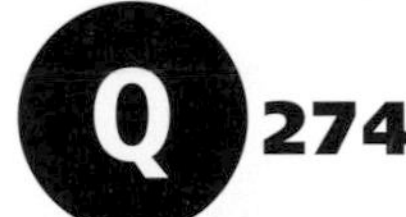

274

Both my young children dislike 'healthy' foods, like fruit, veg and fish, but aren't overweight and seem fit. Should I worry?

It is fairly common for small children to be fussy/faddy eaters and, as long as you try not to appear too concerned about it, it is something many will grow out of in the next few years. Studies have found that even small children who live on a narrow range of foods tend not to suffer from any great nutritional deficiencies. Bear in mind that foods such as pizzas, burgers – and even ice-cream and chocolate – DO contain a wide range of nutrients, including protein, iron, calcium and all the vitamins (but possibly not enough C).

The downside of such foods is that they are mostly high in fat and saturated fat and/or sugar, and developing a taste for them at an early age may increase the likelihood of children getting fat over the years. It IS harder to 'wean' children off a liking for junk food than it is to prevent it in the first place, but it can be done.

The trick is to build on what they do like, try to stay outwardly relaxed at meal times and be 'firm but kind'. The tips below may help you introduce some of the 'healthier' foods into their diet. Exercise will also help prevent weight gain.

For any prospective parents reading this, the message is to start giving children small amounts of a wide range of fruits, vegetables, fish, and so on straight after weaning (gradually building up the repertoire), along with bread, potatoes, pasta, rice, dairy produce, meat and so on, and try to avoid the 'junk' or convenience foods except for rare occasions.

I know these days most parents ask children what they would like to eat, rather than simply presenting it, but I feel that this encourages 'faddy eating' and it is best to give your child your choice of meal most of the time – you know more about good eating than your child. Don't feel guilty for this – you are doing your children a favour by helping them to build up a liking for 'real' unadulterated food.

Tips for fussy eaters

■ Introduce new foods gradually and in small amounts. If the child refuses a particular food, try again in a few weeks. Offer lots of praise if the new food is tried.

■ Make veg and fruits 'easy to eat' – purées are an ideal way to serve them; blended soups are brilliant for veg and pulses, such as lentils. For ideas on 'easy-to-eat' main meals see Feature 24. Later on, larger pieces can be included stealthily.

- Instead of salad leaves, serve small batons of raw carrot, celery, cucumber and so on, with a tasty dip.
- Make meals colourful and attractive. Choose the brightest vegetables (e.g. carrot, sweet potato, peas, tomatoes) and arrange plates nicely.
- If offering green leafy vegetables, slice them thinly and stir-fry in a little oil – this way they retain colour and don't get that depressing soggy, grey 'cabbagey' way. If leafy greens are a no-no, try broccoli florets and green beans instead.
- Fish cakes may be acceptable if 'plain' fish isn't.
- Try to make your own home versions of the fast foods that children seem to like. For ideas, see Feature 24.
- Try adding fruits and veggies into snacks that are liked – e.g., add chopped dried apricot into a soft cheese sandwich.
- Desserts can be anything based on semi-skimmed milk or yoghurt with fruit – there are plenty of colourful ideas that appeal to children. See Feature 24 again.
- Children who won't eat fruit will usually drink fruit juices or smoothies.
- Remember that no child likes all foods – don't try to force a food that your child really dislikes on to him/her. There is so much choice that some other food that he/she does like will offer similar nutrients. If worried about a very small range of food intake, do see your doctor.

See also:
- Questions: 269, 271, 273, 283–4, 286, 289–90.
- Features: 23, 24.
- Key index entries: faddy eating, fast food, healthy eating for children, junk food.

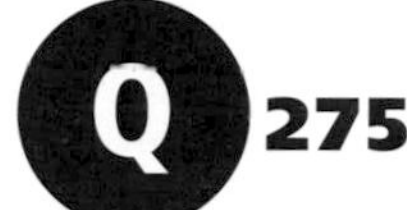

Q 275

Should I worry about my children, both of whom are thin for their age and yet seem healthy enough?

Check out their weights on the charts in Feature 22; if underweight you should visit the doctor for further advice. However, it is likely that they are absolutely fine, slimness may be part of their genetic inheritance and, on balance, it is better throughout life to be slightly slim than too fat. Perhaps your children get more exercise than most – which is nothing but a good thing. If their appetites are healthy and they are basically growing well and their bones are strong, you probably have no need to worry. If their appetites are poor, you can try some of the suggestions in this section.

See also:
- Questions: 274, 276.
- Features: 23, 24.
- Key index entries: appetite, underweight.

FAT FACT

Babies introduced to solid food late are more likely to become fussy eaters, say researchers. Bristol University found that infants not introduced to solids by 10 months later became much fussier eaters.

Research shows that young children tend to have a 'sweet tooth' – probably because breast milk is sweet – but at puberty develop a taste for high-fat foods.

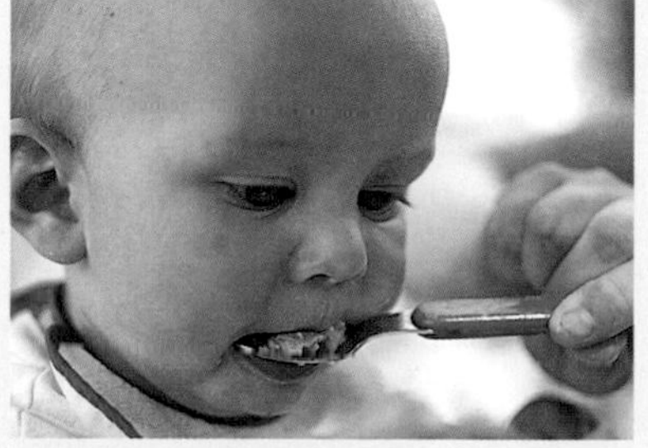

Q 276

What are the best foods for putting weight on a reluctant eater?

All the tips that appear in Q274 may help you to encourage your child to eat – but for the slim child with a poor appetite you may also need to consider ways to tempt him/her with slightly higher-calorie offerings as well. The trick is to give the child a diet containing enough calories for his/her needs while not going overboard on the less healthy items, such as saturated fat and sugar. One of the best ways is to offer small frequent meals or snacks. There is nothing worse than 'overfacing' a reluctant eater with large platefuls. Instead, offer small amounts of nicely presented food and try to get the extra calories consumed between meals. Smooth textures with plenty of taste are most likely to be appreciated. Here are some ideas:

- Milk blended with banana (and other fruits – e.g. strawberries) and a little honey.
- Greek yoghurt and honey.
- Potatoes mashed with butter and cheese.
- Mashed bananas on toasted white bread.
- Ice-cream topped with fruit coulis.

You should, in any case, see your doctor in case there is any medical reason for the poor appetite. If there isn't, plenty of fresh air and good sleep will encourage appetite, as will fun and enjoyment. Depression or worry is a surprisingly common cause of eating problems in children. If quiet and listless, or nervous and 'hyper', this could be the case. In small children, refusing food is a way of showing independence or of getting attention. Build a relaxed atmosphere around meals and never 'force-feed' or make a child sit for hours in front of something they won't eat.

See also:
- Questions: 274–5
- Features: 23, 24.
- Key index entries: appetite, underweight.

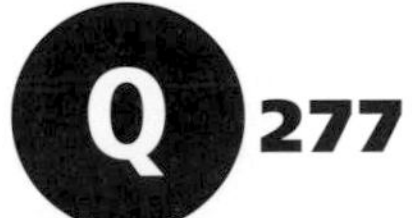

277

How early can you start children on health food?

As you will see in Qs 263–8, 'unhealthy' eating habits are leading children as young as 3 to be obese in record numbers, and so, in one sense, it is important to feed your children healthily right from weaning. The crucial thing, however, is what you mean by 'health food'. Go back to Qs 271 and 273 first, as these discuss the roles of fat and fibre in a child's diet. I assume your concept of health food is perhaps organic – which is absolutely fine for kids. I'm all for organic food for everyone.

Maybe it is also 'whole food'. A whole-food diet may be too high in fibre and bulk and too low in calories for small children, for the same reasons as given in Q273, so you need to introduce foods such as pulses, brown rice, millet, etc. gradually, and watch how your child copes. If he/she is leaving a lot of food on the plate and not putting on weight at a reasonable level, you may need to decrease the amounts of high-fibre, high-bulk, low-density foods and offer more refined items, such as white bread, potatoes, white rice, and slightly more fat – for example, cheese, lean meat, poultry, whole milk.

Some research indicates that children of parents who live on a whole-food-type diet can sometimes suffer from malnutrition, so you have to be careful to find the balance between what is a healthy adult diet and what children need for growth and health. You can quite happily steer them away from all the junk and over-sugared, saturated-fat goodies that children seem to enjoy, but a varied diet based around any meat, fish, poultry, fruit, veg, bread, pasta, rice, pulses and dairy produce is both healthy and offers all necessary nutrients.

It is when you get into restricting choice that you may be more likely to encounter problems with providing a complete range of nutrients and enough calories. If vegan or macrobiotic, for instance, you need to take care that your children get enough calcium, iron, B vitamins, calories and protein. Further parts of this section will help you give your child a balanced diet.

See also:

- Questions: 271–6, 278–9, 287–290.
- Features: 22–24.
- A–Z entries: Macrobiotic diets, Vegetarian diets.
- Key index entries: healthy eating for children, special diets.

FAT FACT

Researchers in America have found that the strongest predictor of weight gain in children aged 11–12 is the consumption of soft drinks. Calories consumed in liquid form appear to blunt the appetite less than those in solids. In America, approximately two-thirds of adolescents consume sugary soft drinks daily – the leading source of added sugar in their diets.

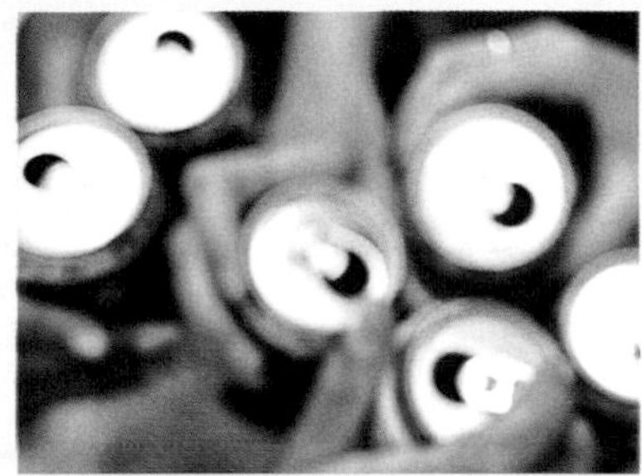

Q 278

Is going vegetarian a good way for children to lose weight?

Vegetarianism means different things to different people. Population studies have shown that a diet based on plant foods, such as pulses, fruit, vegetables, salads and whole grains, is linked with decreased risk of obesity and, as you will see if you read Qs 273 and 277, it may indeed be difficult for a child to get enough calories to maintain weight on such a diet.

However, a vegetarian diet based on full-fat dairy produce, desserts, pastry and so on is no more likely to produce weight loss than the typical non-vegetarian Western diet. I do know many vegetarians who eat a great deal of fat and sugar.

If thinking of persuading a child to become vegetarian in order to lose weight, then remember that vegetarianism doesn't automatically mean slimness, or health. Indeed, true veggies don't eat fish – which has been shown to be linked with many health benefits – and vegetarians who don't eat dairy produce or eggs (vegans) have to be careful in order not to suffer from deficiency in vitamin B12 and iron.

Because going vegetarian restricts food choices, if you have a child who is thinking of going vegetarian (or you want them to do so), you really need to know what you are doing in order to provide them with a balanced diet containing enough of all the nutrients they need for growth and health.

If you can fulfil all these needs, then a vegetarian diet may well be a reasonable option for your child, although it is far from the only way and may not, for most families, be the best way. Contact the Vegetarian Society for more information (see Vegetarian diets in the A–Z).

See also:

- Questions: 194–7, 271–3, 277, 279.
- Features: 16, 23, 24.
- A–Z entries: Vegetarian diets.
- Key index entries: healthy eating for children, vegans, vegetarians.

Nutrition facts for children

Children's food needs vary tremendously over the years, and from child to child, but the information on these pages will help you decide what makes a healthy diet for your offspring.

The chart here gives average nutritional needs for children aged 1–18, based on information from the UK Department of Health and are daily recommended amounts, which will be sufficient for most children. The figures in the fat column represent 35% of total recommended calorie intake for each age group (apart from those aged 1–6) and are based on the DoH's advice that fat intake in those who don't drink alcohol should be 35% of energy intake. I suggest you use these as daily maxima and aim for only one-third of your fat intake to come from saturated fat.

If your child is overweight, the best way to reduce his/her food intake is to reduce calories without reducing the amount of the essential nutrients that he/she needs. The list on the right gives best sources of the main nutrients with their nutrient content per average portion in brackets.

As an example, the typical day's eating opposite shows a sample of a 1,740 cals/day diet for an average 10-year-old girl for weight maintenance, alongside the same diet reduced by about 250 cals/day for slow weight loss of around 1/2 lb (225g) a week. You will see that the diet contains surprisingly high levels of all the listed nutrients (well over the official daily requirements) – showing it isn't all that difficult to ensure your child gets the necessary nutrients. Such a varied diet will also supply enough of all the other nutrients (e.g. vitamins B, E, zinc, etc.).

SELECTED NUTRITIONAL NEEDS AT AGES 1–18

Age	Calories	Fat (g)	Protein (g)	Calcium (mg)	Iron (mg)	Vit C (mg)
Girls						
1–3	1,165	54*	14.5	350	6.9	30
4–6	1,545	68-60*	19.7	450	6.1	30
7–10	1,740	68	28.3	550	8.7	30
11–14	1,845	72	42	800	14.8	35
15–18	2,110	82	45	800	14.8	40
Boys						
1–3	1,230	57*	14.5	350	6.9	30
4–6	1,715	76-67*	19.7	450	6.1	30
7–10	1,970	76	28.3	550	8.7	30
11–14	2,220	86	42	1,000	11.3	35
15–18	2,755	107	55.2	1,000	11.3	40

* Children from weaning to age 5 need more fat than older children. Breast milk is over 50% fat and follow-on milks are 42% fat. The figures for children aged 1–3 are based on 42% fat in the diet, and the figures for children aged 4–6 are based on 40% fat reducing to 35% fat.

WHERE TO FIND THE MAIN NUTRIENTS

Calories The Food Value Charts at the back of the book will help you choose high- or low-cal foods.

Protein Chicken breast fillet portion (42g); 100g (3½oz) of lean roast beef (32g); 175g (6oz) cod (32g); Quarterpounder beefburger (21g); 75g (2¾oz) peeled prawns (17g).
2 medium eggs (14g); 50g (1⅔oz) Cheddar cheese (13g); Small glass (200ml/7fl oz) semi-skimmed milk (6.6g); 150ml (¼ pint) pot of low-fat fruit yoghurt (6g).
100g (3½oz) Quorn chunks (12g); 50g (1⅔oz) dry weight lentils (12g); I medium baked potato (8g); one vegeburger (8g); medium portion of pasta (6g); medium portion of frozen peas (4g); 2 slices of wholemeal bread (5g).

Calcium 50g (1⅔oz) Cheddar (370mg); 200ml (7fl oz) semi-skimmed milk (240mg); 100g (3½oz) ice-cream (130mg); 50g (1⅔oz) muesli (100mg); 175g (6oz) cod (28mg); 50g (1⅔oz) (small portion) of spinach (85mg); 2 slices of white bread (60mg).

Iron 50g (1⅔oz) (dry weight) lentils (5.5mg); 30g (1oz) (medium bowl) Special K (4mg); 100g (3½oz) soya mince (9mg); 100g (3½oz) lean beef (2.1mg); 200g (7oz) baked beans (2.8mg); 2 medium eggs (1.9mg); 100g (3½oz) broccoli (1mg); 25g (¾oz) dried apricots (0.85mg).

Vitamin C (All per 100g/3½oz): red peppers (140mg); blackcurrants, stewed, (130mg); strawberries (77mg); papaya (60mg); kiwi fruit (59mg); mangetout (54mg); oranges (54mg); broccoli (44mg); sweetcorn (39mg); nectarine (37mg); mango (37mg).

SAMPLE DIET FOR 10-YEAR-OLD GIRL
(1,740 CALORIES PER DAY)

FOOD	Calories	Protein (g)	Calcium (mg)	Iron (mg)	Vitamin C (mg)
Day's milk allowance (400ml/14fl oz semi-skimmed)	184	13.2	480	0.2	4
Breakfast					
30g (1oz) Cornflakes (with milk from allowance)	108	2.4	4.5	2	–
Strawberries, 50g (1 2/3oz)	13	0.4	8	0.2	38
30g (1oz) white toast	70	2.5	33	0.5	–
1 tsp (5g) butter	37	tr	tr	tr	–
2 tsp (7g) jam	18	tr	1.5	tr	tr
Packed lunch					
62g (2oz) soft brown bap	135	5.3	62	1.3	–
40g (1 1/3oz) lean ham	67	11.7	4	0.6	–
10g (1/3oz) tomato, cress	5	tr	tr	tr	2
Salad cream, 2 tsp (5g)	17	tr	1	tr	–
50g (1 2/3oz) homemade fruit cake	181	3	42	1	–
125ml (4fl oz) fruit yoghurt (whole-milk)	130	6.3	200	tr	1
150ml (1/4 pint) orange juice	54	0.75	15	0.3	60
Evening meal					
2-egg omelette	160	13.6	62	2	–
200g (7oz) baked potato wedges	150	4.2	10	0.8	5
2 tsp oil for cooking omelette and coating potatoes	90	–	–	–	–
80g (2 3/4oz) peas	55	4.8	28	1.2	10
Medium banana	80	1	5	0.2	8
Snacks					
l apple	47	0.4	4	0.1	6
l crumpet	100	3.3	60	0.5	–
1 tsp (5g) butter	37	tr	tr	tr	–
TOTALS	**1,738**	**72.8**	**1,020**	**10.9**	**134**

The proportions of the main nutrients in the day's eating shown are as follows:
fat 30%; protein 17%; carbohydrate 53%.
The diet reduced by 250 cals/day should produce slow weight loss of around 1/2 lb (225g) a week.

TO SAVE 250 CALORIES:

- Replace the day's butter with low-fat spread: 37 calories saved.
- Replace the jam with low-sugar jam: 9 calories saved.
- Swap the ham for turkey breast: 26 calories saved.
- Use low-fat salad cream: 10 calories saved.
- Replace the whole-milk fruit yoghurt with low-fat diet fruit yoghurt: 80 calories saved.
- Replace the cake with a Harvest chewy cereal bar: 90 calories saved.

TOTAL SAVED: 252.

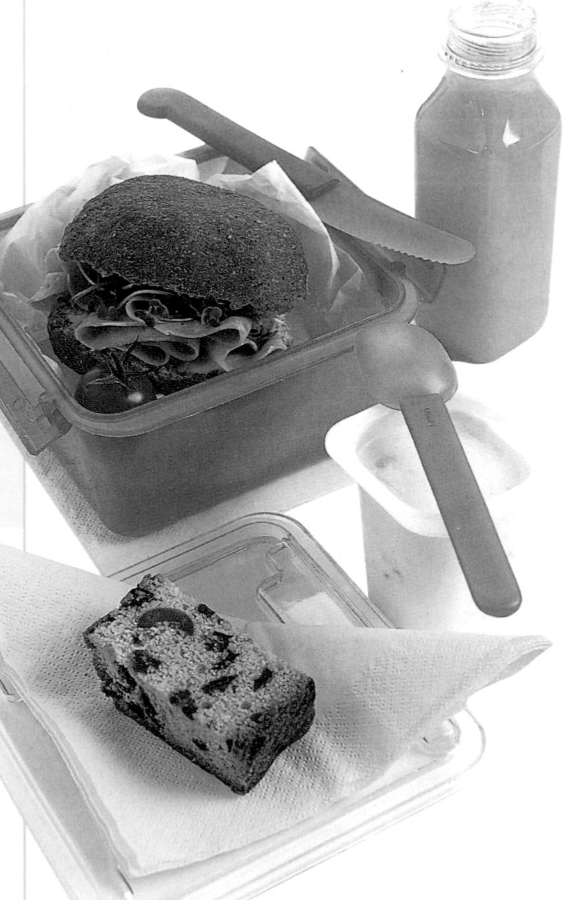

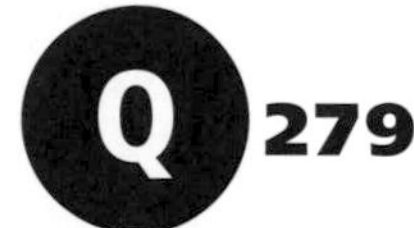

279

My daughter of 13, a lone vegetarian in the family, is overweight and pale. Can you advise me on feeding her?

It sounds as if she's simply given up meat and perhaps other animal-based foods, without learning how to replace the nutrients they provide, or balancing her diet. In truth, she is a little young to know what to do herself, so I suspect she's been overeating sweet and fatty snack foods, and at meal missing out meat and eating whatever else is on the plate. She may be pale because she lacks iron, but in any case I would take her to the doctor and get her checked over, including a blood test.

The Vegetarian Society can offer advice for carnivores who need to cater for a vegetarian. If you can get her started on a healthy, well-balanced veggie diet, including plenty of pulses, fruit, vegetables and whole grains, and cutting back on high-fat or high-sugar items, such as full-fat dairy produce, pastries, pies, cakes, biscuits and chocolate, she should begin to lose a little weight and feel a lot better in herself. In theory, research shows that it should be easier to maintain a reasonable weight while following a vegetarian diet.

If you have a vegetarian to cater for, it has to be said that you will have to spend extra time sorting out meals, but you'll find a list of recommended books at the back of the book to make life easier. The Vegetarian Eating Plan in Feature 16 is a good blueprint for adults, but your 13-year-old may need fewer calories and more iron. Feature 22 explains what nutrients children need for health.

See also:

- ▶ Questions: 194–7, 277, 278, 281.
- ▶ Features: 16, 22, 23.
- ▶ A–Z entry: vegetarian diets.
- ▶ Key index entry: vegetarian children.

FAT FACT

One supermarket survey reveals that children who shop in their stores with their parents score a 68% success rate when they pester for sweets or chocolate to be added to the trolley.

Q 280

How can I avoid my child eating sweets when she starts school and also begins to visit friend's houses without me?

If a child has not been allowed sweets in the first few years of her life it is inevitable that she will be offered sweets when she begins to mix with other children, and she will undoubtedly accept because it is natural for children to be curious about something which a) obviously everybody around her seems to enjoy and b) has for her been banned. Forbidden fruit, as we know, always tastes sweeter. One study at Pennsylvania State University in 2000 found that children whose parents forbade them sweets and fizzy drinks were more likely to have these items in secret.

So she will try sweets. All you can do is impress on her that sweets eaten between meals are not good for her teeth, and avoid buying them. Pester power becomes very strong once children start school, though, so be prepared for some battles.

Eventually you may decide that it is best to limit sweets to a few after a meal, after which she cleans her teeth... a compromise. You can also choose the slightly 'better' sweets, such as good-quality chocolate or liquorice, rather than sweets which are pure sugar and spend a long time in the mouth. You may also cut back on sugar in other forms in her diet – for example, by avoiding over-sweet commercial cakes, biscuits and desserts and opting for fresh fruit or healthier desserts such as those listed in Feature 24.

By the way, research shows that girls under 11 do tend to have a sweet tooth, and after this age it may begin to fade.

See also:

- ▶ Questions: 281, 283, 287.
- ▶ Features: 23, 24.
- ▶ Key index entries: healthy eating for children, sugar, sweets.

281

What is the best way to reduce my child's high intake of sweets and chocolate – banning them altogether or using them as occasional treats?

It is hard, once children reach school age, to police a complete ban on sweets and chocolate – they'll always find some from someone, somewhere... and be more inclined to want to do so if they know that you disapprove. Surprising as it may seem, banning gives children a sweet tooth almost as much as does giving endless sweet treats and rewarding good behaviour with sweets. This is because the child comes to think that if something is so good that it is widely available everywhere (they see sweets on TV, in all the shops, in other children's pockets) and yet so bad that you don't want them to have even one now and then, this has got to be something worth trying – and lying – for.

So I wouldn't ban them, but neither would I use them as occasional 'treats'. Tell your children that you don't like sweets because they are 'empty' calories with virtually no nutrients in them, they are high in calories and that may make them fat, they can contribute to tooth decay, and may contain lots of additives which may not be good for them. Tell them if they would like to try a pack now and then, bought out of their pocket money with your knowledge, then that is up to them, but you think it is a waste of money.

Why give a child the impression that sweets are a special 'treat' when they have such a long list of negatives attached? Try to instil in the children that a real sweet treat would be something truly gorgeous like a bowlful of the new season's strawberries, or a slice of home-made bread with some organic local honey?

See also:

- ▶ Questions: 280, 283.
- ▶ Feature: 24
- ▶ Key index entries: healthy eating for children, sugar, sweets.

FIT FACT

Children who play sport do better in exams and are less likely to have unruly behaviour, say two separate British studies into children and exercise. They are also less likely to take days off school.

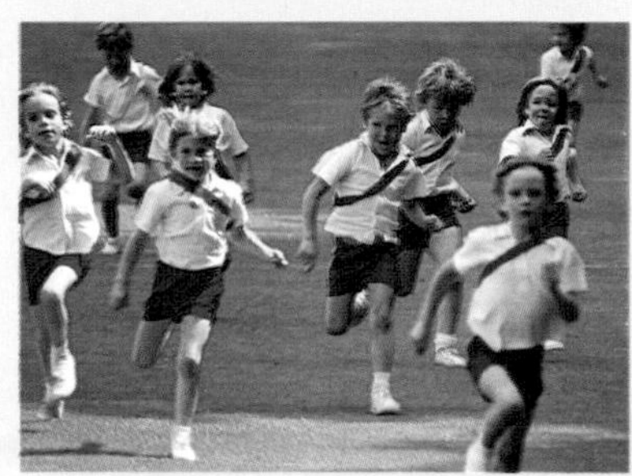

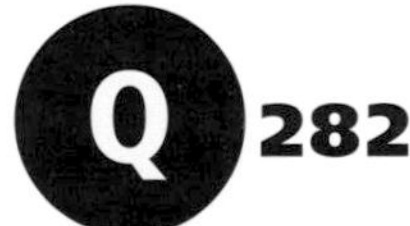

Q 282

I know my children should take more exercise, but it is hard to know what to get them to do, as they refuse even to consider 'going for walks'. Any suggestions?

Most children will get active if there is an element of fun, competition or discovery. I have to admit that most children down the years have loathed 'going for a walk', but if you dress it up as something else (e.g., treasure hunts or orienteering, looking for rare flowers or butterflies) it becomes more acceptable. Even training a puppy on the lead is fun. Of course, you can't always think of ways to make walks more exciting, and older children will turn their noses up at the ideas anyway.

So what else can you do? Here are a few ideas, some of which are more suitable for town than country, others may need some cash (although often not a great deal). Children vary so much in what they enjoy that finding a winning formula to get them moving is a matter of trying several things until you hit the button.

Most of the suggestions will involve you in organizing them, chaperoning and taking part yourself sometimes, especially with younger children. As adults don't tend to get enough exercise either, this can only be a good thing for you too.

- If you have a nearby park or recreation ground, try ball games (football, rounders with a group of friends, cricket, basic tennis, baseball, simple 'catch') followed by a (healthy) picnic in summer.
- Older children will like skateboarding, rollerskating, scootering, cycling if it is allowed in the park.
- Check out the local leisure centre and see what is on offer. Most things are low in cost. You may find such things as badminton, indoor tennis, five-a-side football, gymnastics, trampolining, fencing, cricket. You may find exercise classes for children too. All these are best organized with a group of friends – few children will want to go on their own. Chauffeuring and chaperoning can be shared then with other parents.
- The leisure centre will also offer holiday sessions of rollerskating and dancing and may do short courses in sports, including rugby, cricket, football and tennis.
- The swimming pool is good for children of all ages. If they can't swim well, a course of lessons is a good idea. There should also be courses on offer for lifesaving and diving.
- Sports clubs and similar. Doing a sport with other youngsters makes it much more fun, especially if there are competition days, demonstrations and so on. Your library should have information on what clubs your children could join or the national sports body will help. Nearby there may be orienteering, cycling, athletics, swimming, gymnastics and more.
- Don't forget that dancing is a great calorie-burner and good aerobic exercise, so evenings out at the disco may be good, too. Local youth clubs usually hold regular discos for pre- and young teens. Secondary schools may do something similar.
- Children over 14 may enjoy the Duke of Edinburgh Award Scheme, which involves a high percentage of physical challenges – many schools take it upon themselves to help; www.the award.org, tel 01753 727400.
- Other children might like to join the Cubs or Brownies (later the Scouts and Girl Guides); again, this involves a lot of physical activity (and fun); The Scouts Association, 0845 3001818, The Guides Association, 020 7834 6242.
- Most girls like ponies, as do many boys – riding lessons are expensive, but keen children may offer to muck out and clean the tack in return for free riding (mucking out will get them fitter than the riding).
- Doing chores for a wage. Many children want extra cash – you might consider offering them 'wages for work'. A few hours' digging or mowing at the

weekends, car-cleaning, housework, whatever, will help you and burn off plenty of calories for them.

■ Responsible children over 14 can get themselves a job outside the house for a few hours a week – delivering papers/pamphlets/phonebooks/etc. is ideal as it involves plenty of walking or cycling.

■ Consider sending them on an adventure holiday in the school break – several companies, such as PGL (01989 764211) or Camp Beaumont (01263 576585) do 'two-for-the-price-of-one' breaks. A 'mixed-bag' break – lots of different activities – may help a child to decide what it is that he/she really enjoys and you can then follow this up at home.

Anything you can do that gets them moving, rather than sedentary, all adds up. Don't be put off if your child is overweight – he/she is still likely to be fit enough to start an activity. Many children who begin to take an interest in some form of exercise find that they begin to lose a little weight, and when they see this happening they may also be motivated to eat better.

Lastly – going back to the dreaded walking – consider forgetting the car and walk them to and from school. This really is walking with a purpose – even a 15-minute walk each way means one hour a day, which may well be enough to give your children all the exercise they need.

See also:
- ▶ Questions: 265, 267, 293–5.
- ▶ Feature: 28.
- ▶ A–Z entries: cycling, Fitkids, sports.
- ▶ Key index entries: exercise, metabolism, sports.

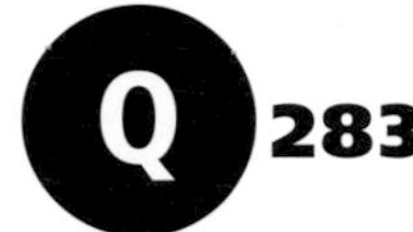

283

Can you give me ideas for healthy, less fattening alternatives to sweets and crisps?

As a between-meal snack, dried fruits such as sultanas, apricots and small stoneless prunes are ideal (they are quite high in calories, but less so than sweets, and they contain a good range of nutrients and fibre). Obviously, fresh fruit would be a good choice. A lot of children don't like 'hard-to-eat-or-peel' fruits, such as oranges and grapefruit, and find apples hard to bite into and this puts them off all fruit.

The fruits that I find children most willing to eat (indeed, to enjoy) are berries such as strawberries, small bananas, kiwi fruit (halved and given in a plastic bag with a little spoon); ready-peeled seedless satsumas and, absolute favourites, seedless grapes.

If it must be something less obviously healthy, then there are a few sweets that are better for them – for instance, good-quality liquorice is not bad; neither is good-quality chocolate, and organic muesli bars are reasonable (though high in sugars).

As an alternative to crisps, you can, of course, get lower-salt, lower-fat crisps, and health food shops stock organic crisps, also often lower in salt and fat. I'd also recommend fresh nuts for children over 5 who aren't allergic – they aren't low in calories, but they contain healthy essential fats which have been shown to help children to health and brainpower. Avoid walnuts as most kids find them too bitter.

Over-5-year-olds may also like two of my own children's favourites – pumpkin seeds and pine nuts. A small plastic bag filled with a variety of nuts, seeds and dried fruit is a great stand-by for a hungry child between meals – or indeed, as a dessert. Children who eat these regularly and then try commercial sweets find the sweets so cloying they can hardly eat them.

See also:
- ▶ Questions: 272, 280–81, 287.
- ▶ Features: 23, 24.
- ▶ Key index entries: healthy eating for children, junk food, sugar, sweets.

284

My 10-year-old is very overweight but goes into terrible tantrums if I don't give him what he wants. How can I cope?

I think you should start by reading through all of this section to date, to see if any suggestions I have made in answer to other problems triggers some solutions for you. It could be, for instance, that you are trying to 'diet' him on too few calories, so he is hungry – this will make him worried and bad-tempered. It may be best simply to try to ensure he doesn't put on more weight while he grows taller. It could

FAT FACT

Most UK children are allowed to access food in the fridge and larder between meals. Only 7% of parents operate a no-eating-between-meals policy and 25% of children are allowed unlimited 24-hour access without having to ask first, according to a supermarket survey.

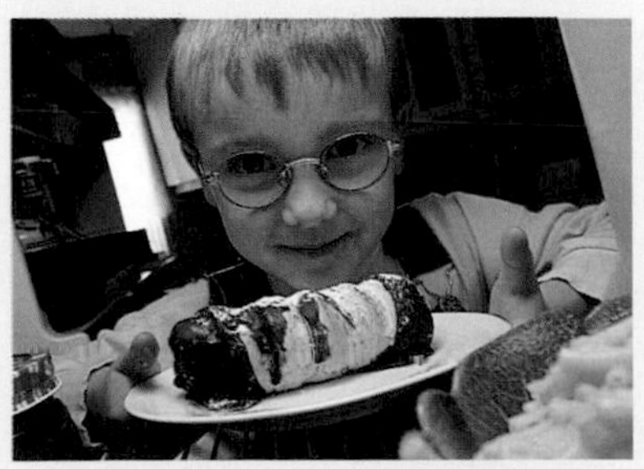

also be he is suffering some sort of 'withdrawal symptoms' from sweet or salty foods. In that case, try the suggestions in Feature 13 for adults – the retraining course. It could be that you are coming on too strong, maybe nagging a bit when more encouragement might work.

It could be that he feels isolated (especially if you have other children who are eating different food from him – see the answer to the next question in that case), because what children eat in front of each other can be almost as important as, say, what trainers they wear. It will help if you – and maybe other members of the family – could eat the same as him. Of course, it could be that he just doesn't like whatever food it is that you are offering him. Children's tastes do take a while to alter, even if they want to be co-operative.

At 10 he should be old enough to talk to you about how he feels and why he feels it – so try to encourage him to tell you what the main problems are and see if you can solve them using some of the tactics described in this section. You too need to explain why he needs to watch his weight and give him nice reasons for doing so – e.g., a new wardrobe of clothes, etc.

You need to break the pattern of these tantrums, which are him trying to 'get round you' and hoping that if he makes life difficult enough for you, you will succumb – and his policy seems to be working. You need to make sure he knows that you want him to be slim and fit, but try to stay relaxed at mealtimes.

It would be an idea to talk to your GP first to tell him or her the problem and then take him in to see the GP, who, it is to be hoped, will reinforce the message– if indeed he DOES need to slim down – and may give you a diet sheet or refer you to a dietician. If your child receives instructions from an outsider he may feel more like complying without a fight, especially if he has to make return visits regularly to be weighed. Some slimming clubs also allow children in, and they have a good success rate in helping to motivate kids. You could also try a 'fat camp' for kids, and take on board some of the exercise ideas in Q282.

Don't despair. If you can offer him meals that satisfy his hunger and contain at least mostly foods that he doesn't dislike, and if you can help to motivate him, things should improve. As soon as he begins to look slimmer, and gets his first new pair of jeans, I am sure you will find that his attitude will improve tremendously.

See also:
- ▶ Questions: 263–83, 285–95.
- ▶ Features: 13, 22–24.
- ▶ A–Z entries: fat camps, Fitkids, sports.
- ▶ Key index entries: motivation, weight control for children.

FOOD FACT

According to the UK National Food Survey, the daily average of calories consumed in the home has fallen from 1,940 in 1989 to 1,740 in 2000, but this excludes calories eaten outside the home, including sweets, alcohol and fast food. As 4 out of every 10 pounds spent on food in the UK goes on food eaten outside the home – takeaways, ready meals or meals in cafés, bars and restaurants – an average calorie intake may actually be 2,436 (1,740 plus 40%).

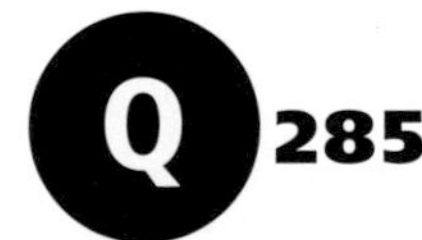

285

I have 3 children, but only one is overweight; this causes endless problems at meal times and the overweight child feels bad. Is there a solution?

I suggest that you feed the whole family a good, healthy diet along the lines suggested in Features 9 and 23, and simply give your slim children bigger portions than average, and your overweight child slightly smaller portions, especially of the high-density, high-fat foods, such as butter and oils, cheese and cream and so on, and give him extra veggies to fill up his plate.

As Feature 23 shows, you can cut calories surreptitiously, a little here and there, to save enough to help him lose weight slowly. If the basic meal is the same as everyone else's, he'll probably be fine with reduced-fat, reduced-sugar products elsewhere. Here are some examples:

- ■ Swap butter for low-fat spread.
- ■ Swap full-fat milk for skimmed milk.
- ■ Swap full-fat yoghurts for low-fat, low-calorie yoghurts.
- ■ If he has packed lunches, use this as a good opportunity to reduce the fat content (see Q287).
- ■ It would be best if all the children have healthy desserts, rather than very-high-sugar, high-fat ones, so use the ideas in Feature 24 and elsewhere in this section to reduce calories in the desserts. If the slim children are still hungry at the end of the meal, they can fill up on bread and honey or similar. Alternatively, the slim children could have full-fat cream on their fruit salad, for instance, while he could have 8%-fat fromage frais, which tastes nice.
- ■ Save calories on drinks – see Q272.

Try to limit occasions when the other children tuck into pizza and he can't – of course this will make him feel he is missing out. Make your own lower-fat version of pizza and let him tuck in too. I am sure the answer mostly lies in 'portion control' and saving a few calories here and there. You're going to have to be more vigilant, but not cooking separate meals for him.

See also:
- ▶ Questions: 263–8, 272, 287–90.
- ▶ Features: 9, 23, 24.
- ▶ Key index entries: healthy eating for children, weight control in children.

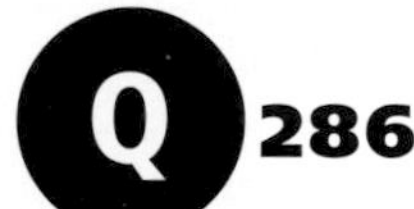

286

My 12-year-old always picks the most fattening and unhealthy items; how can I persuade him to make healthier choices?

I can think of several examples of the kind of situation you probably mean – the school café, where he goes for sausage and chips rather than chicken salad; the morning out with friends in town, when he goes to the burger bar; the pocket money spent on chocolate and sweets; the cola or fizzy orange picked instead of the mineral water from the vending machine; the family lunch out where he chooses steak, chips and sticky toffee pudding; the hand in the biscuit tin rather than the fruit bowl when he gets home from school.

I have had one such boy myself and I can tell you two things. One, it is hard as they get older and start having a life of their own and money of their own to control what foods and snacks they buy, so it is best to try to give them a taste for decent food before they get into double figures, and to talk to them about what makes a healthy diet, and why. When all around him are eating rubbish food he is not likely to pick salad and water, so you have to be realistic about what can be achieved. Maybe we should encourage our children to be friends with the ones who like healthy food, as well as the ones who don't swear, do their homework and say 'please' and 'thank you'! We should also encourage our children not to be afraid to be individual – to lead rather than follow.

Two, you have to exert what influence you can and feel sure it will make a difference to the overall calorie content and nutritional quality of his diet. For example, you could make sure that at least at home there are no fizzy drinks and biscuits and that whatever meals you give him are fairly low in fat and sugar, and not too calorific (unless he is underweight).

FOOD FACT

Food advertising aimed at children – for example, during kids' TV programmes – is 70% for fatty and sugary foods, 16% for cereals and other carbohydrates, 10% for milk and dairy produce, 4% for fish and meat products and 0% for fruit and vegetables.

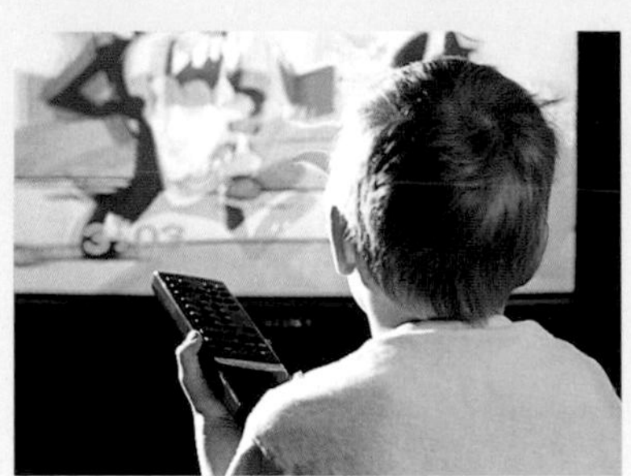

You could also go down the vanity route, and tell him that a healthy diet will give him better skin, more admiration from the girls, or whatever you think may spark his interest. But I don't see any point in turning yourself into the diet police – this will just antagonize him and make him eat all the more of everything you despise.

Lastly, remember that if he isn't overweight he can actually eat more food than you as he goes through his teens – from 15 to 18, boys have higher calorie needs than any other group – and that most food does have some nutrients in it. If he looks as if he is starting to put on too much weight, be extra-vigilant about not offering sugary drinks and high-fat, high-sugar things at home, and encourage him to take more exercise.

With regard to school meals, in the UK new rules insist that school canteens are required to meet certain nutritional standards, for instance offering fish at least twice a week and fruit and veg every day. This still leaves the problem of choice, and chips are still allowed on the menu for over-11s every day. But at least it is an improvement. Life could be worse after all!

See also:

- Questions: 265, 269, 272.
- Features: 23, 24.
- Key index entries: healthy eating for children, junk food.

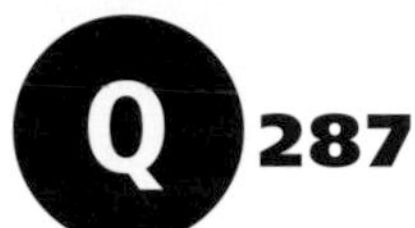

287

Can you advise me on healthy packed lunches for my children, with an eye on calorie reduction?

A good basic packed lunch will contain a carbohydrate element, a protein element, some fresh fruit and/or vegetables, something semi-sweet, and a drink. None of these are high in calories or fat:

Carbs: brown, white, wholemeal or rye bread, rolls, bagel, pitta, cooked rice, couscous or pasta.

Protein: medium- or low-fat cheeses, such as Edam, half-fat Cheddar, egg, extra-lean ham, breast of chicken, turkey, prawns, tuna canned in brine, tinned pink salmon.

Any fruits and vegetables.

Semi-sweet items: malt loaf, home-made fruit cake, teabread (e.g. date and nut, bara brith), digestive biscuits.

Drinks: water, diluted fruit juice, semi-skimmed milk (or home-made milk shake with blended fresh fruit).

For a slightly hungrier child you could add an extra or two – for example, some dried fruit, some fresh nuts (if he/she isn't allergic to them) or seeds, or some low-fat, low-salt crisps. To help keep the fat content of the lunch down for weight-watching children, use low-fat spread or low-calorie mayonnaise to spread on the bread, rather than butter or full-fat margarine.

In winter, you could buy an individual-sized, wide-necked soup vacuum flask and the child can take a home-made soup to school with some bread, instead of the sandwich. In summer, you can use leftover cooked brown or white rice, couscous or pasta shapes to make a salad which he/she can take to school in a lidded plastic container, with a plastic spoon and fork, again instead of the sandwich. The advantage of soups and salads is that you can work in fresh vegetables and salad items in greater quantities than you can get inside a sandwich – and in my experience, a lot of children won't eat salad items inside bread, in any case.

A moderate-calorie lunch for an average child should contain around 500–600 calories and all the following examples contain around that.

- White bread sandwich with half-fat Cheddar and pickle; I satsuma, I small banana, I slice of malt loaf; diluted apple juice.
- Mini pitta filled with flaked tuna, chopped cherry tomato and low-fat mayonnaise; I apple; I slice of fruit cake; semi-skimmed milk.
- Soft brown bap filled with cooked chicken breast and crisp lettuce with low-fat mayonnaise; 3 whole cherry tomatoes; I slice of teabread; I small bag of raisins and cashews (not for nut allergy sufferers); water.
- Leftover cooked brown rice mixed with chopped cucumber, celery, nuts (not for nut allergy sufferers), apple and dried apricot, plus some chopped cooked chicken or cheese and French dressing (or whatever dressing the child will eat); 2 digestive biscuits; diluted orange juice.
- Leftover cooked pasta shapes mixed with chopped tomato, red onion, cucumber, cooked broccoli florets mixed with chopped mozzarella cheese and some mayonnaise thinned down with a little skimmed milk and seasoning; I satsuma; I slice of fruit cake; water.

See also:

▶ Questions: 263–8.
▶ Features: 22–4.
▶ Key index entries: healthy eating for children, weight control for children.

Q 288

What is a good breakfast for a child who is mildly overweight?

It is a good idea for all children to start the day with a breakfast. Research shows that it improves concentration and brain power in the morning. If they skip it, as with adults, their blood-sugar levels will be low until lunchtime.

A good breakfast should contain plenty of fast- and slow-release carbohydrate (explained in more detail in the answer to Q84), for instant and more sustaining energy, as well as some protein, a little fat and something to provide vitamin C (e.g. fruit).

Carbohydrates could include bread, cereal, porridge, bananas, dried fruit. Protein could include milk, yoghurt, nuts, seeds, baked beans, egg.

Vitamin C could be provided by fresh fruit or fruit juice.

A little fat will be provided by a spread on the bread, and from fat within foods such as milk, yoghurt (depending on what type is used), nuts, seeds.

If the child enjoys a hearty breakfast, he/she could have a bowl of cereal with milk and chopped fruit, followed by a slice of bread with spread and some low-sugar jam or marmalade, otherwise the bread element could be skipped. If the child doesn't like breakfast, you could simply make a milk shake from semi-skimmed milk, banana, berry fruits and honey, and blend it all up.

Here are some ideas for good healthy breakfasts:

- Greek yoghurt topped with a handful of muesli or crumbled-up Weetabix and some sliced strawberries or halved seedless grapes; small slice of bread with low-fat spread and low-sugar jam or Marmite.
- Slice of toast with low-fat spread and baked beans.
- Boiled egg with toast and low-fat spread; orange juice.
- Porridge made with milk and topped with extra milk and honey; orange juice.
- Cornflakes with milk and chopped strawberries; slice of bread and honey.

Adjust the size of the packed lunch according to how much breakfast your child prefers to eat.

See also:

▶ Questions: 263–8, 272.
▶ Features: 22–4.
▶ Key index entries: healthy eating for children, weight control for children.

FAT FACT

We live in a fast-food world. The average length of time an adult spends preparing the main meal of the day is now 15 minutes – as opposed to 2½ hours 60 years ago, according to a survey by the University of London.

The balancing act

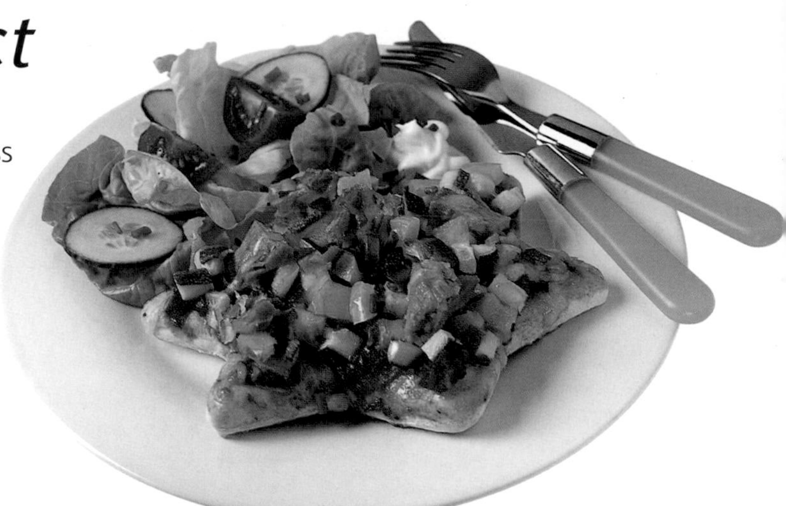

Whether you need to work new foods or less favoured items, like fruits and veg, into your child's diet – or if you need to know how to provide modified versions of their favourite high-fat meals, there are plenty of ideas here to help feed your kids healthily without protest.

Meals for fast-food addicts

Make your own 'fast food' to save on calories and fat.

■ Make home-made burgers with extra lean mince or ground steak, breadcrumbs, seasoning, Worcestershire sauce and egg white to bind; serve in baps with tomato ketchup; potato wedges coated in ready-made Nacho Cheese coating (Schwartz) and baked until golden; and baked beans, peas or sweetcorn.

■ Make chicken nuggets by cutting skinless chicken breasts into bite-sized chunks and coating them in beaten egg then golden breadcrumbs; bake, turning once, until golden and cooked through. Serve with tomato ketchup and large-sized oven chips.

■ Top a pizza base with some home-made or ready-made tomato sauce (see opposite), choice of vegetable toppings plus, if liked, one other topping (see below) and some grated half-fat Mozzarella; bake until bubbling, then serve on its own or with a small side salad and low-fat mayonnaise.

Vegetable toppings, all thinly sliced or chopped small: red onion, mushroom, red, orange or yellow pepper, broccoli, tomato, courgette, baked beans, celery, spinach.

Other toppings, thinly sliced: extra-lean ham, cooked chicken, turkey ham, prawns, tuna, extra-lean minced beef (pre-cooked), extra-lean back bacon, pastrami.

■ Make potato wedges by cutting the potatoes into eighths lengthwise, brushing lightly with vegetable oil, seasoning and baking for 30 minutes until golden. Serve with low-fat sausages or griddled eggs and peas, baked beans or sweetcorn.

Meals for children who won't chew

■ Pasta with home-made tomato sauce (see opposite) either basic or with one of the following chopped in: mushrooms, grilled, peeled and sliced red peppers, halved and grilled courgettes.

■ Poached eggs on mashed potato with a glass of orange juice or some sweetcorn.

■ Cottage pie, preferably bulked out with finely chopped vegetables instead of too much mince.

■ Lasagne made with extra-lean mince and low-fat cheese sauce topping (either ready-made – many brands available – or home-made, using sauce flour and no fat).

■ Fish pie made with white fish, prawns, petit pois and hard-boiled egg, low-fat cheese sauce and a mashed potato topping, served with carrots.

Tasty ways to serve fish

■ Fishcakes made with equal parts white fish or salmon and mashed potato, adding whatever seasoning you think your child will like – just salt and pepper, or you can include herbs or chilli. Fry in a non-stick pan coated with low-calorie cooking oil spray and serve with peas, baked beans or sweetcorn.

■ Fish nuggets – follow the same principle as for chicken nuggets. Choose a sturdy white fish such as cod or monkfish.

■ Tuna bake – bake tuna (fresh or drained canned) in a low-fat white or cheese sauce mixed with petit pois, chopped tomato, sweetcorn and seasoning with a little half-fat Mozzarella to top, until bubbling. Can be served with potatoes or pasta, or you mix pasta into the dish before cooking.

■ Smoked haddock kedgeree – microwave or poach the fish and flake into cooked saffron rice with cooked petit pois and sweetcorn and a little fish or chicken stock.

■ Many children who won't eat basic white fish like the frozen portions of fish fillet in a cheese or parsley sauce, which are usually quite low in calories and fat; good with mashed potato and peas or carrots.

Ways to serve vegetables

- In stir-fries with a favourite meat, e.g. chicken or beef.
- Puréed (by hand or in a blender) and served with roast meats, chops, baked chicken, etc. Try peas, carrots, swede, parsnips, chickpeas, sweet potato, spinach.
- Mixed with potato. Mash the potato and stir in puréed or finely chopped green vegetables, e.g. spinach, pak choi, spring greens.
- In soup – make vegetable soup and purée in a blender until smooth. Choose vegetables your child is most likely to enjoy. Carrot and tomato are two favourites.
- In composite dishes. When making cottage pie, lasagne or stews, add in plenty of vegetables chopped to a suitable size. Once cooked and with lots of sauce or gravy, most children are quite happy to eat them. Baked beans or other cooked pulses are also very good served this way.
- Inside burgers, pittas, tacos, sandwiches, flat breads. Finely sliced crisp lettuce, cucumber, tomatoes, red onion, radish, etc. can be mixed with your child's favourite meat, fish or poultry or cheese and maybe some low-fat mayonnaise.
- As a sauce. Home-made tomato sauce can be used for many dishes; good with meat or poultry as well as pasta. See recipe on the right.
- Crudités and dips. Some children who don't like cooked vegetables will happily eat crunchy colourful raw vegetables, such as carrot, red pepper and celery, especially if served with a tasty creamy dip (fromage frais mixed with low-fat mayo, seasoning and a little grated cheese is good).

Ways to serve fruit

- Cooked, puréed and served with ice-cream or yoghurt – good for apple, pear, peaches and more.
- Puréed raw and served similarly – good for strawberries, raspberries and any soft fruit. Sieve with icing sugar for an easy coulis to go with ice cream.
- Fresh fruit salad – often acceptable when whole fruit isn't.
- Smoothies. Blend chopped peeled fruits with a little water as necessary, or blend fruits and yoghurt, or fruits and milk for added calcium and for a good breakfast substitute. Sweeten with a little honey if necessary. Good fruits: banana, strawberry, raspberry, tinned pineapple, melon, mango, pawpaw.
- Juice: Use a press to extract juice from citrus fruits. They can then be used as a component of home-made smoothies.

Lower-calorie desserts

- Any of the fruit ideas, see above.
- Low-fat custard with sliced banana.
- Layers of Greek yoghurt and fruit slices in a glass.
- Layers of Greek yoghurt and crunchy granola in a glass.
- Banana baked in its skin and served with fruit coulis or a little chocolate sauce.
- 8%-fat fromage frais beaten with a little icing sugar and served with sliced strawberries or other fruit.
- Greek yoghurt or 8%-fat fromage frais layered with crushed strawberries and crushed meringue.
- Low-fat rice pudding swirled with fruit coulis or low-sugar jam.

Home-made tomato sauce

(Serves 4: 60 calories and 3.5g fat per portion)

Heat 1 tbsp olive or vegetable oil in a non-stick saucepan and stir 1 finely chopped medium onion in it over a medium heat until softened Add 1 large crushed garlic clove, if you like, and stir for a minute or two, then add one 400g (14oz) can of chopped tomatoes with their juice, 1 level tbsp tomato purée, 1 tsp sugar and the juice of 1/2 lemon. Stir well and simmer for 30 minutes, stirring from time to time and adding a little extra tomato juice or passata if the sauce looks too thick. When you have a rich sauce which has darkened in colour, season to taste. It will freeze, or keep in the fridge for a day or two.

Variations: add chopped mushrooms with the tomatoes (good with pasta or on baked potatoes); add grilled, peeled, chopped red peppers (ditto); add chopped parsley or coriander for grown-ups; add more garlic or less to taste; add a selection of chopped courgette, aubergine and red onion, ready stir-fried (good with couscous or bulgar wheat); add chopped red chilli (deseeded) and some cooked red kidney beans for a non-meat chilli (good with rice).

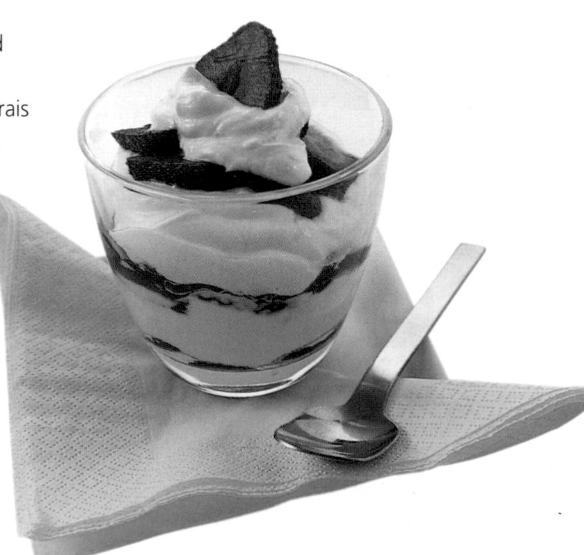

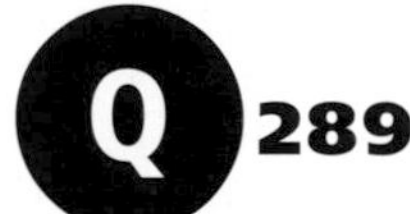

Q 289

Can you give me ideas for main meals for overweight children who only really like burgers, chips and baked beans?

You have to take the evolutionary, rather than revolutionary, approach and work new foods into their diet over the months. Borrow ideas from the Retraining Programme for adults in Feature 13, and a look at some of the rest of this section will give you ideas too. (e.g., Qs 269, 270, 274 and 290) Feature 24 provides ideas for all meal situations, which may help you to work new foods into their diet without protest.

However, I need to make the point that a healthy eating diet and a weight-loss diet aren't the same thing. If your children are overweight they could, in theory, lose weight even while still eating burgers, chips and beans most days. You would simply have to cook the meal in the lowest-fat, lowest-cal way possible, i.e. extra-lean burger, large-cut oven chips or home-made potato wedges, and plenty of baked beans (low in fat and calories), but avoid giving too big a portion of chips, and then make sure the rest of the day's food is not too high in calories and fat either.

As I have said, a lot of the foods that we regard as 'junk' do, in fact, have good points and you shouldn't worry about avoiding all red meat, all chips, etc. You may just need to do some 'tweaking' to make their food intake both healthy and non-fattening. For overweight children it's best to start by cutting sugary drinks, fatty/sugary desserts and similar snacks.

Feature 23 has all you need to know about feeding a child, for health and for slimming, and Q267 has more information.

See also:

- Questions: 263 270, 274, 290.
- Features: 13, 22-24.
- Key index entries: healthy eating for children, weight control for children.

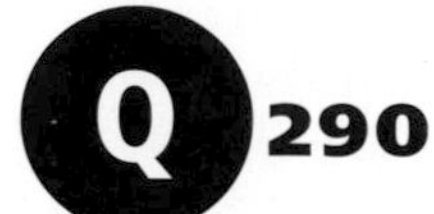

Q 290

How do I present reduced-fat/calorie meals to my children without them realizing? The doctor says they need to lose weight but his diet sheet is full of foods they hate.

Mention a 'diet' to most children and they immediately get uncooperative. So, it's best simply to provide them with reduced-cal meals as outlined in this section, without making a big issue of it. Adapting what you currently give them is usually all that is needed. Ideas appear in Feature 24.

You don't need to mention words like 'low-calorie', 'slimming', or 'can't have'. In fact, it's better not to. The trick is to think of plenty of tasty things that they can have and couple that with slight portion control to get the desired effect over time.

With overweight children, there is no hurry to lose weight and, as we saw in Q267, you could even simply keep them at their current weight and wait while they grow into their weight by getting taller.

In one way it is a pity they were made aware of having to 'diet'. In another, however, having won the battle of the diet sheet, they may be willing to co-operate on small changes to their diets. Also, the more exercise they do, the more they can eat.

See also:

- Questions: 263–89.
- Features: 22–4.
- Key index entries: healthy eating for children, junk food, weight control for children.

Q 291

Is there such a thing as puppy fat?

According to the World Health Organization, the onset of adolescence predisposes a child to increased risk of overweight or obesity. This is partly because of social factors, such as more opportunity to choose their own food, more money to spend on snacks or drinks. Studies reveal that there is also a marked increase in preference for fatty foods at this time, and appetite often increases.

There are physiological changes at adolescence which predispose to increased fat deposition, especially in girls. Genetically, these will be the increased deposits of fat on the breasts, hips, bottom and thighs, which is normal for the average female. The laying down of surplus fat can act as a trigger to the onset of puberty, hence the increased appetite.

These factors all combine to make some children, especially girls, put on body fat fairly rapidly during from age 12 to 14, which is sometimes called 'puppy fat'. Before deciding whether weight loss is necessary, it is important to establish whether the extra weight is within the normal range for your child's age and height (see Feature 22), perhaps with the help of a doctor. Obviously, when a girl matures and gets curves, this is normal and shouldn't be confused with overweight. A good indication is if her waist is still well defined, then she's probably not overweight.

See also:

- Questions: 263–8, 292.
- Features: 22, 23.

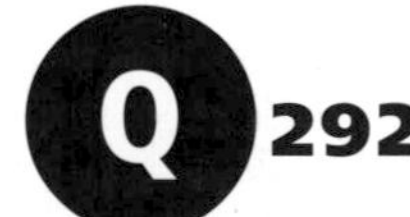

Q 292

Will puppy fat naturally go with age?

'Puppy fat' is a colloquial term used to denote weight gain at adolescence (see the answers to the previous questions) that, it is often said, will naturally disappear in the later teens. If a child has had a sharp increase of appetite around puberty, sometimes the appetite naturally decreases later and the weight problem resolves itself. However, in many more cases, this doesn't happen and the child continues to put on weight and may easily become fat.

If your child does become truly overweight or obese during the early teens (as defined in Feature 22) then unless he/she takes steps to moderate food intake (particularly of high-fat, high-sugar items, snacks and drinks) and to increase exercise output, it is unlikely that all the weight will disappear as he/she gets older.

However, it is true to say that most adolescents will become several inches taller by the time they are fully grown and so the 'weight maintenance and wait for extra height' policy outlined in Q267 may be a good idea for all but the most obese. That is, you may not need to encourage them to follow an actual slimming diet to lose weight, but just strive to maintain their current weight, and their increasing height will slim them down naturally.

See also:

- ▶ Questions: 263–8, 291.
- ▶ Features: 22, 23.

Q 293

Why won't my local gym let my 13-year-old son join and use the exercise equipment?

Many gyms aren't insured for children under 16 to use their equipment, although they may be allowed to join in exercise classes. Traditionally exercise physiologists have thought resistance training with gym equipment an unsuitable form of exercise for children and young teenagers, as their bones and bodies are still growing. Indeed, the UK Physical Education Association still says that no one under 14 should do any such training because of the risk to bones. There is also a feeling that for children exercise should be about natural physical expression, fun and sociability, not a lonely, focused workout on a machine. There is also a policy within some gym chains that members come to work out away from kids, not surrounded by them, and so they deliberately limit membership to adults.

However, despite all this, there is a growing number of gyms catering specially for children from 7 to 14 or 15, where you will find resistance equipment scaled down in size and weight increments to be suitable for children's size and strength, and professionals in the US encourage children to do all forms of exercise – aerobic, strength and flexibility (see Q295).

It also has to be said that, as time allocated to PE and sport in UK schools diminishes (down 50% in the last 5 years), as long as it is done responsibly, anything that encourages children to take exercise safely and happily must be good.

See also:

- ▶ Questions: 294–5.
- ▶ A-Z entry: Fitkids.
- ▶ Key index entries: exercise for children, fitness and health, gyms.

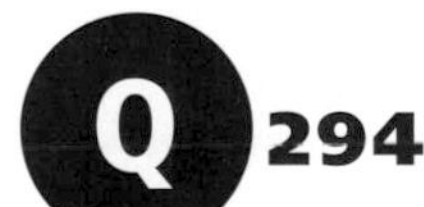

294

What is the best exercise for an exercise-shy child?

This depends mainly on the reason for the dislike of exercise. If it is because they find it boring, then the suggestions in Q282 will probably help you think of solutions. If he/she finds it difficult, then you should encourage him/her to develop confidence with family activities such as cycling, swimming or perhaps adventure walking. Avoid competitive sports or situations where he/she is forced to exercise with children he/she doesn't know well, and encourage rather than bully them.

Perhaps the best solution is to begin a 'walk to school' regime. The 2001 report on obesity from the UK's National Audit Office recommended more children should walk or cycle to school and that schools should coordinate supervision of walking for safety.

Most children who can be persuaded into exercise seem quite quickly to find that they actually enjoy it. Being overweight isn't a contra-indication for exercise, but if your child is clinically overweight (see Feature 22) take him/her to the doctor for a physical check-up.

See also:

- ▶ Questions: 282, 292–3, 295.
- ▶ Features: 22–4.
- ▶ Key index entry: exercise for children.

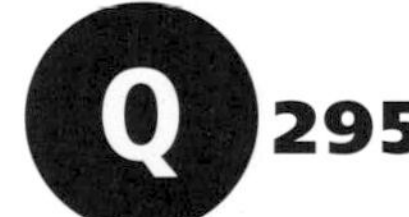

295

Are any forms of exercise dangerous for children?

As explained in Q293, some professionals feel that it isn't a good idea for very young children to perform resistance exercise with weights, or with gym equipment, for example. This is because their bones and bodies are growing rapidly and there is some evidence that such exercise could cause injury and other problems.

However, in the US, the Kid's Activity Pyramid – guidelines for exercise used by health professionals, teachers and so on – suggests that regular muscle-strengthening exercise is important for all children, as it not only helps to build a good physique and burns calories, but can also reduce the risk of osteoporosis later in life. They say that weight-bearing exercise can be carried out, as long as the weight is moderate and muscle strength is increased through additional repetitions. They also recommend push-ups (see Feature 6) and other floor exercises.

What the American Academy of Pediatrics say shouldn't be attempted until the body has completed growth are lifting heavy weights, power-lifting, bodybuilding and repetitive use of very high weights. As a rule-of-thumb, most girls don't finish growth until 16 and most boys until 18.

The AAP also say that children under 6 shouldn't participate in team sports as they don't understand teamwork until that age, and they recommend that young children may not be suitable for distance running or intensive training as there may be musculo-skeletal and other damage.

Their message is that if any child is participating in endurance running and/or intensive training then they should be monitored regularly by a health professional and nutritional intake adjusted accordingly. If you want to know more about what is and isn't suitable exercise for children, you could visit the AAP's website on http//:www.aap.org.htm/.

When it comes to sports, obviously some forms of activity are more dangerous than others – for example, horseriding has one of the highest rates of accident of all sports and is also one that many youngsters enjoy. Climbing, football, even cycling, all have fairly high rates of injury and no doubt there are many more sports that cause accidents and occasional injury to children. All children and adolescents should be properly supervised when undertaking any potentially dangerous sports or exercise – including using free weights or gym equipment.

With sensible precautions, however, I would say it is always better to let your child live an active life with some excitement via exercise than to keep him/her locked inside watching TV where he/she is safe in the short term, but at much higher risk of obesity, disease and shorter lifespan in the long term.

See also:

▶ Questions: 282, 293–4.
▶ A–Z entry: Fitkids.
▶ Key index entry: exercise for children.

FIT FACT

A US obesity expert in New York has invented an exercise bike called the TV cycle, electrically connected to the TV, which when pedalled creates the energy to keep the picture on the TV screen. In a 10-week test of children aged 8-12, the TV cyclers watched TV for only one hour a week because they had to pedal hard to keep the screen on, but children who didn't need to use the bike to keep the TV on watched 20 hours of programmes and exercised for only 8 minutes during the week.

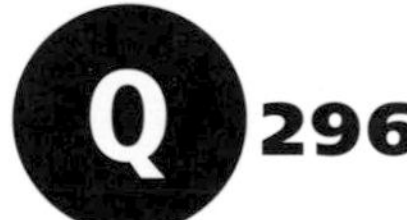

How does one stop a child from getting obsessive about dieting?

Research seems to show that young girls (and boys too, to a lesser degree) are largely influenced in attitude to food, their bodies and 'diets' by their mothers' (and sometimes their fathers') own attitudes.

Eating disorder centres see children as young as 8 for treatment and even 3- and 4-year-olds can be made over-anxious and conscious of food by parents' attitudes. The Human Nutrition department at Glasgow Royal Hospital for Children has found that, ironically, parents over-anxious to give their children a healthy diet, and for them not to be overweight, may in fact encourage eating problems. Parents who are too strict, banning a range of perceived 'unhealthy' or 'fattening' foods are, they believe, inviting problems with eating disorders or, conversely, encouraging obesity by having the opposite effect to that intended. (If you can't have something, you may want it all the more.)

In particular, parents who are obsessive slimmers, calorie-counters or health-food fanatics may find their children are more inclined to diet, be figure-conscious and have a poor self-image than others even when not overweight. A mother's worries about her figure and diet are particularly likely to be emulated by her daughter, according to a study in Boston. Another, published in the *British Journal of Clinical Psychology*, found daughters whose appearance had been criticized by mothers were more likely to diet and 'yo-yo'.

So – after all that, what to do? As we've seen in the rest of this section, obesity is a major problem, and so a real weight problem in a child shouldn't be ignored. BUT the idea of eating as a pleasant, relaxed event and food as an enjoyable part of living should be encouraged throughout a child's life, and overemphasis on calorie-counting and dieting should definitely be avoided.

Equally important is that the parents should show a similarly relaxed attitude – eating well and healthily, but not obsessive about food in general, particular foods, diets, etc. They should be comfortable in their own bodies, taking adequate (not obsessive) exercise, and a healthy (not unhealthy) interest in their appearance. In other words, moderation is the key.

Be a good role model and, hopefully, your children will not become obsessive or suffer eating disorders now or later in life. Your attitude until they're around 12 is the most important. After that, peer pressure to be slim and chats with friends about food and diet, size and weight, may play an equally – or more – important role in how your child views her/his body and eating habits. At this time you need to carry on with the same 'good role model' philosophy and keep a discreet eye on your child's feelings on the subject, while being as positive as possible re their appearance.

It is also worth noting that many anorexics and bulimics come from homes where there are very high standards expected in terms of academic achievement. If you feel you may be inclined to expect too much of your child, try to moderate your attitude there too.

A survey by the Schools Education Unit showed over half of all girls aged 12–15 wanted to lose weight, though most of them weren't clinically overweight at all.

See also:

- Questions: 149–57, 297–99.
- Key index entries: children and weight control, eating disorders, healthy eating.

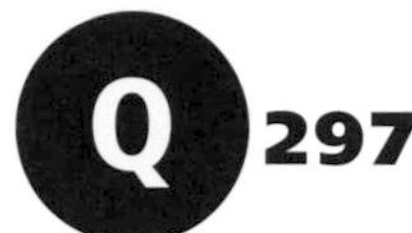

297

What are the signs of anorexia or bulimia in teenagers?

The signs may be similar to those for adults listed in Qs 151 and 155 in Section Four. An anorexic, or pre-anorexic, teenager might refuse to eat with the family and lie about what food she/he has eaten. She/he may talk about food and dieting a lot – one survey reveals that dieting is the strongest indicator of eating disorders. Meals may be skipped – particularly breakfast and lunch at school. She/he may try to disguise a thin body with layers or baggy clothes; may seem withdrawn and may also do a lot of exercise.

Many teenagers with eating disorders become obsessive about food – cooking food for you, taking cookery lessons at school and even wanting a career in catering. Bulimics may lie or steal to get money for food, or steal food. Both potential anorexics and bulimics may be over-anxious, often about schoolwork or performance, and have high standards.

It is estimated that up to 10% of teenagers have a 'pre-anorexic' mild eating disorder when they skip meals and are thinner than they should be, while saying they are fat. At this stage, with care and attention, the problem is easier to solve.

Busy working parents with children in a household where meals are rarely taken together, are at higher risk of having an anorexic or bulimic in the household without anyone noticing, so do involve yourself in your child's life and meal times.

See also:

- Questions: 149–58, 296, 298–9.
- Key index entries: eating disorders, healthy eating for children.

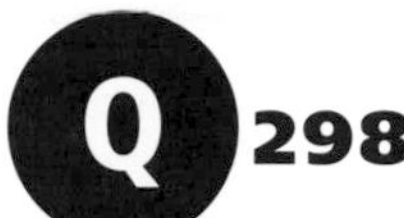

298

What should I do if I think my child may have an eating disorder?

If you suspect a child has an eating disorder, do what you can to discover the truth – many children will deny there is a problem, but a talk with the school or college head, or even with worried friends, may bring the problem to the surface. Although teenagers do talk a lot about diets, body image and so on, when a friend actually succumbs to an eating disorder they are understandably worried and may be relieved to confide in an adult.

Do take your child to the doctor if you suspect an eating disorder. You can also contact one of the helplines in Q151 and you'll be offered counselling for the child or whole family, as well as medical help. Eating disorders are notoriously difficult to self-treat and unlikely to go without professional help.

See also:

- Questions: 149–57, 296–7, 299.
- Key index entry: eating disorders.

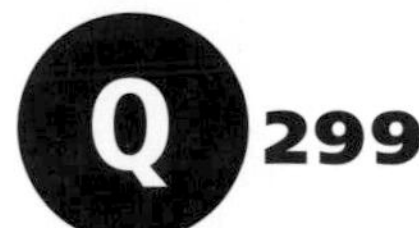

299

My 15-year-old daughter refuses to eat any food from animals. Is this a good thing, or faddy eating that should be discouraged?

If your child has been a committed animal rights follower and has been a vegetarian for some time, then it would seem that she is simply continuing with her beliefs and this isn't a fad. However, if she has suddenly decided to forgo all animal produce for a less altruistic reason – for example, she says she is allergic to it, or feels it's making her fat – then it sounds like something she's decided to do in order to get thin, and may not be a good idea.

A high percentage of teenage girls are vegetarian and in many it is a way of cutting calories without parental dissent, although I don't doubt many are also committed veggies. If your daughter is insistent, turn to Qs 278 and 279, where you will find advice on making sure that she eats a healthy diet. You should also read the previous three questions, which may help you decide whether your daughter has an underlying eating disorder, or at least a potential one.

See also:

- Questions: 194–7, 278–9, 296–8.
- Feature: 16.
- A–Z entry: vegetarian diets.
- Key index entries: eating disorders, healthy eating for children, vegans, vegetarianism.

FAT FACT

A survey of 36,000 pupils by the UK Schools Health Education Unit in 2000 found that 60% of girls aged 14–15 and 28% of boys believed that they needed to slim. In the same survey, a fifth of girls said they missed breakfast and 15% said they missed lunch.

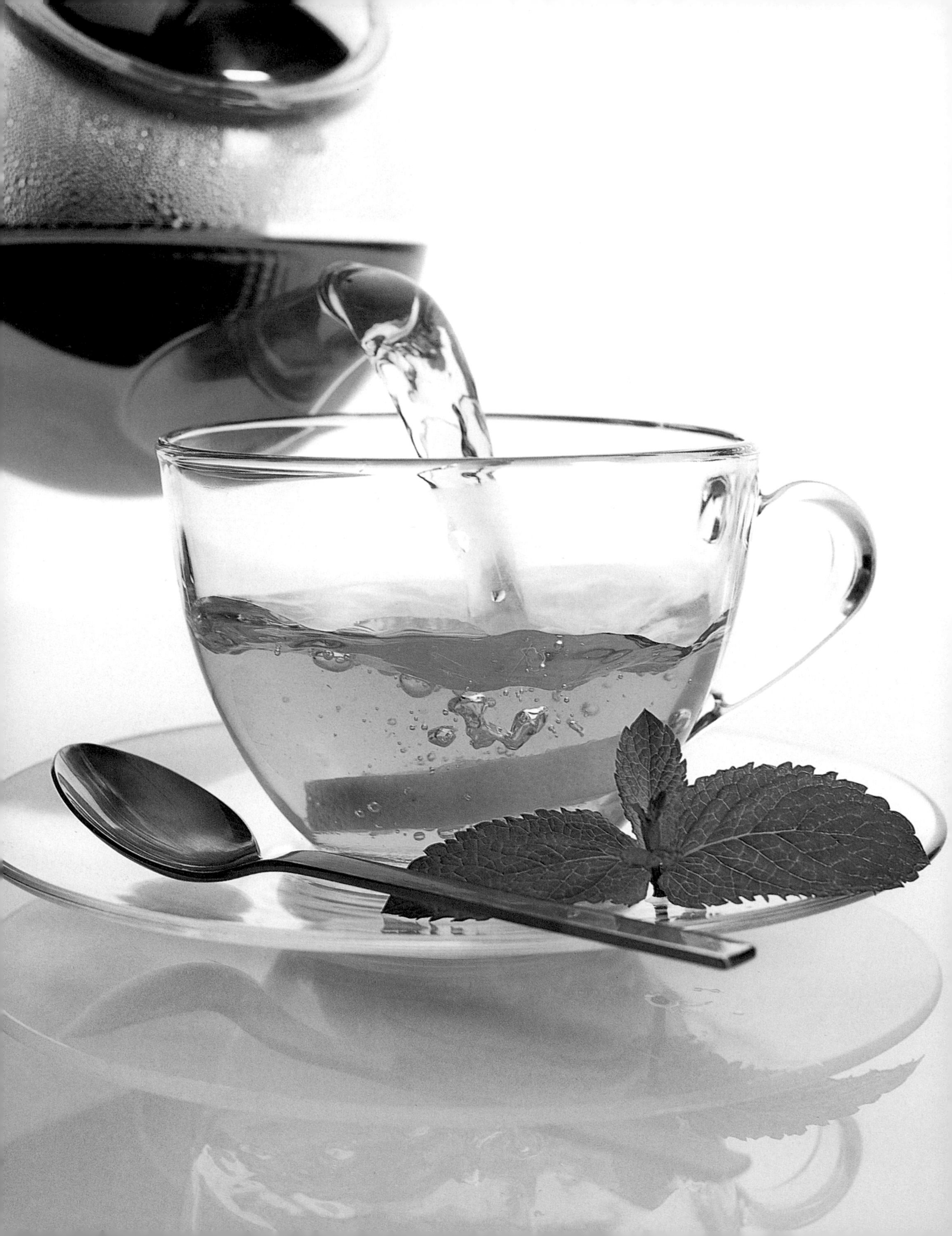

Section Nine

Your weight, your health

It is said that most people who diet to lose weight do so for reasons of vanity rather than health. It should be the other way round, as obesity is one of the major causes of, or contributing factors to, a long list of health problems, with over 30,000 people dying each year from obesity-related illness. The World Health Organization describes the health consequences of obesity as 'many and varied'. They also say that it may affect psychological health by having an adverse effect on the quality of life and creating psychosocial problems.

A high Body Mass Index is linked with coronary heart disease and cardiovascular disease, also with type-2 diabetes, high blood pressure, arthritis, some cancers, back pain and more. Many overweight people are also unfit – as fatness doesn't predispose to exercise – which is another negative health factor.

The cost to the nation of obesity is vast. According to the National Audit Office, the direct cost to the NHS of dealing with obesity via consultations, drugs and other treatments is £500 million, and if the indirect costs, such as lost working days and treatments for problems occurring because of obesity, are included the cost soars to £2.1 billion.

Yet even small losses in weight by obese people can result in a better health profile for them. A relatively small percentage reduction in body weight can improve blood pressure, for example, and 5–10% losses in the obese can reduce the risk of mortality considerably.

In this section we look at all the many aspects of how your weight affects your health.

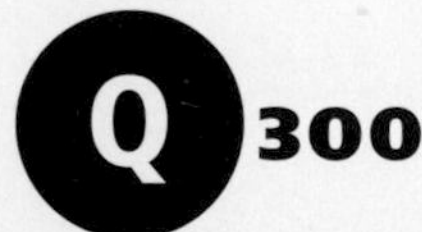

Q300

What are the main links between weight and health?

An average body weight (BMI between 20 and 25) is associated with your highest chance of good health. Both overweight and underweight can affect health in various ways. Qs 25 in Section One and 319 in this section give you some background on underweight and health, and Q26 and Feature 25 later in this section describe the links between overweight and health in detail.

Here are a few more facts and figures:

- Each year nearly 10,000 people in the UK and 70,000 in Europe develop cancer because they are fat, according to a study published in the *International Journal of Cancer* in 2001, with breast and colon cancers most closely linked with overweight.
- The Institute of Cancer Research reported in 2001 that obesity is the second biggest cause of cancer (after smoking) and that 10% of cancers in non-smoking Americans are attributable to weight.
- Middle-aged adults who have diabetes and/or high blood pressure (a high proportion of whom will also be overweight) are more likely to suffer from dementia. In tests on people aged 47 to 70, mental decline was greater in all those who had diabetes and in those with high blood pressure aged over 58.
- A rise in diabetes in the USA of 33% in the last 10 years is linked with a similar rise in people with obesity.
- A body weight only 10% above average has been shown to increase the risk of death from coronary heart disease.

The fact is that obesity is increasing across the world at such an alarming rate, and is so closely linked with so many illnesses and health problems, that finding ways to stem its progress is a priority for health organizations everywhere.

See also:

- Questions: 26–31, 301–6, 319.
- Features: 3, 25.
- Key index entries: Body Mass Index, obesity, weight and health.

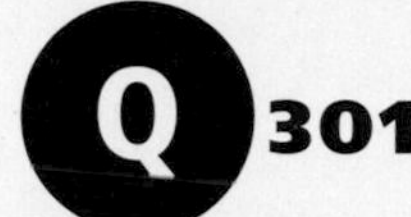

Q301

If I put on weight, how soon will it begin to affect my health?

For most of us, keeping a BMI around 20–25 offers the greatest protection against weight-related disorders. Your risk of health problems due to increased weight rises gradually almost in line with the amount of weight you put on, rather than exactly how long you have been at a particular weight, though it is reasonable to conjecture that the longer you have been overweight the more likely it may be that you will have weight-related problems, even if you keep your (over)weight stable.

FAT FACT

Obese lorry drivers stand more chance of having accidents at the wheel due to falling asleep while driving than non-obese drivers, because their weight makes them vulnerable to sleep disorders, according to the British Sleep Foundation.

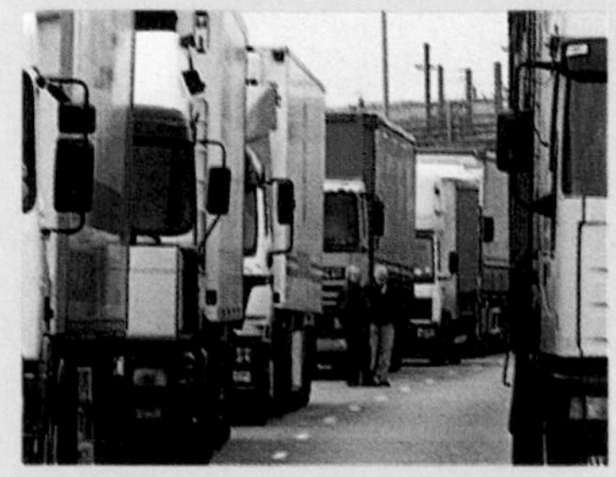

Obviously, if you put on a stone or two for a few months and then lose it, you are unlikely to suffer health problems related to your short period of being overweight. As another example, if you have always been slim and only in the last few weeks put on half a stone or so, again it is unlikely that any weight-related health problems will result from that. You need to check out your current BMI (using Feature 3) to see what your current risk of health problems is, before considering whether you need to lose weight.

In fact, if you repeatedly put on weight and then lose it (the 'yo-yo syndrome'), that also increases your risk of health and heart problems, so many experts believe that it is better to maintain a slightly high stable weight than to keep 'yo-yoing'.

See also:

- Questions: 302–6, 313–14, 325–6.
- Features: 3, 25.
- Key index entries: Body Mass Index, obesity, weight and health.

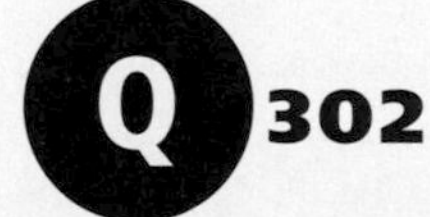

Q302

How overweight do you have to be before you get health problems?

The general consensus of opinion is that once your BMI reaches about 27–8, your risk of getting ill health begins to increase considerably and over 30 you are officially classed as obese. Feature 3 shows you the different bands of body mass index and what each means.

However, different professionals with different specialities do disagree on what exactly an ideal weight is, and the starting point for weight-related problems. For instance, one report published in the *European Heart Journal* in 2001 concluded that, for middle-aged women, the healthiest BMI in order to have the least chance of metabolic risk factors for coronary heart disease is 22 or less, and another report found that women who gained only 20lb (9kg) from their teens through to middle age doubled their risk of heart attack. And yet for prevention of osteoporosis and, indeed, to avoid the yo-yo dieting syndrome, many experts believe that for middle-aged women a BMI of 22 is too low.

A good indicator of health risk is having a large waist measurement, with or without a high BMI. For more information on that, see Feature 3 and Qs 56, 324 and elsewhere.

See also:

- ▶ Questions: 26, 28–31, 56, 300, 301, 303–6, 324–6.
- ▶ Features: 3, 25.
- ▶ Key index entries: apple shape, body mass index, health and weight.

FAT FACT

According to one recent study on diabetes care conducted in the USA, on average, for every 2lb (1kg) in weight that a person puts on over the normal range, their risk of developing diabetes increases by about 9%.

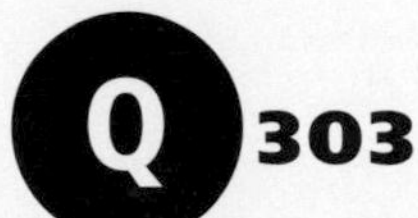

Does overweight shorten lifespan?

We know that obesity is linked with a wide range of illnesses and health problems (see Feature 25) and, as some of these are life-threatening, then obesity can be indirectly responsible for shortening life for people who develop these illnesses. We do also have some concrete evidence of exactly how obesity can shorten lifespan.

For instance, one US study of over 300,000 people by the University of North Carolina, published in 1999, found that obesity increases the risk of death from natural causes for a man aged between 40 and 50 to that of a male nearly 6 years older, and the risk for a similarly aged woman increased to that of a woman 6.4 years older. As another example, the survey found that a 5ft 10in (1.75m) man weighing 20lb (9kg) over the ideal BMI has a 20% higher risk of death.

A further study published in the *New England Journal of Medicine* also in l999, this time using over 1 million US adults, also supported an increase in risk of death from all causes, including cardiovascular disease and cancer, throughout the range of moderate to severe overweight for both men and women in all age groups.

Studies by the US National Center for Toxicological Research, approaching the subject from the reverse angle, have indicated that people who cut their calorie intake down to a maximum of 1,800 a day show large improvements in the biochemistry of their cells, and similar tests on animals have shown that they can increase their lifespan by 50%, although this work needs to be investigated further.

The World Health Organization, in its 2000 report on obesity, states that obese people face 'increased risk of premature death'. The consensus worldwide seems to be that risk of premature death increases on a reasonably level curve upwards once BMI goes over 25, with a much steeper curve after 30. At moderately high BMIs, abdominal obesity (central fat distribution) is an additional factor (see Feature 3 and Q324) – i.e. if you have much of your surplus fat around your middle even though your BMI is only moderately high (say 26–9), risk of early death is increased.

Problems are also increased if you have other risk factors for premature death as well as obesity – for instance, high blood pressure, high cholesterol, and/or you smoke or have diabetes. If you also take no exercise, with an official classification of sedentary (see Feature 1), then that too may increase risk of shortened lifespan.

HOWEVER! There is always some research that will come out and seem to prove the opposite to the bulk of evidence. The Cooper Institute for Aerobic Research in Dallas claims that a study of 22,000 men has discovered that it is fitness, not fatness, that matters when it comes to prolonging life. They say that unfit, lean men are more likely to die young than fit, fat ones.

Certainly, I don't doubt that being unfit may shorten your life span – so whether you are fat or lean, it is important to take regular exercise, particularly for aerobic fitness.

See also:

- ▶ Questions: 26–31, 300–302, 304–6, 324–6, 328–32.
- ▶ Features: 1, 3, 25, 27.
- ▶ Key index entries: apple shape, body mass index, weight and fitness, weight and health.

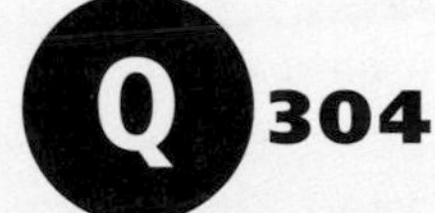

I am overweight but I feel perfectly healthy, so why should I worry?

There are, no doubt, many overweight people who are currently healthy and feeling fine. If you are young, you are especially likely, outwardly at least, not to be showing any signs of ill health due to your weight. Sadly, were your arteries to be examined, they may well shows signs of unhealthy fatty deposits, or were you to have a thorough all-over check-up, problems might show up (e.g. raised

FAT FACTS

- The number of adults worldwide who have diabetes has risen to 151 million – 5% of the world's population. Experts blame the rise – 11% in 5 years – on our unhealthy lifestyles and the fact that many countries are adopting typical Western habits.
- High-fat, high-sugar diets, coupled with inactivity, lead to obesity, which is closely linked with type-2 diabetes.
- In the UK, 8% of all hospital admissions are due to diabetes and related conditions.

cholesterol, high blood pressure, early wear and tear on the joints, insulin resistance and so on, see Feature 25).

There is also, no doubt, a percentage of overweight people who reach a ripe old age with hardly a day's illness – figures quoted in this book deal with populations and averages, and some are bound to be the lucky ones who aren't average. As they say, it is the exception that proves the rule, but please don't forget that a BMI over 30 (about 20% overweight) IS a predictor of ill health later in life and so, if you are young, don't think that you will necessarily 'get away with it' for the rest of your life.

However, you reduce your chances of ill health due to obesity if you have no other negative symptoms or risk factors – i.e. if obesity is the single risk factor that you have. For example, if you don't smoke, if you have good cardiovascular fitness (you take plenty of exercise), if you have normal blood pressure and blood cholesterol levels, if your surplus weight is evenly distributed rather than being mostly around your middle, if your close family are all healthy, then your chances of continuing to be healthy are much higher.

I'd suggest a twice-yearly check-up to make sure that you are still defying the odds as you get older.

See also:

- ▶ Questions: 300–303, 324.
- ▶ Features: 3, 25.
- ▶ Key index entries: obesity, weight and health.

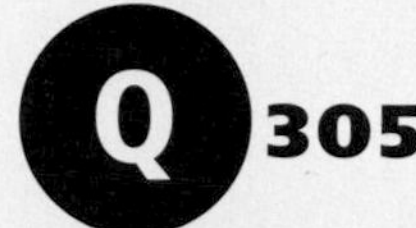

Is it true that it is better for your health to put on weight as you get older?

Go back and read the answer to Q27, which will give you some background to the debate. As you will have now read, the consensus seems to be that a small weight gain into mid-life is okay, some say beneficial. There are, however, experts who believe that no weight gain is better (mostly because it seems to lower the risk of heart disease – and for more on this you need to check out the answer to Q 326).

What everyone is agreed on is that large weight gains as you get older definitely aren't good news. Again, the reasons why being overweight or obese is not generally a good idea are discussed in detail elsewhere in the book (e.g. Q300), and this applies just as much, or even more, to older people. A report published in 2000 by the UK Office of National Statistics found that, although our general life expectancy is more than it was in previous generations, people retiring now will suffer four extra months of ill health, mostly due to the rise in obesity.

And, as incidence of obesity rises year on year, experts already predict that our lifespan will, indeed, begin to shorten again, and by the time the current generation of youngsters is old they shouldn't expect to live as long as their grandparents.

See also:

- ▶ Questions: 27, 300–304, 326.
- ▶ Feature: 25.
- ▶ Key index entries: weight and health, weight in mid-life, weight in old age.

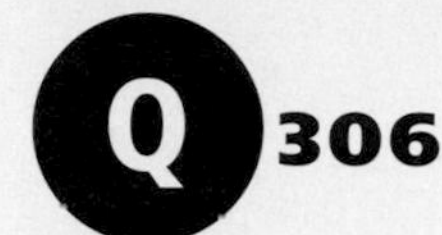

If I have been fat for a long time, can I reverse ill health if I lose weight, how much do I need to lose, and can I really do it?

You are never too old to lose weight and improve weight-related symptoms, and your surplus fat is never so entrenched that it will not respond to a reduced-calorie diet and some activity.

Studies have shown that, in an obese person weighing 16 stone, a reduction in body weight of around 10% affords significant improvement in health, and may reduce risk of premature mortality by about 25%. The Royal College of Physicians says that, with a 10% weight loss, blood pressure comes down, cholesterol levels reduce and diabetes is less likely or, if present, better controlled. A report published in the *British Medical Bulletin* in 1997 says that with a 22lb (10kg) weight loss, deaths from diabetic complications are reduced by 30–40%, deaths from obesity-related cancers by 40–50%, the number of cases of diabetes type-2 can be reduced by 50%, blood pressure falls by 10 points on average and LDL cholesterol in the blood reduces by 15% on average, while symptoms of angina are reduced by 91%.

As examples, a 10% weight loss translates as 21lb (9.5kg) for a 15-stone person or 2 stones (12.75kg) for a 20-stone person. If you are very overweight, you would probably notice improvements in health with losses smaller than that – for example, high blood pressure begins to reduce almost as soon as you begin to lose weight.

As we have seen in the answers to the previous questions, an ideal weight range is a body mass index of around 20–25, but it is much better to lose at least SOME weight and reduce your BMI somewhat than to not even try because you think you would never get near this ideal range.

Weight loss for health is relative – as examples, someone with a BMI of 40 reduces their risk of ill health and premature death by lowering their BMI to 35; someone with a BMI of 35 reduces the risk by getting down to a BMI of 29; someone with a BMI of 29 reduces their risks by lowering their BMI to 25. The slimmer you can get, down to a reasonable BMI, the greater your chances of living a long and healthy life – but, in practice, professionals find that people have more chance of maintaining a weight loss if they aim for small losses. And it is, after all, the maintenance of your new weight that is more important than actually getting there.

Check out other parts of the book for advice on how to lose weight and keep it off.

See also:

- ▶ Questions: 28–9, 300–305, 307–10.
- ▶ Features: 3, 25.
- ▶ Key index entries: body mass index, healthy slimming, weight and health.

FAT FACT

In the USA in 2000, 12% of the cost of illness related to excess body fat, and in 1998 obesity became one of the American Heart Association's primary risk factors for coronary heart disease, along with smoking, high blood pressure, raised serum cholesterol levels and physical inactivity.

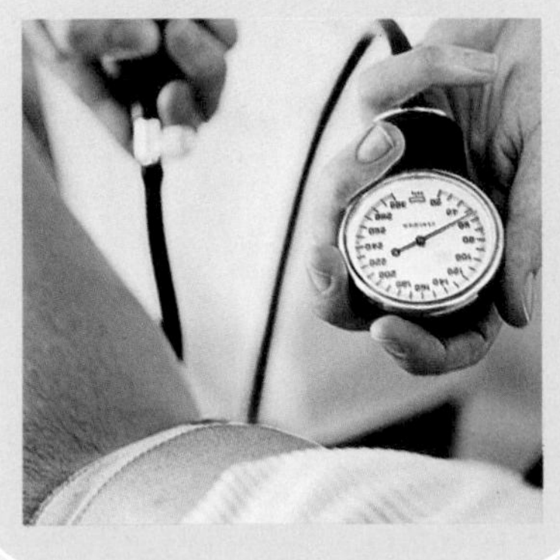

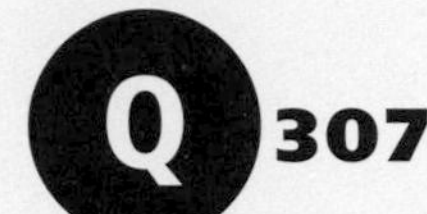

Q 307

What is the healthiest slimming diet in the world?

In general terms, a healthy slimming diet is one that is similar to a normal, healthy eating diet – high in natural foods, such as fruit, vegetables, whole grains and pulses, and with sufficient protein and a little fat – but with the calories it contains reduced to a sufficiently low level to produce slow to steady weight loss. A basic healthy diet is explained in detail in Section Three and in particular in Qs 81–104 and Features 8 and 9. For many people, a calorie reduction of about 500 a day will be sufficient to produce the desired weight loss and, again, for many people, the best way to reduce the calorie content of a basic healthy diet is to reduce portion sizes slightly, particularly of the high-density, high-fat foods.

One of the great advantages of slimming on a really healthy type of diet is that as you lose weight, you also reduce your risk of various modern Western diseases associated with poor diet. For example, up to 80% of bowel and breast cancer may be preventable through diet changes, and scientists have found that women who follow a healthy diet such as that outlined in Feature 9 cut their risk of dying from heart disease by 30%. Problems such as diverticulitis, constipation, fatigue and dry skin – to name but a few – can also be helped with good diet.

As for the healthiest slimming diet in the world, perhaps there is not really such a thing. For one, we have so many different foods to choose from, not only in this country, but from country to country. The choices vary so much that THE perfect healthy slimming diet would be very hard to define in terms of which actual foods should be eaten, in what quantities. All I can do is show you examples of what 'a' healthy diet looks like, rather than 'the' healthy diet – and leave the fine-tuning of the diet up to you. People do also vary in their nutritional needs, according to a variety of factors – their current health, their age, their activity levels, and so on. So pinpointing a perfect diet for everyone is not possible.

Unless you have a particular health problem, though, I wouldn't worry too much about the 'fine tuning' aspect of your slimming programme. If you bear the general healthy eating principles in mind (particularly with regard to choosing whole, natural foods and keeping a watch on your fat intake) and also watch portion size and between-meal snacking, you should do well. Until you feel confident, why not try one or more of the eating plans that appear throughout the book? You could also get your doctor to refer you to a dietician for personal help.

See also:

- ▶ Questions: 74–122, 308–27.
- ▶ Features: 8–16.
- ▶ A–Z entries: calorie counting, diet coaches, low-fat diets.
- ▶ Key index entries: dieting and health, healthy slimming, high-carbohydrate diets, nutrients.

Health links with overweight

Being overweight or obese increases your risk of getting thirty or so different diseases or health problems – some fairly minor, but most serious or even life-threatening. Here you can see at a glance the risks you run. (For more on how overweight you have to be before these increased risks begin, see Qs 300-306.)

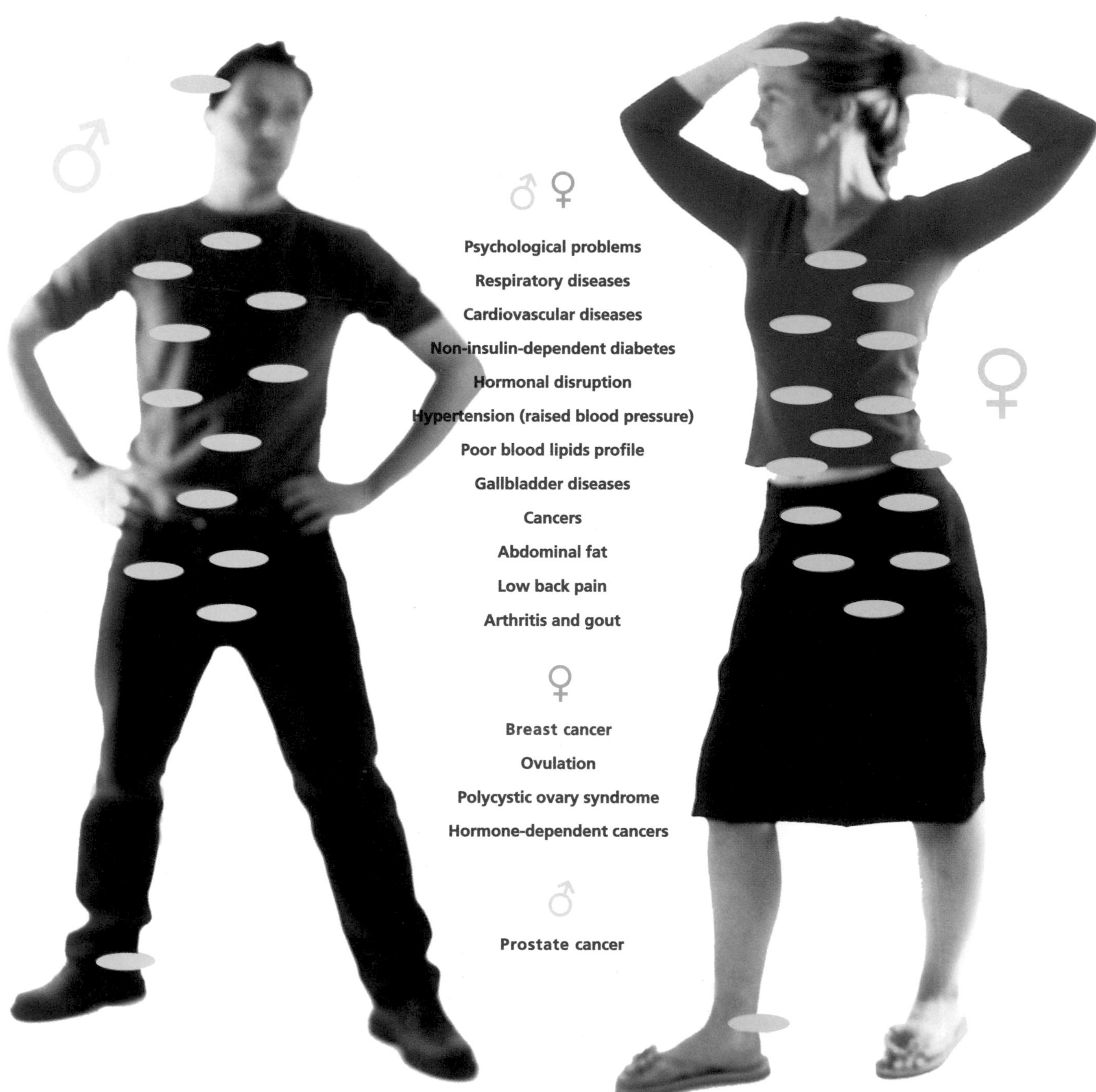

 Men and Women

Psychological problems
Obesity is associated with social prejudice, discrimination in the workplace and elsewhere, and with body dissatisfaction. This can lead to low self-esteem, depression and other psychological disorders.

Respiratory diseases
Obesity impairs respiratory function and makes breathing harder work. An average of 70% of people with 'obstructive' sleep apnoea (repetitive cessation of breathing during sleep) are obese. Snoring is almost always present and tiredness and headaches are other symptoms.

Cardiovascular diseases
These include coronary heart disease, stroke and other associated diseases. Even at body weights only 10% above average, deaths from CHD are increased, and consistent data on the relationship between overweight, obesity and heart disease have been produced over several decades. It is now thought that obesity is an independent risk factor, as well as increasing the incidence of other risk factors for CVD, including high blood pressure, raised cholesterol, abdominal fat and insulin resistance.

Non-insulin-dependent diabetes (NIDD)
The link between type-2 diabetes and overweight is very strong. For example obese women aged 30–55 have a risk of developing the disease that's 40 times greater than women with a body mass index of less than 22. Another study overview indicates that 64% of male and 74% of female cases of NIDD could have been prevented if none of the cases had had a body mass index over 25.

Hormonal disruption
Obesity is associated with various hormone abnormalities, including insulin resistance (a 'pre-diabetic' state in which body tissue requires greater than normal insulin for glucose regulation which may, in turn, lead to glucose intolerance), increased cortisol production and decreased growth hormone levels. In men, testosterone levels may decrease; in women, progesterone levels may decrease and testosterone increase.

Hypertension (raised blood pressure)
Obesity increases the risk of developing high blood pressure and the incidence of high blood pressure in overweight adults is nearly three times higher than in non-overweight adults. High blood pressure is a risk factor for heart disease.

Poor blood lipids profile
Cholesterol and triglycerides are fats (lipids) found in the blood. Obesity is associated with reduced levels of HDL cholesterol (the 'good' cholesterol) in the blood, increased levels of LDL cholesterol (the 'bad' cholesterol) and increased levels of triglycerides, a pattern which is associated with heart disease.

Gallbladder diseases
Obesity raises the risk of pancreatitis, gallstones and gallbladder cancer. Even moderate overweight may increase the risk of gallstones.

Cancers
Cancers of the colon, rectum, gallbladder and pancreas, and hepatic and renal cancers have a higher incidence in obese people. In one large study, 750,000 people were followed for 12 years and deaths from cancers were 33% higher in obese men and 55% higher in obese women.

Abdominal fat
Intra-abdominal fat (IAF–central fat distribution) is a particular risk factor for a variety of conditions and premature death. For example, in some studies it has been even more closely linked with NIDD than overall overweight, and it is closely linked with insulin resistance. People with excess abdominal fat have a higher risk of coronary heart disease and high blood pressure than those with fat on their hips and thighs. IAF is also associated with increased risk of hormonal cancers, especially breast cancer, ovulatory dysfunction and sleep apnoea.

Low back pain
Overweight and obesity place undue stress on the joints and muscles of the lower back and hip area, and low back pain is a common result, with the risks of suffering from low back pain increasing as weight rises.

Arthritis and gout
The symptoms of osteoarthritis – particularly in the knees – are generally increased in the overweight and obese. Although fat intake and metabolic changes may be partial causes, it is likely that the mechanical results of the excess weight are the main link. Gout is a form of arthritis affecting single joints, usually the big toe, and there is increased risk in overweight people.

 Women

Breast cancer
Obesity and, in particular, abdominal fat increase risk of post-menopausal breast cancer. Weight gain in adulthood is also associated with increased risk of breast cancer.

Ovulation
Obesity can disrupt ovulation, which may mean that a woman's chances of becoming pregnant are diminished.

Polycystic ovary syndrome
Obesity can make this condition – repeated or multiple cysts on the ovaries which, it is estimated, account for 20% of all cases of infertility – and its effects worse, and losing weight can improve them.

Hormone-dependent cancers
As well as breast cancer, incidence of endometrial, ovarian, uterine and cervical cancer may all be increased in obese women, although not all studies agree how great the increased risk is.

 Men

Prostate cancer
There is some evidence of increased risk of prostate cancer in obese men.

SYNDROME X

Also often referred to as the 'metabolic syndrome', this is a 'clustering' factor of five overweight-related symptoms that act in combination to increase the risk of cardiovascular disease significantly. They are intra-abdominal (central fat) obesity; insulin resistance, impaired glucose tolerance, high blood pressure and poor blood lipid profile. People with two or more of these symptoms can be classed as having 'syndrome X'.

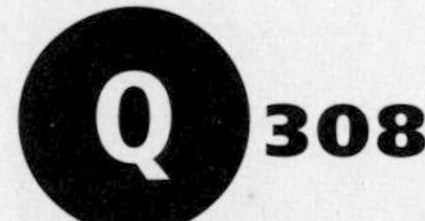

While slimming, should I eat organic food?

Organic versions of non-organic food are no more 'slimming', in that they contain about the same number of calories – some may even contain more. As an example, an organic free-range chicken may have denser flesh than a battery chicken, because it has been allowed to grow normally and it will have a smaller percentage of water by weight. Water is calorie-free, so, ounce for ounce, the organic chicken will probably contain a few more calories. However, don't let that bother you. It's not a big enough difference to stop your slimming campaign in its tracks! I am just trying to say that you don't need to buy organic to lose weight.

I must admit, though, that I do prefer organic food, not only because I perceive it to be better for me, but also because the organic food I buy usually tastes better. Although governments and other experts are always claiming that organic doesn't taste better and doesn't contain extra nutrients, some trials show it does, and some trials even show that some organic foods have a better nutrient profile.

I am very lucky in that I can purchase local organic foods from neighbours, and can also grow some of my own, and I would defy anyone to tell me these don't taste and eat better than mass-market stuff from the supermarket; I've tried both and I know which I prefer.

The difference I think buying the best you can afford in the way of fruits, veg, salads, meat, poultry, fish, even bread, may make to you if you're trying to slim is that slimmers have generally cut back on fat, salt and sugar and are missing the taste hit these gave them. Superb-tasting organic food can go a long way towards filling the gap. Also, it can seem more satisfying; e.g. a slice of stoneground organic wholemeal bread keeps you feeling full for longer than a slice of wrapped white bread.

If you have a choice, spend money on your food rather than on alcohol, clothes and so on. I'm sure it'll make you happier!

See also:

- A–Z entry: whole foods diet.
- Key index entries: calories, healthy eating, weight control, whole foods.

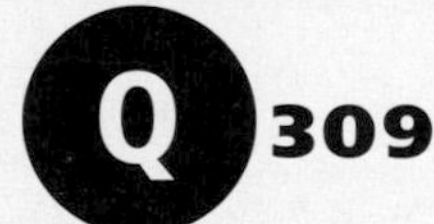

Are all slimming diets healthy?

No. Typical examples of potentially unhealthy slimming diets are any that reduce calories too low for optimum nutrient intake and may also cause other problems such as low blood sugar – i.e. 'crash' diets. Other examples are diets that limit the types of food you can eat, so that you may suffer nutrient deficiencies that way – e.g. an 'egg and grapefruit diet'.

There is evidence that the fashionable high-protein, low-carbohydrate diets may be unhealthy, and even vegetarian diets can be unhealthy if the dieter isn't careful to choose a suitably wide range of foods. High-fat, low-carbohydrate diets are generally unhealthy and even calorie-counting can be a poor way to slim if you aren't sensible – you might lose weight on 1,250 calories a day of chocolate, but it wouldn't be good for you.

The US Department of Agriculture has produced a report on the efficacy and health of a number of popular dieting methods and comes out in favour of the basic low-fat, high-carb diet as the best and healthiest way to slim. The World Health Organization also endorses this.

The A–Z at the back of the book has detailed analyses of all the most popular diets and gives each a score and a percentage rating. Go for those that did well and you'll know you have a healthy diet. If you have any specific queries on particular types of food and health, many individual questions in this book deal with them (see the cross-references). However, I would always advise you to visit your doctor and get referred to a dietician, especially if you have any health problems.

See also:

- Questions: 80–109, 115–21, 307–18.
- Features: 8, 9, 26.
- A–Z entries: calorie counting, crash diets, low-fat diets, vegetarian diets, (plus many named diets).
- Key index entries: food value charts, healthy slimming, high-carbohydrate diets, high-fat diets, high-protein diets, low-carbohydrate diets, Top 20 popular diets.

FAT FACT

An American doctor has coined the term 'orthorexia nervosa' for health food junkies who become so obsessed with eating a pure, natural diet and avoiding all things artificial or 'bad for them' that food dominates their behaviour and ruins their social lives. People who are hooked on health foods may become as thin as people with anorexia nervosa.

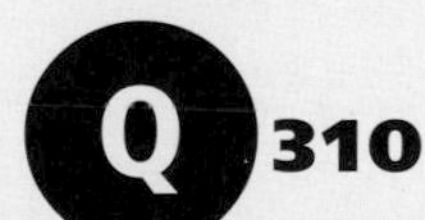

Are all healthy diets slimming?

No. There is more potential to lose weight on a healthy diet, mainly because it is harder to eat too many calories on a diet that contains the recommended amounts of fruits, vegetables, salads, complex carbohydrates, lean protein and so on. A healthy diet is high in 'bulk' but fairly low on density (calories per gram weight). However, if you don't pay some attention to portion size, or if, say, you snack on hefty amounts of healthy nuts, seeds or bread between meals, you could easily exceed your required number of calories and end up putting on weight.

The only way to lose weight is to create an energy deficit in your body (see Q18) – by burning up more calories than you take in. There is some small advantage to be gained by the type of food that you eat (e.g. protein and carbohydrate will tend to store fewer calories on you than fat does), but in the total scheme of things the difference won't be huge.

I hope I haven't put you off following a healthy diet while you slim. There are many other advantages to eating a perceived healthy diet – for example, you are less likely to suffer from hunger pangs. And, of course, you'll be doing your body more good by slimming on a healthy diet than on a ridiculous one, as Q307 explains.

See also:

- Questions: 18, 79, 307–9, 311.
- Feature: 9.
- Key index entry: healthy slimming.

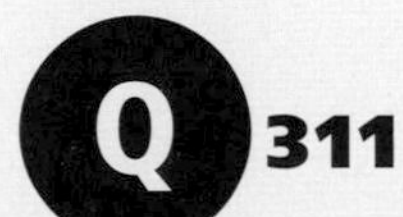

311

Are there any healthy fats that can help you lose weight?

Fats are discussed in detail in Qs 89 and 90 and in Feature 8, so go back and read them. There is a type of fat called CLA, found in meat and dairy produce, which trials have shown to effect increased weight loss over a period of weeks. You do, however, need to eat vast quantities of these products in order to get enough CLA, so that blows that one (although supplements are available).

Oils expert Dr Udo Erasmus also believes that an adequate intake of the essential fatty acid omega-3 group may also help weight loss, and certainly, these healthy fats are in shortfall in many of our diets, and so getting extra of them will be of benefit to many people, even if weight loss doesn't result. These oils are found in oily fish, flaxseeds and, to a lesser extent, in pumpkin seeds and various plant oils. Fish oils are particularly important for keeping your heart healthy.

See also:

- Questions: 89–90.
- Feature: 8.
- A–Z entry: low-fat diets.
- Key index entries: essential fatty acids, fats, healthy slimming.

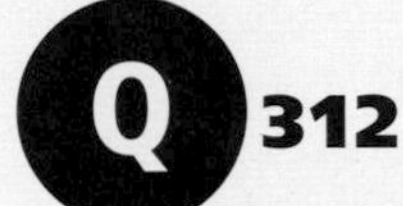

312

If crash dieting isn't healthy, why has his doctor put my very overweight husband on a very-low-calorie liquid diet?

Obese people with life-threatening conditions (or sometimes before an operation) may be put on a monitored VLCD diet to get their weight down and thus reduce the risk of early death or problems during anaesthesia or surgery. It is often a 'last resort', when attempts to get the patient to lose weight on a normal calorie-controlled diet have failed.

Obesity specialists recognize this as a valid and useful way to slim patients, and the World Health Organization says VLCDs should be reserved for rapid weight loss on medical grounds in patients with a BMI over 30. I assume your husband meets these requirements, hence the treatment. VLCDs aren't recommended otherwise.

For more on very-low-calorie diets and liquid meal replacements, see the A–Z.

FAT FACT

An unhealthy slimming diet can affect looks as well as health. All the following symptoms may result from a diet low in calories and/or nutrients: dull eyes, bloodshot eyes, bleeding gums, dry skin, rough skin, weak nails, dry hair, shedding hair, dull hair, dandruff.

See also:

- Questions: 105–9, 300–306, 320, 327.
- Features: 3, 25.
- A–Z entry: very-low-calorie diets.
- Key index entries: crash diets, healthy slimming, very-low-calorie diets, weight and health.

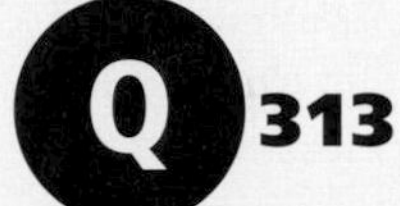

313

Why is yo-yo dieting bad for your health?

This is explained in some detail in Q206. The good news is that even if you have been yo-yo dieting for some years, if you stop and begin a healthy eating regime to stabilize your weight, you shouldn't have done yourself any lasting damage, although you'll need to do some strength (resistance) exercise to build up lean tissue (muscle) and thus build up metabolic rate.

You should also avoid crash dieting in the future, and one of the most important points is that you should never aim for too low a body weight. Although we have seen in other questions in this section that maintaining your BMI below 25 has a good health profile, for past persistent yo-yoers, it may be best to aim for a level above that if it means it is one you can maintain. The increased risk to health of a BMI of, say, 26 or 27 compared with 25 is not great.

See also:

- ▶ Questions: 105–6, 205–7, 314.
- ▶ Features: 1–3.
- ▶ Key index entries: Body Mass Index, crash diets, healthy slimming, metabolism, yo-yo dieting.

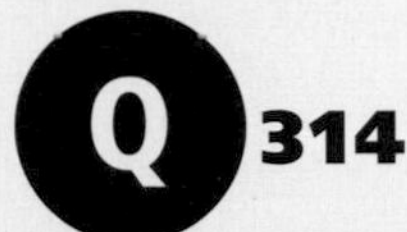

314

Which is worse – to be permanently overweight or to yo-yo diet?

Neither is desirable, but it is probably better to be slightly overweight than to keep losing weight then regaining it, for reasons outlined in Qs 205–7 and 313. A BMI up to 27 may be considered acceptable. However, if your body mass index is creeping up over that level, it would be best to try to lose some weight, with professional advice so that you don't fall into the yo-yo trap again.

Ironically, medics may put very overweight people (BMI 30-plus) on to VLCDs (see Q312) which effect rapid weight loss – but weight regain after such a regime is very common. So it is better for you to seek help now before your problem gets any worse, rather than waiting until drastic measures need to be taken.

See also:

- ▶ Questions: 28–9, 205–7, 313,
- ▶ Features: 3, 25.
- ▶ Key index entries: Body Mass Index, weight and health, yo-yo dieting.

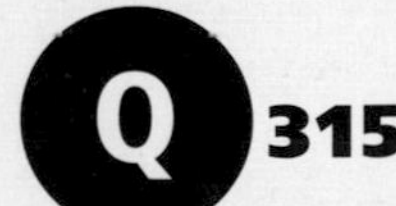

315

How do I keep 'regular' while slimming?

Some diets do predispose to constipation, but you should be able to avoid it if you follow these guidelines:

■ Don't diet on too few calories. If you don't eat enough, your system won't process your food properly. Aim to diet on no fewer calories than your own basal metabolic rate (see Feature 1).

■ Don't follow a high-protein, low-carbohydrate diet. A low-carbohydrate diet will also be a low-fibre diet, and inadequate fibre is strongly linked with constipation. Instead choose a high-carbohydrate, moderate-fat diet, such as that in Feature 9, and make sure that most of the carbohydrates you eat are whole (e.g. fruits, vegetables, roots, pulses, brown rice, wholewheat pasta, wholegrain bread) rather than refined (e.g. white bread, white rice), because refined carbohydrates have had a great deal of their fibre removed.

■ Eat at least your five portions of fruit and vegetables a day and drink plenty of water – for fibre to work properly you need adequate fluid. Fruits and veg are very high in water (e.g. an apple is 84% water, cabbage is 90% water). Six glasses of water a day should work well.

■ If these measures alone aren't enough, also try adding more foods that seem to have a particularly good laxative action to your diet. These include citrus fruits, rhubarb, spices, cabbage, prunes, figs and garlic, although people do vary in their own reactions to these. Don't start using strong laxative pills, as you can get dependent upon them so that when you stop using them you will be more constipated than ever.

■ Lastly, take half an hour or more of vigorous exercise a day – this seems to boost all the body's systems, including digestion and elimination. Stomach exercises, too, can help.

See also:

- ▶ Question: 83.
- ▶ Feature: 9.
- ▶ A–Z entries: The F-Plan, whole-food diets.
- ▶ Key index entries: fibre, healthy slimming, whole foods.

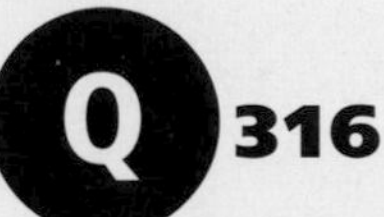

316

What is 'low blood sugar' and why do dieters apparently often get it?

The official name for 'low blood sugar' is hypoglycaemia, a condition that can arise for various reasons. Its symptoms may include feeling dizzy, feeling weak, palpitations, hand tremor, lethargy/fatigue, irritability, feeling 'spaced out' and perhaps hungry.

Blood-sugar levels are influenced mainly by food intake – when you eat something, levels rise – and by insulin, which is released by the pancreas to convert the sugar to fuel or to help convert it to fat for later use. Once the insulin has done its job, blood-sugar levels should be normal, but this isn't always the case. Hypoglycaemia can occur in diabetes when the diabetic doesn't match their food intake with their insulin levels; this can be a serious condition and is relieved by immediate intake of glucose or sugary food.

In non-diabetics, hypoglycaemia can occur frequently or occasionally, mildly or more strongly, depending upon the individual, their diet and the circumstances. Or, of course, in many people symptoms may never be experienced. Here are the usual reasons that you may experience low blood sugar when you are slimming:

■ Long periods of fasting. If following the type of diet generally not recommended in this book (or, indeed, by many obesity experts), in which you go for many hours without eating, low blood sugar is likely simply because you've had nothing to eat. A suitable snack (see opposite) or meal will restore the blood sugar levels.

■ Not enough to eat. Periods of surviving on very-low-calorie meals, even if they are regular, may induce low blood sugar simply because you aren't giving yourself enough to eat and the energy in the food you are eating is absorbed by the body too quickly.

It is important not to diet on too few calories (see Q104) and also to eat the right types of food when trying to lose weight (see below).

■ Bingeing on sugary foods. It is quite common for dieters to get a physical/psychological urge for something sweet to eat, especially during strict diets as just outlined. This may be more apparent in women before a period, or even when people are under stress and extra stress hormones are produced, as hormones can affect insulin production and blood sugar levels.

Here is the typical scene: you have been trying to be extra-'good' on your diet and haven't eaten much. Your blood-sugar level is low. Suddenly, you feel ravenous and/or the uncontrollable urge for something sweet. You give in, eating a chocolate bar or two, a bag of sweets, or several biscuits, say. You carry on eating, in fact, until you feel satisfied. Your blood-sugar levels will rise quite quickly as the sugars in most of these refined products are quickly absorbed into the bloodstream. Your pancreas then goes into 'panic mode' and releases a great deal of insulin to cope with this sudden influx of sugar. Within an hour or more, the insulin has done its job, maybe over-efficiently, and once more all that sugar has been converted into energy or fat and your blood-sugar level is low again and you may have that classic sense of dizziness, weakness and so on as described earlier. You may be tempted to eat yet more sweet food – and the cycle begins again.

■ Hard exercise. If you are not only trying to lose weight, but also indulging in long periods of exercise to burn off more calories, you may suffer low blood sugar, because your body will be using the readily available sugar for energy. Think of the marathon runners who are fed sugary drinks or bananas along the road – this is to keep their blood-sugar levels up. If they didn't do this, hypoglycaemia would probably set in and they would feel terrible and have to give up. If you are doing more exercise than usual, you need to eat properly (see below).

The answer to avoiding all these situations is to eat properly. This means:

■ Eating regular meals – a breakfast, a lunch, a main meal and two small between-meal snacks is ideal. The Basic Diet in Feature 9 is a typical ideal diet. As you will see, you can still lose weight on such a regime and your blood-sugar levels will remain much more constant.

■ Eating plenty of foods low on the Glycaemic Index (see Q84). These are the foods which are absorbed less rapidly into the bloodstream and will help your body to produce insulin gradually, in moderate amounts, and keep your blood-sugar level even throughout the day, thus avoiding all the symptoms of hypoglycaemia. As a bonus, slimmers will also feel less hungry by eating a diet rich in these foods.

■ Avoiding simple carbohydrate foods, particularly sweets, biscuits, cakes and sugary drinks, and especially when eaten as a snack/without low GI foods to counteract their effect. If you feel the urge for a sweet snack, have one with fibre – e.g. a piece of fresh or dried fruit.

■ Avoiding caffeine (it can cause the pancreas to release extra insulin, thus making low blood sugar situation worse).

■ Avoid alcohol on an empty stomach as alcohol acts like sugar and will send your blood sugar levels high, then dip them low because of the insulin effect.

■ Avoid smoking as this, too, disrupts the body's regulation of blood sugars.

■ Eat adequate amounts of chromium-rich foods, such as broccoli, shellfish, wheatgerm, nuts, cheese, fruits and vegetables, as chromium is another important factor in the regulation of blood sugar. However, I wouldn't advise a chromium supplement as, if you follow the above tips and cut down on your sugar intake, this won't be necessary.

■ Regularly eat oily fish, flaxseeds and other sources of omega-3s. Research shows they may help regulate blood-sugar levels by increasing insulin sensitivity.

■ Before exercising, make sure you have had a small meal or decent snack containing complex carbohydrate plus a medium- or low-GI fruit or other item. *Examples:* slice of wholemeal bread with a banana; rye crispbreads with hummus; small bowl of pasta with tomato sauce.

All these measures should help to keep your blood sugar levels even while you lose weight and, indeed, afterwards.

See also:

▶ Questions: 83–7, 104, 108.

▶ Feature: 9.

▶ A–Z entries: chromium, The F-Plan, Glycaemic Index diets.

▶ Key index entries: fibre, Glycaemic Index, healthy slimming, low blood sugar.

FIT FACT

A study published in the *Journal of Epidemiology* has found that moderate consumption of alcohol is three times more beneficial for men than for women, but that much of the protective factor of just four units a week for men, and three for women, occurs in men over 55 and women over 65.

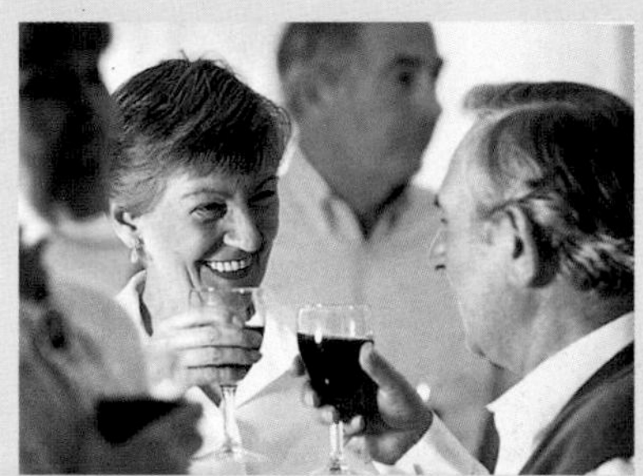

The facts on detoxing

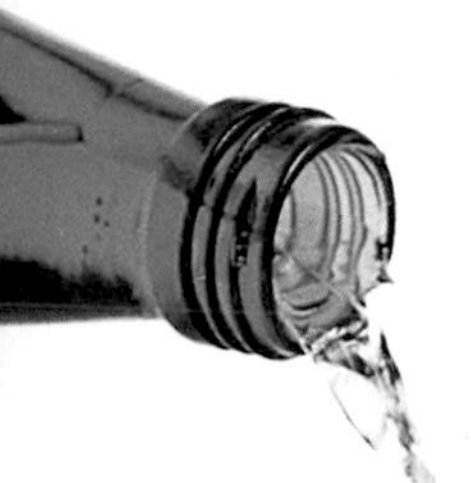

If you have ever thought about trying a 'detox' regime but aren't sure either what they are for or what they consist of, here are the answers.

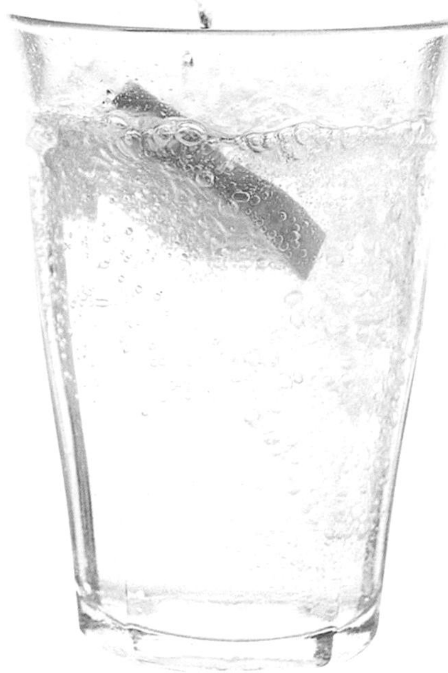

What 'detox' means

To 'detoxify' is, literally, to remove toxins, or poisons, from within your body.

Who might need a detox

Anyone who has been living on a poor diet (high in 'junk' or food that may be contaminated with 'pollutants', such as artificial ingredients, pesticides, herbicides, hormonal residues or antibiotics, etc.), anyone who has an unbalanced diet, or one high in alcohol or caffeine (both toxins), anyone who smokes or lives in a polluted atmosphere, or has been ill recently (viruses and bacteria are toxins), or taking medication long-term, including over-the-counter things like paracetamol.

You may also benefit if you have been under long-term emotional and or physical stress, perhaps with symptoms such as skin outbreaks, headaches, fatigue or irritability, because stress reduces the body's ability to cope with an overload of pollution. However, some people aren't suitable for a detox regime – see Q318.

Detecting the signs that you need a detox

Apart from being able to say 'yes' to several of the pointers in the previous question, signs that you might benefit from a detox are bloating around the stomach area and perhaps around the eyes; tired, dull eyes; enlarged glands up the sides of your neck and perhaps elsewhere; irritable bowel syndrome or constipation; frequently feeling run down.

How a detox should work

When you are fit, healthy, stress-free and, possibly, young, your body has its own efficient defence and filter system to help break down, neutralize or eliminate pollutants and toxins before they can do you a great deal of harm – the lymphatic system, the liver, the kidneys, the bowels and the skin.

With their help, toxins should be removed via the sweat, urine, breath, and faeces. However, when these organs become overloaded with work (too many toxins) or aren't working as well as they should (when you are ill, stressed, old), they may need some help, otherwise toxins may be stored in the body fat.

The idea of a good detox diet is to eat a pure and natural diet, high in foods and drinks that will actively help remove toxins and aid the function of the lymph, liver and kidneys. The good detox will also avoid all foods likely to hinder the programme and, of course, all sources of toxicants. Backing this up, you will also choose a healthy lifestyle during the detox.

What is a good detox programme?

One that contains

- Only organic foods and drinks. By choosing organic, you remove most of the possibility that your food contains traces of added toxins, e.g. pesticides, fungicides.
- Only 'whole', unrefined foods as far as possible, including whole grains, nuts, seeds, high-quality plant oils.
- A high proportion of fruits and veg.
- About 3½ pints (2 litres) of water or similar drink a day (see box opposite).
- Regular items to aid detox (see opposite).

One that avoids

- Fasting – fasting isn't necessary to detox and I would advise against it, especially if you suffer from hypoglycaemia.
- All highly processed and refined foods.
- All animal food except organic live yoghurt.
- Alcohol, caffeine, tobacco, drugs.
- I would also avoid vitamin and mineral supplements, as these can contain a long list of artificial ingredients, sweeteners, etc.

One that ensures that you –

- Take regular gentle to moderate exercise: for example, walking coupled with yoga or stretching exercises.
- Eat regularly and drink regularly.

- Avoid stress and stress-related work, including heavy exercise.
- Go to bed early and sleep with an open window.
- Get outdoors as often as you can and learn to breathe deeply.
- Take time for yourself and relax as much as possible.

Side effects of detoxing

You may have a headache for the first few days, but this can be minimized by eating regularly on the allowed foods. It is said that the headache is due to the toxins being released, but it is more likely to be because of the reduction in calories and carbohydrate, and caffeine withdrawal. You'll lose weight, much of which will be water, so you'll go to the toilet more often. You may also have a much looser bowel.

How long to stay on a detox

Very short detox regimes are not as effective as you might think, as your body stores toxins in the fat, and fat stores can't be mobilized in a day or two. I suggest you try a mild detox similar to the one here when you have a quiet week (preferably at home, not working), and see how you get on. You can add extra food if you feel too hungry, but follow the guidelines above.

If you then incorporate ideas from the detox into your regular habits, even when you increase calorie intake, you should be giving yourself long-term protection against external pollutants that you can't control – like poor atmosphere, smoky rooms, etc. – and also helping your body to be strong in defence and elimination. As a bonus, you should also easily be able to maintain a reasonable weight.

Helping detox by exercise

Regular exercise is important because this enhances the work of the lymph and increases toxic elimination via the sweat and breath, and also encourages urine and faeces excretion. During exercise, liver activity is also increased.

Detox sample plan

(Don't forget the guidelines – everything organic, plenty of water, eat regularly)

Day 1

On rising: glass of water, cup of dandelion tea.
Breakfast: apple, live yoghurt.
Snack: pumpkin seeds.
Lunch: vegetable soup made by peeling and chopping a mix of carrot, parsley, leek, tomato, onion and garlic, plus herbs of choice, and cooking with water or home-made vegetable stock (no salt) to cover until tender, then blending until smooth.
Snack: orange, sunflower seeds, aloe vera juice.
Evening: red pepper, cucumber and herb (e.g. chives, parsley, dill, tarragon) salad with olive oil dressing and a small portion of organic poached salmon which is optional – otherwise have some live yoghurt as a dessert, or some seeds with your salad.

Day 2

On rising: water with fresh lemon juice.
Breakfast: blueberries and live yoghurt.
Snack: walnuts.
Lunch: fresh fruit salad with sunflower seeds and tahini paste.
Snack: apple, cup of dandelion and burdock tea.
Evening: Vegetable Soup as Day l.

Day 3

On rising: freshly squeezed fruit juice or a fruit smoothie.
Breakfast: fresh fruit salad with sunflower seeds.
Snack: almonds.
Lunch: tomato, cucumber and herb salad with a small piece of grilled fresh tuna, which is optional – otherwise have some live yoghurt for dessert or some fresh nuts with your salad.
Snack: apple, cup of green tea.
Evening: large mixed leaf salad with olive oil and balsamic vinegar dressing; live yoghurt to follow.

HELPING THE DETOX EFFECT THROUGH DIET

A good detox diet provides items in the diet that will help the work of the lymph, liver and kidneys, as well as encouraging regular bowel function. It will also provide plenty of antioxidant phytochemicals , vitamins A, C and E, and zinc to deoxidize the body and neutralize harmful free radicals which are produced in greater amounts during a detox regime.

Some good detox foods and drinks are:
To help liver function: dandelion root, marigold, parsley, burdock, milk thistle, peppermint, dock root, globe artichoke, apples, olive oil, cucumber, onions.
To help the lymphatic system: angelica, lovage, marigold, oregano, rosemary, dock root, echinacea, ginger, cayenne.
To help fluid elimination: dandelion, nettle, parsley, tarragon, apple, cucumber, onion, dock root.
To help purify the blood: garlic, chives, onion, leek, dandelion, nettles, echinacea.
Laxative effect: olive oil, burdock, dock root, aloe vera juice, citrus fruits, liquorice root. Also all high-fibre foods, fresh fruits, vegetables and water will help elimination.
To increase perspiration: marigold, thyme, garlic, onion, chives, mustard, green tea, chilli.

Many of these can be taken as a herbal drink, chopping the herb and infusing in boiling water for 5 minutes, then straining. Use instead of water once or twice a day. Dandelion and burdock tea is widely available in health food stores. Milk thistle and echinacea can be taken in tincture form.

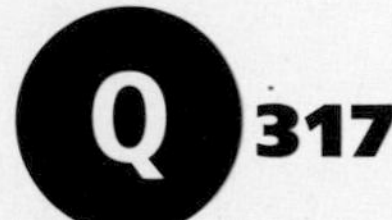

What are the health advantages of a detox diet?

Sometimes there are few advantages, if any, as many of the 'detox' regimes that are offered in the newspapers and magazines are of little benefit to most people. A detox is supposed to rid your body of all the pollutants that you, or your environment, have been putting into it – e.g. 'bad' foods containing additives, preservatives or too much fat, pesticides, herbicides, hormones, heavy metals, smoke and air pollution, alcohol, tobacco, medicines... and more.

The idea with most detoxes is that you eat or drink natural – and naturally detoxing – items and avoid everything likely to add to your body's pollution levels. If you choose a good detox, you may indeed be able to help your body to rid itself of some of these pollutants and you may indeed feel better. However, a bad or wrongly carried-out detox may have you feeling worse. Some detoxes are little more than fasts, and others ask you to spend a lot of money on bottled potions, pills and so on, which really isn't necessary.

Feature 26 answers your most asked questions about detoxing and provides a simple regime if you wish to try a detox. And the Detox section in the A-Z examines well-known detox regimes more closely.

See also:

- Questions: 77, 92, 107, 318.
- Feature: 26.
- A–Z entry: detox diets.
- Key index entries: detoxing, healthy eating, healthy slimming.

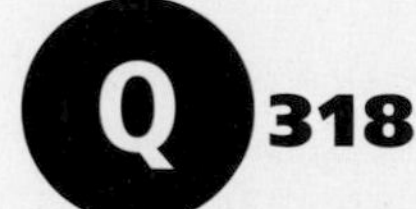

Will a detox diet actually help me to lose weight?

I would say that it will. All detoxes that I have come across reduce your calorie intake significantly and would thus almost certainly help you to lose weight – but NOT because the toxins have been keeping you fat, incidentally. Much of the weight loss will be fluid, not fat. Detoxes tend to be very low on carbohydrate, which acts to retain water in the body. A low-carbohydrate diet therefore encourages water elimination and in a week-long detox you might lose several pounds of fluid and as well as a pound or two of fat.

I wouldn't recommend that you stay on a detox-type regime for long periods as they are too low in calories, so they are not much use for long-term weight loss, unless you use them on a 'one week on, three weeks off' basis (one week on the detox and three weeks of normal healthy eating). I would also not advise people prone to yo-yo dieting to follow a detox, nor people prone to low blood sugar. A detox is a kind of crash diet by any other name, and ordinary gentle calorie reduction is best for both these sets of people.

For many people, however, a good detox gets them into the right frame of mind for healthier eating and weight loss in the long term, if necessary. In other words, it can be a very good start. Feature 26 will give you all the advice you need.

See also:

- Questions: 211, 317.
- Feature: 26.
- A–Z entry: detox diets.
- Key index entries: carbohydrates, cellulite, detox, fluid retention, healthy slimming.

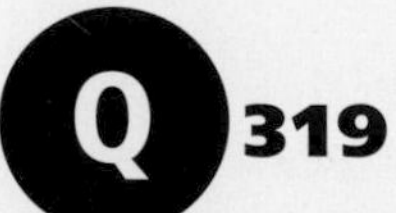

Can you be too thin for good health as well as too fat?

Yes. The recommended healthy weight falls between a Body Mass Index of 18.5 and one of 25. If your BMI (see Feature 3) is lower than this, you are considered to have an unhealthily low weight, which may predispose you to the health problems listed in Feature 3. Some experts believe that a BMI lower than 20 is too thin, and as you get older it may be best to consider a BMI of around 22–3 as a good lower level to aim for. Thin people are more prone to osteoporosis in later life. Also, maintaining a low BMI (say, 20–23) may not be a good idea later in life for women, as fat has been described as 'nature's HRT', helping maintain oestrogen levels.

If you check out your BMI and find you are too thin, see your doctor for advice, both on whether your thinness may be a symptom of a medical condition and on nutritional help. If you feel you may have an eating disorder that is making you thin, you can also check out the answers to Qs 149–57 for further advice and contacts.

See also:

- Questions: 27–9, 149–57, 233, 319.
- Feature: 3.
- Key index entries: body mass index, hormones, osteoporosis, weight and ageing, weight and health.

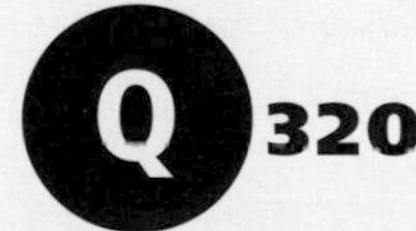

Why do surgeons dislike performing operations on very overweight people?

There is a higher degree of risk of anaesthesia complications if you are obese, and also it is literally harder for the surgeon to perform operations when you have layers of fat which may impede the progress and finesse of the process.

Obese people are often asked to lose weight before an op, and sometimes given a weight above which the operation won't be carried out. If you need to lose weight for an operation, the Basic Diet in Feature 9 may be suitable, but if you have any medical problems it is best to discuss diet with your doctor, who should refer you to a dietician for further help.

See also:

- ▶ Questions: 38, 327.
- ▶ Features: 3, 9.
- ▶ A–Z entry: slimming surgery.
- ▶ Key index entries: healthy slimming, obesity, operations.

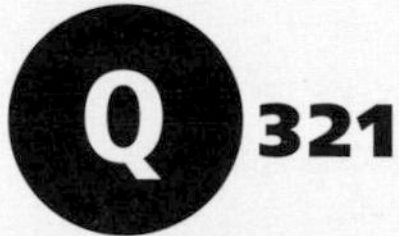

321

Can you recommend a good slimming diet for a diabetic?

Diabetes UK says that it doesn't provide a special diet for diabetics, as the diet they should follow is similar to the kind of healthy diet that is appropriate for most people. The Basic Diet in Feature 9 should therefore be fine for a diabetic. This diet is for both slow-to-moderate weight loss and weight maintenance, as explained in the feature. It is important for diabetics to try to control their weight, or lose weight if necessary. Type-2 diabetes may be improved or even cured via weight loss.

It is worth mentioning a few extra nutritional facts which may help if you are diabetic and trying to lose weight:

- ■ Eating 'little and often' really IS the way to go for you, to help keep blood sugar levels even. Don't go more than 2½ hours without something to eat during waking hours.
- ■ Be extra sure to get plenty of foods with a low Glycaemic Index into your diet (see Q84). These will also help stabilize your blood sugars and help keep hunger at bay.
- ■ Don't try dieting on a plan very low in fat. The 25–30% level in Feature 9 is low enough. A little fat with your meals helps the meal take longer to be absorbed and, again, will help maintain even blood sugar levels. The same applies to protein. So, at every meal aim to get some low-GI carb, some fat and some protein. Section Three will help you find out more about these food groups.
- ■ Diabetics may have kidney problems, so drink enough water to help them work well (but not too much, which can overtax the kidneys – about 6 glasses of water a day will be good in normal circumstances).
- ■ Diabetics may be more prone to infections, so get plenty of fresh fruits, salads and vegetables in your diet for the antioxidant carotenes and vitamin C, which help to protect you. Get the antioxidant zinc from foods such as nuts, seeds and lean red meat, and get vitamin E, another antioxidant important for diabetics, from nuts, seeds and plant oils.
- ■ Research shows that a diet rich in oily fish, nuts, seeds and plant oils may help to regulate the blood-sugar levels.
- ■ Don't be tempted to try dieting too quickly – aim for a weekly weight loss of no more than half a pound (225g) (after the first week of slimming), which should be possible by reducing your daily calorie intake by only 250 or so. If you try to reduce your calories down too low, you may create problems in maintaining even blood-sugar levels.

Diabetics should always discuss diet with their doctor and not follow any new diet without their knowledge.

Diabetes UK (formerly the British Diabetic Association), 10 Queen Anne Street, London W1G 9LH; tel 0207 323 1531; www.diabetes.org.uk.

See also:

- ▶ Question: 316.
- ▶ Features: 3, 9.
- ▶ A–Z entry: Glycaemic Index Diets.
- ▶ Key index entries: blood-sugar levels, Glycaemic Index, healthy slimming.

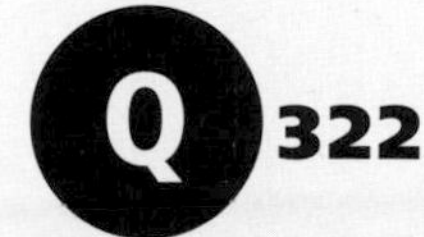

322

What is the best slimming diet for someone with arthritis?

There are two types of arthritis: osteoarthritis and rheumatoid arthritis. Osteoarthritis is a degenerative condition of the joints that often occurs with age, and is sometimes called 'fair wear and tear', giving stiffness and pain in the affected joints, such as the hips, knees or spine. Overweight can make the problems of osteoarthritis worse, as the joints have to bear a greater load, so losing weight can help.

Sufferers can follow the Basic Diet which appears in Feature 9, and which contains reasonably high amounts of the antioxidant vitamins C and E, which have been found in some trials to help osteoarthritis. Cod liver oil and other fish oils may also help, and the Basic Diet is also adequate in oily fish. You could also take a daily supplement of 10ug cod liver oil if you like.

Rheumatoid arthritis is most common in adult women and is a chronic inflammatory condition involving multiple joints, when the immune system appears to overreact to some stimulant within the body. Joints may swell and there may be pain, and there are often periods of remission. The causes of rheumatoid arthritis aren't fully understood.

Various foods have been cited as making rheumatoid arthritis worse, but the list of foods which may affect some people (but don't affect others) is quite long and the research is anecdotal rather than scientific. These foods include all members of the 'nightshade family' (potatoes, tomatoes, aubergines and peppers), all foods high in saturated fat (full-fat dairy produce, fatty cuts of meat and poultry, baked goods, etc.), coffee, alcohol, citrus fruits, all dairy produce, wheat, corn, and nuts.

You could follow the Basic Diet in Feature 9, but if you feel that any of the above foods do seem to aggravate your rheumatoid arthritis, when these foods appear in the diet plan, they could be replaced with other, similar foods. For example, rice instead of potatoes, any other vegetables instead of the nightshade ones, pulses and fish instead of meat (although lean meat should be fine), water and herb tea instead of coffee and alcohol, other fruits instead of citrus, soya products instead of dairy, and rye bread or rice crackers instead of wheat and corn products. Instead of nuts you could try seeds, or a little extra of good-quality plant and fish oils in your diet.

If you are not sure which foods may make your arthritis worse, you could go through the list, eliminating one type of food at a time for a period of two months to see if symptoms improve. If they seem no different, you can reintroduce that item into your diet; if they improve, you may avoid that item in future. However, elimination diets are always best undertaken with the help of a trained dietician, so ask your doctor to refer you to one. The problem with trying to diagnose a food intolerance is that, as we have seen, rheumatoid arthritis tends to go through periods of remission and so it is hard to be sure whether an improvement in your condition may be due to removing a food from your diet, or because coincidentally you have entered a remission which would have happened anyway.

Foods that may help the symptoms of rheumatoid arthritis are oily fish, which contain the essential fats omega-3s, and fruit and vegetables, again probably because of the antioxidants they contain. Blood tests on people with rheumatoid arthritis show low levels of the mineral selenium, so it could be that a diet with adequate selenium may help too – find it in nuts, seeds, lentils, fish, pork and whole grains.

In other trials, the spice turmeric has been found to help – add it to curries, soups, stews and so on – and some people say that evening primrose oil helps them.

Lastly, a completely vegetarian or vegan diet has been found to help prevent rheumatoid arthritis in some people, or minimize its symptoms, so you might like to try the Vegetarian Diet in Feature 16. As a compromise, you could take fish-oil supplements while you do this or, if you prefer, try flaxseed oil, which is also omega-3 rich.

The good news is that if you follow a healthy diet, such as any adaptation of that mentioned above, weight loss should almost naturally follow.

See also:

- Questions: 300–306, 327.
- Features: 8, 9, 25.
- A–Z entry: vegetarian diets.
- Key index entries: omega-3, weight and health.

FAT FACT

Research shows that men from all cultures are most attracted to women with a waist-to-hip ratio of about .70, no matter whether they are slim or plump. For example, both Audrey Hepburn and Marilyn Monroe had WHRs of .70, though one was a size 10 and the other a size 16.

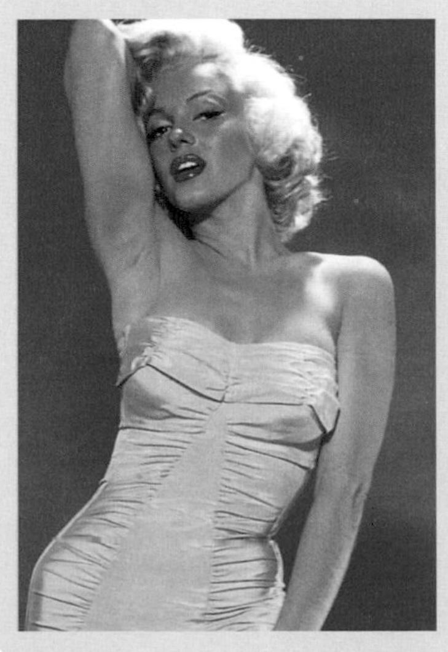

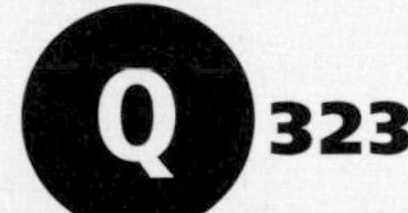

323

What is the best slimming diet for someone with high blood pressure?

If you have high blood pressure you can almost immediately reduce it by losing weight (if you are overweight). The Basic Diet in Feature 9 is a good healthy diet to follow, but for high blood pressure you can bear the following adaptations and notes in mind:

- Aim to lose weight steadily rather than yo-yoing. There is research to show that yo-yo dieting can make high blood pressure worse.
- Limit your salt intake to no more than 4g a day – this is about a level teaspoon of salt, equivalent to 1.8g of actual sodium. Don't forget that salt occurs in many ready-made products, so you have to cut right back on these as well as avoiding salt added in cooking and at the table. For more on salt in the diet, see Feature 13. The Basic Diet is naturally fairly low in salt. There are salt substitutes such as LoSalt available, and you can use herbs and spices to add flavour to your meals instead.

THE ASHWELL SHAPE CHART

Although a simple measure of your waist circumference (see Feature 3) can give you a very good indication of the health risk your midriff poses to you, this chart, devised by Dr Margaret Ashwell, may be even more accurate. It measures your waist against your height.

Simply read off your height (in inches or metres) and your waist measurement (in inches or cm) and find the point at which the two measurements meet, then read off your 'risk factor'.

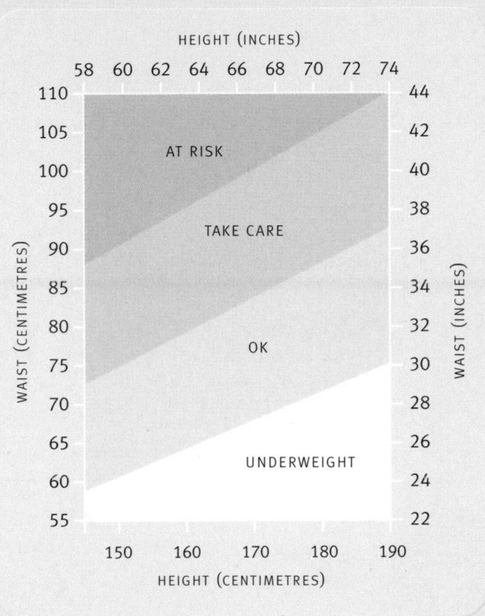

■ Eat plenty of potassium-rich foods, as a high potassium intake can help to lower blood pressure. These include most fruits and vegetables, dried apricots, nuts and pulses.

■ Other nutrients that may lower blood pressure include calcium (low-fat dairy produce, dark leafy greens), magnesium (nuts, seeds, whole grains, green vegetables), omega-3 fats (oily fish, flaxseeds).

■ Garlic and soluble fibre (found in fruits, pulses and vegetables) may also lower blood pressure.

See also:

▶ Questions: 300–306, 325–27.
▶ Features: 9, 13.
▶ Key index entries: heart, weight and health.

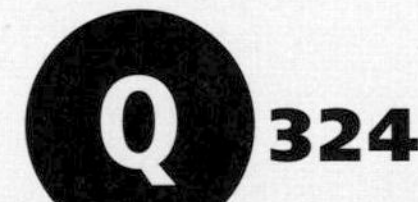

What causes an apple shape, why is it unhealthy and how can I beat it?

The apple shape (surplus weight stored mainly around the abdomen and waist – also called intra-abdominal fat or central fat distribution) is linked with health problems such as coronary heart disease, diabetes and other Syndrome X factors (see Feature 25), whereas the pear shape (heavy hips, bottom and thighs) does not appear to present the same level of risk.

This shape is predominantly a male phenomenon, although women are more prone to develop an apple shape in mid-life, particularly after menopause. This is because the female hormones are present in much smaller amounts and so the shape tends to become more 'male'. There is also evidence that abdominal fat develops when you are under long-term stress. The hormone cortisol is released during stress, and it seems that high levels of cortisol in the body tend to encourage central fat to accumulate. Researchers at Yale University studied 60 women and found that the more stress they were under, the more fat they stored around their stomachs. In other words, the people most likely to develop an apple shape are stressed men of any age, and older stressed women.

The apple effect can be minimized with a sensible diet (e.g. the Basic Diet in Feature 9), regular exercise and stress-reduction techniques (in fact, exercise is a good stress-buster anyway). The cross-references below will give you a lot more detail on 'apples and pears', particularly Qs 55 and 56 and Feature 3, which discusses how to tell if your pot really is too big for your health by doing the Waist Circumference Test. The panels on this page also gives you two other methods of judging your apple shape – the Ashwell Shape Chart and the Waist-to-hip Ratio.

See also:

▶ Questions: 14, 48, 55–6, 248, 250–302.
▶ Features: 3, 9, 25.
▶ Key index entries: apple shape, exercise, healthy eating, intra-abdominal fat, pear shape, stress, waist circumference.

THE WAIST-TO-HIP RATIO

A third and final way of assessing whether or not you are a healthy shape is to discover your waist-to-hip ratio. This is simple to do – just divide your waist measurement by your hip measurement, using a calculator. The result is your WHR (waist-to-hip ratio). For men, a figure over 0.95 and for women, a figure over 0.80 indicates excessive intra-abdominal fat and increased risk to health.

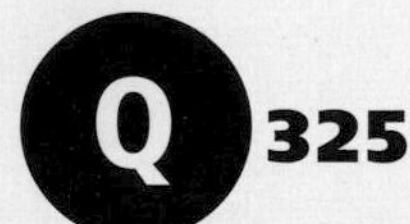

Why does overweight increase your risk of heart disease?

Until recently, the consensus of opinion was that overweight increases your risk of heart disease (or coronary arterial disease, as some medics now prefer to call it), as well as other cardiovascular diseases, including stroke, because it predisposes you to other cardiovascular risk factors, including high blood pressure (hypertension), raised total cholesterol and impaired glucose tolerance and diabetes.

However, several long-term studies now seem to show that obesity is what the experts term an 'independent' risk factor – meaning that, even if you had none of the health problems listed above, it could still increase your risk of cardiovascular disease and premature death. These studies – including the famous Framingham Heart Study – positively link weight gain with the risk of developing CHD, and the fatter you are, the greater the risk becomes. Also, intra-abdominal fat is more closely linked with CVD than any other distribution of body fat. The evidence is so strong that the American Heart Association has listed obesity as one of the primary risk factors for CHD.

If you already have heart disease and are overweight, it is important to try to reduce your weight, say specialists, to within 10% of a normal weight range (i.e. to get down to a BMI of around 27–8 maximum), as excess weight increases the load on your weakened heart, especially during exercise, which is generally encouraged for heart patients.

See also:

- Questions: 55–6, 250, 302, 324, 326.
- Features: 3, 9, 25.
- A–Z entries: 'British Heart Foundation' Diet, The Eskimo Diet.
- Key index entries: apple shape, healthy eating, heart, intra-abdominal fat, weight and health.

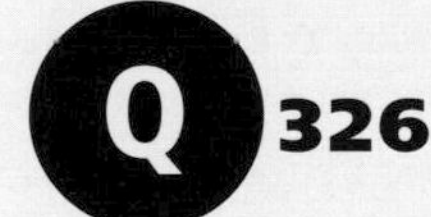

What is the ideal weight and diet for a healthy heart?

First – ideal weight. Most research seems to show that the people with the healthiest hearts are actually quite thin. The World Health Organization says that death from heart disease is increased in individuals only 10% above average weight, while recent research published in the *European Heart Journal* suggested that, for middle-aged women at least, a healthy BMI is only 22 – less, I would say, than most middle-aged women currently manage by quite a few pounds, and less than most experts would cite as a healthy weight in mid-life for the prevention of osteoporosis. Other research appears to concur with this surprising result.

However, when we look at the prevention of premature death from all causes, the consensus is that your BMI has to get well over 26 before your chances of early death begin to increase significantly. So, as you can see, the subject of ideal weight for health, and for a healthy heart, is currently being hotly debated.

Once again we need to bring in the 'central fat distribution' factor – if you are apple-shaped, but yet within a normal range BMI, your risk of getting heart disease increases. This is discussed in detail elsewhere, see the cross-references below. If you are at the heavier end of normal-range body mass index – i.e., around 25 – but don't have an apple shape, you are probably don't have much of an increased risk. If you are young, though, I suggest that you do try to maintain your BMI around 22 for women and 23 for men, especially if there is a history of heart disease or stroke in your family – this will ensure the highest protection possible against future heart disease. Much more research needs to be done on the subject – but even so, one thing is certain. The fatter you are, the greater your risk of getting a cardiovascular disease.

An ideal diet for maintaining a healthy heart is one that doesn't make you put on too much weight. If you need to lose weight, the Basic Diet in Feature 9 is a healthy way to do so and includes plenty of the foods that are thought to help you to a healthy heart in other ways. These are:

- Oily fish and fish oils – the special omega-3s (DHA and EPA) that fish contain is good at preventing blood clots, lowering the levels of blood fats and helping to reduce blood pressure. Interestingly, there is a lot of research to show that the kind of diet people are

FAT FACT

Researchers at the Duke University Medical Centre in the USA studied 9,000 heart patients over 12 years and worked out that, on average, overweight people develop heart disease seven years earlier than people of normal weight. The average age of normal-weight people who came to the clinic over these years was 64, while in obese people it was 57, the researchers revealed in l999.

normally told to follow to help prevent heart disease (or improve health and/or weight if you already have heart disease) – very low in fat and high in carbohydrate – although reducing the 'bad' LDL cholesterol in the blood, actually tends to increase the levels of harmful triglycerides in the blood, but if you regularly eat oily fish (or take supplements) and take regular exercise, the trigylceride levels tend not to increase.

This is a complicated subject for the layperson and much more research needs to be done, but let me just advise you to include plenty of oily fish (or omega-3 supplements) in your healthy, reduced-fat diet – and cut back on saturated and trans fats, rather than polyunsaturated fats and monounsaturated fats, as explained in Feature 8.

■ Antioxidant-rich fruit and vegetables. Vitamins A, C and E and the minerals zinc and selenium help to protect your heart by helping to destroy the 'free radicals' produced via oxidation in the body. Find vitamin beta-carotene, which converts to vitamin A in the body, in orange, red, yellow and dark-green fruits and vegetables; find vitamin C in most fruits and vegetables; and find vitamin E in plant oils, nuts, seeds, dark greens, avocados and sweet potatoes. Nuts, seeds and fish contain selenium and zinc, while red meat is also a good source of zinc. Tea and red wine also contain beneficial antioxidants, but wine should be limited to one or two glasses a day (see Q186).

■ Plant chemicals. Special 'phytochemicals' called flavonoids can help your heart – find them in citrus fruits, blackcurrants, melon, berry fruits and red peppers.

■ B vitamins including folate – find them in liver, whole brains, pulses, leafy vegetables.

■ Soluble fibre – find this in oats, pulses and many fruits and vegetables.

See also:

- ▶ Questions: 28, 55–6, 186, 250, 300–306, 325.
- ▶ Features: 3, 8, 9, 25.
- ▶ A–Z entries: 'British Heart Foundation' Diet, The Eskimo Diet, low-fat diets, very-low-fat diets.
- ▶ Key index entries: essential fats, healthy eating, heart, omega-3, weight and health.

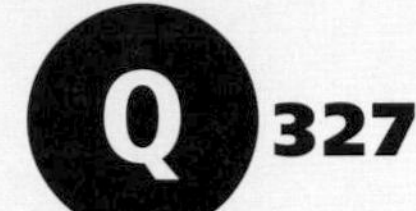

Should I go to the doctor for help with losing weight?

Doctors won't thank me for advising everyone who needs to lose weight to go to the surgery for advice – they would be overrun and unable to cope, as up to half of us are overweight! I think you need to use common sense to decide whether a visit to the doctor is wise. Here are some occasions when it may be so:

■ If you have been putting on weight and you feel that you haven't altered your eating or exercise patterns. If you have other symptoms (e.g. tiredness, lethargy, coldness), you should certainly go. Unexplained weight gain may be a sign of an underlying health problem.

■ If you are very overweight – with a body mass index over 30 – I think you should see the doctor. You should get a thorough check-up and the doctor will probably want to give you advice on lifestyle changes you could make – diet, exercise and so on. He/she may refer you to a dietician. He/she may even give you a prescription for visits to your local gym – in the UK, a standard prescription charge allows you a monitored course of exercise at the leisure centre, gym or swimming pool in participating areas.

Obese people are at increased risk of all kinds of health problems, which is why it is important to involve your doctor. Many obese people have tried to lose weight themselves and find it too difficult, so seeing the doctor may help you to lose the weight this time.

■ If you think you may have an eating disorder, it is a good idea to see your doctor, who may refer you to a specialist for help.

■ If you are pregnant or thinking of becoming pregnant and are overweight, you should see your doctor.

■ If you have repeatedly tried to lose weight and failed. Your doctor may be able to give you advice – or may even suggest a slimming pill such as sibutramine.

Some doctors are not as sympathetic as they should be with overweight people – such unsympathetic doctors should realize that a few minutes' helpful consultation with an overweight person now may save much NHS money (half a billion pounds a year of it) and much of their time in future years. Also, in my experience, some doctors don't know a great deal about sensible slimming or nutrition, although some, of course, do. Which side yours falls into is a bit of a lottery. If you feel you aren't getting good advice, ask to be referred to the community dietician.

So when is it NOT necessary to visit your doctor about a surplus weight problem? I'd say if you are in good health otherwise and have decided, using Feature 3, that you need to shed a stone or so, then you may follow one of the plans in this book, which also contains much practical advice, or you may like to join a slimming club (discussed in the A–Z) for support and advice, or choose one of the high-rating diets discussed in the A–Z.

See also:

- ▶ Questions: 36–7, 102–4, 307.
- ▶ Features: 3, 8–13.
- ▶ A–Z entries: calorie counting, low-fat diets, slimming clubs.
- ▶ Key index entry: healthy slimming.

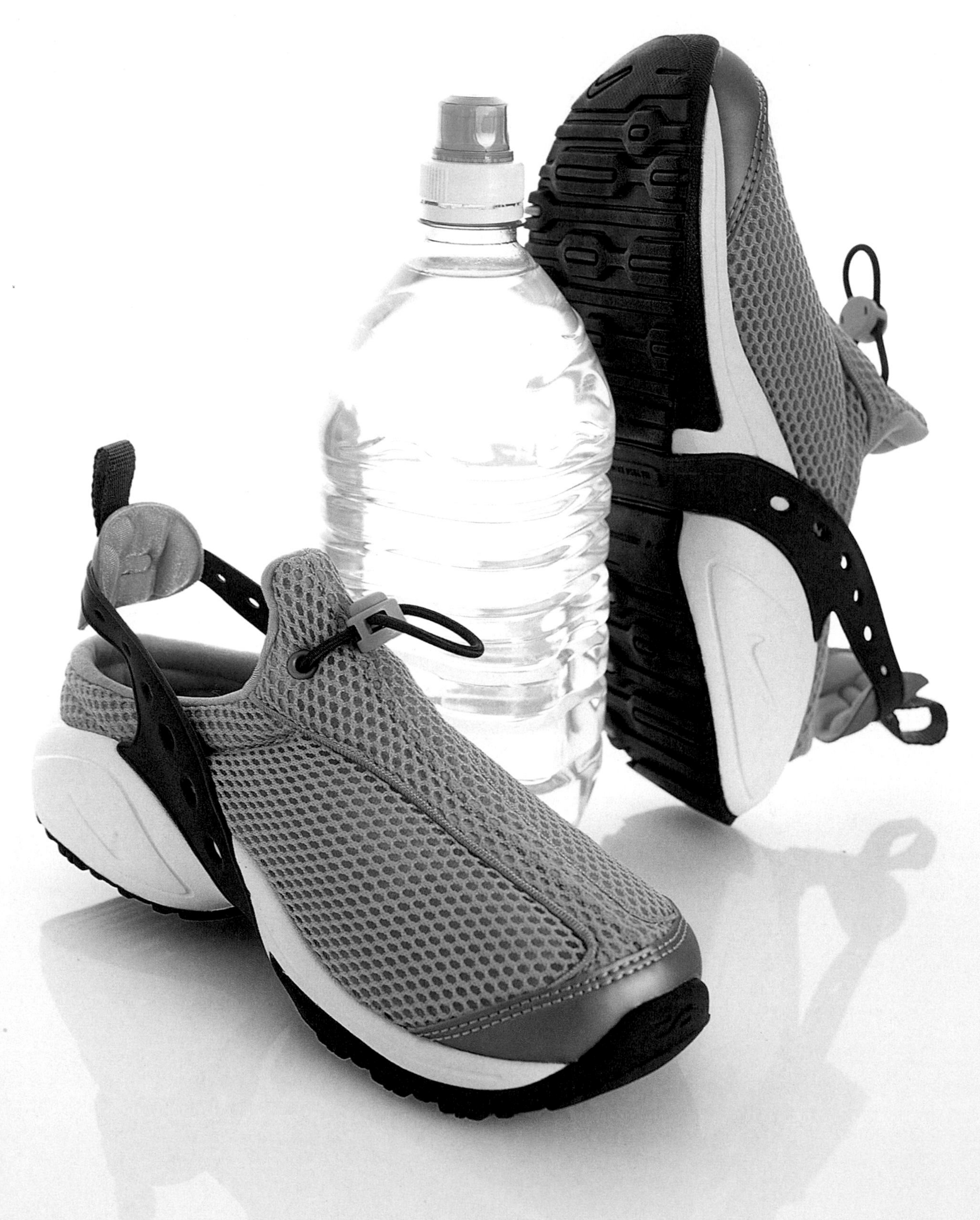

Section Ten

Your weight, your fitness

As you will discover throughout this book, regular exercise is a vital and indispensable part of both weight maintenance and weight loss. Aerobic exercise helps to burn calories, while resistance exercise maximizes lean tissue and therefore helps to keep the metabolic rate high.

Exercise is also vital for good health – hundreds of studies all over the world have concluded that regular activity protects against many diseases, illnesses and health problems, including high blood pressure, cardiovascular disease, osteoporosis, Alzheimer's disease, depression, insomnia and stress. It may also reduce disability from arthritis, help to prevent breast and other cancers, increase concentration and memory, and can help minimize symptoms of PMS. Regular exercise also increases average lifespan – so people who exercise are slimmer, healthier and live longer than non-exercisers.

Extraordinary, then, that it is estimated that only 30% of British adults do regular aerobic exercise. Even young adults avoid exercise – with only one in 20 women aged 16 to 24, and one in five men of the same age range doing an hour a day of physical activity. Our children are the most sedentary generation there has ever been.

We need to get moving. This section answers your questions on weight, fitness and health.

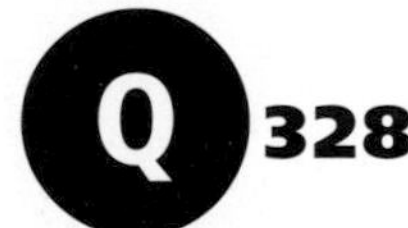

Is it possible to be overweight and yet be fit?

Yes, it is possible. You can achieve both cardiovascular (heart-lung) fitness and muscle fitness (strength) while carrying too much body fat around (see Q30). I expect many young people – some rugby players and field sports enthusiasts, for example – are fit while clinically overweight. As you get older it becomes less and less likely that if you are very overweight you will be fit, as studies show that the more obese you are, the less exercise you do, and it is exercise that keeps you fit.

The other point is that certain people who have excellent muscular strength, if not excellent cardiovascular health – for example, body builders – may be overweight according to their Body Mass Index (BMI, see Feature 3) but not according to their body-fat percentage. However such people may not be 'all-round' fit – their heart-lung fitness might not be top-notch and their suppleness is likely to be poor. True fitness is not just being aerobically fit, but also fit in terms of strength and flexibility, and perhaps also in balance, that great harmonious state of well-being when you feel not only fit but also healthy and happy, and look good.

So, although you may have a satisfactory level of fitness, if you are carrying too much body fat, you are predisposing yourself to ill health later in life (maybe not too much later), and you may not be happy with your body at all. The harmony is spoilt, and therefore my instinct would be not to class you as 100% fit. However, research shows that people who take regular cardiovascular exercise tend to lose weight over time, so if you are CV fit, you may lose the weight quite naturally.

Your own current fitness level can be assessed in a basic way – see Feature 27.

See also:

- Questions: 1, 2, 26, 30, 240, 329–32.
- Features: 3, 27.
- Key index entries: fitness, overweight.

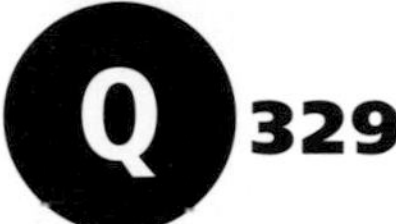

In what ways do overweight and underweight affect fitness?

Many top athletes and sportspeople have a low BMI, well towards the bottom end of what is normally considered desirable (around 18.5), but they are fit. However, if your body weight goes too low, so that health is affected, then in turn fitness levels will suffer, as fitness maintenance training is neither effective nor desirable when you are unwell. The line between being thin and fit and too thin for real fitness is also very fine.

I would suggest that the person with a low BMI and low body fat but with average or above average lean tissue (muscle) is almost bound to be fitter than someone with a low BMI, low body fat and a low lean tissue profile as well. In other words, if you are thin but well-muscled, then you're okay! For a discussion on overweight and fitness, see Q328.

See also:

- Questions: 25, 28, 30, 66, 319, 328.
- Features: 3, 25, 27, 30.
- Key index entries: weight and fitness, weight and health.

FIT FACT

Even if you are not exercising enough to produce weight loss, it can lower cholesterol levels, researchers have found. One hour's aerobic exercise four times a week lowers 'bad' LDL cholesterol by up to 15% after three months, and increases 'good' HDL cholesterol.

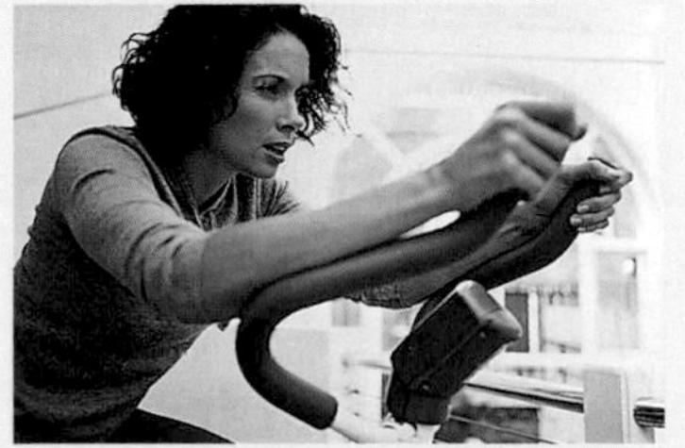

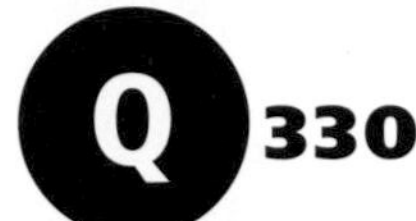

Large size seems a requisite for success in some sports – e.g. sumo wrestling, weight-lifting – so does this mean that these sportspeople are unhealthy and/or unfit?

Fitness is a word often used to describe cardiovascular fitness (fitness of heart and lungs) but in fact to be truly fit you need to be fit in three areas – CV, strength and flexibility. The answer to Q328 explains that it is possible to be overweight and yet fit in terms of strength, cardiovascular fitness and even flexibility. However, it is also possible to take part in some types of sport and be unfit, at least in some areas. For example, the sumo wrestler and the shot-putter may not have particularly high cardiovascular fitness. Not all sports, by any means, keep one fit in all corners of the fitness triangle, whether one is fat or slim.

More examples – running may keep you CV-fit and keep your legs strong, but does nothing for flexibility or upper body strength. Weight-lifters may have incredible strength but their CV-fitness may not be brilliant and neither may their flexibility profile. (Weight-lifters, by the way, can't be classed as overweight using the BMI, because so much of their weight is lean tissue, so you can't really include them in your list of fat sportspeople.)

Most sportspeople and athletes are

average weight or slim, so what the sumo wrestlers, shot-putters and weight-lifters prove is that different sports require different physiques. I can't find any scientific analysis of the health or life expectancy of sumo wrestlers, but I can say that as they are much more physically active than many obese people they are probably healthier and fitter than most of them.

See also:

- Questions: 328–9.
- Feature: 25.
- Key index entries: weight and fitness, weight and health.

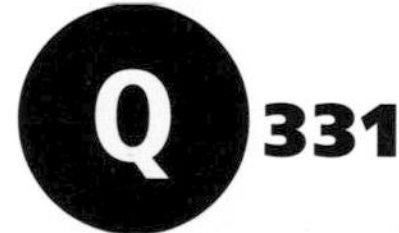

331

In what ways does fitness affect weight?

In general, if you are cardiovascular fit, that means you take regular aerobic exercise, which is a good calorie-burning occupation, and this should mean you don't have as much trouble as a non-exerciser in keeping weight down. If you have good muscle strength, that means that you have a high proportion of lean tissue, which is more metabolically active than fat tissue, so you burn more calories even when you are not active, during the course of a day. This also, then, will help you to keep your body fat down. However, as muscle weighs more than fat, some people find that when they do a long-term healthy eating and exercise programme including weight training, they lose body fat and reshape, but don't actually weigh less on the scales. Flexibility doesn't have any particular effect on your weight.

See also:

- Questions: 328, 332–3.
- Features: 1, 2, 28–30.
- Key index entries: aerobic exercise, metabolic rate, strength exercise, weight and fitness.

FIT FACT

More than 70% of people in the UK currently take too little exercise to protect their health. Experts estimate that your risk of stroke or heart disease could be roughly halved with only 20–30 minutes of moderate aerobic exercise, such as walking, four times a week. The British Heart Foundation reckons that at least 10,000 British lives could be saved a year if people only kept fit.

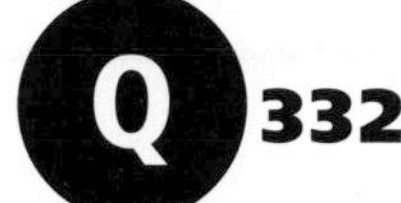

332

In what ways does being fit affect health?

It is generally held that if you are physically fit then you are better able to ward off illness because your immune system may be fitter, too. Numerous studies conclude that you are also at less risk of contracting cardiovascular disease and some cancers, arthritis and other health problems. Also some forms of exercise can lower blood pressure. If you exercise to keep your weight down, you will also be less at risk from all the health problems which affect overweight people listed in Feature 25. Research also shows that exercise helps ward off depression, lifts mood and helps mental fitness.

However, if you over-train, you may suffer poor health as a result, with a lowered immune system. The key, as always, is balance and common sense. The rest of this section will help you to decide upon an optimum level of exercise to get you fit and maintain good health.

See also:

- Questions: 328–31.
- Features: 25, 27–30.
- Key index entries: fitness and health, weight and health.

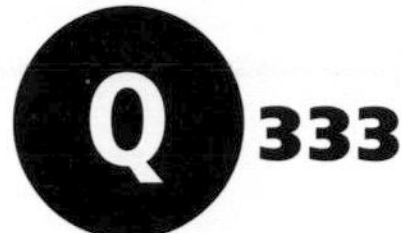

333

How does exercise help with weight control when it increases appetite?

Exercise doesn't automatically increase appetite, at least not in the short term. Indeed, there is good evidence to show that if you feel hungry after a workout, it is either lunchtime, or it is a psychological hunger rather than a physiological need. 'I've just burnt 300 calories in the gym – good, I deserve a chocolate bar!' In fact, one study came to the conclusion that people overestimate how many calories they are burning in the gym and tend to eat more calories than they have burnt to reward themselves. Obviously, in this case exercise won't help you to lose weight. The trick is to know how many calories you really are burning and refuel sensibly (see the end of this answer), and if gym work makes you eat more, choose other, more moderate forms of exercise.

There is also some anecdotal evidence that you are more likely to feel the need for food after a fairly short exercise session (half an hour or so) than after a longer one – as, at least for some people, the appetite seems to be dulled by longer exercise periods.

In the long term, with regular exercise the body may try to match food intake to energy expenditure but, according to US research, this coupling is weak and in the long term it is possible to create an energy deficit and lose weight.

If you do tend to feel hungry after exercise, first drink plenty of low-calorie drink, to avoid dehydration. This will help to give you a feeling of fullness, too. Then eat a small carbohydrate-rich snack such as a slice of bread or a banana, which will restore your blood-sugar levels if you have been working out vigorously. After a long and vigorous session (especially if you feel dizzy or fatigued), you could take a sports energy drink.

However, with sensible diet, overall your calorie intake needn't increase because of exercise. For example, a session done after breakfast means that you can use your mid-morning snack as your post-exercise energy booster, adding no extra calories to your day's intake at all. Or a late afternoon session after your mid-afternoon snack can be followed by your evening meal. Planning is all!

In general, exercise helps with weight control by burning calories – both aerobic exercise and strength (resistance) training does this. Aerobic exercise burns calories (or actual body fat) while you are doing it, and for a while afterwards, while strength training burns calories, and, by increasing your body's proportion of lean tissue, which is metabolically active, you also raise your metabolic rate long-term and burn more calories that way too. One study published in the *American Journal of Clinical Nutrition* found that weight training 3–5 times a week raises the metabolic rate by 15%.

See also:

- Questions: 6, 21–3, 35, 331, 334–65.
- Features: 1, 2, 27–30.
- A–Z entries: exercise classes, weighted workouts.
- Key index entries: appetite, exercise.

FIT FACT

Music plus exercise gives you a 'double whammy' of mood-enhancing hormones – the exercise itself increases endorphin release, and so does music, which, study shows, helps avoid exercise pain and strain on the heart.

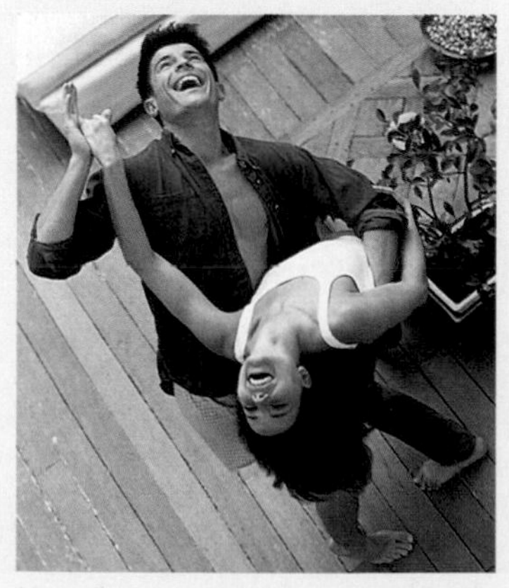

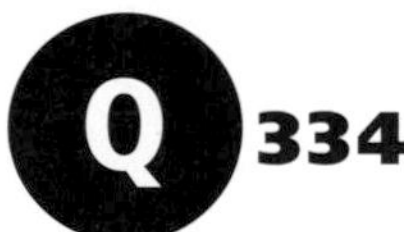

Q 334

I hate exercise – what is the best calorie-burning activity for me?

If by 'exercise' you mean formal exercise, such as classes, gyms or organized sport, then there is plenty left that you can do. Walking is the best all-purpose exercise and you might like to read Q282, which, although it is aimed at encouraging children to exercise, actually has many good ideas for reluctant adults too.

Should you genuinely dislike all physical activity, from getting out of bed in the morning to brushing your teeth, then you have a more serious problem. As you will see if you read Feature 1, all activity, even standing or washing up, uses more calories than complete inactivity, so the more active you can make your day-to-day and hour-to-hour (minute-to-minute, even) life, then the more calories you will burn without having to do any 'proper' exercise at all.

So make an effort to build extra bits of movement into your routine. The Berlin Health Education Centre found that housework is every bit as good as a moderate workout for calorie burning and fitness – dusting, vacuuming, polishing, mopping, carrying things, all burn good quantities of calories (see Feature 28 for approximate amounts). Also think about gardening, mowing, carrying shopping, running up and down stairs, parking the car a little further from where you want to be and walking the extra distance, etc.

If that all sounds too much like hard work, or too boring, then think of some fun ways to burn calories. How about dancing (even to a CD in your own sitting room), line-dancing, long sessions of lovemaking, or in-line skating. Alternatively, go for some of the less competitive, non-team sports, such as orienteering or cycling.

Don't condemn all 'real' exercise out of hand. I know four confirmed 'exercise haters' who, when dragged along screaming to Ashtanga yoga, kick-boxing, jazz dance and step classes respectively, ended up hooked, now look forward to their classes, and have also taken up other forms of exercise. Exercise releases hormones that make you feel better. So keep an open mind, grab a friend for moral support and give some things a try.

See also:

- Questions: 282, 338–46.
- Features: 1, 28.
- A–Z entries: dancing, sports.
- Key index entries: exercise, metabolism.

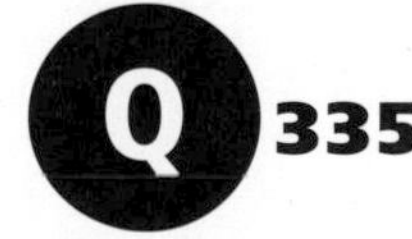

Q 335

What is aerobic exercise?

Aerobic exercise may also be called cardiovascular exercise, stamina building exercise, or endurance fitness. Aerobic exercise is exercise which achieves the following:

■ It increases cardiac fitness, strengthening the heart muscle and making it more efficient, thus reducing the number of beats per minute it has to do to pump the blood around your body. There is thus less strain on the heart during exercise and at rest.
■ It increases lung capacity – increasing the volume of usable air sacs in the lungs, and it increases the efficiency of the exchange of oxygen and carbon dioxide – if you are fit, you can get more oxygen from a breath, and your breathing rate slows down.
■ It burns up calories and/or body fat as you perform the exercise and can increase your metabolic rate slightly after the exercise is over.
■ It may increase the strength in the used muscles (e.g. legs in running or cycling, arms in rowing) and build a small amount of extra lean tissue.

The type of exercise that counts as aerobic is that which gets your heart rate up into the 'training zone', which is normally between 60% and 80% of your maximum heart rate (for more on this see Q353) and what you can continue to do for a period of time without having to stop.

Research shows that unfit people can gain benefits in their cardiovascular fitness with only short periods (e.g. 10 minutes) of aerobic exercise, done regularly. The fitter you get, the longer or harder you have to work to keep improving, and most experts say that you need to do aerobic exercise for a minimum of 3, and preferably 5, times a week, whatever your level of fitness.

Types of aerobic exercise include brisk walking, running, cycling, rowing, swimming and dancing. Feature 28 lists the aerobic potential of all types of exercise.

See also:
▶ Questions: 6, 331, 333–4, 336–56.
▶ Features: 1, 2, 27–9.
▶ A–Z entries: exercise classes, exercise equipment, sports, walking.
▶ Key index entries: aerobics, cardiovascular health, exercise, fitness.

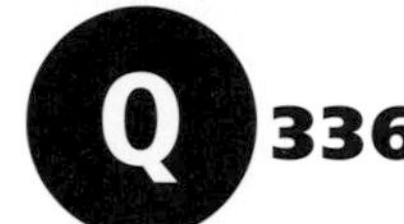

Q 336

How often do I have to exercise to lose weight?

Feature 28 shows you how many calories you are likely to burn off during various activities. For example, you would burn around 180 in a half-hour's walk or 400 in an hour's cycle ride. To lose a pound (0.5kg) of fat you need to burn off about 3,500 calories in excess of your normal weight maintenance needs. So to lose a pound of fat via, say, brisk walking, you would need to do around 10 hours of walking.

I always say that if you can lose half a pound of body fat a week through exercise, you are doing well. That would translate into seven 40-minute walking sessions at 240 calories each, which equates to the recommendation from the American College of Sports Medicine that 30 minutes or more of moderate intensity exercise, such as walking, is done on most, or preferably all, days of the week.

As you can see, how often you need to exercise to lose weight depends upon how much weight you have in mind to lose via exercise, what type of exercise you choose, and how long your session lasts. For maximum weight loss, then, one would have to do regular daily exercise of high aerobic intensity (e.g. running, fast cycling, crawl swimming) for long periods of time, and add resistance (weight) training into your schedule too (see Q333). If you are unfit, however, you need to begin any exercise programme gently and build up fitness gradually, so such a hard regime would be neither wise nor possible.

Even in the long term, though, most of us aren't that keen, or haven't that amount of time to spare to carry out an extreme regime, and will be happy with slow body-fat reduction thanks to a sensible, more attainable exercise programme and a moderate calorie-reduction diet (see Feature 9).

A research paper published in the *International Journal of Obesity* in 2001 concluded that 'a substantial but manageable amount of exercise is required for weight control', equating to about four hours' walking a week. Two recent studies have also found that in the battle against surplus weight, it is regular moderate exercise that achieves better results than intensive bursts of exercise. One of the studies, from Maastricht University in Holland, found that people who do a weekly intense session at the gym end up expending less energy over the course of a week than people who regularly do moderate exercise such as walking or cycling. Adding extra activity into your daily life in the form of non-formal exercise (see Q334) will also help create an energy deficit.

See also:
▶ Questions: 6, 18, 331, 333–5, 337–65.
▶ Features: 1, 2, 9, 27–30,
▶ A–Z entries: exercise classes, sports, walking.
▶ Key index entries: exercise, metabolism.

FIT FACT

Bristol University has discovered that men halve their risk of heart attack if they have sex three or four times a week. Doctors now believe that sex is as good for you as running or other aerobic activity.

Fitness assessment

The tests here will give you an assessment of your all-round fitness, including aerobic fitness, upper- and lower-body strength, and upper- and lower-body flexibility. Do a three-minute warm-up before all the tests (see Feature 6).

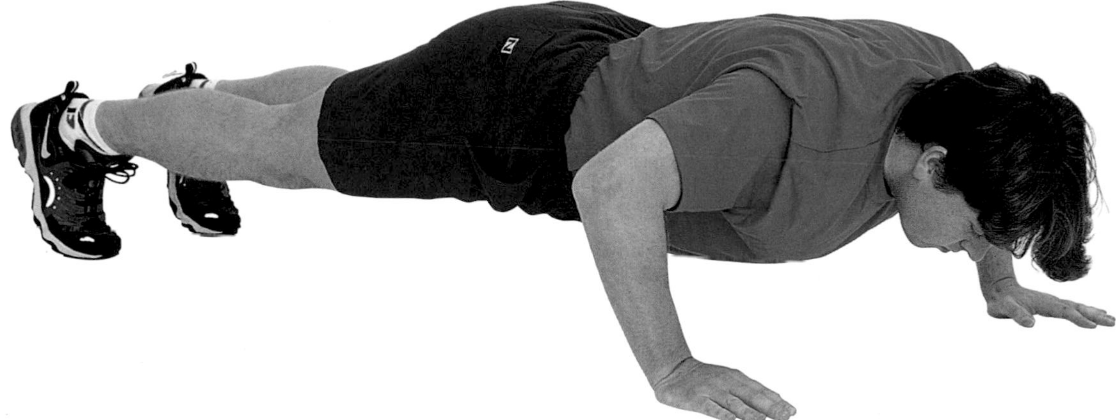

Aerobic fitness – The Step Test

The Step Test assesses your cardiovascular fitness, sometimes known as stamina or aerobic fitness. The assessment categories are non-scientific but will give you a good approximation of your fitness. For a more accurate, scientific assessment based on pulse rate, you will need to visit a gym or health centre, where cardiovascular fitness can be tested by a professional using suitable equipment. Alternatively, if you wish to buy a personal heart rate monitor (see the A–Z, heart rate monitors) you can do an accurate test at home, based on your pulse rate during or immediately after exercise, which will be explained in the accompanying leaflet. I find that trying to count your pulse rate yourself, using your fingers, during or after exercise is hard and rarely presents an accurate reading.

The test

You need just a step or stair, or similar solid structure, about 8in (20cm) high for women, 12in (30cm) high for men, and a watch. All you have to do is step up and down for 3 minutes precisely. The technique is to stand near the base of the step, and step up with your right foot, then up with the left foot, then down with your right foot and down with your left foot. That completes one step. Alternate the leading foot with each step (i.e., on your second step, you begin with the left foot). As soon as you have finished the 3 minutes (or can't complete any more steps), check down the list here to find the state that most closely matches your own and read off your probable level of fitness:

■ The exercise was very easy and you feel fine and not at all breathless.
You are extremely fit#.

■ The exercise was moderately easy and you are only slightly breathless.
You are very fit.

■ The exercise was slightly hard and you are fairly out of breath.
You are of average fitness.

■ The exercise was hard and you are very out of breath.
You are less fit than average.

■ The exercise was very hard and you are extremely out of breath.
You are unfit.

■ The exercise was too hard and you couldn't complete the 3 minutes.
You are very unfit.

Cardiovascular fitness only.

Upper body strength – The Press-up

Wearing trainers and suitable clothing, lie on your stomach on the floor (preferably on an exercise mat) with your hands beneath your shoulders and palms flat on the floor. With spine strong, stomach tucked in and head and neck in alignment with your back, lift your body off the floor until your weight is supported by your hands and toes (see illustration left). Lower your body back down by bending your elbows until your chest is about 5in (12.5cm) off the floor and then raise it again, using your arm strength and keeping spine strong. Continue, counting each press-up, until you can't do any more. Rest.

■ 30 or more (men); 20 or more (women).
Your upper body is very strong.
■ 20 or more (men); 15 or more (women).
Your upper body is fairly strong.
■ 10 or more (men); 7 or more (women).
Your upper body is averagely strong.
■ 3-9 (men); 2-6 (women).
Your upper body is weak.
■ Less than 3 (men); less than 2 (women).
Your upper body is very weak

Lower body strength – The Chair

Wearing trainers and suitable clothing, and with a watch, find an empty space of wall and stand with your back against it. Move your body down while you move your feet out from the wall until your thighs are parallel to the floor and your shins are parallel to the wall. Put your hands on your thighs and stay there as if you are sitting on a chair; begin timing yourself. Maintain the position for as long as you can. How long can you stay there?

■ 90 seconds or more.
Your lower body is very strong.
■ 60 seconds or more.
Your lower body is strong.
■ 45 seconds or more.
Your lower body is average.
■ 30 seconds or more.
Your lower body is weak.
■ Less than 30 seconds.
Your lower body is very weak.

Upper-body flexibility – The Fingertip Test

You may need someone to help you assess your success in this test. Don't do this exercise when your body is cold. Wearing flexible, non-baggy clothing, stand upright with your back straight, your knees soft. Raise your right arm and bend at the elbow so that your right hand drops down behind your back. Bend your left arm at the elbow behind your back and try to reach your left fingertips up to meet your right fingertips; go further if you can and clasp the hands together. How did you do?

■ I could clasp my hands together.
You have excellent upper-body flexibility.
■ I could touch my fingertips together easily.
You have good upper-body flexibility.
■ I could barely touch my fingertips.
You have average upper-body flexibility.
■ My fingertips were a few centimetres apart.
You have poor upper-body flexibility.
■ My fingertips were more than 4 in (10cm) apart.
You have very poor upper-body flexibility.

Lower-body flexibility – The Sit and Reach Test

Don't do this exercise when your body is cold. To test your hamstrings and lower back, sit on the floor with your legs together out in front of you, your toes pointing towards the ceiling, your arms at your sides, your lower and upper back not slumped (sitting with your bottom and back against a wall will help you retain the correct posture). Slowly lean forward with your arms, reaching for your toes. Don't hunch your shoulders over in order to try to reach further and don't strain your neck. How far can you reach?

■ Beyond your toes.
You have excellent lower-body flexibility.
■ Easily to your toes.
You have good lower-body flexibility.
■ Nearly to your toes.
You have average lower-body flexibility.
■Around your ankles.
You have poor lower-body flexibility.
■No further than mid-shin.
You have very poor lower-body flexibility.

YOUR RESULTS

If you scored poor on cardiovascular (aerobic) fitness, begin a regular exercise programme, starting gently and gradually increasing in difficulty. Feature 29 offers graded aerobic programmes. Also see Qs 334–7 and the rest of Section Ten for more information on other aerobic activities. Feature 28 rates many activities for aerobic benefit and calories burnt.

If you scored poor on strength, begin with the programme in Feature 6 and then progress to that in Feature 30. Also see Qs 333–4 and 350, and the rest of Section Ten for more information on other muscle-building activity. Feature 28 rates many activities for strength-enhancing.

If you scored poor on flexibility, do the programme in Feature 7 every day, and also try to include regular activities in your life which may increase your suppleness, such as swimming or yoga. Also see the activity chart in Feature 28 to see which activities are good for flexibility.

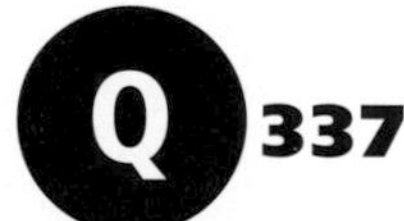

337

How long do I have to exercise for at a time to lose weight?

The important factor is how long in total you exercise for over the course of, say, a week, not how long each individual session is. Much recent research shows that both short sessions and long sessions burn equal amounts of fat or calories if they add up to the same time in the end. A study at Loughborough University found that three 10-minute sessions of brisk walking a day, five days a week, achieved the same rates of calorie burn and fitness levels as five half-hour walks a week and a similar study at the University of Virginia in the USA found the same thing.

The crucial thing is that you can't go for three 10-minute walks a week and expect to burn many calories. So it's either 'short and very frequent' or 'longer and less frequent'. The choice is up to you and what fits in best with your lifestyle. Also see the answer to the previous question which discusses the importance of the type of exercise you choose to do.

See also:

- Questions: 333–6, 338–65.
- Features: 27–30.
- Key index entries: exercise, fitness, metabolism.

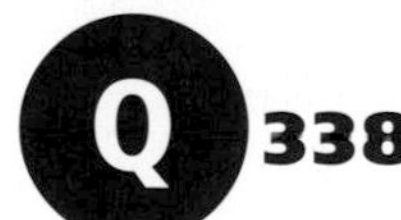

338

How much weight can I lose through exercise?

You have to work quite hard to lose more than about half a pound of body fat (225g) a week through exercise, but as long as you do exercise regularly, over and above your previous levels, then you should continue to lose weight and/or body fat down to a weight that is optimal for you, particularly if you manage to increase your muscle (lean tissue) through resistance exercise as well. When you are at or near that weight, it should then be possible to maintain a suitable weight via an exercise and diet maintenance programme.

The best combination is to exercise regularly and cut down your calorie intake slightly, to produce a weight loss of about 2lb (1kg) a week if you are very overweight, or 1lb (0.5kg) a week if you are not so overweight. The answers to Qs 336 and 337 give you more information on the duration, frequency and intensity of the exercise that you should do.

FIT FACT

A study of 3 million gym-goers has revealed that there is an increased risk of heart attack during exercise in those who only go occasionally and then work out hard. Going less than once a week increases the risk.

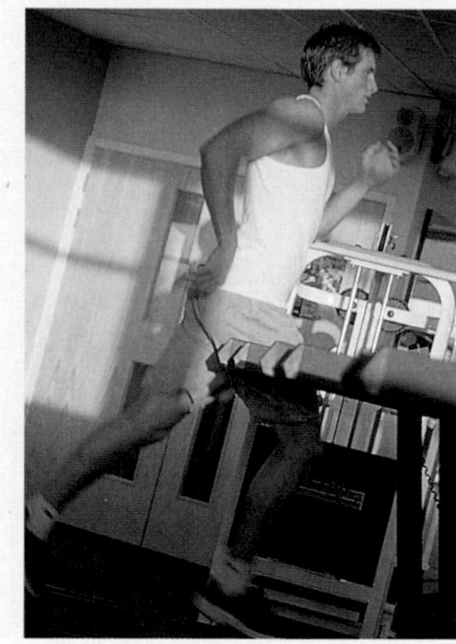

See also:

- Questions: 331, 333–7, 339–65.
- Features: 27–30.
- Key index entries: exercise, metabolism, weight.

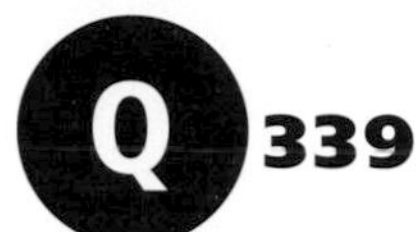

339

I exercise for 40 minutes every day by walking my child to and from school, but I don't lose weight. Why?

You would find that if you gave up the five-days-a-week walk and didn't alter your eating habits, you would slowly put on weight, which would prove that the walking is affecting your weight control, but not in the way you want. When we discuss how you can lose weight through exercise (see Qs 333–8), I am talking about new exercise, over and above what you have habitually been doing. You are currently exercising enough to maintain your current weight, and to lose weight you would need either to increase the amount you are doing and/or cut your calorie intake a little.

Even if you have only recently started walking your child to school, and so therefore it IS a 'new' activity, you are probably not burning up enough calories to show anything other than a very slow weight loss. If this sounds hardly believable, let me explain.

I expect your child is quite young (if he or she needs walking to school), and therefore, having done a similar thing myself for years, I know that you are probably walking to school at a leisurely pace rather than a brisk walk. In that case, you are not burning anywhere near as many calories during the daily 40 minutes as you might if you were walking alone or with an adult. You're walking 10 minutes each way, 4 times a day. A single 10-minute walk from your home to school with a child may be a distance of only about a quarter of a mile, perhaps a little more. That means you are walking perhaps a mile a day, or 5 miles a week. Research shows that you burn about 100 calories for every mile you cover (whether you walk slowly, briskly, or even run). So you are burning only about 500 calories a week in your school walks. Even if this was a 'new' exercise, it would still only produce a weekly weight loss of about one-seventh of a pound, or a pound every seven weeks.

Walking quicker on the half of the journey when you aren't with the child won't up the calories burnt – as we've seen, if you are walking a quarter of a mile, it doesn't matter what pace you go at. You need to find a longer route home and burn more calories off that way. Walking on your own, you should be able to cover about 2½–3 miles in 40 minutes – burning nearly three times the calories of your walks with your child and burning off nearly half a pound a week. Even if extra walking isn't possible, don't get disheartened and abandon your daily walks – they will be doing your health good even if weight loss isn't apparent.

See also:

- Questions: 333–8, 340–65.
- Features: 27–30.
- A–Z entry: walking.
- Key index entries: exercise for weight control, fitness, metabolism.

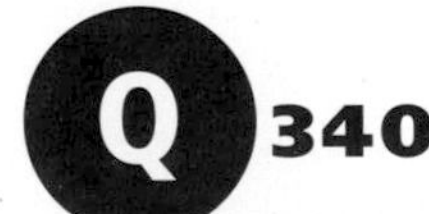

Is the best exercise for weight control 'short and sharp' or 'slow and long'?

First go back and read the answers to Qs 336–8 to give you the background. What matters for calorie burning is the total amount of time you spend and the intensity of the exercise. As we've seen, around 4 hours a week of moderate-intensity exercise, like brisk walking, should result in weight loss over time. A similar length of time spent on a harder exercise, such as running or an advanced aerobics class, would result in more calories burnt in the same length of time. Alternatively, a shorter length of time spent on the harder exercise would result in the same calories burnt as the 4 hours' walking.

There is some evidence that short bursts of exercise are more easily fitted into people's lives and therefore they may stick with it, and there is also some evidence that people who do long, infrequent bouts of hard exercise (e.g. a weekly session of circuit training at the gym) end up eating more calories than they expend, so on balance it would seem that short, frequent sessions of moderate-intensity exercise are the best way to go. How you split the time up is really up to you. Do what fits best with your life.

See also:

- Questions: 333–9, 341–65.
- Features: 27–30.
- Key index entries: exercise, weight.

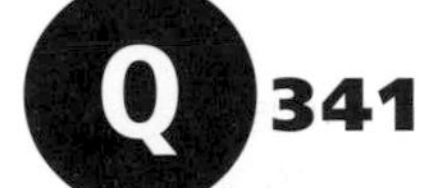

What low-cost exercise can I do to lose weight?

The cheapest aerobic exercise is walking, and it is also the simplest and easiest, so I would go for that. Cycling is also quite inexpensive, although obviously you have to buy the bike. If you have a music system, you could put on some upbeat music and dance away the calories.

Simply getting more active in your everyday life can burn plenty of calories without costing you anything – you could even save money. For instance, you could walk to work instead of taking a car or bus, which would save petrol or fare. You could sack the cleaner and do housework instead of watching TV three or four times a week. If you have a garden, you could get out there and dig a patch to grow your own vegetables, thus saving money again.

You could also consider doing sponsored walking or cycling to raise money for charity – a great motivator.

See also:

- Questions: 334, 336–40, 342–65.
- Features: 27–30.
- A–Z entries: cycling, walking.
- Key index entry: exercise.

FIT FACT

Our motorized lives mean we walk an average of 8 miles less a day than 50 years ago. We cycle much less too – in 1949, 34% of non-walking miles travelled were by bike, now less than 2% are. Studies at the University of California found walking an extra mile a week reduces chances of mental decline by 13%.

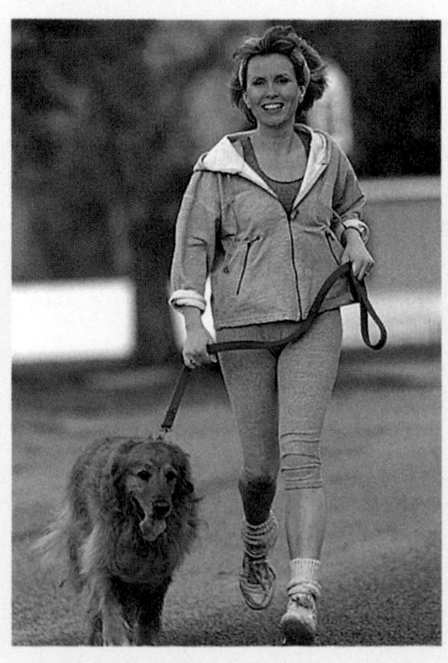

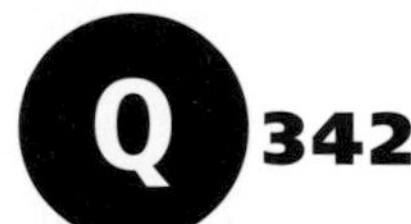

What's the best calorie-burning programme for a beginner? I am quite unfit.

The three aerobic fitness programmes in Feature 29 offer levels to suit all abilities – just start on the first level and follow the instructions. Of the three, I would advise you to start on the walking programme, which is the easiest. For calorie-burning inside your own home, see Q344.

If you want to burn the maximum calories you should also begin doing some resistance work – i.e. something that will strengthen your muscles and add bulk to them so that your overall metabolic rate is raised. Again, you need to start gradually and build up the resistance and number of times you repeat each move.

I suggest that you start with the 10-minute Tone in Feature 6 and do this for a few weeks, then move to the programme in Feature 30, which uses weights. Alternatively, you could join a gym for professional machines and advice, or you could think about getting some 'posher' equipment for home use. In that case, read Q361.

If you are starting out at rock-bottom unfitness and have never done any formal exercise before, you should think about getting a check-up from your doctor to make sure you are in good enough health to begin, and you should always obey the instructions about safe exercise. The most important thing is to go at your own pace – you're not in competition with anyone – and build up fitness gradually. Though for most people – even elderly beginners – results are remarkably quick. You won't lose weight rapidly through exercise alone, but you will notice a different in your shape, particularly around the midriff at first, your muscle tone and your energy levels. That is the great thing about exercise – it has benefits all across the board.

For more noticeable weight loss, combine your calorie-burning regime with a slightly reduced-calorie diet such as that in Feature 9.

See also:

- ▶ Questions: 331–41, 343–65,
- ▶ Features: 6, 9, 27–30.
- ▶ A–Z entries: exercise equipment, gyms, sports, walking, weighted workouts.

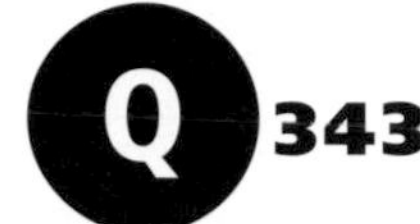

I can spare 10 minutes a day and am reasonably fit. Which exercise will burn up the most calories in that time?

With just 10 minutes you need something that you can do 'instantly' without having to travel or prepare, and yet you need something more intense than walking. At home, you could skip or rebound (7 calories a minute), or step (9), all of these have an inbuilt facility for warming up and cooling down – just do gentle marching on the spot before and after skipping and stepping, and do gentle mini-jumps on the rebounder at either end of your programme.

If you fancy more expensive equipment, a rower burns up about 8 calories a minute, a Stairmaster 9 calories a minute and an elliptical trainer 9 calories a minute. Most of these machines come with a built-in calorie readout, but some experts say that these give optimistic views of how many calories you are actually burning. Even so, a 10-minute session using any of the ideas here will be enough to burn around 100 calories and will keep you at a basic level of fitness.

Generally, any exercise that works both arms and legs at once will burn more calories than one that just works one or the other, so a rower is better than an exercise bike, for example. Also, anything that involves you standing rather than sitting is harder work (e.g. a treadmill rather than a bike). Lastly, any work on an uphill incline is harder than on the flat, and so will increase calorie burn (e.g. a stepper or a treadmill on incline is harder work than a flat treadmill).

Whatever you do, try to maximize your time by 'doubling up' – for example, when you step, carry hand weights or use wrist and ankle weights. If you can increase your muscle mass, you will burn more calories as you workout (and indeed, all the time).

In the long term, do try to make some small changes in your lifestyle so that you can afford to spend a bit more time on yourself. You should build in time for flexibility work three times a week and don't forget always to warm up and cool down to prevent injury, aches and pains.

Unfit people please note – these high-intensity, short-burst exercises aren't suitable for you. You need to build up fitness gradually with a moderate intensity activity like walking, which will also burn calories, albeit more slowly.

See also:

- ▶ Questions: 336–8, 340, 344, 348, 353.
- ▶ Features: 27–30.
- ▶ A–Z entry: exercise equipment.
- ▶ Key index entries: calorie burning, exercise, fitness.

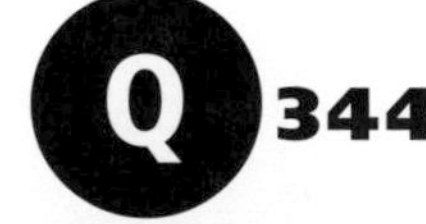

Can you recommend any home exercise equipment which will help me burn calories?

There is a huge range of equipment that you can buy, from a basic skipping rope to a top-of-the-range treadmill costing thousands of pounds. The exercise equipment section in the A-Z will help you decide what is right for you. The main consideration, apart from cost, is where you will keep the item(s) that you buy.

If you have to keep a folding treadmill or bike in a cupboard or an outhouse, for example, it is unlikely that you will use it. If you haven't a room to set aside where any large equipment can be left out ready to use, I'd think twice about buying anything large and settle for the rope or, at most, a rebounder, which is lightweight and set down ready to use in a second.

Bear in mind that for optimum calorie-burning you need to do some strength training as well as aerobic training, so investing in a set of dumbbells or resistance bands (more info in the exercise equipment section in the A–Z) would be a good idea.

See also:

- ▶ Questions: 335–38, 340–43.
- ▶ Features: 27–30.
- ▶ A–Z entries: exercise equipment, weighted workouts.
- ▶ Key index entries: calorie burning, exercise, fitness.

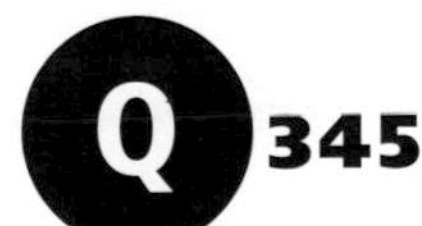

345

When you exercise, what is the difference between burning calories and burning fat?

When you exercise, you can use both carbohydrate (stored as glycogen in the body) or fat for fuel. In the early stages of an exercise session, more carbohydrate than fat is burnt (particularly with high-intensity exercise, where carbohydrate is the body's 'preferred fuel'), but as the session progresses beyond 20 minutes, the percentage of fat burnt increases. Towards the end of prolonged exercise – an hour or more – when glycogen reserves are low, fat will be supplying about 80% of your energy requirements. The fitter you are, the better your body is at burning fat for energy during exercise.

However, if you want to lose weight, it doesn't really matter whether you are burning up body fat while you are exercising or using your glycogen stores or blood sugars. Whatever type of fuel you are using, you are still 'burning' calories. Any exercise that you do – whether it is housework, jogging for an hour or skipping for five minutes, for example – will use up calories for energy and, over time, if you create an 'energy deficit' – burning up more calories than you take in (see Q18), your body will have to use its own fat stores for fuel. Whether this happens while you exercise or while you sleep, over time you will still 'burn' the fat and lose weight.

As you will see if you read the answer to Q337, you burn just as many calories in three 10-minute sessions of exercise as in one 30-minute session. So don't worry too much about this fat-burning thing, and just concentrate on being as active as you can, taking regular aerobic exercise and doing some resistance (strength) work, and as long as you don't overeat to compensate for the extra calories burnt, you should lose body fat over time.

Feature 28 gives average calories burnt in a variety of activities, Feature 1 helps you find out how many calories a day you burn on average (your metabolic rate), and Feature 9 gives you a sensible calorie-reducing diet. Use all these to help you formulate a suitable exercise and diet programme.

See also:

- ▶ Questions: 18, 335–44, 346–65.
- ▶ Features: 1, 2, 6, 9, 28–30.
- ▶ A–Z entries: exercise classes, exercise equipment, sports, walking, weighted workouts.
- ▶ Key index entries: calorie burning, energy equation, fat burning, metabolic rate, weight loss.

FIT FACT

Research shows that the more intense (hard) the exercise, the more the metabolic rate is raised when you have finished exercising. One study found that, after an average moderate-intensity exercise session, an extra 12–35 calories are burnt, but after an average high-intensity session, up to 180 extra are burnt.

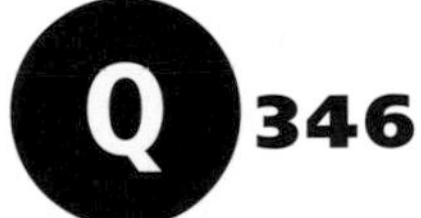

346

What's the best all-round programme to keep me fit and help me lose a little weight?

You need to do regular aerobic work (see Q335) to burn calories and keep heart and lungs fit; regular resistance training (strength work), which tones your body, keeps lean tissue (muscle) intact (or even increases it), helps boost metabolic rate and burns calories; and regular flexibility exercise to keep joints supple.

The aerobic programmes in Feature 29 are graded for fitness; the 10-minute Tone in Feature 6 will provide basic toning work – once mastered, progress to Feature 30; and the stretching programme in Feature 7 will keep you flexible. I suggest you do the aerobics programme on alternate days, the strength work on the days you aren't doing aerobic, and that you do the stretching every day after your workout.

See also:

- ▶ Questions: 335–45, 348–65.
- ▶ Features: 6, 7, 27–30.
- ▶ A–Z entries: exercise classes, exercise equipment, gyms, sports, walking, weighted workouts.
- ▶ Key index entries: aerobics, exercise, metabolism, weight loss.

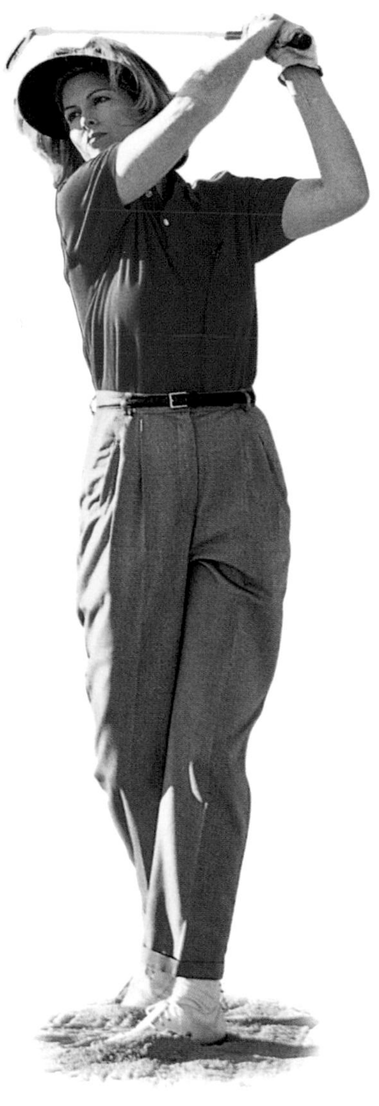

Activities chart

If you want to know the benefits of any particular form of activity, including the amount of calories it burns, this is the place to look.

Before you begin a new activity, it pays to make sure that your choice will help you to achieve what you want.

The chart explained

The chart lists over 50 activities each with star ratings for their benefits on different aspects of fitness and calories burnt.

The stars mean:

* Little or no benefit;

** Moderate or good benefit;

*** Very good or excellent benefit

So, for example, cycling has a very good aerobic effect, very good lower body strength effect, and little or no benefit for your upper body and flexibility.

For good all-round fitness you should choose activities, or a mix of activities, that will give you benefit in all areas.

The calorie columns

The 'calories per minute' column is based on how many calories a minute this activity burns for a person weighing 10½ stone or 147 lb (67kg). If lighter, you will burn less; heavier you burn more. To work out a more exact figure, use the next column 'calories per lb (0.5kg) of body weight per hour'.

EXAMPLE: You weigh 8½ stone or 119lb (54.5kg). To find out how many calories you burn walking at 3.5 mph, you multiply your weight in pounds by the cals/lb(0.5kg)/hr, which is 2.4. This comes to 285 calories burnt per hour. If you want the calories per minute, divide this by 60, and the result is 4.76 rounded up to 5.

The fitness rating column

The last column gives you an assessment of the suitability of this activity for your own current fitness level.

1 = suitable for fairly unfit people/beginners.

2 = suitable for reasonably fit people/ people who are used to exercise.

3 = suitable for fit or very fit people who have been exercising for some time.

Activity	Aerobic benefit	Upper-body strength	Lower-body strength	Flexibility	Calories per minute	Cals/lb(0.5kg) /hour	Fitness rating
Aerobics class	***	**	***	**	6.5	2.6	2
Badminton	**	**	**	*	5.8	2.4	1
Basketball	**	**	**	*	6	2.4	2
Bowling	*	*	*	*	4.5	1.8	1
Circuit training	***	***	***	*	5.5	2.2	2
Cricket, average	*	**	**	*	3	1.2	2
Cycling, 10mph	***	*	***	*	6.6	2.7	1
Dancing, slow	**	*	**	**	4.5	1.8	1
Dancing, fast	***	*	**	**	9	3.7	2
Digging	*	**	**	*	5	2	1
Elliptical trainer	***	**	**	*	9	3.7	2

Activity	Aerobic benefit	Upper-body strength	Lower-body strength	Flexibility	Calories per minute	Cals/lb(0.5kg) /hour	Fitness rating
Fencing	**	**	**	*	5	2	1
Football, forward, average	**	*	**	*	5.5	2.2	2
Golf	**	**	**	*	4	1.6	1
Gymnastics	**	***	***	***	5	2	2
Handball	**	**	**	*	4	1.6	1
Hockey	**	**	**	*	5.5	2.2	2
Horse riding, trot	**	*	***	*	6.8	2.8	2
Housework	*	**	**	**	4	1.6	1
Jogging, 5.5mph	***	*	***	*	8	3.2	3
Judo	*	**	**	***	4	1.6	2
Mowing (not self-propelled)	***	**	**	*	5	2	1
Rowing (leisure)	**	***	*	*	5	2	2
Rower (gym)	***	***	**	*	8	3.2	3
Running, 6.5mph	***	*	***	*	10.3	4.2	3
Running, 7.5mph	***	*	***	*	14	5.7	3
Running, 10mph	***	*	***	*	17.6	7.2	3
Scootering	**	*	**	*	4	1.6	2
Sitting	*	*	*	*	1.1	0.4	1
Skating, ice	**	*	**	*	4	1.6	2
Skating, in-line	***	*	***	*	5.2	2.1	2
Skiing, cross-country	***	**	***	*	9	3.7	3
Skiing, downhill	**	**	***	*	6.4	2.6	3
Skipping (rope)	***	*	***	*	7	2.8	2
Squash	**	**	**	*	9	3.7	3
Stairclimbing/ stairmaster/step	***	*	***	*	9	3.7	2
Standing	*	*	*	*	2.1	0.85	1
Stretching	*	*	*	***	2.2	0.9	1
Swimming, slow crawl	***	***	**	*	8.5	3.5	2
Swimming, slow breast	***	***	**	**	7	2.8	1
Table tennis	**	*	*	*	6	2.4	1
Tennis, singles	**	**	**	*	7	2.9	2
Trampoline/ rebounder	***	*	**	*	7	2.9	2
Volleyball	**	**	**	*	5.8	2.4	1
Walking, 2.4mph	***	*	**	*	5	2.1	1
Walking 3.5mph	***	*	**	*	6	2.4	1
Walking, 4.5mph (powerwalking)	***	*	**	*	7	2.8	2
Walking uphill (15% incline/2.4mph)	***	*	***	*	6.7	2.7	2
Weight training	*	***	***	*	4.6	1.9	2
Yoga, Ashtanga	**	**	**	***	7.3	3.0	2
Yoga, static	*	**	**	***	4	1.6	1

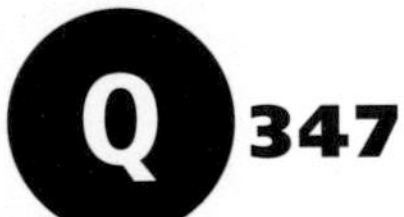

347

Does everybody burn calories at the same rate during exercise?

No. The less you weigh, the fewer calories you will burn, and the smaller your percentage of lean tissue (muscle), the fewer you will burn. As an example, at an average cycling pace, a 13-stone person with a high lean-tissue percentage may burn around 9 calories per minute, while an 8-stone person with a low lean-tissue percentage may burn about 5 calories per minute.

This is true whatever the exercise. The 'calories per minute' given in Feature 28 are therefore based on an average weight person of 10½ stone (67kg), as explained, but if you want to work out the exact number of calories you are burning for your weight you can do so using the 'calories per pound of body weight per hour' column.

Below are other examples of the difference in calorie burning between the light and heavy person.

See also:

- Questions: 4–6, 13, 32.
- Features: 1, 2, 28.
- Key index entries: calorie burning, metabolism, weight.

AVERAGE CALORIES BURNT PER MINUTE

	8 stone (51kg)	13 stone (83kg)
Cycling 10mph	5	8
Tennis	5.5	9
Swimming, crawl	6.5	10.5
Running, 6.5mph	8	13

Q 348

Which is the better exercise – walking, running or swimming?

An almost impossible question to answer, as it all depends on you, how fit you are, what you want to achieve, how much time you've got, etc. Each of the activities you mention is good in a different way.

Walking is a great calorie-burning and fitness tool, particularly for beginners and the unfit, and those looking for something low-cost and easy, but does little for upper-body strength, or overall flexibility.

Running burns many more calories than walking or swimming, but you can't really just go out and do it if you are unfit. It also makes you hot and sweaty, so you need to have a shower and change after you've done it. Running on a hard surface may also, in time, affect weight-bearing joints and there is a generally higher risk of injury than with walking. It also is no good for upper-body strength or flexibility.

Swimming burns calories and is also a better all-round exercise for balanced body strength and flexibility – but you have to like water, be able to swim, be fairly near a pool, have the money and time to go swimming regularly. Also, swimming is non-load-bearing and, therefore, is not good for maintaining bone density.

All this proves that choosing the right exercise for you should be done with care. Think about what you want to achieve and how fit you are, and how any exercise will fit in with your life. If you start one activity and find you don't enjoy it, pick another – there is plenty to choose from and we can't always get it right first time.

Feature 27 will help you decide on your fitness level and Feature 28 will help you find activities to suit you.

See also:

- Questions: 334–47, 349–65.
- Features: 27-29.
- A- Z entries: running, sports, walking.
- Key index entries: exercise, fitness.

FIT FACT

If you are exercising to maintain healthy bones, go for high-impact exercise, such as jogging, tennis, squash, or step aerobics. People who take part in such activity are likely to defer bone density problems for four years longer than people who don't, according to a study in the *British Medical Journal*.

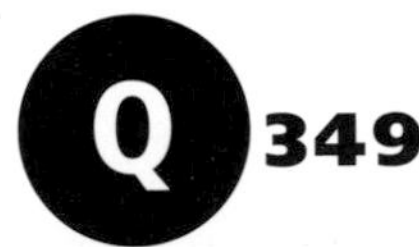

349

How much exercise is too much?

Another impossible question, as it depends upon your level of fitness and many other factors. In general, the less fit you are, the less exercise you can (or should) do. For example, a 20-minute walk will be plenty in one day for an unfit person, whereas a trained marathon runner will run several hours in a day without suffering.

You need to pace your activity programme to suit your level of fitness, and, as you get fitter, to how fit you want to be. If you use common sense and follow the guidelines in the exercise features in this book, it is unlikely that you will be doing too much work – what is termed 'overtraining'. Indeed, if you are very fit, the programmes in this book will probably be too easy for you.

However, let's look at what 'too much' exercise is, and how it can adversely affect you. Overtraining or 'burnout' is something that may occur (usually in competition-standard athletes) when they become stale, find performance declining, feel sluggish and tired and may have other symptoms. This is unlikely to happen to you, the beginner or moderate exerciser.

You are more likely to suffer from problems if you don't have the right technique, or try to overtax yourself slightly at the gym. You may then get aches, pains or strains, which are your body's way of telling you that you have not been going at a suitable pace for your level of fitness.

Then there are people who aren't trained athletes but become dependent on exercise – obsessional about it – and seem to spend almost every spare minute at the gym or out running. This is called 'exercise addiction' and may be linked with eating disorders in some. One study in 2000 by the University of Birmingham and published in the *British Journal of Sports Medicine* found that 18% of women studied, who were all regular exercisers, showed signs of exercise addiction.

The causes of this addiction are not certain, but one theory is that obsessional exercisers become hooked on the endorphins released when you exercise, giving the classic 'exercise high' – and withdrawal symptoms if exercise is stopped. Addicted exercisers may also be laying themselves open to a wide range of health problems. These include a reduction in the efficiency of the immune system, predisposition to osteoarthritis in the worked joints, possible cessation of periods in women, fatigue and excessive thinness.

As with most aspects of life, sensible exercise is balanced and forms part of your life, rather than the major part of it. Just as carrots are good for you but too many carrots can make you ill, so exercise is good for you but not to excess. For most people, an hour a day of formal exercise would be plenty for fitness, calorie burning and health benefits, if the hour includes aerobic/strength and flexibility work and if you get other forms of activity during your normal day. People who exercise a lot should always take sufficient time to rest between sessions to allow the body to recover, and all but very experienced athletes shouldn't do high-intensity exercise for more than 90 minutes at a time to avoid suppressing the immune system.

See also:
- Questions: 336–37, 340, 346, 353, 365.
- Features: 6, 7, 27–30.
- Key index entries: exercise, fitness.

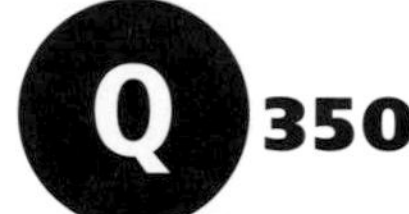

350

Which exercise apart from weight training is good for building muscles?

Any aerobic exercise that works one of the major muscle groups will help to build muscle in the group worked. For example, running, cycling and step aerobics will help to build strong leg muscles. Plyometrics – jumping, bounding, hopping and leaping – have also been shown to be good for muscle building in the legs. Swimming and rowing, for example, will help to build strong arm muscles. The Activity Chart in Feature 28 shows which exercises are good for building upper- and lower-body strength.

See also:
- Questions: 331, 333, 348, 351, 356–8, 361.
- Features: 28, 30.
- A–Z entries: exercise equipment, gyms, sports, weighted workouts.

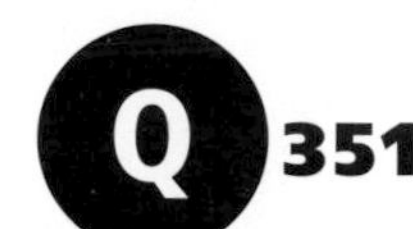

351

Which aerobic exercise is good for tone?

See the previous question, as 'tone' is similar to 'strength' – you get good body tone when you work muscles. Aerobic exercise can help give your body a streamlined look by burning calories and helping shed fat (a covering of fat won't allow even toned muscles to show) and also by strengthening muscles, depending upon which aerobic exercise you choose.

For general toning, one of the best aerobic exercises is swimming, as it works all the muscles in the body. Up- and downhill walking are also good for the lower body, and rowing for upper-body

FIT FACT

Jogging for 2 hours a week may decrease your risk of premature death by 60%, researchers in Denmark found in 2000. A 22-year-study of 4,658 Danish men found that even if joggers smoke or have high cholesterol, they live longer than non-joggers with similar habits.

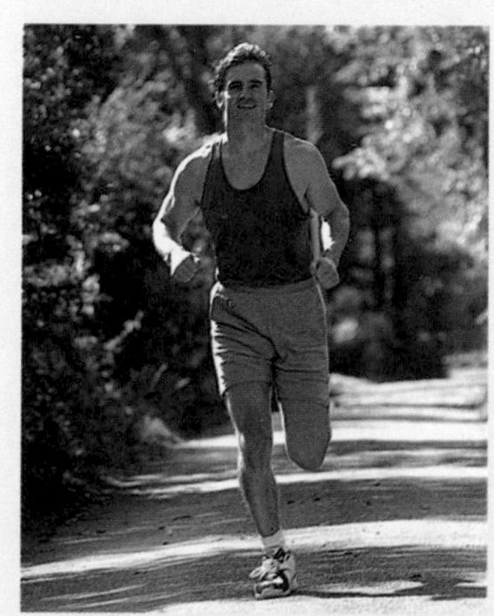

tone. Specifically for leg muscles, choose cycling or brisk walking, including hillwork.
See also:
- ▶ Questions: 348, 350, 352, 360.
- ▶ Features: 28, 29.
- ▶ A–Z entries: sports, walking.
- ▶ Key index entries: exercise, fitness, toning.

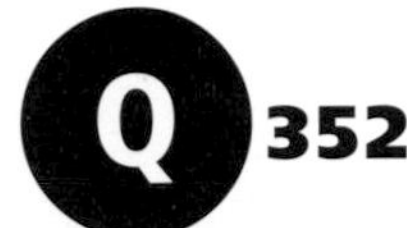

352

Which is the best exercise for flattening my stomach, apart from floor exercises?

Swimming is excellent, as your abdominal muscles are used all the time. Other good exercise includes hillwalking, dancing and Ashtanga yoga. Static yoga is great, as are digging and weight training.
See also:
- ▶ Questions: 48, 58, 351, 360.
- ▶ Features: 5, 27–30,
- ▶ A–Z entries: sports, walking, yoga.
- ▶ Key index entries: body tone, stomach.

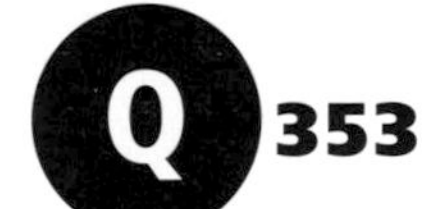

353

What are my 'training zone' and my 'maximum heart rate'?

Maximum heart rate is the greatest number of pulse beats/minute your heart should beat. The standard way of gauging MHR is to subtract your age from 220. Your training zone is the heartbeat range at which you will gain the most benefit from aerobic exercise, and most experts give it as 60–85% of MHR, with 75% often cited as ideal – though I suggest 60% for unfit people and beginners. EXAMPLE: You're 40. Your MHR is 180 (220–40) and training zone is 108–53 (60–85% of 180).

The aim is to keep your pulse rate (heart rate) at this level throughout your workout. If you go over the upper end of the training zone, slow down, and if you go under the lower end, work a bit harder.

At the gym the cardiovascular (aerobic) equipment comes with built-in heart-rate monitors. For home work you can buy portable heart-rate monitors. Another way to gauge you're working within a suitable training zone is the 'perceived exertion test' – if you feel you're working but can still talk, then you're probably at a suitable intensity.
See also:
- ▶ Questions: 335, 337, 340, 345–7.
- ▶ Feature: 27.
- ▶ A–Z entry: heart-rate monitors.
- ▶ Key index entries: cardiovascular exercise.

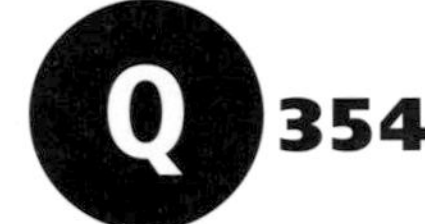

354

What's the best time to exercise to burn fat?

Studies on athletes show their peak time for training is in the evening, when body temperature, heart rate, reaction times and even flexibility are all 'at their best', so this is probably your best time to exercise as you may find the work easier. One recent study found the hormones cortisol and thyrotropin were higher in exercisers at that time, indicating that the body is adapting better to training.

However, if you happen to be an 'early bird', leaping out of bed full of energy, you could also use this time, after suitable warming up, to do some low-intensity aerobic work, like walking, and save the harder stuff, such as running, for later in the day. But don't leave it too late – if you do anything other than winding-down yoga or stretching too close to bedtime, you may have trouble getting to sleep, as adrenaline levels may be high.

All that said, most people fit workouts in with their lifestyles and exercise at all times of day or night. If you find a time that suits you, stick with it – the time of day isn't the most important consideration.
See also:
- ▶ Questions: 336–8, 342–3.
- ▶ Feature: 28.
- ▶ Key index entries: exercise, fitness.

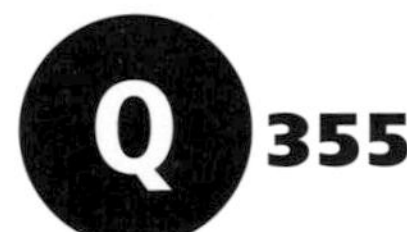

355

What is the best food and drink to help me improve my exercise performance?

For the average person following a moderate exercise programme, a normal, healthy diet such as that in Feature 9 is fine, containing as it does adequate carbohydrate, protein and fat. You don't need special supplements, vitamins or extra protein. If you're trying to lose weight with a combination of diet and exercise, you should not necessarily eat extra food after a normal workout session as research shows you may end up taking in more calories than you've burnt. Do make sure that you drink enough water so that you

FIT FACT

Honey is the latest 'buzzfood' for fitness. The Sport and Nutrition Lab at Memphis University in the USA has found that not only does regular intake of honey increase the speed and endurance of athletes, but it also significantly helps recuperation after a workout and acts to keep blood sugar levels much more stable than intake of some other forms of sugar.

are not dehydrated during or after exercise. For normal moderate exercise sessions, sports drinks containing glucose shouldn't be necessary. For more, see Q364.

See also:

- Questions 333, 364.
- Feature: 9.
- Key index entries: Glycaemic Index, healthy eating.

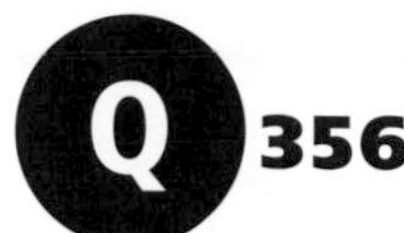

356

Which is best for weight control – weight training my muscles, or aerobic exercise?

Most forms of aerobic exercise tend to burn more calories per minute than weight training (see Feature 28) and so, until recently, slimmers were advised to do a lot of aerobics and weight training was hardly mentioned. However, much recent research has concluded that weight training may be vital in slimming. Not only does it use calories while you are actually doing it, it raises metabolic rate afterwards, in a similar way to aerobic work.

Lastly, regular weight training increases lean tissue (muscle) and as muscle, even at rest, burns up more calories than body fat, it increases metabolic rate and helps you slim, or maintain weight.

So the ideal exercise programme is one combining aerobic work and resistance training. Try a programme from Feature 29 plus, at first, the 10-minute Tone in Feature 6 if you are a beginner, then moving on to the weights programme in Feature 30.

See also:

- Questions: 6, 13, 30, 35, 333–55, 357–65.
- Features: 27–30
- A–Z entries: exercise classes, gyms, sports, exercise equipment, walking, weighted workouts.
- Key index entries: exercise and slimming, lean tissue, metabolism.

FIT FACT

Researchers have found that runners who have a high-caffeine drink, such as a can of cola, before a race, can actually run for longer, because the caffeine helps to mobilize the body's fat stores so that they can be used for energy – but it only works as a booster in this way if you aren't actually an habitual caffeine drinker.

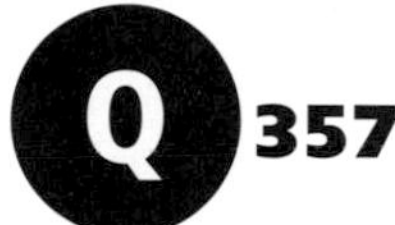

357

How does strength training help weight loss?

It can help to burn calories while you do it; it can raise your metabolic rate afterwards and can also raise your metabolic rate full time, as your increased muscle mass, gained through the strength (weight/resistance) training, is more metabolically active than body fat.

I should also point out that if you add a lot of muscle through strength training you may actually find that you don't lose weight at all, even though you may alter your body composition and appear slimmer. The extra muscle weighs more than fat and so this effect may 'cancel out' the fat loss as far as weight goes. However, having a higher muscle percentage and lower body-fat percentage is great to aim for, as it makes you look slim and toned, and is healthier than being slim with a low lean tissue percentage – for example, you are at less risk of osteoporosis.

See also:

- Questions: 356, 358.
- Features: 6, 27–30.
- A–Z entries: exercise equipment, gyms, weighted workouts.
- Key index entries: exercise and slimming, lean tissue, metabolism.

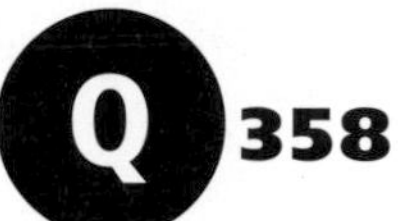

358

Is it true that muscle converts into fat when you stop exercising?

No. Muscle can't 'convert into' fat as they are two completely different substances; muscle is mostly water and protein, whereas body fat is – well, fat. The body can convert surplus dietary fat, carbohydrate or protein into body fat if you eat too much of any of these for your energy needs. The body can also do the reverse – use stored muscle and stored fat as energy if you don't eat enough calories for your needs – converting these stores into carbohydrate and usable energy through a series of processes, but it can't actually make muscle into fat.

What may happen if you stop exercising is that the muscles will lose 'tone' and bulk; they will 'atrophy'. If, at the same time, you continue to eat as much as you did when exercising, you will be creating a calorie surplus, because without exercise and with decreased muscle, your body won't need so many calories to maintain its weight. So eventually surplus calories will be stored as body fat – and there you have it, muscle replaced with fat. However, definitely not, muscle 'converted' into fat by some strange chemical process in the body, and the new body fat will not necessarily appear in the same places as the muscle – it's more likely to end up around your waist.

To avoid this, the ex-exerciser needs to reduce calorie intake to meet their new needs. Best of all – don't stop exercising at all, though I know sometimes it is inevitable, through injury, illness and so on.

See also:

- Questions: 1–2, 18, 22, 30, 76–8, 331, 333, 357.
- Key index entries: body fat, the energy equation, exercise, metabolism, muscles, weight gain.

Aerobic fitness programmes

Whatever your level of fitness, you can choose a walking, cycling or swimming programme to help you improve fitness and burn calories.

There are only two rules:

1 Whatever your chosen programme and whatever level you are on, you should do a session at least 3 times a week, and preferably every other day.
2 You should work within your Training Zone.

Training zone

To be aerobic, your work needs to raise your heart rate (pulse rate) into a suitable training zone. This is between 60 and 85% of your maximum heart rate, which is 220 minus your age.

For example: you are 30, so your MHR is therefore 190, and your training zone is between 114 and 161. Very unfit people should train at the lower end of the training zone, i.e. 60–70%. Fitter people can train in the centre, about 75%. Very fit people can train at the higher end, 80–85%.

WALKING

	Distance	Time
Level 1	1 mile	20 minutes
Level 2	2 miles	40 minutes
Level 3	2 miles	35 minutes
Level 4	2 miles	30 minutes
Level 5	3 miles	45 minutes
Level 6	4 miles	55 minutes

CYCLING

	Distance	Time
Level 1	3 miles	20 minutes
Level 2	6 miles	40 minutes
Level 3	6 miles	30 minutes
Level 4	6 miles	24 minutes
Level 5	9 miles	30 minutes
Level 6	12 miles	40 minutes

Notes for all programmes

The programmes are divided into 6 levels, with Level 1 for beginners, up to Level 6 for more advanced exercisers. Choose which programme you prefer (if very unfit, choose walking) and start at Level 1, progressing through the levels in your own time. If you are also doing a resistance programme (e.g. Feature 30), you may prefer to do this on alternate days to your aerobic work.

General guidelines

- Wear suitable clothing and footwear (if appropriate) for your chosen programme.
- Warm up with the warm-up routine described in Feature 6 and cool down with the stretching programme described in Feature 7. Warm-up time is extra to that listed for your chosen activity.
- Don't exercise if you are over-tired or ill.
- See Q364 for eating and drinking before, during and after exercise.

Walking

- You need a pedometer, or measure your distances by car.
- Walk with an even gait, tummy tucked in, head up, arms swinging, shoulders relaxed, breathing naturally and evenly.
- Walk on fairly level ground unless otherwise stated.
- Stay on each level for as long as it takes for you to reach the standard stated. Walk for the time given until you can manage the distance given in that time. When you can do that, move on to

the next level and repeat the process.
■ Once you've reached Level 6, continue to improve by more uphill walking or, if you like, you can begin jogging.

Cycling

■ You need a reliable bicycle with a distance gauge, and a helmet.
■ Take a drink and a puncture kit with you and always be safety-conscious.
■ Cycle on fairly level ground if possible, unless otherwise stated.
■ Stay on each level for as long as it takes you to reach the standard stated, cycling for the time given until you can manage the distance given in that time, then move on to the next level.
■ Once you've reached Level 6, continue to improve by adding more uphill cycling or continue increasing speed and distance covered in the time.

Swimming

■ You obviously need a handy swimming pool, preferably 25m, as it is harder to train properly in a small pool. A waterproof watch would be an advantage, unless your pool has an easily seen clock.
■ If you have not swum in a long time, consider getting some lessons to improve your stroke technique.
■ Stay on each level until you can swim CONTINUOUSLY for the time stated, then move on to the next level.
■ After Level 6, improve by increasing the distance covered with each stroke, by increasing the number of laps you do in the same time, and by increasing the length of time you swim and by introducing backstroke and butterfly as liked.

To keep track of your heart rate during exercise it is best to wear a heart rate monitor (see A–Z), but otherwise the Perceived Exertion Scale here gives you a good idea of how hard you're working. The work should be moderate-to-hard, and you should be able to talk if you are working at the right level. Don't train outside your correct zone – if the work is too light it isn't aerobic, and if it is too heavy it also isn't aerobic, and may also be dangerous. If you have to keep stopping, the work is too hard. Make a note of your own percentage training levels here:
60%: 75%: 85%:

SWIMMING

	Time	Stroke	Notes
Level 1	10 minutes	breast	3 mins may be all you can manage at first. Concentrate on technique and do pool exercises in between laps while you build up fitness.
Level 2	15 minutes	10 mins breast; 5 mins front crawl	Concentrate on trying to increase distance covered with each stroke. Alternate different strokes if you like (e.g. 2 mins breast / 1min crawl).
Level 3	20 minutes	10 mins breast; 10 mins crawl	Concentrate on trying to increase speed as you improve.
Level 4	30 minutes	15 mins breast; 15 mins crawl	Concentrate on technique, particularly breathing correctly.
Level 5	30 minutes	15 mins crawl; 15 mins back crawl	Concentrate on technique.
Level 6	30 minutes	Crawl with ankle and wrist weights	Concentrate on technique and breathing

THE PERCEIVED EXERTION SCALE

Decide how the exercise feels while you are working	The heart rate equivalent	Aerobic training effect
1 Very, very light		None
2 Very light		None
3 Light		None
4 Fairly light		Warm-up
5 Moderate	60%	Beginners' zone
6 Quite hard	70–75%	Average training zone
7 Hard	80%	Fit training zone
8 Very hard	85%	Maximum aerobic training zone
9 Very, very hard		Anaerobic
10 Much too hard		Anaerobic

Mixing it

You can mix and match your aerobic programmes if you like – e.g. two sessions of swimming a week and two sessions of walking a week – as long as you work through the levels as stated.

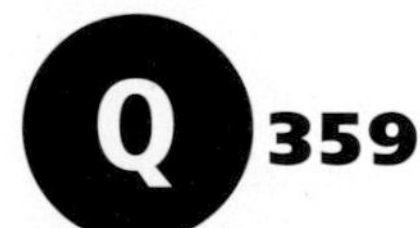

Will isometrics get me slim?

Isometrics are a static form of conditioning your muscles – normally a muscle is contracted and held for several seconds before being released. Done regularly, this can help you to look more toned up, as a floor toning programme can, but it is it is not a major calorie-burning exercise, like aerobic activity or weight training. Yes, you'll burn a few extra calories doing it, but hardly enough to make any difference to your weight. Isometric exercise needs to be carried out properly and there is some evidence that it can increase blood pressure, so take advice from your gym or exercise teacher before using it to tone up.

See also:

- Questions: 333, 336–38.
- Features: 6, 30.
- A–Z entries: gyms, weighted workouts.
- Key index entries: exercise and weight, toning.

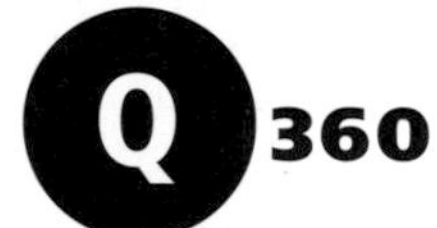

Can you get fit and slim through gentle exercise, such as yoga?

Much yoga is deceptively not gentle and so, if you are looking for gentle exercise, be sure to check out your yoga class to make sure it really is that. Yoga can be as relaxing or as tough as you want. The A–Z gives more information about the different kinds and where to find classes.

If you want gentle, you should join a beginners' hatha yoga class, for example. If you do it regularly, it will improve certain aspects of your fitness – particularly flexibility and perhaps strength. At any rate, you should find your body shape improving because yoga elongates the muscles and helps tone them. What gentle yoga won't do, though, is improve your cardiovascular fitness as it isn't aerobic, or build up a great deal of muscle, and therefore it won't burn many calories or increase your metabolic rate a great deal.

If you want to lose weight via exercise you need to couple aerobic work with strength training, as explained elsewhere.

See also:

- Questions: 65, 66, 333–59, 361–65.
- Features: 27–30.
- A–Z entries: exercise classes, exercise equipment, gyms, weighted workouts, yoga.
- Key index entries: exercise, exercise and weight, fitness.

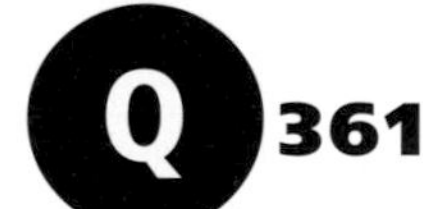

Can you give me advice on building muscle at home?

Many people have managed to increase their muscle mass by simply lifting weights in their bedroom once a day, and so a decent set of dumbbells is all you need to buy to begin with. An alternative – very popular with women – is a set of resistance bands. You also need to know what exercises to do – Feature 30 is a starting point, and you can also buy various books, charts and so on to help (see under Gyms, exercise equipment in the A–Z).

When weight training, it is important that you do the moves correctly so as to avoid injury or strain. To build muscle you need to keep increasing the weight increments, rather than worrying about the number of repetitions. Low weights with lots of reps tends to 'tone up' the worked muscle, rather than building bulk.

If you have more room and more money to spend, there is a wealth of resistance training equipment you can buy to help build muscle. There are 'home' versions of all the big machines you will find in the gym, from leg presses to pec decs – again, see the A–Z for more information. However, be wary of spending too much on equipment that takes up too much space, or that involves a lot of altering pins, screws, etc. to train different parts of the body.

See also:

- Questions: 350, 356–7.
- Feature: 30.
- A–Z entries: exercise equipment, gyms, weighted workouts.
- Key index entries: book list, exercise, muscle, strength training.

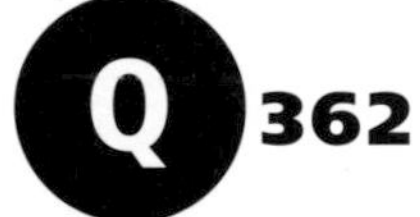

How much weight can I expect to lose if I join a gym?

This largely depends upon how often you go and what you do when there. Most people visit their gym 2 to 3 times a week, and spend an average of 1 to 1½ hours using the equipment. Assuming 1 hour on cardiovascular work (e.g. treadmill, bike, Stairmaster) and half an hour on the resistance machines, you would probably (depending upon your weight, how hard you work, and how much time you spend gossiping in between stations) burn about 500 calories, though this is a very rough estimate. You could probably work out a more accurate total by adding up the calories burnt at the disciplines you actually do, using Feature 28, which also takes account of your own weight. So, saying 500 calories burnt per visit, times 3 – you use 1,500 calories a week at the gym. As a pound of body fat equals about 3,500 calories, then you are in theory burning just under half a pound of fat a week.

However, in my experience, new regular gym-goers very often lose less than this –

nearer a pound a month. If you are unfit, it is hard to burn lots of calories per visit at least for the first couple of months. But, of course, you will be toning up, and gradually building a little more muscle – so, over time, your body-fat percentage and your figure should both improve considerably, as long as you go regularly and gradually increase times/distances/ resistance, etc. The gym trainers should help you build up a safe, effective programme and the fitter you get, the more calories and fat you will burn.

See also:

- Questions: 331, 333, 335–8, 340.
- Features: 27, 28.
- A–Z entries: exercise classes, gyms, weighted workouts.
- Key index entries: exercise equipment, exercise and weight control, gyms.

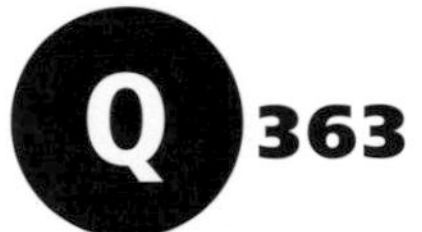

Is there any exercise I should avoid if I am very fat?

If you are very fat and also very unfit, then you should avoid all intense, hard, strenuous exercise and begin a gentle regime, such as Level 1 Walking (Feature 29) coupled with an easy body toning programme, such as that in Feature 6. Over time your fitness will improve and you can make the work you do harder.

In theory, fatness in itself, if you are healthy and fit, doesn't stop you doing any exercise but in practice there are several activities that you would probably find uncomfortable – for example, jogging.

I would take your doctor's advice on what exercise to do other than that suggested above, and get a thorough health check-up at the same time. No doubt you should try to lose some weight, as diet and exercise do go together, and it makes little sense to get yourself fit if you are still carrying enough body fat to put your health at risk. The cross-references give more information on these risks.

See also:

- Questions: 300–306, 327, 328–32.
- Features: 6, 27, 29.
- Key index entries: exercise and weight, weight and health.

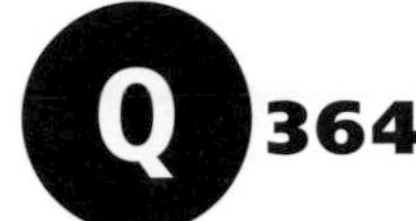

Can I exercise on an empty stomach, or should I wait until I've eaten?

It's not wise to exercise a long time after your last meal, as your blood-sugar levels may be low and this could cause you to feel weak, dizzy, even faint. For normal exercise sessions (e.g. an hour at the gym or an average brisk walk), I'd suggest having a healthy meal about two hours before, or a carbohydrate snack, consisting of both quick- and slow-release carbs, about an hour before. This would be something like an apple and a banana, or a slice of wholemeal bread and honey, or Cornflakes and milk. Eating anything more than a light snack too near exercise time may cause you some discomfort and affect performance, so don't eat a big meal and then go straight into exercise after that.

During anything other than the mildest, shortest of activities, you should have a ready supply of water to keep you hydrated (roughly 2 pints/1 litre of water per hour of moderate exercise) and you should drink plenty afterwards, too.

After a long and/or strenuous bout of exercise, you can have a snack consisting of a quick-release carbohydrate (e.g. a banana or a slice of white bread and honey) to restore blood-sugar levels. But slimmers should note that after short or moderate exercise sessions, refuelling may not be necessary – you may end up taking in more calories than you have burnt.

See also:

- Questions: 84–6, 333, 355.
- Key index entries: eating and exercise, healthy eating.

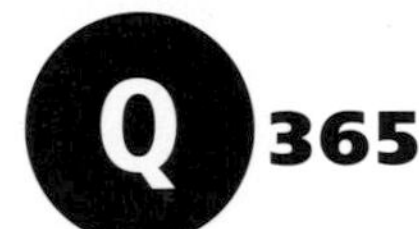

When is it unwise to exercise?

If you are ill you shouldn't exercise at all. If you are convalescing, you should take exercise on doctor's advice (perhaps gentle walking would be good but running would be bad, for example). If you have done a lot of exercise in a short space of time, you should rest and give the body a chance to recuperate – overtraining damages the immune system and has other drawbacks.

Research at the University of Colorado found that rats that exercised when they wanted to were healthier, with better immune systems, than the rats forced to exercise against their wills. So if you really aren't in the right frame of mind to exercise, perhaps it may be wise to leave it until later or tomorrow.

You should also take exercise at a pace and intensity to match your current level of fitness – so attempting too hard an exercise is unwise. If you feel unusually tired after a workout, or have seriously aching muscles, then you have been over-exercising. It is also unwise to do any high-intensity exercise infrequently – e.g. going to the gym after a month's absence and doing a hard workout on the Stairmaster. Research shows that you may be putting yourself at risk of a heart attack.

People with long-term health problems, e.g. angina, or who are pregnant should ask their doctor's advice before exercising.

See also:

- Questions: 353, 363.
- Feature: 27.
- Key index entries: exercise and health, fitness.

Simple strength training

Once you find the exercises in Feature 6 easy, you can progress to these fairly simple exercises using either dumbbells or a barbell. They will help develop your muscles and strength – but read the safety tips first. For advice on equipment see the A–Z (exercise equipment).

SAFETY FIRST

- At first, do the programme 3 times weekly. You can increase to 5 times as you get fitter.
- Warm up before training, using the warm-up for Feature 6 and cool down afterwards, using the stretches in Feature 7.
- Follow the instructions for each exercise.
- Keep stomach tucked in, good posture and 'soft' knees, unless otherwise stated.
- Exercise in a warm room with some source of fresh air and wear suitable clothing and non-slip footwear.
- If you feel pain or the worked muscle feels exhausted, stop.

Upright Rows
(for shoulders, upper back, chest and biceps)

Stand with your feet hip-width apart, holding a barbell with your palms facing your body, hands in front of each thigh. Now breathe in and raise the bar up to neck height, keeping your elbows high and the bar close to your body. Slowly lower as you breathe out.

What weight to use?

The standard criteria for what weight to use is this: by trial and error, find the maximum weight you can lift to do just ONE repeat of each exercise, and then use 50–60% of that weight for your routine. E.g. if you can do ONE upright row (see right) with a 10kg weight, then use 5–6kg weight for that exercise.

How many repeats?

At first, repeat each exercise 8–10 times or as many as you can if less than that. As you get stronger, pause for 1 minute, then do another set of 8–10 reps, and finally, a third. When you can do 3 sets without trouble, increase the weight by a small increment (5–10%), start back on 1 set and build up back to 3. Gradually increasing weights builds strength safely.

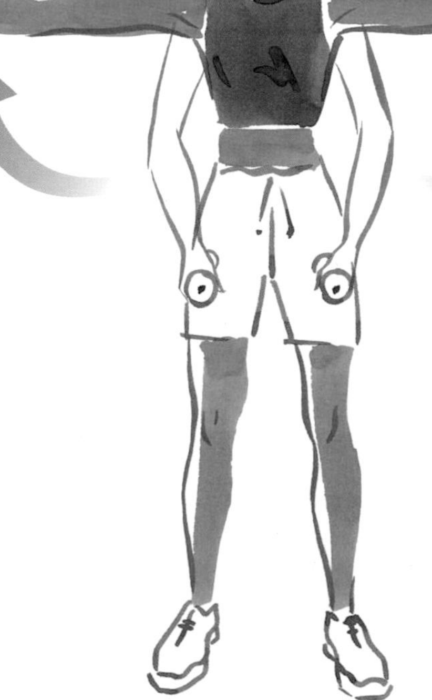

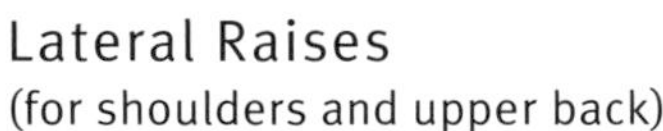

Lateral Raises
(for shoulders and upper back)

Stand with your feet hip-width apart and a dumbbell in each hand, palms facing inward. Breathe in and slowly raise your arms up and outwards to your sides, keeping your arms straight, until the dumbbells are just above shoulder height. Slowly lower as you breathe out.

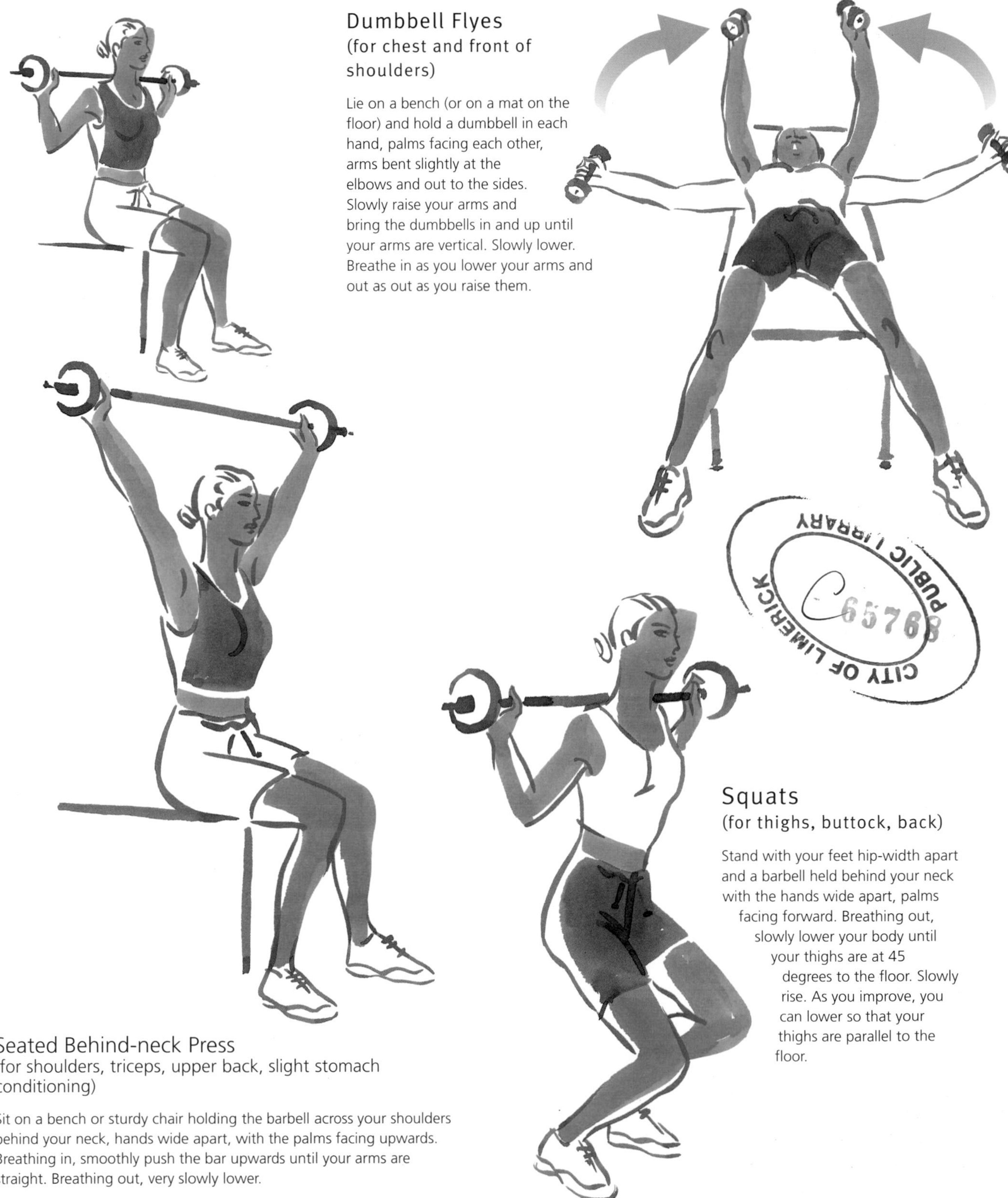

Dumbbell Flyes
(for chest and front of shoulders)

Lie on a bench (or on a mat on the floor) and hold a dumbbell in each hand, palms facing each other, arms bent slightly at the elbows and out to the sides. Slowly raise your arms and bring the dumbbells in and up until your arms are vertical. Slowly lower. Breathe in as you lower your arms and out as out as you raise them.

Squats
(for thighs, buttock, back)

Stand with your feet hip-width apart and a barbell held behind your neck with the hands wide apart, palms facing forward. Breathing out, slowly lower your body until your thighs are at 45 degrees to the floor. Slowly rise. As you improve, you can lower so that your thighs are parallel to the floor.

Seated Behind-neck Press
(for shoulders, triceps, upper back, slight stomach conditioning)

Sit on a bench or sturdy chair holding the barbell across your shoulders behind your neck, hands wide apart, with the palms facing upwards. Breathing in, smoothly push the bar upwards until your arms are straight. Breathing out, very slowly lower.

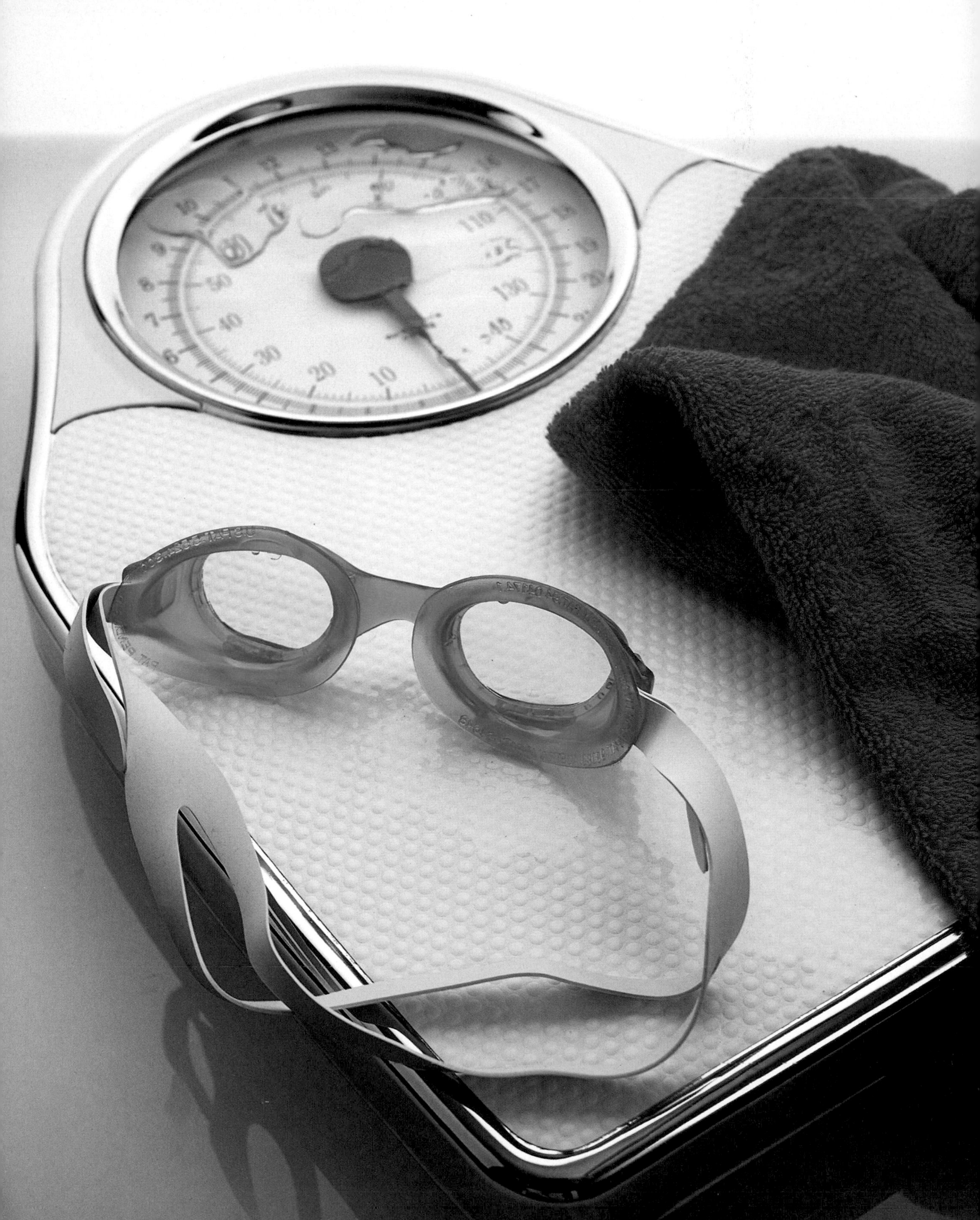

A–Z of diet products, methods & programmes

For the unwary slimmer or would-be exerciser, the world is full of help in many forms – hundreds of different diets, pills, supplements, gadgets, treatments; thousands of consultants, coaches, trainers and classes. Sadly, not all the help available is any good.

This A–Z section aims to help sort the good from the bad, or the indifferent.

From cellulite treatments to negative calories, from cabbage diets to slimming surgery, from blood group diets to fat magnets, over 100 diet and fitness programmes, aids, methods and products are evaluated in an unbiased fashion.

The 'Top 20' most popular diets of the past twenty years are analysed for health and efficacy, and given a percentage rating – an at-a-glance list of these ratings is given overleaf. So, if you are planning to invest in something to help you to slimness or fitness, start here and you could save yourself a lot of time, expense – and frustration.

TOP 20 POPULAR DIETS

The twenty diets analysed in detail throughout the A–Z are those that I consider have been the most popular and/or famous over the past few decades; they are not necessarily the best from the point of view of either nutrition or dieting. The results of the analyses are given here as percentage ratings. When choosing a diet plan, the higher its rating the better. No diet will be as effective in the long term without regular exercise.

Place	Rating	Diet
1=	80%	Low-fat diets
1=	80%	Glycaemic Index diets (e.g. The Glucose Revolution)
3	77.5%	Calorie counting
4	75%	The F Plan
5=	70%	The Hip-and-thigh Diet
5=	70%	Replacement meals (e.g. Slim-Fast)
5=	70%	Very-low-fat diets (e.g. Eat More, Weigh Less; Pritikin)
8=	67.5%	Diuretic diets (e.g. The Waterfall Diet)
8=	67.5%	Raw food diets
10	65%	Sugar Busters
11	57.5%	Food combining (e.g. Hay system; Eat Great, Lose Weight/Somersizing)
12	55%	Cabbage Soup Diet
13	52.5%	Scarsdale Diet
14	50%	Atkins Diet (also Protein Power; Carbohydrate Addicts' Diet)
15=	47.5%	Eat Fat, Get Thin
15=	47.5%	Eat Right 4 Your Type
15=	47.5%	Rotation Diet
15=	47.5%	The Zone
19	42.5%	Crash diets
20	35%	Beverly Hills Diet

Acupuncture

Acupuncture is the ancient Chinese medical treatment in which needles are inserted in the body along 'meridians' (channels of energy) according to what the practitioner decides is necessary. It is a recognized method of controlling pain and has been used instead of anaesthesia throughout the world, and is also useful for many other conditions, including headaches and infections, but its success in controlling body weight, or acting as an aid to slimming, is much less well documented.

Some people who go for acupuncture do lose weight, but this may be because it can be successful at treating stress and therefore eating less may be a knock-on. Some practitioners believe the needles stimulate 'acupoints' that make the brain produce extra endorphins (the 'pleasure' hormones), which may reduce appetite or psychological need for food. There may also be a degree of 'placebo effect' – you want it to work, so it may.

Qualified acupuncturists are members of the British Acupuncture Council.

■ The British Acupuncture Council, 63 Jeddo Road, London W12 9HQ; tel 020 8735 0400; www. acupuncture.org.uk

■ Acu-Medic Centres, 020 7388 5783.

Alexander Technique

Created a hundred years ago by an Australian actor, The Alexander Technique helps heighten body awareness and co-ordination, teaching optimum ways to move and be still. Improved posture is one of the major physical benefits, and this can make the body look slimmer – and make you look more confident and, indeed, feel more confident. The technique has also been shown to reduce stress levels, which may help you control poor eating habits, and may improve health in many other ways – for example, muscular or skeletal problems, including arthritis and backache.

■ Society of Teachers of the Alexander Technique, 20 London House, 266 Fulham Road, London SW10 9EL; 020 7284 3338; www.stat.org.uk

See also: Book List.

Aromatherapy

A regular aromatherapy session (hand massage using essential plant oils mixed in an oil base) may help a slimming campaign in a peripheral way – by increasing your sense of well-being, relaxing you, or providing satisfaction for a sense (the sense of smell) other than the taste buds, for example. However, aromatherapy cannot produce weight loss without you creating your own calorie deficit (see Q18). A properly trained aromatherapist meets criteria laid down by the Aromatherapy Organizations Council. A list of these practitioners can be obtained from the address that follows.

■ The International Federation of Aromatherapists, 182 Chiswick High Road, London W4 1TH; 020 8742 2605; www.int-fed-aromatherapy.co.uk
See also: Massage; Q146.

Atkins Diet

To give it its complete name, *Dr Atkins New Diet Revolution* (Dr Robert C. Atkins, Vermilion, £6.99) is the most famous high-protein diet of all. The original *Dr Atkins Diet Revolution* was first published thirty years ago, based on the same high-protein, low-carbohydrate, high-fat principles, and this updated version was published in 1992.

The Atkins diet goes against the healthy eating advice given by the World Health Organization, the American Dietetic Association, and the USA and UK Departments of Health, which is that we should eat a diet high in carbohydrates, moderate in protein and moderate in fat. Dr Atkins' diet contains 55–65% fat (compared with the healthy maximum of around 30%), less than 20% carbs (compared with the healthy level of 50–55%) and about 25% protein (as opposed to 15–20% in a normal healthy diet).

Atkins claims that a high-fat, high-protein, low-carb diet automatically ensures that fat is burnt and, he claims, avoiding carbohydrate means that insulin production is decreased, and insulin resistance (see Feature 25) – and therefore obesity – is avoided. Both of these claims are not strictly true.

Firstly, you can get overweight on a high-fat diet, as dietary fat converts to body fat when too many calories for your needs are eaten, from whatever kind of food or drink the calories come. Secondly, insulin resistance doesn't actually cause weight gain, it is simply an associated symptom of obesity in many people. Being obese is more a cause of insulin resistance than vice versa.

Thirdly, Atkins claims that eating a low-carbohydrate diet causes ketosis, which in turn reduces appetite, and this, at least, is true. However ketosis (the production of ketone bodies that replace glucose as a source of energy in the blood when carbohydrate intake is very low) is not a desirable state for the body to be in and can be dangerous. Lastly, the diet claims to boost the metabolic rate, which indeed it may do – eating a high-protein diet increases the metabolic rate through dietary induced thermogenesis (see Q88).

Two other diets which fit into a similar mould are Protein Power and the Carbohydrate Addict's Diet, which aren't rated separately but would receive similar scores to the Atkins diet.

The Diet

There is a 14-day induction diet on which you can eat all meat, fish, poultry, eggs and most cheeses, cream, butter, vegetable oils, mayonnaise, plus small quantities of various salads and vegetables up to 20g of carb a day, while you must avoid all fruit, bread, pasta, grains, starchy vegetables, milk and yoghurt, as well as some other items.

After the 14 days you are perhaps allowed a little more carbohydrate (from 15-60g a day) for the ongoing diet, depending upon your own level of what Atkins terms 'metabolic resistance to weight loss', but amounts are still tiny – Atkins describes grapefruits and apples as high-carbohydrate foods and calls all fruit 'risky'. A weight maintenance diet allows small amounts of certain grains and perhaps a piece of fruit or a potato now and then, and nuts and seeds.

Typical calorie count for a day's eating: 1,400–500.
Weight loss promise: Average of 4–12 lb (1.8–5.4kg) in the first 14 days.
Typical day's eating on the induction plan:

■ ***Breakfast:*** Ham, fried egg; decaffeinated coffee; water.
■ ***Lunch:*** Salad of 1/2 medium avocado, 1 small tomato and chicken with olive oil dressing; water.
■ ***Evening:*** Prawn cocktail with a little Iceberg lettuce and mayonnaise dressing; steak, 6 slices of cucumber and 1/2 small onion salad with sour cream; soda water.

Short-term effectiveness: Because of the drastic reduction in carbohydrate (which causes fluid loss from the body) and calories (which causes fat loss), weight loss may be rapid. ● **Score: 5**

Long-term effectiveness: If strictly adhered to, weight loss will continue and may be rapid, tailing off as ideal weight is neared. ● **Score: 5**

Ease of use: The major part of the diet is easy as you don't have to weigh or measure foods that don't contain carbohydrate (e.g. meat, oils, eggs), but for the small amounts of carbohydrate allowed in the diet it is best to count the grams (chart provided in the book) to make sure you don't go over your limit – this can be fiddly. Eating out may be a problem, and overall the diet requires a high level of dedication. ● **Score: 2**

Cost: Animal protein foods can be expensive, as can many of the salad items and allowed vegetables. Many low-cost foods, such as bread, potatoes, rice and pasta, are all but banned. ● **Score: 1**

Palatability: Of little use to vegetarians and far from ideal for anyone who enjoys fruit, vegetables, and carbohydrate foods, has a sweet tooth or enjoys a glass of wine or, indeed, unrestricted access to a wide variety of healthy foods. Has been described as boring. Could be painless for committed carnivores and vegetable-haters. ● **Score: 2**

Satiety: A diet very low in carbohydrates produces ketosis, which gives a feeling of fullness, but psychological hunger may be a problem as food choices are so restricted. ● **Score: 3**

Health factor: Hard to find any health professionals who endorse a high-protein, high-fat, low-carbohydrate diet, with the levels of total fat, saturated fat and cholesterol so out of kilter with current recommendations. At such a low carbohydrate intake, fibre content is very low indeed and there may be shortfall in the vitamins, minerals and plant chemicals found in these foods. The US Department of Agriculture, in its recent review of popular diets, found that high-fat, low-carb diets are low in vitamins E, A, thiamin, B6, folate, calcium, magnesium, iron, zinc and potassium; may produce higher than average lean tissue loss and may cause feelings of weakness or faintness. Ketosis may produce nausea, bad breath and a nasty taste in the mouth. Diets high in protein can accelerate calcium loss from the body and may increase risk of osteoporosis. Low-carbohydrate diets are contraindicated for sportspeople and other very active people. Nutrition Australia has described the diet as unsuitable for use in either the short or long term, and the USA Physicians' Committee for Responsible Medicine in its 2001 review of diets gave the Atkins diet no stars – an 'unsafe' rating, describing high-protein diets as 'dangerous over the long run'. ● **Score: 0**

Scientific basis: However much insulin there is in the blood, you won't store food as fat unless you create a positive energy balance (i.e., eat more than you need). The USDA reports that diets such as the Atkins Diet work because, when carbohydrates are so restricted, the calories from ingested fat and protein are 'self limiting', thus overall calorie intake is decreased. In other words, there is little scientific magic to the diet – it is a calorie-restricted diet by another name. There may also be an increase in metabolic rate due to raised dietary-induced thermogenesis and fluid loss. ● **Score: 2**

Total score 20

Percentage rating 50%

■ *Dr Atkins New Diet Revolution* (Robert C Atkins, 3rd revised edition, Vermilion p/b, £6.99, January I999, ISBN 0 09186783 5)

■ www.atkinscenter.com

■ Atkins Nutritionals 001 516 563 9280.

See also: Q88, Carbohydrate Addict's Diet, High-fat diets, High-protein diets, Protein Power, Top 20 Popular Diets.

Ayurveda

Ayurveda is an ancient Indian system of natural, holistic medicine. Treatments include diet, herbs, exercise, meditation and detoxifying. There are three basic body types in Ayurveda – Vata, Pitta and Kapha – and the Kapha type strongly correlates with the endomorph in Western body typing (see Feature 4). According to Ayurvedic principles, the Kapha has a slow metabolism and a large appetite, and may put on weight easily.

To control this tendency, a Kapha-pacifying diet should be followed; this is, basically, one which avoids sweet and salty foods, dairy produce and fried foods, and which is high in vegetables, salads, light and 'dry' foods. Indeed, on such a diet, most people would lose weight as overall calorie intake would be low to moderate. For more information on Kapha types and Ayurveda, see the address below.

■ Ayurvedic Medical Association UK, 59 Dulverton Road, Selsdon, South Croydon, Surrey CR2 8PJ; 0208 657 6147.

See also: Q146.

Bathroom scales

Although it isn't completely necessary to weigh yourself to find out whether or not you're overweight – an honest look in the mirror can usually give you a pretty accurate idea – bathroom scales are a useful tool.

Choose bathroom scales to match your income and needs. I would opt for a set that measures weight in both metric and imperial, as most of us have a job understanding our weight in kilos. Many modern scales only measure in kilos, so beware. If your eyesight isn't good, go for a set with an eye-level readout or with an extra-large dial and print. Check how much the scales weigh up to – some only weigh to 18 stones (115 kg). In any case, if you are over 20 stones I recommend that you get a professional-quality scale for accuracy and robustness (e.g. Salter Professional model 200). If you have very big feet, you may find lots of modern scales are too small for you to stand on.

Some scales come with a built-in body fat monitor. There is even a scale which, when programmed with your height, gives you your Body Mass Index (Salter Body Mass Index Scale Model 992).

How accurate are most scales? In one test I ran several years ago, not one set of scales was 100% accurate when compared with weight recorded by an official weights inspector. However, this may not matter. Few scales are more than a half stone (3kg) or so out either way, and if you always weigh yourself on the same scales then you will still know whether or not you are maintaining your weight. You should also keep the scales in the same place, as they will weigh differently on different surfaces.

Brandsmall.com (click on health and beauty products) has an extensive range of discounted bathroom scales from a few pounds up to top-of-the range, or try www.scalesexpress.com.

The BBC Diet

This book, following a TV series, was a big hit in 1988 for Dr Barry Lynch and the follow-up, *The Complete BBC Diet*, is still available. It was often acclaimed as a healthy and sensible diet plan, with recipes, exercise, advice on weight maintenance and so on.

■ *The Complete BBC Diet* by Dr Barry Lynch (BBC Books, revised edition January I994) ISBN 0 14023722 4.

Beverly Hills Diet

The original Beverly Hills Diet, published in 1981, was a huge success in the US and UK, and its author, Judy Mazel, recently published *New Beverly Hills Diet*, which is similar to the first in concept. Ms Mazel believes that the body needs the enzymes found in particular foods in order to digest food and convert it to energy. For example, her theory is that the enzymes found in fruit will break that fruit down in the body but won't allow other forms of carbohydrate foods to be digested, or those that contain protein or fat. We become overweight, she says, when our food isn't digested, but turns to body fat.

This theory is fantasy – no food can make you fat until it has been digested, and it is the body that makes its own digestive enzymes, and enzymes found in food will be broken down by the digestive system.

The Diet

Based on what Mazel calls 'conscious combining' (this is not quite the same as the Hay system of food combining), the diet contains a great deal of fruit. There are fruit-only days (e.g. up to 5lb/2.25kg of grapes on a grape day is not excessive, says Mazel), vegetable days, and days when you are allowed some starchy carbohydrate or some protein (but little else). The rules are quite complicated, considering how little there is to eat.

Typical calorie count for a day's eating: 800.

Promised weight loss: Up to 15lb (6.75kg) in 35 days.

Typical day's eating:

- ***Breakfast:*** 8oz (225g) prunes.
- ***Lunch:*** Unlimited strawberries.
- ***Evening:*** Baked potato.
- ***To drink:*** Water, coffee or tea.

Short-term effectiveness: This is a crash diet by another name, and initial weight loss will usually be high, much of which will be fluid and lean tissue. ● **Score: 3**

Long-term effectiveness: Few people can sustain such a restricted and low-calorie diet for long, which is just as well. For long-term maintenance Mazel relies upon limiting types of food at one meal – e.g., three proteins, or three carbs, or fruit only with Champagne, with mono meals (one food only) interspersed to keep overall calorie count low. Compliance would be difficult over time. ● **Score: 1**

Ease of use: Only limited weighing and measuring, but diet ingredients may be hard to find and the diet is very antisocial – eating out or at friends' houses would be hard. ● **Score: 2**

Cost: Many of the ingredients are expensive. ● **Score: 2**

Palatability: If you like fruit and vegetables you may like the diet, but the one-food-only meals would become very boring for many people, and starches such as baked potato are not very palatable when served alone. ● **Score: 2**

Satiety: Unless specified, you can eat all you want of the food allowed at a particular meal until you are full! she says. But it is surprisingly hard to eat a great deal of a single food, as all research has found. On fruit-only days (particularly with pineapple or watermelon, both high on the Glycaemic Index), blood sugar levels are likely to fluctuate and you may feel hungry. ● **Score: 2**

Health factor: With such a restricted range of foods, especially in the early stages, nutrient shortfalls are likely, including some vitamins and minerals, protein and essential fats. People unused to high amounts of fruit may suffer from stomach cramps, diarrhoea and wind. The faddy element of the diet may encourage a poor relationship with food. Calorie content is likely to be too low for short- or long-term use and, on some days, blood sugar levels may fluctuate and cause lethargy/dizziness/weakness. ● **Score: 1**

Scientific basis: The diet may work to help weight loss because it is low, or very low, in calories. The 'scientific' theories behind the system show a lack of understanding of nutrition and how the body works. ● **Score: 1**

Total score 14

Percentage score 35%

■ *The New Beverly Hills Diet* by Judy Mazel (Health Communications, November 1996, ISBN 1 55874431 2).

See also: Top 20 Popular Diets.

Body-clock Diet

There are two body-clock diet books currently available. The earliest is *The Body-clock Diet* by Dr Alan Maryon Davis (Network Books, l996 ISBN 0 56337159 5), which is a diet for women geared to the cycles of the monthly period. The second is *The Body Clock Diet* by Sidney MacDonald Baker and Karen Baar (Vermilion, 2001, ISBN 0 09185656 6), which provides a diet based on the theory that we should eat to suit our day and night rhythms. By timing our consumption of protein (in the morning) and carbohydrate (in the evening), we can control our weight and prevent disease.

Scientific research shows that there is some benefit to be had by eating in this way, as higher-protein meals in the morning keep us more alert and high-carbohydrate meals in the evening help us to relax and sleep well – but if you are to lose weight, the success of the diet depends upon its total calorie intake and whether or not this is low enough to help you slim.

Body fat monitors

Although your Body Mass Index can give a very good indication of whether or not you need to lose (or gain) weight, the most accurate gauge of whether or not you have a true weight problem can be found by measuring your body fat percentage.

Body fat can be measured using simple skin fold callipers, although results can be inconsistent, especially with the cheaper plastic callipers. The callipers grip two layers of skin in various places on the body (e.g. triceps, abdomen and thigh), the distance between them is measured and the amount of subcutaneous fat can then be calculated. You really need to get someone else to use the callipers on you.

Buy callipers that come with a booklet explaining how to work out body fat percentage from the measurements taken. The most expensive and accurate type is the Harpenden at around £200; but basic plastic callipers plus booklet (e.g. AccuMeasure) are around £15.

You can also purchase electronic body fat monitors. These work by 'bioelectrical impedance analysis', where electrode pads are placed on the wrist and foot and a current passed through the body, from which body fat percentage can be estimated (e.g. Maltron Bioimpedance Monitor, from about £165). These are normally used in gyms and health centres. There are also monitors in the form of scales – where you get a readout while standing on the platform (Tanita TBF-551, about £90, Tanita BF350, about £420), and handheld simple versions (Omron BF300, about £76).

It is debatable whether it is worth investing a lot of money in a machine to measure your body fat, as a combination of the BMI and Waist Circumference (see Feature 3) can tell the average person almost as much. See also Q30.

■ Proactive Health sells a range of callipers and body fat monitors: 0870 8484842; www.proactive-health.co.uk

Body for Life

This bestselling book by US fitness guru Bill Phillips claims to be able to transform your shape and your fitness in 12 weeks, and there is a strong bodybuilding element. The book urges you to buy supplements from Bill Phillips' own organization. The recommended diet is high-protein, which isn't in line with current nutritional thinking. The workout programmes in the book are reasonable – but, if you are an absolute beginner, I'd start on something easier first (like the exercise programmes in this book).

■ *Body for Life* by Bill Phillips, (HarperCollins, November l999) ISBN 0 06019339 5.

'British Heart Foundation Diet'

A one-sheet diet to lose 10lb (4.5kg) in three days has been passed around – usually via fax – in the UK in recent years, often attributed to the British Heart Foundation and sometimes called the Greenlane Diet. This faddy diet is, in fact, nothing whatsoever to do with the British Heart Foundation, who don't endorse diets. And if they did, I am sure they wouldn't endorse this one! Where it actually did start, I can't find out, though as the diet uses 'cups' as a measure it looks like it must be from the USA.

The diet itself is a strangely old-fashioned and unpalatable one, similar to crash diets of the 1970s, containing grapefruit, dry toast, cottage cheese, 'snax' biscuits (whatever they are) and quite a lot of tuna and beetroot. There seems to be no logical reason behind the choice of foods and there is no magic chemical reaction likely here to make you slim. The calorie content is very low – at about 700 a day – which is why you would lose weight on it, but such a low-calorie intake is best avoided unless under medical supervision. In other words – bin the diet if you ever get a copy.

Sample day's eating:

■ ***Breakfast:*** 5 'snax' biscuits, l slice of Cheddar cheese, l small apple; l cup of black tea/coffee/water.

■ ***Lunch:*** l boiled egg, l slice of dry toast; black tea/coffee/water.

■ ***Dinner:*** l cup of tuna, l cup of beetroot, 1 cup of cauliflower; 1/2 melon, 1/2 cup of diet vanilla ice-cream; black tea/coffee/water.

■ Most of the comments and ratings under the entry on Crash diets will apply to this diet.

Cabbage Soup Diet

This is a very-low-calorie, low-fat diet based on a mixed vegetable soup and a few other foods, including fruits, vegetables and restricted carbohydrates and protein. The usual advice is to follow it for a week, then eat normally for two weeks, before following it again as necessary. The rumour that it was recommended by American heart organizations is completely false; it was spread mainly through the Internet, and isn't endorsed by any health professionals as far as I know.

The Diet

The soup (enough for about 6 portions) is made from 3 onions, l green pepper, l head of celery, half a cabbage, 2 tins of chopped tomatoes, l pack of onion soup mix and 3 pints of vegetable stock from cubes.

Typical calorie count for a day's eating: 800–1,000.

Promised weight loss: Up to 10lb (4.5kg) in 7 days.

■ ***Day 1:*** Unlimited cabbage soup; unlimited free fruits (most allowed except bananas); tea, coffee (black, unsweetened), water, cranberry juice.

■ ***Day 2:*** Unlimited cabbage soup, raw or plainly cooked vegetables (most except potatoes allowed); one large baked potato with butter in the evening; drinks as Day l.

■ ***Day 3:*** Unlimited cabbage soup; free fruits and veg; drinks as Day 1.

■ ***Day 4:*** Unlimited cabbage soup; up to 6 bananas; up to 8 glasses of skimmed milk, drinks as Day 1.

■ ***Day 5:*** Unlimited cabbage soup; up to 500g (1lb 2oz) lean beef (or chicken); 1 large tin of tomatoes or 6 fresh tomatoes; drinks as Day 1.

■ ***Day 6:*** Unlimited cabbage soup; unlimited lean beef (or chicken), unlimited free vegetables; drinks as Day 1.

■ ***Day 7:*** Unlimited cabbage soup; unlimited boiled brown rice, unlimited free vegetables; drinks as Day 1.

Short-term effectiveness: As average daily intake would be 800–1,000 calories, weight loss is virtually guaranteed. ● **Score: 5**

Long-term effectiveness: Not recommended as a sole long-term diet, but used one week in three might result in long-term weight loss or weight maintenance. ● **Score: 2**

Ease of use: Not too much to remember and little cooking involved, but involves preparing separate meals from non-dieting household members. ● **Score: 3**

Cost: Inexpensive. ● **Score: 5**

Palatability: Small range of foods allowed; won't be appreciated by people unused to a very high intake of fruits and vegetables; the soup is fairly boring with no herbs or spices recommended. ● **Score: 2**

Satiety: No need to feel hungry as various items are unlimited on each day, but people used to a more balanced diet may well feel cravings for other types of food. ● **Score: 2**

Health factor: Most days very low in protein, carbs, calcium and essential fats. The soup is high in salt (and probably monosodium glutamate)

because of the onion soup mix and stock cubes. Averaged out over the week, the fruit and veg content is reasonable, probably representing 6–7 portions a day. However, the diet encourages the idea of avoiding a whole range of foods, encourages faddy eating and is probably much lower in calories than experts recommend. It is, in effect, a crash diet. ● **Score: 0**
Scientific basis: Claims no miracles, works via low calorie content – although, if the 'unlimited' soup and other unlimited items were eaten to excess, calorie content might not be low and a correspondingly low weight loss result. ● **Score: 3**
Total score 22
Percentage rating 55%
The New Cabbage Soup Diet by Margaret Danbrot (Blake, £5.99 ISBN 1 85782 4105) modifies the above diet to improve its nutritional profile.
See also: Crash diets, Top 20 popular diets.

Caffeine/caffeine supplements

Caffeine is not only a stimulant which keeps you alert, but has been shown to enhance sports performance in certain conditions. Studies found that 3–13mg of caffeine per 2 1/4 lb (1kg) of body weight (about 180–780mg for a 135lb (60kg) person – or the equivalent of 2–6 cups of coffee, depending upon strength) taken an hour before exercise, such as running or cycling, improves endurance by prolonging time before exhaustion. An average of 2 1/2 cups produces about 20% better performance in moderately strenuous exercise. It probably does this by increasing production of epinephrine, which in turn mobilizes the body's fat stores that can then be used for energy, thus sparing glycogen stores.

In strength training, caffeine mobilizes calcium, which improves muscle strength, but not mass. With constant use, however, these effects diminish (i.e. if you take caffeine regularly, it won't work) and consuming a high-carb meal at the same time (as many sportspeople do) also diminishes the effect. Caffeine is a diuretic, so may cause dangerous dehydration during prolonged exercise.

Caffeine has also been cited as an aid to slimmers because of its stimulating effects on the nervous system and hence the metabolism – unless you drink a lot of coffee (which isn't advisable), though, overall effect will be small. The fat-mobilizing effect described is of no use unless you burn the mobilized fat off with exercise. If you don't, it will simply be restored as body fat.

In the USA, caffeine hasn't been present in over-the-counter diet supplements for several years, as the Food and Drug Administration stated there was no evidence for its efficacy. Caffeine is widely available in many drinks, including coffee, tea, hot chocolate, cola and energy drinks. It is also available in various sports supplements which are sold on the Internet.

Caffeine over-consumption can have negative side effects (see Q101). My advice for slimmers and normal exercisers (not athletes) is that dallying with supplements or increasing levels by other means is not a good option.
See also: Q101, Sports supplements.

Calorie Counting

One of the most universally recognized ways to lose weight, calorie counting involves deciding upon a suitable daily calorie intake for weight loss – which can be varied according to the individual's needs – and then keeping food intake within that calorie level, with the help of a guide to the calorie content of all food and drink or with calorie-counted menus. For accuracy, most foods will need to be weighed or measured. (Note – all diets that work rely upon creating an energy deficit through reduction of calories, but are listed under their more typical headings, e.g. high-fibre, low-fat, high-protein.)

The Diet

A sample day of calorie-controlled eating at approx. 1,500 calories:
■ ***Skimmed milk allowance:*** 250 ml (9fl oz)
■ ***Unlimited:*** Tea or coffee (with milk from allowance), salad greens, herbs and spices.
■ ***Breakfast:*** 30g (1oz) bowl of cornflakes with 5 tbsp skimmed milk (extra to allowance) and l tsp sugar; l slice of toast from a medium-cut large sliced loaf with 7g (1/4oz) low-fat spread and 7g (1/4oz) low-sugar marmalade.
■ ***Mid-morning snack:*** 125ml (4fl oz) tub of diet fruit yoghurt.
■ ***Lunch:*** Sandwich of 1 x 100g (3 1/2oz) can of tuna in brine, drained, in 2 slices of bread from a medium-cut large sliced loaf with 7g (1/4oz) low-fat spread, green salad items and l dessertspoon reduced-fat mayonnaise; l apple.
■ ***Mid-afternoon snack:*** 2 fingers of Kitkat.
■ ***Evening meal:*** l x 150g (5oz) chicken breast, baked, with 1 x 150g (5oz) baked potato and 10g (1/3oz) knob of butter; 100g (3 1/2oz) mixed frozen peas and carrots; 2 1/2dsp instant gravy; 70g (2 1/2oz) low-fat vanilla ice-cream with 1 dsp strawberry sauce.

Short-term effectiveness: Will work to produce weight loss if the calorie level chosen is large enough to create an energy deficit. ● **Score: 4**
Long-term effectiveness: A calorie-controlled diet can be followed indefinitely and because of the variety of foods allowed may be easier to follow long-term than many other diets. However, the necessary weighing and measuring is a chore which often causes people to 'slip'. ● **Score: 4**
Ease of use: A lot of weighing and measuring of foods involved in order to stay within calorie limit, which is not always practical, but fits in well with normal eating patterns. ● **Score: 3**
Cost: Varies according foods chosen, adaptable. ● **Score: 4**
Palatability: Dieter can choose foods and drinks to suit and therefore is likely to choose those he or she enjoys. ● **Score: 5**
Satiety: Varies with foods chosen; may be low. ● **Score: 3**
Health factor: Offers the chance for a varied diet, which is good, but plenty of room for abuse as poor food choices may be made. The

sample diet listed above offers adequate protein, simple carbohydrates, minerals and most vitamins, but is low on complex carbohydrates, essential fatty acids, fibre and vitamin C. ● Score: 3
Scientific basis: Scientifically proven method of losing weight. ● Score: 5
Typical weight loss: 1–2lb (0.5–1kg) a week.
Total score 31
Percentage rating 77.5%
Comprehensive calorie guides to branded and non-branded foods and drink are produced in booklet form and updated regularly; these are on sale in newsagents shops (e.g. *A–Z of Calories*, Octavo, £1.99, *Your Greatest Guide to Calories and Fat*, Slimming Magazine, £1.99).
See also: Section Three, Qs 74–104; Feature 9, Top 20 popular diets.

Carbohydrate Addicts' Diet

Richard and Rachael Heller wrote this diet in the 90s and have produced a follow-up with 475 hefty pages. Basically it is a low-carb, high-fat, high-protein programme not of the kind currently recommended by health organizations and similar in style to all the other low-carb diets mentioned in the A–Z, including the Atkins Diet and Protein Power.
■ *The Carbohydrate Addict's Lifespan Programme* by Rachael Heller and Richard Heller (Plume Books, January 1998) ISBN 0 45227838 4.
See also: Qs 80, 88; Atkins Diet, High-protein diets, Protein Power.

Cellulite treatments

As Qs 210–14 explain, beating cellulite is a long and slow process, to be won only through a combination of diet and exercise, with regular vigorous massage also helping to improve the look of the skin. Despite this, there are thousands of 'cures' and treatments available. Here are just some.
Cellulite creams: Creams (often sold with massage mitts) are rubbed into the areas of cellulite daily. These creams contain a variety of ingredients said to stimulate fat metabolism – for instance xanthines – in laboratory conditions, but recent studies have not shown them to be effective with cellulite. They may also cause an allergic reaction. Cellulite creams were tested in a double-blind study published in the *British Journal of Plastic and Reconstructive Surgery* (September 1999) and, after 12 weeks, only 3 of 17 women reported even slight improvements. What creams will do, when used with massage, is help to improve the texture of the skin and therefore the appearance.
Massage: Manual massage can increase the circulation and lymphatic drainage, reduce muscular spasms, and can improve the appearance of the skin over cellulite, smoothing its appearance somewhat. Massage with a mechanical device (such as those used in beauty salons) may be more effective as the force used may be stronger.

One mechanical system of massage called Endermologie, carried out in salons, has been approved by the US Food and Drug Administration as 'temporarily' reducing the appearance of cellulite – note the word 'temporarily'. This system uses a double-headed rolling and suction action. In the same British study that evaluated the massage creams, Endermologie was tested and one-third of the women said that they felt there was an improvement in their cellulite while two-thirds did not feel this.
Herbal supplements: Herbal supplements sold as aids to cellulite reduction often contain a similar range of plant extracts, frequently including bladderwrack (for thyroid function/fluid retention), gingko biloba (said to stimulate circulation), horse chestnut, grapeseed extract, and so on. The selling literature promotes these supplements as aids to circulation and fluid drainage, and some claim to stimulate metabolism and reduce localized fats – without the need to diet or exercise. There are also herbal patches on sale that are said to work in a similar way.

However, these products don't have to be properly scientifically tested. In one well-known case in 2000, the US Federal Trade Commission charged the importers of the most popular brand, Cellasene, with making false claims for the product. And in November 1999 British research was published in the *Journal of Psychotherapy* in which neither women who tried a placebo pill nor women on Cellasene noticed any improvement in their cellulite. Some supplements contain high levels of iodine, which could be dangerous. My advice: your money is probably better spent on healthy food and exercise.
Liposuction: Liposuction is best for deep fat, rather than that near the skin, and thus isn't an effective treatment for cellulite.
Electrotherapy: Electricity passed through pads on the skin stimulates the muscle under the pad. However, this form of 'toning' isn't suitable for the treatment of cellulite (which is fat, not muscle) and the US Food and Drug Administration considers promotion of muscle stimulators for cellulite reduction fraudulent.
See also: Qs 210–14, Salon treatments.

Chewing gum

There are several brands of chewing gum made for slimmers, most of which contain the trace mineral chromium (see next entry) and are said to help curb sugar cravings and control blood sugar levels. Others contain hydroxycitric acid, which is said to make you feel full. If you tend to overeat because you need something to 'chew on', then chewing gum (any sort, not just for slimmers) might help you eat less. There is, however, little scientific evidence that these special gums can help you to lose weight because of their ingredients.

Chromium picolinate

Chromium is a trace mineral found in greatest quantities in broccoli, brewer's yeast, wheat germ, nuts, liver, prunes, egg yolks, apples, cheese and many other foods. In the body, chromium acts as an insulin 'helper', transporting nutrients to where they are needed. Supplements of chromium, in a form with picolinic acid (said to aid absorption), are promoted as aids to weight loss, fat burning and muscle building.

Athletes in training, with diets producing less than 200mcg of chromium a day, may benefit from a supplement. Research from the American Department of Agriculture also indicates that glycaemic control in diabetics may be helped with supplements, but the scientific evidence for the remaining claims appears to be unsubstantiated.

Indeed, one trial showed that sedentary overweight people actually gain weight when using the supplement, and another that chromium picolinate was no more useful than a placebo in enhancing lean tissue levels or promoting fat loss while exercising. In addition, chromium supplements may accumulate in the body to dangerous levels, and may also interfere with the working of iron to produce iron-deficient anaemia.

Cider vinegar

Cider vinegar is often claimed to have special properties in aiding weight loss – but other than the fact it is virtually calorie-free and can be added to the list of 'unlimited' items on your slimming plan, it has no magic slimming properties at all. It won't put fat on – but won't take it off, either.

CLA

CLA, or conjugated linoleic acid, is a compound that occurs naturally in the diet, mainly in the fat of meat and dairy produce, and is showing exciting promise in the field of weight control and body composition. The British Nutrition Foundation's definition of the compound is 'a collective term for metabolic by-products resulting from the conversion of linoleic acid to oleic acid by rumen bacteria'.

Since its accidental discovery in l979 by Professor Michael Pariza (Food Research Institute, University of Wisconsin), CLA has been the subject of many scientific trials. The first trials on 20 men and women in Norway in l997 using CLA capsules showed an average reduction of 7lb (3kg) of body fat over 3 months, while the control group had no reduction. *The Journal of Clinical Nutrition* reported another 60-person Norwegian trial in which the volunteers who took CLA lost an average of 6lb (2.75kg) over 12 weeks without dieting or exercise.

According to researchers in Ohio, CLA supplements increased arm girth, enhanced muscle strength and boosted lean tissue in bodybuilders. In 2000, the American Chemical Society therefore concluded that CLA can help people to lose weight and improve the ratio of fat to muscle.

How does it work? CLA appears to work by regulating enzymes in the fat cells, reducing the rate at which the body deposits fat and helping to break down stored fat. Also by tending to increase lean tissue, which is more metabolically active than fat, it can increase the metabolic rate and increase weight loss that way.

Scientists have estimated that 3.4g a day is enough CLA to get these beneficial effects. Such an amount is almost impossible to get from a normal diet. However, supplements appear to be 100% safe. Currently available supplements provide varying amounts of CLA, from as little as 800mg per capsule. These are expensive – one brand is £44.95 for a month's supply. However the US Department of Agriculture is looking at ways of increasing the CLA in our diets by producing CLA-rich milk, eggs and pork, which may render supplements unnecessary for all but vegans.

In the UK, supplements can be obtained from Biocare (brand-name Lipotone; tel 0121 433 8710); Reflex Nutrition Ltd (brand-name Reflex CLA; tel 0870 757 3353). CLA is also known to control type-2 diabetes in adults and as well as several types of cancer and atherosclerosis.

Co-enzyme Q10

Q10 – also known as ubiquinone – is a substance similar to a vitamin, the role of which throughout the body is to facilitate the conversion of food to energy and act as an antioxidant. Scientific tests over 15 years have shown that supplements of co-Q10 can be helpful for people with heart conditions such as angina pectoris, in aiding oxygen uptake by the heart when they exercise, meaning they can exercise for longer. There is also solid research that shows co-enzyme Q10 can improve the condition of the gums and help to prevent gingivitis.

It is contained in offal, spinach and pulses, as well as a variety of other foods, but it is thought that ageing and illness may reduce the body's ability to synthesize it. Recently, co-enzyme Q10 has been touted as an aid to slimming, but scientific proof is not forthcoming. However, there is plenty of anecdotal evidence of improved energy levels and reduction in chronic tiredness through taking supplements. This could result in a greater willingness to take regular exercise, which could have a knock-on effect in creating enough calorie deficit to help weight loss indirectly. There are no known toxic effects. A supplement of 30mg a day is typical, and these can be bought in pharmacies, health food shops and via all the major supplement mail order companies.

Counselling

Some people find that one-to-one counselling can help them with their food- or weight-related problems. Compulsive or binge eaters, in particular, can respond well to counselling sessions. The organizations listed below can put you in touch with counsellors in your area, or you could try counselling one-to-one on one of the Internet websites.

- The British Association for Counselling and Psychotherapy (BACP), 1 Regent Place, Rugby, Warks CV21 2PJ; tel 0870 4435252; www.bad.co.uk
- The British Association for Behavioural and Cognitive Psychotherapy, PO Box 9, Accrington, Lancs BB5 2GD; 01254 875277.

■ The Eating Disorders Association helpline: 01603 621414 (9am-6.30pm); www.edauk.com
■ The National Centre for Eating Disorders (offers one-to-one counselling); 01372 469493; www.eating-disorders.org.uk
■ Mind (National Association for Mental Health) 020 8519 2122; www.mind.org.uk
■ www.psychologyonline.co.uk
■ www.friendly-ear.com

Crash diets

Sometimes called 'fad' diets, these diets are very low in calories (normally well under 1,000 cals/day) and are usually based on a restricted selection of foods – e.g., fruit or eggs, or cheese or juices, or combinations of two or three of these. The name derives from the fact that the weight is supposed to come 'crashing' off. Such diets are usually followed for a short period of time and most are 'set' diets – stating exactly what and when you should eat each day and at each meal. Very popular in the 70s and 80s, they now appear to be having a revival.

Sample two-week diet
■ ***Breakfast:*** Boiled egg, crispbread; apple juice.
■ ***Mid-morning:*** Apple juice.
■ ***Lunch:*** Cheddar cheese, lettuce, tomato, cucumber; apple juice, black coffee.
■ ***Mid-afternoon snack:*** Apple juice or lemon tea.
■ ***Evening:*** Mug of Bovril, boiled egg, crispbread, tomato.
(Further 13 days repeated similarly with a few minor variations and one liquids-only day.)
(Ratings and comments below apply to crash diets in general and not specifically to the one above.)
Typical day's calorie intake: 6–800
Promised weight loss: Some promise up to 14 lb (6.5kg) in 2 weeks.

Short-term effectiveness: As calorie count is very low on crash diets – e.g. the one above is about 650/day – weight loss is inevitable. Most crash diets are low in carbs and initial weight loss will be quite drastic as much of loss is fluid. ● **Score: 3**
Long-term effectiveness: Weight loss will continue but slow down (for explanations on this, see Sections 1 and 3). Compliance – how well you stick to the diet – with such a restricted diet would be low in the long term, but in the medium term, one interesting study conducted by the world-famous obesity expert Professor John Garrow and colleagues found that 15 obese patients lost on average 1 1/2 stones (9.5kg) on a 16-week milk-only diet of approximately 800 calories a day. Professor Garrow reported that these weight loss results were significantly better than for the people in the trial following a conventional diet, and were comparable with treatment by obesity drugs. He concluded, 'We are not advocating milk only as a general long-term reducing diet ... because in the long term it will cease to be novel and compliance will fall. Probably the best strategy is to rotate diets...' Surprising – and very interesting – comments. However, these patients were monitored and the picture may be very different for someone dieting alone. Health organizations worldwide are unanimous in saying that in the long term, crash diets don't work (because people don't stick to them and/or regain the weight afterwards). ● **Score: 1**
Ease of use: Most crash diets are easy and quick to prepare, and take away the element of choice and dilemma. As Garrow found with his milk diet, patients found it 'novel and simple'. However, such diets may not fit in well with normal family and social eating. ● **Score: 3**
Cost: Depends on which diet is being followed, but usually fairly low-cost as the amount of food that needs to be purchased is low. ● **Score: 3**
Palatability: Again, depends on choice, but if the dieter picks foods he or she enjoys, then the diet may be palatable. ● **Score: 3**
Satiety: Most of these diets are so low on calories and carbs that – at least for the first week – they will cause hunger pangs and probably other symptoms of deprivation. ● **Score: 1**
Health factor: A small range of foods will almost inevitably give a small range of nutrients. For example, the diet above is low on carbs, fibre, some vitamins and minerals, including C and calcium, the essential fats and fluid. On a milk-only diet, Garrow reports that over 24 weeks the dieters didn't become deficient in iron or vitamins – again, surprising news – but did become constipated (a likely outcome on many crash diets).

It is widely accepted that crash/fad diets frequently lead to weight regain – the yo-yo dieting syndrome – no reassessment of long-term eating habits and no long-term weight control, all of which is good for neither physical nor mental health. However, for people with life-threatening obesity, monitored crash diets have a place. ● **Score: 1**
Scientific basis: Crash diets work to produce weight loss by reducing calorie intake. However, many are promoted using bogus science or nutrition. ● **Score: 2**
Total score 17
Percentage rating 42.5%
See also: Cabbage Soup Diet, Fasting, Meal replacements, Top 20 popular diets, Very-low-calorie diets, Qs 32–40 & 105–11.

Cycling

Cycling is an excellent form of aerobic exercise, suitable for most fit or fairly fit people, which will help to increase cardiovascular fitness, build lower body muscle, increase metabolic rate, burn calories and thus help with weight loss.
■ British Cycling Federation, National Cycling Centre, Stuart Street, Manchester, M11 4DQ; tel 0161 230 2301; www.bcf.uk.com
See also: Exercise equipment – static bikes; Sports; Feature 29.

Dancing

Dancing is an enjoyable and good way to burn calories as it can be strenuous or less strenuous, depending on the type you choose to do. There are classes for all levels of ability throughout the country.

Further information:

■ For ballroom-type dancing – Dancesport UK 0208 568 0083; www.dancesport.uk.com. For line-dancing classes in your area – www.linedancing.org.uk

See also: Feature 28, Exercise classes.

Detoxing diets

If you want to try a detox you could either follow the simple plan outlined in Feature 26 and Qs 317 and 318, or you could try another method:

Books: There is a plethora of detox books available, almost all of which would help you to lose weight but some are not hot on scientific fact. Amongst the best and/or most popular are:

■ *The Detox Plan* by Jane Alexander (Gaia, May 2000) ISBN 1 85675156 2. Complete decluttering for mind and body including a 10-step body detox. No nonsense; good section on the importance of breathing correctly. My favourite.

■ Jan Scrivner's *Total Detox* (Piatkus, December 2000) ISBN 0 74992153 6. Six types of detox offered from a 30-day 'ultimate detox' to a quick weekend detox.

■ *The Liver Cleansing Diet* by Sandra Cabot (Women's Health Advisory Service, July l996) ISBN 0 64627789 8. One of the first detox books by the Australian doctor, a huge bestseller. Strict early diet, recipes, supplements recommended, all vegetables to be eaten raw.

Detox supplements: The most famous detox aid is probably Bio-Light, a three-day detox in a bottle. It comes in 4 flavours and you take it alongside a reduced-calorie diet to 'feel great, look good and curb weight', so the makers say. The concoction contains items such as cloves, liquorice, kelp, juniper, boldo and fruit juices, and will have a diuretic effect. However, just following a typical low-carb, high-fruit and vegetable detox diet would also have this effect.

Bio-Light, from chemists nationwide, telephone info line: 0239244 9312; www.bio-light.co.uk

There are many other detoxing supplements available, mostly in pill or tincture form. Typical contents include milk thistle (liver detox), artichoke (diuretic) and dandelion (diuretic), but many herbs or antioxidants may be included. There is little scientific evidence for the efficacy of these supplements as aids to a healthy liver, but they may aid fluid elimination. However, they shouldn't be taken for long periods as important minerals can be removed from the body, and in any case they may not offer a great deal more help than the basic detox diet. Taking such supplements without altering your eating and lifestyle habits certainly won't do the trick.

Some of the best supplement companies in the UK are:

■ BioCare Ltd: 0121 433 3727; www.biocare.co.uk

■ The Health and Diet Company: (FSC supplements) 0870 7504527; www.gnc.co.uk

■ Higher Nature Ltd: 01435 882880.

■ Solgar: 01442 890355; www.solgar.com

■ Healthspan: 0800 7312377.

■ Nature's Best: 01892 552176; www.NaturesBestOnline.com

■ Neal's Yard Remedies: 0161 831 7875.

See also: Feature 26; Qs 317, 318; Cellulite treatments, Diuretics.

Diet aromas

Particular aromas are said to blunt the appetite and manufacturers have taken advantage of this idea to produce patches, pens, inhalers and so on, which you sniff when you get the urge to eat. Typical scents are vanilla and chocolate. Some people find them effective, others don't; but one research trial at St George's Hospital in London found people wearing vanilla patches lost twice as much weight as people wearing no patches (but this could have been the placebo effect).

See also: Slimming patches.

Diet coaches

Personal coaching to help you eat healthily and lose weight is becoming more popular in the USA and is beginning to catch on in the UK.

Many personal fitness trainers also offer diet advice, but ask them for their qualifications and references if possible. For reliable diet advice, you would probably be better off visiting a British Dietetic Association nutritionist; their dieticians are all state-registered (SRD) or qualified nutritionists. Be aware that 'nutritional therapists' aren't qualified by the BDA and that they will almost always be keen to suggest supplements you should be taking. With a balanced diet of real food, this should not often be necessary and may cause you unnecessary expense.

Obviously, personal advice can be fairly expensive, although postal advice isn't. A cheaper option with similar benefits, but slightly less personal attention, would be to join a slimming club. An even cheaper option, if you have a serious problem, would be to visit your doctor and get referred to a dietician.

■ British Dietetic Association: for a list of private practitioners in your area, send a SAE, marking your outward-going envelope 'Private Practice', to the British Dietetic Association, 5th Floor, Charles House, 148/9 Great Charles Street, Queensway, Birmingham B3 3HT; 0121 200 8080; www.bda.uk.com

■ SlymRyte: 0870 7280606; www.slymryte.co.uk. In-person visits in some areas, or diets by mail (high-protein only at the moment – see High-protein diets).

■ Total Health Personal Training: 01784 469996.
■ British Association of Nutritional Therapists: 0870 606 1284.
See also: Internet slimming, Personal trainers, slimming clubs.

The Diet Cure

This book by Julia Ross claims to end food cravings, mood swings and weight problems by 'rebalancing' your body's chemistry through what she describes as natural food supplements. The dietary advice in this book goes down the 'high-protein' route, with fairly small amounts of carbohydrate (rarely wheat) allowed. Although she says you should eat at least 2,100 cals/day, totting up the menu suggestions the daily total appears to come out on average at about 500 less than that, using average portion sizes.

With a healthy diet, a long list of dietary supplements (which may include items like amino acids, thyroid boosters, aloe vera and others) should rarely be necessary in order to control your weight or beat other symptoms such as hypoglycaemia (low blood sugar).
■ *The Diet Cure* by Julia Ross (Michael Joseph, 2000) ISBN 0 71814397 3.

Dine Out and Lose Weight

This is the title of a book by French dieting guru Michel Montignac which was very popular in the 90s with business people in France and the UK as it described how you could eat out regularly and still slim. It is a fairly high-fat, high-protein, low-carb diet, with alcohol allowed.
■ *Dine Out and Lose Weigh*t by Michel Montignac, revised September l996 (Montignac Publishing) ISBN 2 90623634 9. Also by Michel Montignac, *Eat Yourself Slim – and Stay Slim!* (Montignac Publishing August l999) ISBN 2 91273700 1.

Diuretics

Diuretic foods or supplements won't help you shed body fat, only fluid. Certain foods and herbs – such as melon, celery, watercress, asparagus, artichoke and dandelion – are natural diuretics and regularly including them in your diet may help alleviate fluid retention. A range of diuretic supplements is available from almost all major supplement manufacturers and these often include celery seed, juniper berries, parsley and dandelion. Diuretic supplements shouldn't be taken for more than a few days as they can flush important minerals from your body, and in any case it is always best to aim to relieve fluid retention via diet and exercise. Diuretic drugs (prescription only) are mainly prescribed for reducing fluid retention in people at risk from high blood pressure, heart disease, liver or kidney disorders.
■ See the list of supplement manufacturers under Detoxing diets.
See also: Feature 17, Q203, Cellulite treatments, Detoxing diets, Diuretic diets, Slimming pills.

Diuretic diets

Feature 17 contains a basic safe diuretic diet of especial use for pre-menstrual fluid retention. If you are retaining a lot of fluid (or think you may be) at other times, you should see your doctor for advice as it could be caused by a medical condition. There are various diuretic diet books. The best-selling and most well-known one at the moment is *The Waterfall Diet* by Linda Lazarides (Piatkus September 2000) ISBN 0 74992155 2.

The Diet

Linda states that it isn't a low-calorie diet, but for the first two months all the following are banned: sugar, honey, syrup and all foods containing them, bread and all wheat products, dairy produce, eggs, yeast, red meat of all types, salt and all highly salted foods including ham, bacon, smoked fish, hard cheeses, bought pies, quiches; commercial soft drinks; fatty foods including burgers, sausages, chocolate, crisps, butter, margarine, fried food, cream, cheese, mayonnaise, pastry, sauces, dips and fatty desserts, white flour, alcohol and foods containing artificial additives – all the foods that Lazarides says may be causing your fluid retention.

Avoid that lot and you are almost certain to be reducing your calorie intake significantly, even if you eat your fill of the non-banned foods, which include soya milk and yoghurt, fruit, vegetables, seeds, nuts, oats, brown rice, pulses, lean organic poultry and fish. To drink you can have water, homemade juices, herb teas and other low-caffeine drinks.
Approximate calorie content: 1,000 calories a day.
Weight loss promised: up to 14lb (6.4kg) in a week.
Typical day's eating (first 2 months)
■ ***Breakfast:*** Soya yoghurt with apple compote and nuts; fruit juice.
■ ***Lunch:*** Salad of cooked brown rice, chopped vegetables and tofu or sardine chunks in French dressing; herb tea.
■ ***Evening:*** Mixed vegetable and lentil soup using salt-free stock; homemade oatcakes.
■ ***Snacks:*** fresh fruit, nuts.
The diet goes on to Phase 2, which sets out to find which, if any, foods you are allergic to (as Lazarides says that allergies may cause fluid retention). Phase 3 is a long-term plan with only a few banned foods.

Short-term effectiveness: Avoiding all foods that may encourage fluid retention – particularly refined carbohydrates and salt – will cause the body to lose several pounds of fluid – the amount will vary from person to person. Some body fat will also be lost. ● **Score: 4**
Long-term effectiveness: The diet is likely to continue to produce weight loss and there is a long-term strategy explained, but for many people I fear it will be hard to stick to this diet for life. ● **Score: 3**
Ease of use: For most people who have been eating a typical Western diet, this would be particularly hard to adapt to; major changes need to be made, but some recipes and meal suggestions are given. ● **Score: 1**

Cost: If you shop wisely, choosing fruit and veg in season and cheaper items like pulses and tofu, it needn't be too expensive. Also you won't be buying all those added-value foods like cakes, nor alcohol. ● **Score: 4**
Palatability: Again, for the Western palate, this will be a shock. But, if it is persisted with, the palate should change and the fresh flavours of this basically natural diet should begin to win. ● **Score: 3**
Satiety: There is no portion control, so you can eat all you want of the allowed foods, which should keep you feeling full as there is plenty of fibre and foods low on the Glycaemic Index. ● **Score: 5**
Health factor: The diet has the potential to be quite a healthy one, though items such as wholemeal bread are banned at first, as are lean red meat, wholewheat pasta, eggs and cheese – all staples in most people's diets, and all good foods as part of a balanced diet. This may cause nutritional imbalances over time unless you're very careful and I don't think Lazarides gives enough guidance/menus for a balanced diet. There is plenty of fruit and veg, and the diet is very low in saturated fat, but the tone of the diet is slightly predisposing to encourage faddy eating. ● **Score: 3**
Scientific basis: You will lose fluid on this diet, at least at first, because of the low carbohydrate and salt content – and if you have mild intolerances to one or more of the foods you are required to give up, then that may reduce bloating. You will almost certainly also lose fat as it really is hard to eat a lot of calories. The promised weight loss of up to 14lb (6.4kg) in a week seems excessive. ● **Score: 4**
Total score 27
Percentage rating 67.5%
See also: Q203; Feature 17, Detoxing diets, Diuretics, Low-carbohydrate diets, Top 20 popular diets.

The Doctor's Quick Weight Loss Diet

Over 3 million copies of this diet book by Dr Irwin Stillman were sold between l967 and the 80s, and it was probably the first modern high-protein diet, after which Atkins et al followed. However it was even more strict, allowing not even vegetables – it was basically meat, poultry, fish, cheese, eggs and water. Now you are unlikely to find a copy, except in second-hand bookshops or on the Internet. Probably just as well as it would have rated 0 for health on my system.
■ *The Doctor's Quick Weight Loss Diet* by Dr Irwin Maxwell Stillman and Samm Sinclair Baker (Pan, l970).

Eat Fat, Get Thin

This book by Barry Groves offers a high-fat, high-saturated-fat, high-protein, low-carbohydrate diet which basically goes against all current official (some would say commonsensical) nutritional thinking. It differs slightly from typical high-protein diets, such as the Atkins diet, by allowing a little more (60g per day) carbohydrate, but is still woefully low in fruit, vegetables, grains and other complex carbohydrates, and fibre. Groves urges you to leave all visible fat on meat, says that you may eat up to 3,000 cals/day and you needn't exercise if you don't want to.
Typical calorie count for a day's eating: 1,500–2,000 (see below).
Promised weight loss: Up to 2lb (1kg) a week (more initially).
Typical day's eating:
■ ***Breakfast:*** Fried bacon, eggs and kidneys (unlimited quantities); starch reduced bread with butter; coffee with cream.
■ ***Lunch:*** Cheddar cheese omelette with salad dressed with mayonnaise; coffee with cream; apple.
■ ***Evening:*** Steak with the fat band left on; broccoli and green beans dressed with butter, small portion (100g) new potatoes; piece of Brie, 2 cream crackers.
■ ***Other drinks throughout day:*** Water, tea, low-calorie soft drinks.

Short-term effectiveness: Low carbohydrate will cause fluid loss of several pounds; low calorie intake may cause reasonable fat loss. ● **Score: 3**
Long-term effectiveness: Not ideal as a long-term diet but, if followed, weight loss may continue slowly. ● **Score: 2**
Ease of use: Fairly easy to understand and follow. ● **Score: 4**
Cost: Could be expensive, depending upon choices made – in general you are encouraged to eat a lot of animal protein, such as red meat, which can be expensive. ● **Score: 2**
Palatability: If you love meat, eggs, cheese, etc., it could be fine in the short term. Not one for vegetarians! In the long term even hardened meat eaters may get frustrated with the lack of much carbohydrate to add to the plate. ● **Score: 2**
Satiety: As Groves points out, research shows that if you eat fat just on its own (without accompanying sugar or carbs) you quickly reach a point at which you don't want any more. High-fat, high-protein foods will also keep hunger at bay between meals quite well. He uses this fact to say that you can eat as much as you like of the high-fat, high-protein foods – knowing that you won't be able to. ● **Score: 4**
Health factor: Not a diet that fits in with current international healthy eating advice. No exercise tips given. Potentially unsafe diet couched in scientific terms. ● **Score: 0**
Scientific basis: There is no magic slimming potential in eating high amounts of fat. Also, Groves' citings of scientific evidence for his claim that a high-saturated-fat, high-cholesterol diet is not unhealthy are very selective. As explained, the 'eat all you like' advice is based on the knowledge that you can only eat so much high-fat, high-protein food before feeling full. In other words, the diet limits calorie intake for you. Groves' estimate that you may be eating 3,000 calories a day is probably a huge overestimate. ● **Score: 2**
Total score 19
Percentage score 47.5%.
■ *Eat Fat Get Thin* by Barry Groves (Vermilion, 1999) ISBN 0 09182593 8.
See also: Qs 88–90, Feature 8, High-protein Diets, Top 20 popular diets.

Eat Great, Lose Weight

This is the title of a best-selling book in the USA, now available in the UK, by American actress Suzanne Somers. She coined the phrase 'Somersizing' for going on her diet, which is basically a food-combining diet.

■ *Suzanne Somers' Eat Great, Lose Weight* (Running Press, September 2001) ISBN 0 76241160 0.

See also: Q 91, Food combining.

Eat More, Weigh Less

This book by Dr Dean Ornish has been a bestseller in America and is a very-low-fat, high-carbohydrate diet with virtually no animal produce allowed. We look at it in more detail in the entry on Very-low-fat-diets.

Eat Right 4 Your Type

This book by Peter D'Adamo has sold over 2 million copies worldwide and is based on the idea that you should eat according to your blood type. If you do, he claims, you will lose weight, fight allergy, ward off infections and increase your energy levels. It could also help you fight the major diseases and the deterioration of old age, D'Adamo claims. This is apparently because your blood type reflects your body chemistry and how you absorb and deal with nutrients.

The Diet

In precis, blood type O should eat a diet high in meat and fish, low in carbohydrates and low in dairy produce, avoiding various foods, including lentils, brazil nuts, avocados and oranges; blood type A should eat a high-plant, low-dairy, high-fish diet, avoiding red meat. Types B should eat most meat, except chicken and bacon, some fish, and most dairy foods, as well as plenty of fruit and vegetables, while the rare type AB combines the diets of both A and B type. Exercise varies according to your type, too; for instance, only type O should engage in vigorous exercise, while type A should only do light activity, such as golf and yoga.

Typical calorie count for a day's eating (group O): 1,200–500.

Promised weight loss: Not specific.

Typical day's eating (for Blood Group O):

■ ***Breakfast:*** Slice of 100% rye bread, plums, walnuts; pineapple juice.

■ ***Lunch:*** Mackerel fillet, spinach, red pepper and onion salad with olive oil; fresh figs; dandelion tea.

■ **Evening:** Lamb chops with garlic; broccoli, parsnips; rosehip tea, apple.

(Comments refer to Blood Type 0 diet)

Short-term effectiveness: This high-protein, low-carbohydrate diet will result in initial fluid loss and fat loss in most people. ● **Score: 4**

Long-term effectiveness: Small amount of fat loss should continue if the regime is stuck to. ● **Score: 3**

Ease of use: Complicated diet with lots of things you must eat and can't eat, which is not at first easy to follow. ● **Score: 1**

Cost: Will vary according to which foods you choose, although the high meat element may make it more expensive than average. ● **Score: 3**

Palatability: Large range of foods on the banned list include most dairy products, various cereals, most breads, most grains and pasta, many veg, potatoes and fruits, coffee and tea. Have to enjoy meat and fish. ● **Score: 2**

Satiety: Average to good. ● **Score: 4**

Health factor: As so many foods are banned you have to be careful to get a varied balanced diet to provide a complete range of nutrients. Faddy eating can encourage an unhealthy attitude to food. Fairly low-carbohydrate/high-fat content goes against current nutritional thinking. The exercise advice is unbalanced. ● **Score: 1**

Scientific basis: The idea that you should eat according to your blood type is the author's idea and not based on any scientific research. In any case, the A, B, O blood grouping classification is just one system of blood grouping. The ability to break down and digest food is not related to your blood type, and neither is optimum eating for weight loss.

As the diet is largely based on natural foods, and all blood types are encouraged to cut highly processed foods down or out, it may reduce calories naturally. Most people have blood in group O, and the O group diet is basically a high-protein, low-carbohydrate one which would be self-limiting in calorie content. D'Adamo also gives specific low-calorie diets for weight loss which will work whatever blood type you are. ● **Score: 1**

Total score 19

Percentage rating 47.5%

■ *Eat Right 4 Your Type* by Peter D'Adamo (Century, reissued February 2001) ISBN 0 71267716 X.

See also: High-protein diets, Top 20 Popular Diets.

Eskimo Diet

This best-selling book of l990 set out to explain how eating a diet high in fish oils could protect against heart disease. Not a weight loss book as such, but much of the research and advice is still appropriate today. Now not available to buy new, but you may find copies in second-hand bookshops or on the Internet auction sites.

■ *The Eskimo Diet* by Dr Reg Saynor and Dr Frank Ryan (Ebury, l990) ISBN 0 85223809 6.

Exercise classes

Attending an exercise class regularly can be a good and fairly inexpensive way to keep or get fit. You don't have to join a private gym – local leisure centres have inexpensive classes, or the YMCA (which runs one of the best-regarded fitness instruction training programmes in the country) has 81 clubs nationwide. Some classes in local halls may also be fine. These tips will help you get the most out of a class:

■ Pick something that you think you will enjoy and which you think will be within your capabilities.

■ Try to watch a class before you join.

■ Make sure the place in which the class is taken is warm and dry, with adequate ventilation and suitable sprung floor.

■ Talk to the instructor. Ask for their credentials – a RSA, NVQ or YMCA qualification is ideal. Don't be afraid to ask for a written CV and check it out at your leisure. Unqualified teaching may do you more harm than good. The Fitness Industry Association has a list of approved instructors in the UK.

■ Wear comfortable clothes and non-slip training shoes.

■ Always stop if the work is too hard for you, and don't be afraid to ask questions before/after a session, or put your hand up during a session for assistance.

A selection of classes on offer

■ ***Basic aerobics*** – from beginners to advanced, these are the most popular and common exercise classes of all. Low-impact aerobics is more gentle (telephone the Fitness League on 01932 567566; www.thefitnessleague.com). Dance aerobics may be more highly choreographed and may be for those already experienced in basic aerobics. Good for cardiovascular fitness, calorie burning and some toning effect.

■ ***Step*** – hugely popular for 10 years, a Step class, where you step up and down on a platform, will get you cardiovascular fit, burn up lots of calories and tone lower body, particularly buttocks and thighs. More fun than you might imagine; widely available.

■ ***BodyPump or BodyMax*** – aerobics with weights, so in effect you are doing double the work in the same time. Leave for later if you are unfit. Great for improving cardiovascular fitness in the already fairly fit; terrific calorie burner and for all-round strength.

■ ***Boxercise*** – circuit training with boxing moves, though no one gets hit. Good fun if bored with aerobics or want more of a challenge.

■ ***Body conditioning*** – umbrella term for a session of toning and stretching. A little light aerobic work may be included.

■ ***Tums and bums*** – for toning tums and bums, often including legs; or abs only.

■ ***Core training*** – latest buzzword in exercise, to strengthen the body 'core' – abdominals and back – tel Reebok 0800 305050 or find this at all Cannons health clubs, 08707 808182.

■ ***Stretching*** – for increased suppleness and relaxation. Body Balance classes include principles from several methods including yoga and Pilates.

■ Phone Fitness Professionals on 0870 5133434; or Scoot on 0800 192192; or the YMCA on 0208 520 5599 or 0207 343 1850.

■ On the web, try www.fitnesswebsites.co.uk, www.gymuser.co.uk, www.health-club.net. www.feelingfat.co.uk and www.thefitnessleague.com

Yellow Pages and libraries are also good sources of information.

■ For a register of accredited teachers, contact the Fitness Industry Association, 02076200700; www.fia.org.uk

■ Finding the particular class you want, if it is one of the less common ones, is not always easy – Reebok (0800 305050) originates many of the cutting-edge classes. Fitness Professionals can help with BodyPump.

See also: Dancing, Fitkids, Gyms and Health Clubs, Pilates, Yoga.

Exercise equipment

If you want to buy exercise equipment for use at home, there is a huge choice in all price brackets. It can be broadly categorized into cardiovascular equipment (exercise bikes, treadmills, rowers, etc.), strength training equipment (benches, weights, multigyms, etc.) and toning and flexibility equipment (bands, balls, rollers, toning pads, etc.).

Tips

■ Before you buy any equipment, spend time working out what you want to achieve (strength or tone or flexibility or aerobic fitness, or all of these). Send off for several catalogues from the reliable mail-order firms listed below, or visit their websites and browse. Also use the guidelines below. Then try to visit an outlet in person to try out the equipment you are thinking of buying.

■ Work out where you are going to use the equipment. Even if it folds/rolls away, if you have to move it every time you use it, you may not do so. For people short of space, small pieces of portable equipment are best. Very heavy equipment may not be suitable for upstairs rooms.

■ Buy the best-quality equipment you can afford. This is especially true of cardiovascular items and large pieces like multigyms. Cheap equipment can be undersized so that you can't do a full range of movement (e.g. treadmill bases short/narrow, rowing range too short), or they may be uncomfortable and/or unstable, or may not carry a large weight, and often frustrating because as you get fitter, you soon reach the machine's maximum capability.

■ To stave off boredom, go for cardiovascular machines with as much built-in electronic wizardry as you can afford. At the very least, choose a machine with a display showing calories burnt, speed, time and distance. This way you can easily monitor your own improvement, which is a good incentive to continue. A machine with a built-in heart rate monitor is a good idea and doesn't cost much more; varied training programmes are another good option.

Cardiovascular equipment

■ ***Exercise bikes:*** Choose from traditional upright or recumbent bikes (reclining position said to be better for people with bad backs), which can be electronic (mains required), magnetic, air fan or friction-powered. Look for fully adjustable seat and pedal, and sturdy build. Price range: £150 to £2,000+.

Good brands: Tunturi, Kettler, Reebok.

■ ***Treadmills:*** Motorized treadmills are among the best bets for less fit people. Best ones come with automatic elevation, maximum speeds of at least 10mph (16kph), a walking area of at least 17 x 50in (37.5cm x 1.25m), and with a full electronic display. Built-in heart rate monitor makes working within your training zone easier. Handy if they fold for moving. Prices from about £750 up to £4,000+. *Good brands:* Tunturi, Kettler, Reebok, Powerjog, Spirit.

■ ***Rowers:*** Hard workout not always suitable for the unfit and/or people with back problems, but great all-round strength and cardiovascular exercise. Avoid rowers in the £100 or so range, which won't give you a good workout. Cheapest decent machines (about £400) work on friction-belt resistance; dearer models work on air fan, water or magnetic resistance. Need a lot of space (up to 8ft/2.5m in length). *Best regarded* are the Concept 11 Rower (about £800) and the Water Rower (about £850). *Other good brands* are Tunturi and Kettler.

■ ***Elliptical trainers:*** Cross trainers with a skiing-like action, which work upper and lower body simultaneously with no impact on legs. Models available with and without mains. Prices from £250 to £2,000+. *Good brands:* Reebok, Eclipse, Kettler, NordicTrack.

■ ***Steppers and climbers:*** Use fairly small floor area and work the buttock and leg muscles while burning off plenty of calories. Simulates hill-walking or climbing. Non-motorized steppers work on hydraulic resistance – a good bet for an inexpensive machine. Prices from £250 to £2,000+. *Good brands:* Tunturi, Stairmaster.

■ ***Rebounders:*** Mini-trampoline useful for low-impact exercise; stores easily, low cost. *Good brands:* PT Cross-Trainer, about £60.

■ ***Steps:*** Platform to step up and down on, with up to three adjustable heights. Good basic piece of equipment, stores easily, lightweight but robust. Builds lower-body strength as well as cardiovascular fitness. Prices from about £25. *Good brands:* The Step, Reebok Step.

■ ***Skipping ropes:*** Cheapest home cardiovascular equipment – but skipping is hard work and for indoor work you need a high ceiling and enough space. Various ropes come in leather, nylon or graphite-coated, with or without weights and skip counters. From about £2. *Good brands:* ProCanadian Speedrope, Reebok Jump Rope.

Strength Training Equipment

■ ***Multigyms:*** Compact mini-gyms with a variety of 'stations' or exercises that you can do on them for total-body toning/strength. Or that is the idea! DO go for the best you can afford. Some lower-cost multigyms don't suit taller people and you may also need to make fiddly adjustments between each different exercise. Because there are no free weights involved, multigyms may be safer to use than barbells/dumbbells. Look for one that will fit into the space you have available and which offers a lat pull down, pec dec, leg press, leg extensions, bench press and other exercises, and with total resistance of at least 200lb (90kg). Prices from £300 up to £6,000+ for large gyms that more than one person can use at a time. *Good brands:* Body-Solid, Kettler, Vectra.

■ ***Mini-gyms:*** Workout benches that rely on body weight and pulleys as resistance (Total Gym, about £150; Body Sculpture Total Ultra Gym, about £120). Quite good for the price.

■ ***Benches and free weights:*** With a basic bench, a barbell and a set of dumbbells, you can do a fairly comprehensive strength workout and you don't have to spend a lot to get a decent bench set. Buy a bench with a barbell rest incorporated (you can't work out on a bench with a barbell unless you have a rest) and a leg curl/extension attachment. You will also need an exercise wall chart or a book (photocopy the pages and pin them on the wall). Start with the lightest weights and be sensible. Prices from about £60 up to £750 for a luxury bench. *Good brands:* Marcy, Weider, Prorange.

For serious training you will need a barbell with one or more sets of weights from 2.5lb (1.2kg) to 10lb (4.5kg) and a pair of dumbbells with similar weights. Adjustable weights are so much more versatile than fixed weight dumbbells. Prices from about £20 for a barbell set, £25 for a dumbbell set. *Good brands:* Golds, Weider, York.

■ ***Other weight training equipment:*** You can buy individual pieces of training equipment such as a lateral pull-down station, a pec dec, a pull-up station, a leg extension and curl set, a bicep/tricep machine, and so on. Bear in mind that these take up almost as much space as a small multigym and will only help you perform one (or at most a few) exercise. You need to buy weights as well with many of these. Prices from about £75 to £250. *Good brands*: York, Body-Solid.

You can also buy a weighted vest, useful for runners (Reebok Ironwear Vest) and ankle, knuckle, waist and wrist weights to add resistance to floor exercises; mini hand weights, weighted barbells (no extra weights necessary).

Toning and Flexibility Equipment

■ ***Abdominal exercisers:*** An ab cage makes doing crunches easier on the neck and can help you do the exercise correctly. From £15. Ab rollers have made a comeback – you kneel and slide them along the floor. From about £20. The Torsotrack 11 has been voted a 'best ab buy' by professionals and seems less hard than other abdominal exercise work – you kneel and slide your upper body along a track. From about £80; tel 0800 975 8904; www.tvshop.com

■ ***Resistance bands and tubes:*** Ideal for toning work when you travel, and are low in cost. They come with exercise instructions and you can do a whole-body workout. From about £2.50 for a set.

■ ***Balls:*** Fitballs are large inflatable balls that can be used for toning and flexibility work and to improve core stability. From about £10.

■ ***Electronic toning pads:*** These you attach to your flabby bits, switch on, lie back and let the machine tone you up. If used regularly (up to 40 minutes a day), they have a small toning effect on the muscles underneath the pads, but do nothing for actual fitness. You can also buy a toning band which you wrap around your middle and is less fiddly to put on. Slendertone 0845 0707777, www.slendertone.co.uk; Cleo 0113 2527744, www.club-cleo.com

■ ***Toning tables:*** A bed-like table with separate pieces that move, moving a part of your body at the same time. Might be useful for people with particular physical difficulties, the elderly or those in convalescence. Slim Images 0800 7312799.

All the following companies do a wide range of equipment.
■ Fitness Network, 0208995 7700; www.fitnessnetwork.co.uk
■ ProActive Health, 0870 8484842; www.proactive-health.co.uk
■ Gym World, 0800 0189836; www.gymworld.co.uk
■ Fitex, 0800 616179; www.fitex.co.uk
■ Active Fitness, 020 89607891; www.activefitness.co.uk

False Fat Diet

A book whose author, Elson M. Haas, believes that we can appear much fatter than we really are due to sensitivity to certain foods. This book is a cross between a detox, a diuretic diet and a wheat- and dairy-free diet – you may lose weight on the system but it would be mostly fluid and probably some fat too, as your calorie intake is likely to reduce if you follow the eating guidelines.
■ *The False Fat Diet* by Elson Haas and Cameron Stanth (Bantam, April 2001) ISBN 0 55381348 X.

Fasting

I don't recommend fasting as a good way to lose weight (although you undoubtedly would) as it could be unsafe, especially if continued for long. However I realize that people worldwide do fast, and swear it helps them to feel better, with more energy. Check with your doctor before beginning any type of fast, however short.
■ *The Fasting Diet* by Steven Bailey (Contemporary Books, May 2001) ISBN 0 65801145 6, described by the publishers as 'Risk-free fasting'.
■ *Fasting and Eating for Health* by Joel Fuhrman (St Martin's Press, May l998) ISBN 0 31218719 X.
See also: Qs 77 and 107, Juice diets.

Fat acceptance groups

There are a number of 'fat acceptance' groups throughout the world whose main aims are to improve quality of life for fat people, and to promote their acceptance by others. These are commendable, but the waters get muddied by their aversion to helping obese members to shed weight even for health reasons. Fat acceptance groups are anti-slimming almost across the board – which is a shame, as not all overweight people necessarily want to stay fat. Anyway, I certainly think they offer help and support, and there are plenty of spin-offs, like events, friendship and more.
■ USA – National Association to Advance Fat Acceptance (NAAFA); 001 916 558 6880; www.naafa.org
■ International – Largesse, the Network for Size Esteem; www.eskimo.com/-largesse
■ The International Size Acceptance Association (ISAA); www.size-acceptance.org, whose UK branch is www.big-people.org.uk/ISAA
■ UK – Size Net, www.sizenet.com; who are also a member of ISAA.
■ UK – The National Size Acceptance Coalition, tel 020 700 0509; email freesize@size.fsnet.co.uk

Fat burner diets

The premise behind fat burner diets is that they encourage the body to burn its own fat for fuel and the conversion of food to energy rather than fat. One of the most popular in recent years is Patrick Holford's *30-Day Fat Burner Diet*, which works, he says, by creating the ideal blood sugar and insulin balance on a diet of 50% carbs, 25% protein and 25% fat. In fact, a typical day's eating (porridge for breakfast, a 'fatburner' sandwich for lunch with some carrot soup, and an evening meal of kedgeree with steamed vegetables, plus two pieces of fruit and a dessertspoon of pumpkin seeds for snacks, and unlimited low-calorie allowed drinks) comes to around 1,250–1,300 calories a day. This will help you lose weight because it is low in calories; and it has the added advantage that many of the foods are low on the Glycaemic Index, so hunger will be less of a problem than on some diets. The diet is a generally healthy one. As we see elsewhere in this book, fat is burnt when you create a calorie deficit on a long-term basis. All slimming diets are, therefore, 'fat burner diets'.
■ *The 30-Day Fat Burner Diet* by Patrick Holford (Piatkus, January l999) ISBN 0 74991920 5.
See also: Q18, Glycaemic Index diets.

Fat camps for kids

The Carnegie International Weight Loss Camps organization runs summer camps for overweight children and their aims are to educate the children in healthy eating and activity, to help them lose weight, in both the short and long term, and to have fun. This USA-based company has also, for the past few years, run a successful camp in the UK for six weeks during the summer via Leeds University.
■ Telephone 0113 283 2600, ext 3560; www.lmu.ac.uk

Fat substitutes

Fat substitutes are manufactured ingredients which have bulk and texture similar to fat, but with fewer calories than fat. They may be used in commercial foods, but aren't for sale otherwise.

The most well known fat substitute is probably Olestra. Although this is made from sugar and oil, it contains no calories because it is not digested by the body – its molecules are too large. In the USA, where it was approved in 1996, it is used in snack items such as crisps, but it isn't approved for use in the UK. Its side effects can be loose stools and stomach cramps, and it may inhibit the body's absorption of the fat-soluble vitamins A, D E and K and carotenes.

The original fat substitute, Simplesse, is approved in both the USA and UK (and elsewhere) and is made from milk or egg protein with a mouth-feel similar to fat. It has a quarter the calories of fat and is used in low-fat margarines, frozen desserts and other commercial produce. It seems to have few, if any, side-effects as it is a 'natural' food.

Unfortunately, research indicates that the use of foods made with fat substitutes doesn't necessarily help with weight control – people seem to eat more calories in other forms.

Fit for Life

This book and eating system by Harvey and Marilyn Diamond, which has been around for several years, offers a regime for weight loss which includes eating nothing but fruit before noon, and eating appropriate combinations of food the rest of the time. If these right combinations aren't eaten, the authors say that the food will rot in the intestines. Much of the diet is fruit and vegetables, and carbohydrates and protein shouldn't be eaten together. Refined sugars are banned, as they also lead to 'putrefaction' and although fruit is good you mustn't eat it at the end of a meal. The system seems to be a combination of the Hay System and Judy Mazel's Beverly Hills diet and is not one that I would recommend, as it is faddy and is not based on nutritional or scientific fact. The amounts of weight loss cited are also unsafe – loss of 50lb (23kg) in a month claimed by Harvey Diamond is excessive.

■ *Fit for Life* by Harvey and Marilyn Diamond (Bantam, April 1987) ISBN 0 55317353 5.

See also: Beverly Hills Diet, Crash diets, Food combining.

Fitkids

Fitkid is an organization in the UK which has 500 clubs throughout the country for 5–12-year-olds. Its aim is to promote activity for health and pleasure in the young population. There are many activities on offer, such as volleyball, spacehoppers and skipping ropes. Telephone 0161 491 6800 or visit www.Fitkid.co.uk. The Fitness Professionals organization has the Fit Club, the association for children's fitness instructors; they offer a kids' PACE exercise circuit. Phone 0990 133434 for more details. Next Generation is a new chain of junior health clubs for children over five, with fully equipped junior gyms and other facilities, such as mini courts for tennis and basketball. Tel 028948 9701; www.nextgenerationclubs.co.uk

The F-Plan

This diet book by British author Audrey Eyton, originally published in 1982, was the first high-fibre slimming diet, and is still the most famous of them all. *The Complete F-Plan Diet* was published a few years later and is still available today. The theory behind this diet is that a high intake of dietary fibre (now correctly called non-starch polysaccharides) quickly fills you up while you are eating – because you have to do a lot of chewing, you reach satiety point before you have eaten too many calories; it offers bulk without calories (because fibre largely passes through the system undigested); and it also keeps hunger pangs at bay between meals as high-fibre foods take longer to digest than their low-fibre, refined counterparts.

The Diet

The diet is low in fat, high in complex carbs, such as whole grains, baked potatoes and pulses, high in fruit, most veg are unlimited and you can have the odd glass of alcohol. Fibre content is about double the recommended daily amount of 18g.

Typical calorie count for a day's eating: 1,250.

Promised weight loss: About 2lb (1kg) a week.

Typical day's eating:

■ ***Breakfast:*** Special recipe 'fibre filler' cereal/nut/fruit mix with skimmed milk from allowance; portion of fresh fruit.

■ ***Lunch:*** Nutty coleslaw; fresh fruit.

■ ***Evening meal:*** Baked potato, baked chicken (no skin); mixed salad; fibre filler with skimmed milk.

■ ***To drink:*** Calorie-free drinks, tea, coffee with skimmed milk from allowance (1/2 pint/300ml a day).

Short-term effectiveness: People unused to a high-carb, high-fibre diet may find themselves retaining more fluid than normal and this may counteract the early effect of the fat loss on the scales, but reasonable amounts of fat will be lost on a 1,250 cals/day diet. ● **Score: 3**

Long-term effectiveness: If the diet is continued, weight loss should continue steadily. ● **Score: 4**

Ease of use: Straightforward diet with not too many rules but some weighing and measuring, plus totting up of your daily calorie and fibre intake is called for. Meals are fairly simple to prepare. ● **Score: 4**

Cost: Fairly inexpensive. ● **Score: 4**

Palatability: Some tasty recipes and some not so tasty. Plenty of variety. The breakfast fibre filler is a bit dry and lacking in flavour. Famous side-effects of flatulence and stomach bloating may occur. ● **Score: 3**

Satiety: For the calorie content, it is certainly filling and should keep you satisfied from one meal to the next. ● **Score: 4**

Health factor: The diet is generally one of the healthiest to be found, even today. Although there is evidence that high intakes of wheat bran (found in the fibre-filler breakfast) can inhibit the absorption of minerals such as iron and calcium, a high-fibre diet is linked with less risk of some cancers – new research suggests there is 40% less risk of bowel cancer with high fibre consumption (from all sources, not just wheat). The F-Plan may be low in essential fats from fish and plant oils depending on food choices made. Plenty of water or other low-calorie liquid should be taken on a high-fibre diet. ● Score: 4

Scientific basis: Most of the rationale for eating a high-fibre diet while slimming is correct. However, it is interesting to note that not all high-fibre foods are low on the Glycaemic Index – the index that measures how quickly foods are absorbed into the bloodstream. For example, baked potatoes, parsnips, wholemeal bread and dates (all feature a lot in the F-Plan) are high on the index and quickly absorbed into the bloodstream. The diet works like any slimming diet – by reducing the total number of calories that are eaten. ● Score: 4

Total score 30

Percentage rating 75%

■ *The Complete F-Plan Diet* by Audrey Eyton (Penguin, January 1987) ISBN 0 14010024 5.

See also: Qs 83–85, High-fibre diets, Low-fat diets, Top 20 popular diets.

Food Combining

This wasn't devised as a weight loss diet, but people who follow the system do inevitably lose weight, at least to begin with, because the system is self-limiting in calories as there are so many rules and restrictions. Many people love eating the Hay way, but many more have tried it and had to give up. Those who do stick with it often report feeling energized, with niggling ailments improved.

Dr William Hay invented food combining (The Hay system) early last century. He believed that disease is caused by accumulation of toxins and acid waste and that we can all have good health if we avoid eating foods that fight. To do this we should not mix protein and carbohydrate foods at the same meal, because starches are broken down by alkaline saliva and proteins require gastric acid. As well as this major rule, there are also banned foods and other rules about how and when to eat.

A potted guide:

■ Fruit should always be eaten alone.

■ Vegetables can be eaten alone, or with any other allowed food.

■ Allowed carbs (breads, grains, pasta, pulses, potatoes) can be eaten with fat and/or vegetables but not with protein foods. And limit yourself to one carbohydrate food at a meal.

■ Protein foods (meat, fish, poultry, dairy produce, tofu) can be eaten with veg but not with fat or carbs. Limit yourself to one protein food at a meal.

■ 70% of your daily intake should be of high-water-content foods.

■ Eat only whole foods; avoid refined starches (white bread, white rice, white pasta, etc.), sugars and artificial additives.

Typical calorie count for a day's eating: 1,000–1500.

Promised weight loss: Nothing promised, but weight loss almost inevitable if you are overweight.

Typical day's eating

■ ***Breakfast:*** Bowl of fresh fruit salad; glass of fruit juice.

■ ***Lunch:*** Salad sandwich on wholemeal bread with mayonnaise.

■ ***Evening meal:*** Grilled steak with selection of vegetables (no butter)

To drink: Water, herb tea.

Short-term effectiveness: As a weight loss diet, should be very effective. ● Score: 4

Long-term effectiveness: If the diet is continued, weight loss should continue if you are overweight and many people use the system as a way of maintaining weight loss. ● Score: 4

Ease of use: Quite hard to learn all the rules to begin with, but once they are grasped the system is fairly easy to use, as there is no weighing or measuring of food and because the rules are so hard and fast, there is little temptation to stray. However, the diet is unsociable and eating out can be a problem. ● Score: 3

Cost: Mid-range. ● Score: 3

Palatability: Few people coming from a typical Western diet would find the food combining system very palatable – no more ham sandwiches, no more baked potato with cheese, no more eggs on toast, no more roast potatoes with your roast beef. ● Score: 2

Satiety: Not high. When carbohydrates such as a baked potato (high on the Glycaemic Index) are eaten without protein, they are not likely to keep you feeling full for long. ● Score: 3

Health factor: Surprisingly, if you choose from a wide range of the foods that are allowed on the diet, it does contain all the food groups necessary for health, although some experts feel it may be too low in calcium and iron for some. The faddy aspect of the diet may encourage, or mask, eating disorders. ● Score: 3

Scientific basis: There is no scientific evidence to support the 'don't mix protein and carbohydrate' theory. The body is perfectly capable of digesting proteins alongside carbs and, indeed, very many foods contain both themselves (e.g. pulses, potatoes). In other words, the whole rationale for the Hay system is nonsense, but nevertheless it manages to be a reasonably healthy calorie-controlled diet. ● Score: 1

Total score 23

Percentage rating 57.5%

■ *Food Combining for Health* by Doris Grant and Jean Joice (HarperCollins, reissued January l993) ISBN 0 72252506 0.

■ *The Complete Book of Food Combining* by Kathryn Marsden (Piatkus, September 2001) ISBN 0 74992217 6.

See also: Q91, Eat Great, Lose Weight, Fit for Life, Top 20 popular diets.

The Formula

A diet book by Americans Gene and Joyce Daoust based on eating 40% carbohydrates, 30% fat and 30% protein (the formula). This ratio is the same as in The Zone. The authors say that the 'formula' is the most important aspect of the plan and that counting calories isn't important, but the plans that they create for different people will all result in weight loss because they will be creating a calorie deficit.

There aren't enough carbohydrates in the diet to rate this as a particularly healthy regime – 50 to 60% is a healthy target. The protein content is also much higher than recommended levels.

■ *The Formula* by Gene and Joyce Daoust (Vermilion, February 2001) ISBN 0 09185744 9.

See also: The Zone.

Glycaemic Index diets

Originally devised for diabetics, the Glycaemic Index is a ranking of carbohydrate foods which measures the rate at which blood glucose levels rise when a particular food is eaten. Glucose itself has a rating of 100, so the nearer to 100 a food is, the higher its 'GI' rating and the more quickly it is absorbed – and the more quickly blood sugar levels will drop again. A food with a low GI rating is absorbed more slowly and likely to keep blood sugar levels constant, which may help avoid hunger.

The basis of glycaemic index diets such as The Glucose Revolution is that a diet containing most of its carbs as foods with a low or moderately low GI will help you lose weight by keeping blood sugar levels even and hunger pangs at bay. In the last few years there have been several books based on the index – the most popular are listed below.

The Diet

A typical GI diet is low in fat and high in carbohydrates, with the emphasis on low-GI carbs, such as pulses, certain fruits and vegetables, yoghurt and whole grains.

Typical calorie count for a day's eating: 1,500.

Promised weight loss: Not usually specified but 1–2lb (0.5–1kg) a week would be average.

Typical day's eating:

■ ***Breakfast:*** Porridge served with apple and raisins and skimmed milk; orange juice.

■ ***Lunch:*** Veg and pot barley soup with pumpernickel bread; 2 plums.

■ ***Evening meal:*** Lentil and lean beef bolognese sauce on wholewheat pasta; green salad; low-fat fruit yoghurt.

■ ***To drink:*** during the day: Water, tea with skimmed milk, herb teas.

Short-term effectiveness: People increasing their intake of complex carbohydrates may find that, in the first few weeks of this diet, they retain more fluid than they are used to, which will result in the fat loss not showing up much on the scales. For most people, however, the moderately reduced calorie regime will produce fat loss. ● **Score: 3**

Long-term effectiveness: Should result in slow or steady weight loss over time and compliance should be good (see Satiety) and weight maintenance good. ● **Score: 5**

Ease of use: A fairly easy diet to follow, with plenty of familiar foods to eat – but people who have followed a typical low-fibre, refined carbohydrate diet may find the increase in pulses and whole grains means that cooking skills need rethinking. ● **Score: 3**

Cost: Can be inexpensive, as GI diets normally ask you to eat only small portions of animal protein foods, which tend to be the most expensive. Choosing out-of-season low-GI fruits and vegetables would make the diet more expensive, but this is up to you. ● **Score: 4**

Palatability: Ideal for vegetarians and people who love starches and plenty on the plate. For some people, the increased intake of pulses and vegetables may be a chore. ● **Score: 3**

Satiety: Very good for a reduced-calorie diet. ● **Score: 5**

Health factor: This is a high-carbohydrate, low-to-moderate-fat, moderate-protein diet which fits in well with current nutritional thinking, albeit with its added dimension of the GI factor. ● **Score: 5**

Scientific basis: To lose weight you need to create an energy deficit, so any implication in the glycaemic index diet books that your fat will disappear no matter how many calories you eat is not true – these diets do reduce the calories enough so that most people would lose weight, because high-fat foods and sugary foods are discouraged. However, the premise that hunger is kept at bay with low GI foods, and blood sugar levels moderated, is backed by a great deal of scientific research. If you are going to follow a high-fibre, low-fat, reduced-calorie diet, you might as well include in the GI principle for its added benefits. ● **Score: 4**

Total score 32

Percentage rating 80%

■ *The G-Index Diet* by Richard N. Podell (Warner Books, March l994) ISBN 0 44636576 9. The first well-known GI book.

■ *The Glucose Revolution: the Authoritative Guide to the Glycemic Index* by Thomas MS Wolever, Jennie Brand Miller, Kaye Foster-Powell and Stephen Colagiuri (Marlowe and Co, June l999) ISBN 1 56924660 2. The definitive guide by Canadian and Australian experts, with GI listings, recipes and information on weight loss and other health aspects.

■ *The Glucose Revolution Pocket Guide to Losing Weight* by Thomas MS Wolever (Marlowe and Co, March 2000) ISBN 1 56924677 7.

■ *The Glucose Revolution* by Anthony Leeds, Jennie Brand Miller, Kay Foster-Powell and Stephen Colagiuri (Coronet, new edition June 2001) ISBN 0 34076826 6. Formerly published under the title *The G.I. Factor*.

See also: Fat-burner diets, SugarBusters, The Zone, Top 20 popular diets.

The grapefruit diet

Grapefruit diets tend to ask you to eat half a grapefruit before every meal, in the forlorn hope that the 'enzymes' in the fruit will help to burn up the calories in the meal. This is a completely false concept. Grapefruits are quite low in calories and contain good amounts of vitamin C, but the grapefruit diet works because the meals add up, on

average, to no more than 800 calories a day – too low for health or sensible slimming.
See also: Crash diets, the Mayo Clinic Diet.

Gyms and health clubs

Joining a gym or health club can be a good way to get and keep fit. There are various types of club you might join – from 'pay as you go', local-authority-run leisure centres, to small gyms where the workout machines are the only facility, to family-type monthly-membership clubs through to exclusive annual-membership clubs. Read this checklist before you sign on the dotted line.

■ *Check that a club is a member of the Fitness Industry Association (0207 620 0700); www.fia.org.uk, and check that the instructors are also on the FIA register (which has three levels of training). Look around the club, including all the facilities; here are some guidelines:*
■ Is there up-to-date cardiovascular and weight training equipment (it's a bad sign, for instance, if one or more of the machines is out of use, if seats or handles are ripped, etc.)
■ Are all exercise areas bright, light, warm, well-ventilated?
■ If you want to do classes, check that the class area has a sprung floor.
■ Ask what fitness assessment you get before beginning – it should be thorough, and you should get a starting programme and a run-through session before using cardiovascular and strength training equipment.
■ Is there enough staff to supervise the people attending? If you see an exercise area with no staff supervision, that is a bad sign.
■ Does the gym area look overcrowded? Are people queuing for machines? Are any classes in progress too full/too empty?
■ Are the changing facilities clean? Is the water warm? Are the lockers working? If you are shy – is there a separate men's/women's area for changing and/or exercising?
■ For families, is there a crèche or other facility for children?
■ Does the club have the facilities you want – e.g. swimming; a yoga class; a particular machine? If you aren't sure what you will want, the more facilities a club has the better. On the other hand, there is no point paying fancy prices for things like crèches, pools, beauty salons and restaurants if all you want is a workout in the gym three times a week. Try to write a list of things you want and questions you have before you go to visit, and after the visit, go home and think about what you've seen – and the membership deals – before signing up.

Costs

Most clubs have various types of membership – peak, off-peak, family, single, couples, etc. Some have a joining fee and a monthly membership (best if you don't know whether or not you will continue to go), others ask you to sign up for a whole year. Local leisure centres may simply want you to pay when you attend, for whichever facilities you use.

There are hundreds of small individual gyms and health clubs across the country as well as several large, and expanding, 'named' chains – those listed below are all well-regarded. For a general picture of what is available near you, check out the websites listed, go to the library or look in local Yellow Pages.

■ ***Health club- and gym-finding websites:***
www.fitnesswebsites.co.uk www.health-club.net
www.feelingfat.co.uk www.gymuser.co.uk
www.scoot.co.uk
■ ***By phone:*** *Talking Pages* 0800 600 900.
■ ***Health club chains:***
Cannons – Infoline: 08707808182; www.cannonsclubs.co.uk
LivingWell – Infoline: 0800 136636; www.livingwell.co.uk
Holmes Place – head office 0207795 4100; www.holmesplace.co.uk
YMCA – 0208520 5599; www.ymca.org.uk

Health farms

A visit to a health spa or farm may give your diet plan a kick-start. Several of the best-known UK farms are listed below, but you will also find that many hotels can offer fitness/beauty or health facilities almost as good, and probably at less expense.

Before you book, send off for the brochures or check out the websites, which will help you decide whether the farm has the right 'feel' for you – some are friendly and relaxed, others less so. Some allow alcohol and higher-calorie diets, others offer a more Spartan regime. The range of classes, treatments and facilities will also vary, as do the prices.

Health farms
■ Cedar Falls Health Farm, Bishops Lydeard, Taunton, Somerset TA4 3HR; 01823 433233; www.cedarfalls.co.uk
■ Champneys, Wiggington, Tring, Herts HP23 6HY; 01442 291111; www.champneys.co.uk
■ Forest Mere Health Farm, Liphook, Hants GU30 7JQ; 01428 726000; www.healthfarms.co.uk
■ Henlow Grange Health Farm, Henlow, Beds, SG16 6DB; 01462 811111; www.healthfarms.co.uk
■ Hoar Cross Hall Health Spa, Yoxall, Staffs DE13 8QS; 01283 575671; www.hoarcross.co.uk
■ Inglewood Health Hydro, Kintbury, Berkshire RG17 9SW; 01488 685111; www.inglewoodhealth.co.uk
■ Ragdale Hall Health Hydro, Ragdale, Melton Mowbray, Leics, LE14 3PB; 01664 434831; www.ragdalehall.co.uk
■ Shrubland Hall Health Clinic, Coddenham, Suffolk IP6 9QH; 01473 830404; www.shrubland.com
■ Stobo Castle Health Spa, Peebles, nr Edinburgh, Border Scotland EH45 8NY; 01721 760600; www.stobocastle.co.uk

Hotel health spas
■ The Celtic Manor Resort, Newport, Gwent, is new, with extensive health and fitness facilities; 01633 413000; www.celtic-manor.com

■ *The AA Hotel Guide 2002* (AA Publishing, September 2001) ISBN 0 74953108 8, and *The Good Hotel Guide 2002* (Ebury Press, September 2001) ISBN 0 09187967 1 list hotels with spa facilities. Both are updated annually.
See also: Exercise classes, Gyms and health clubs.

Heart rate monitors

If you want to know exactly how hard your heart is working during exercise and whether or not you are working within your correct training zone, the best way to tell is by linking yourself up to a heart rate monitor. These have come down in price in the last few years – you put a strap around your chest containing the transmitter, and wear a watch containing the receiver. Most of the exercise equipment retailers listed under Exercise equipment stock a range of heart rate monitors at prices from about £35. For around £100 you can get a monitor which also measures calories burnt, fitness level, and many other things. Polar is the best-known manufacturer.

Herbalife

If you see anyone wearing a badge that says 'lose weight now – ask me how' you'll know he/she is a Herbalife rep. Launched in 1980 in the USA, Herbalife went on to be one of the largest 'pyramid selling' organizations. Herbalife representatives sell a range of diet products and supplements, but the basis of the diet is 'Formula 1', where you replace two meals a day with a shake drink and eat a normal (but low-fat) main meal. To maintain weight, you replace just one meal a day and eat two normal meals. The nutritional composition of the diet is high-protein/low-carbohydrate.

Apart from the shakes, there are bars, soup mixes and drinks. The herbal supplements contain a variety of vitamins, antioxidants, herbs and minerals such as chromium. Although these may ensure that you don't suffer basic nutritional deficiencies while on the diet, they probably won't add a great deal to the calorie-burning effect.

Research reported at the International Congress on Obesity in 2001 claimed that meal-replacement plans have a higher success rate, especially for weight maintenance, than dieters who use ordinary food all the time. Further research is called for to confirm results like this.

Herbalife products are relatively expensive but, if you enjoy meal-replacement-type diets – and do better when the element of choice is taken away – this system is no worse than the others and may be better than some, although replacing two meals a day brings the total calorie count down a bit too low for comfort. If you enjoy real food and/or a healthy natural diet, I'd try another method.

■ Herbalife – reps usually advertise in local papers or will be in the local phone book. USA head office is on (00 1) 310 410 9600. For UK distributors, phone 0800 169 4198.

See also: Herbal diet supplements, Replacement meals, Very-low-calorie diets.

Herbal diet supplements

A read through the small ad sections of the slimming magazines and the tabloid Sunday newspapers will bring forth a wealth of advertisements for herbal preparations said to aid weight loss. Most of these are not worth buying. The following herbs and spices are some of the most researched of the few that may help you to lose weight in conjunction with a diet and exercise programme.

Ma huang: A herb used in China for 5,000 years, containing a natural form of ephedrine which helps to dull the appetite as well as increase the metabolic rate. The *International Journal of Obesity* reported in 2001 that a combination of ma huang and guarana (see Caffeine) helped testers to lose significantly more weight than people receiving a placebo. However, it stimulates the central nervous system and shouldn't be used by people with high blood pressure or heart conditions. Several deaths have been reported from its usage in the USA.

Zotrim: A newly marketed supplement made from three South American herbs which in a double-blind test reduced hunger by slowing down the rate at which the stomach empties.

Kelp: Kelp and other sea greens, such as dulse, are rich in iodine, the mineral which helps the thyroid (which controls metabolic rate) to function efficiently. The World Health Organization says that up to 1.5 billion people may be at risk from thyroid malfunction, often due to an iodine deficiency. Of course you may not be one of those people – and too much iodine can be toxic.

Others: Chilli can speed up the metabolic rate but is best eaten with normal food. Asparagus, artichoke, kelp, celery seed and other plants may be diuretic – reducing fluid retention (see Diuretics). Various other little-known plants are said to speed up the metabolic rate and may be included in herbal preparations or pills. These include garcinia cambogia, said to be rich in the stimulating compound hydroxycitric acid (HCA), which is also supposed to help prevent hunger in dieters. The latest study on hydroxycitrate, published in the *International Journal of Obesity* in 2001, found that supplementation with HCA didn't increase satiety or fat burning, but it might help prevent weight gain.

The problem is that, as food supplements (such as herbal preparations) aren't subject to rigorous testing, you can't be sure that the claims made are accurate, and, as we have seen, taking herbal concoctions ad lib may have unwanted side effects and could even be dangerous. If you feel that herbs may help you slim, you may be best off visiting an accredited Chinese herbalist (The Register of Chinese Herbal Medicine 07000 790332) or someone who belongs to the National Institute of Medical Herbalists (01392 426022).

Otherwise, the supplement distributors listed in the entry on Detoxing diets sell a reliable range of herbal preparations.

See also: Q12, Caffeine/supplements, Detoxing diets, Diuretics/supplements, Herbalife, Slimming pills, Sports supplements, Vitamin and mineral supplements.

The Hip and Thigh Diet

First published in l988, Rosemary Conley's *Hip and Thigh Diet* was embraced by UK women slimmers, staying at No 1 in the bestseller list for years. Its expanded, updated form, *The Complete Hip and Thigh Diet*, has sold over 2 million copies. The title cleverly acknowledges that most women are pear-shaped and sets out to beat this via diet and exercise.

The Diet

The hip and thigh diet is a fairly straightforward low-fat, low-calorie regime with no particular magic except that it cuts the fat down very low. There is no calorie or fat gram counting as such to be done, but the dieter picks meals from lists of breakfasts, lunches, main meals and extras, and much of the content of these has to be weighed, although every day you can have a jacket potato or portion of rice or pasta as big as you like, to satisfy your appetite.

There is a fairly long list of forbidden foods, including all butters and low-fat spreads, all dairy except skimmed milk, low-fat yoghurt, low-fat cottage cheese and low-fat fromage frais (though some of the recipes include small amounts of cheese and egg), all oils and lards, and all nuts and seeds (except tiny amounts for vegetarians), as well as the more obvious things like fried foods, pastry, cakes, chocolate, cakes, biscuits.

Meals include lean meat, poultry and white fish (but virtually no oily fish), pulses, unlimited vegetables and fair amounts of basic carbohydrates such as bread, vegetarian proteins, potatoes, rice and pasta.

Although the amount of fat in the diet each day will vary according to the menus chosen, I estimate you will be getting about 15–20% of your daily calories from fat, which puts this diet at the top end of the 'very-low-fat diets' category. Small amounts of alcohol are allowed and various low-calorie drinks, juices, tea and coffee are allowed. There is a daily 250ml (9fl oz) skimmed milk allowance.

Typical calorie count for a day's eating: 1,200

Promised weight loss: Not specific, but many case histories in the book show losses on average of about 1–3 lb (0.5–1.35kg) a week.

Typical day's eating:

■ ***Breakfast:*** 2 Weetabix with skimmed milk from allowance and l tsp brown sugar.

■ ***Snack:*** Raw carrot and celery.

■ ***Lunch:*** Mixed fresh fruit and chicken breast salad dressed with yoghurt and wine vinegar dressing.

■ ***Evening meal:*** Melon, small lean grilled rump garlic steak with large jacket potato, boiled mushrooms and unlimited vegetables; glass of red wine; rice pudding made with skimmed milk and artificial sweetener.

■ ***To drink:*** Tea with skimmed milk, mineral water, diet cola.

Short-term effectiveness: The reduction in calories via what would be, for most people, the quite drastic reduction in fat intake will undoubtedly lead to good weight loss in the early weeks for most people. ● **Score: 4**

Long term effectiveness: If the diet is continued, weight loss will carry on, probably slowing down. The exercise programme is a bonus which will help maintain weight loss – few diet books have a proper exercise section. ● **Score: 4**

Ease of use: Fairly ordinary, easy-to-find ingredients used. There are a lot of recipes but most are simple. Some people may find cooking without fat strange at first but the instructions are clear. The banned list of foods makes complying with the diet fairly straightforward, but eating out may be a problem and convenience 'ready' meals don't figure at all. The maintenance plan allows extra choice of foods. ● **Score: 3**

Cost: You can choose meals from any price bracket – there are many low-cost meals. No compulsory expensive ingredients. ● **Score: 5**

Palatability: Some recipes make good use of herbs and other flavourings to try to disguise the lack of fat, while others are less palatable – e.g. the fish pie containing only potatoes, cod and seasoning! Plenty of fruit and vegetables. It might be a good idea to use Conley's cookery books alongside the diet to enliven proceedings. ● **Score: 3**

Satiety: People who have followed the diet report finding it easy to stick to without having the urge to binge, however it is not as high in carbohydrates as some low-fat diets and is quite low in calories overall. ● **Score: 3**

Health factor: Most health professionals agree that a low-fat diet is one of the healthiest to follow; however, some would say this plan is a little low in the omega-3 fats from oily fish and seeds, and in the omega-6s found in plant oils. The diet is otherwise balanced if you make wise and varied meal choices from the lists from day to day (though you could pick an unbalanced diet if you chose to, as there is little guidance). Conley recommends a multivitamin pill a day. ● **Score: 3**

Scientific basis: Based on low-fat, low-calorie eating, the premise of which is tried and tested. However, the implication that the diet has any particular special effects on slimming the hips and thighs, as opposed to any other part of the body, is false. Fat is as likely to go from the bust, stomach, arms, etc. as it is from the hips and thighs. ● **Score: 3**

Total score 28

Percentage rating 70%

■ *Rosemary Conley's Complete Hip and Thigh Diet* (Arrow, 1993) ISBN 0 09911011 3.

See also: Qs 89, 90, Low-fat diets, Top 20 popular diets.

Hypnosis

Hypnosis has been described as a form of therapy which works on the subconscious to change thought and behaviour patterns. The state of hypnosis is a deeply relaxed state somewhere between waking and sleeping – the depth of the hypnotic trance can vary. Hypnosis may help some people to control overeating and therefore to lose weight. Usually at least four sessions may be needed, sometimes more.

■ The National Register of Hypnotherapists and Psychotherapists, 12 Cross Street, Nelson, Lancs, BB9 7EN; 01282 716839.

See also: Counselling.

Internet slimming

If you have a computer and are connected to the worldwide web, several companies aim to ensure that diet books, magazines and slimming clubs are a thing of the past. Several new sites offer a combination of all these things to help you lose weight without leaving home or spending any money.

They do vary in the quality of their advice, user-friendliness and the extent of available information. Some offer a great deal of interaction with other slimmers, and even the possibility of having your own personal diet or fitness programme devised on line. There may be a recipe library, reviews of products, exercises – and more. They can do almost anything except actually weigh you in person to make sure you aren't cheating.

The sites listed here are those I have found most interesting but a search engine, such as Google, will no doubt come up with more you will like. Tip – go for sites ending in co.uk to get British-based advice, which you may find more usable than the US-based advice you are likely to find with .com sites (though some .coms are UK-based). There is one exception – I found the official 'Shape Up America! site very good for assessing fitness.

■ www.feelingfat.co.uk – just like a chatty magazine online with everything you would expect from a slimming magazine.

■ www.realslimmers.com – plenty of real-life success stories to inspire you and the advice and diets are written by leading dieticians and experts.

■ www.shapeup.org – Shape Up America; plenty of fitness and food advice, with the chance to test your own fitness levels.

■ www.slimtime.co.uk – run by a successful slimmer, with lots of success stories, plus advice on food, exercise, the psychology of weight loss and more.

■ www.weightlossresources.co.uk – for a small monthly fee you can be given a personalized diet and exercise plan, complete with nutrition advice and customized meals. Also offers a members' forum, news, etc.

See also: Diet coaches, Personal trainers, Slimming clubs.

Isometrics

This static exercise method was very popular in the '60s and '70s. The muscles are contracted, held (usually against a resistant force) for several seconds and then released. Done several times a day, this is a quick way to improve muscle tone and strength. Isometric training has largely fallen out of fashion and is rarely on offer in fitness centres, etc. It isn't suitable for people with high blood pressure and/or heart disease.

Juice diets

A juice-only fast or detox programme will result in rapid initial weight loss, much of which will be fluid. Juice fasts contain vitamin C and other vitamins and minerals, but few calories, almost no protein and no fat, and as such shouldn't be undertaken as a slimming regime and shouldn't be followed for more than a day or so on an occasional basis.

While fruit and vegetable juices contain all the vitamins and minerals of the whole plant they contain little fibre, which may be a disadvantage. Slimming on a diet of whole fruits and veg as part of a balanced reduced-calorie diet is a better long-term idea. All the books below will provide ideas for juicing.

The latest hyped juice diet is the Hollywood 48-Hour Miracle Diet – available through many US outlets on the Internet – a packaged mix of juices, vitamins, minerals, antioxidants and essential oils. This will help you to shed weight as described above, but contains no miracle ingredients. As it is about $30 a time, you'd be better off with a glass of fruit juice, a multivitamin pill and a couple of omega-3 supplements.

■ *Juice Blitz* by Leslie Kenton (Vermilion, January 2000) ISBN 0 09182585 7.

■ *Juicing for Health* by Catherine Wheater (HarperCollins, new edition February 2001) ISBN 0 00710691 2.

■ *Juice Fasting and Detoxification* by Steve Meyerowitz (Sproutman Publishing, April l999) ISBN 1 87873665 5.

See also: Fasting.

Kitchen scales

If you like to cook or want to weigh that last gram of fat, you need a good set of kitchen scales. Choose ones with small increments (down as low as 1g is ideal) for fine weighing, but make sure they will take at least 1kg, 2kg is even better. Make sure they weigh in ounces and grams, and have an 'add and weigh' facility. Scales on which you can put a plate are handy. You can buy special dieters' scales which will weigh a tiny one-tenth of an ounce, but they tend not to take the heavier weights.

■ www.scalesexpress.com

■ www.trade-web.co.uk

Laxatives

Laxative pills shouldn't be used as a method of weight control as overuse can be dangerous and long-term use upsets the mechanism of the colon, and dependence could result. Laxatives may also prevent absorption of some of the nutrients in food. Some low-calorie slimming diets – particularly those low in dietary fibre, including crash diets and high-protein/low-carb diets – may result in constipation, in which case fruit, vegetable, whole grain and pulse intake should be stepped up and eight glasses of water a day should be taken with food and between meals. Some foods and herbs have a naturally laxative action and it is generally better to include these in your diet than rely on laxative pills. They include rhubarb, spices, aloe vera, citrus fruits, psyllium husk, linseeds and olive oil. Supplements of acidophilus, available at health food stores, may also help. *See also:* Qs 151, 155.

Lecithin

Lecithin is a substance found in all our body cells and is present in large amounts in the brain and liver, as well as in some foods, particularly egg yolks, nuts, liver and whole grains. Lecithin acts as an emulsifier, turning large fat particles in the body into smaller ones and thus making it easier to digest.

Lecithin supplements – in the form of granules or liquid – are widely available and are of use to people who don't tolerate fats well in the diet, for example, people who have had their gall bladder removed. It may also help with memory and help keep blood cholesterol levels under control.

Its reputation as a slimming aid probably came about because of the way it deals with fat in the body. However, it is of no use whatsoever for slimming; it can't rid your body either of dietary fat or body fat – you need to create a calorie deficit to do that (see Q18).

Low-fat diets

Low-fat diets aim to reduce total fat in the diet and usually concentrate on getting saturates down as low as possible, while foods with essential polyunsaturated fats (and/or monounsaturated fats) are usually allowed in fairly small quantities. Some low-fat diets are much lower in fat than others, and diets with a total fat content of less than 20% are discussed under Very-low-fat diets. Here we look at the pros and cons of reduced-fat diets, moderately low in fat at 20–30%. Surprisingly, there are few well-known dieting regimes that come into this category, although most Glycaemic Index diets do, as does Patrick Holford's Fat Burner Diet.

The Diet

A low-fat diet may have around 25% fat, and most have around 20–25% protein and about 50–55% carbohydrate. The premise is that, as fat is the most energy-dense nutrient that you can eat, with 9 calories per gram, reducing the fat in the diet is an easy way to cut calories. As the diet is also high in carbs – and most low-fat diets recommend high consumption of 'complex' carbs, like whole grains, potatoes and pulses, plus plenty of fruit and veg – it is said to satisfy hunger.

Typical calorie count for a day's eating: 1,500.
Promised weight loss: Most low-fat diets offer steady weight loss of 1–2lb (0.5–1kg) a week.
Typical day's eating:

- ***Breakfast:*** Small bowl of muesli with skimmed milk and chopped fresh fruit; slice of wholemeal toast with very-low-fat spread and marmalade.
- ***Lunch:*** Tuna in brine with a large mixed salad dressed with a little olive oil French dressing; low-fat fruit yoghurt; handful of dried apricots.
- ***Evening meal:*** Stir-fry of lean pork fillet with a selection of chopped veg, cooked in a small amount of groundnut oil, served with boiled egg-thread noodles, banana, glass of wine.
- ***To drink:*** Tea, coffee, (with skimmed milk), water, fruit juice.

Short-term effectiveness: As high in carbohydrates, immediate weight loss won't be so noticeable as with a high-protein regime, as it doesn't have the same diuretic effect. But fat loss will begin straight away if the low-fat diet is also moderate in total calories. ● **Score: 3**
Long-term effectiveness: The World Health Organization has come to the conclusion that a moderately reduced-fat, high-carb diet produces better results for long-term weight maintenance than basic calorie counting, and the US Department of Agriculture states that such diets produce weight loss even when they are consumed 'ad libitum' (i.e. with unlimited carbs). Other studies conclude that people are more likely to stick with diets which reduce calories moderately (as most moderate low-fat diets do) than those which reduce calories more drastically. ● **Score: 5**
Ease of use: The moderate nature of most low-fat diets means that they may be easier to follow than others. Food used are generally familiar. ● **Score: 4**
Cost: No special high-cost foods needed and the complex carbs such as grains, root vegetables are low in cost. ● **Score: 4**
Palatability: People used to a high-fat diet may find the reduction in fat hard to get used to at first. ● **Score: 3**
Satiety: Diets high in carbohydrate tend to offer a high degree of satiety. Fruit and vegetable consumption is encouraged on most low-fat diets. These will add to the bulk on the plate and have been shown to increase the length of time it takes to eat a meal, also adding to satiety value. Total calorie content is usually not too low, again ensuring satiety. However, not all low-fat, high-carbohydrate diets make full use of carbohydrate foods that are low on the Glycaemic Index, which would be an additional satiety bonus. ● **Score: 4**
Health factor: Most international heart associations and authorities recommend a diet low in saturated fat and high in carbs as a good way to prevent heart disease and other health problems (see Section 9 and Q90). A moderate amount of unsaturated fat, present in most moderate low-fat diets, may be a positive health factor, and the US Department of Agriculture stated in 2001 that the moderate fat-reduction diet is optimal for ensuring adequate nutrition levels in dieters. ● **Score: 5**
Scientific basis: Low-fat diets work to help people lose weight by reducing the total number of calories they consume, creating a

calorie deficit which should produce slow to steady weight loss. However, it is possible to consume a low-fat diet and still eat too many calories in the form of carbohydrate foods and low-fat protein foods (or alcohol). So, unless the total calorie content of the diet is moderated, a low-fat diet may not work. ● **Score: 4**

Total Score 32

Percentage rating 80%

■ The Diet Bible Basic Diet in Feature 9 is a 25%-fat, high-carbohydrate diet.
See also: Qs 80, 83–5, 89, 90, Glycaemic Index diets, Top 20 popular diets, Very-low-fat diets.

Low-fat foods

Supermarkets are filled on the one hand with high-fat, high-sugar foods designed to help make us fat, and on the other hand with all kinds of low-fat products, designed to get us thin again. Low-fat foods are big business – you can get low-fat cakes, biscuits, desserts, sauces, and many more.

Research has shown that, in the long run, people who buy commercial low-fat foods don't tend to eat any fewer calories than people who don't buy them, and don't in the long run become slimmer. One reason may be that a lot of the sweet low-fat foods tend to be quite high in sugar and so, although total fat may be reduced, the calorie count may still be high. Another reason is that when we eat a 'low-fat' item, we feel we are allowed to indulge ourselves in something else that IS high in fat. If you are going to treat yourself, therefore, you may be just as well off choosing the original high-fat version.

However, regularly choosing skimmed milk, low-fat yoghurt and low-fat spread rather than the full-fat is probably a good idea, as the perception of these foods is more that they are staples, rather than reduced-fat versions of 'treat' items.
See also: Qs 89, 90, Fat substitutes.

Macrobiotic Diet

Despite its 'nothing but brown rice' reputation, in fact the dietary element of modern macrobiotics can be a very healthy regime. Macrobiotics is based on an ancient Far Eastern philosophy of holistic living, but the current macrobiotic food guidelines have evolved over the past 120 years.

The basic diet contains of 50% whole grains; 25% seasonal vegetables, cooked or raw, 10% protein foods such as fish or pulses; 5% sea vegetables, 5% soups and 5% fruits, nuts, seeds, and drinks such as herbal teas. Sugars, spices, alcohol, meat, eggs and cheese are not allowed, as the first three are too yin (cool) and the rest too yang (hot).

There is much more to the macrobiotic diet and way of life than this, of course, but viewed as a potential diet for slimming, macrobiotic eating has many plus points, being high in natural unrefined foods, complex carbohydrates and vegetables. Allowing, as it does, fish, nuts and seeds, it is low in saturated fat but high in essential fats and fulfils just about all of the modern criteria for a healthy slimming or maintenance diet for adults, although it could be a little low in calcium. You would still need to watch portion sizes of the denser foods in the diet to keep calories to a reducing level for weight loss, but this would be unlikely to be a problem as the diet contains so many high-bulk, low-calorie items. The advantages of this type of diet are described in more detail under Low-fat diets.

■ The Macrobiotic Association, 99 Yeldham Road, London, W6 8JQ; www.macrobiotic.co.uk

■ *An Introduction to Macrobiotics* by Oliver Cowmeadow (Thorsons, August 1988) ISBN 0 72251414 X.

■ *Macrobiotic Diet* by Michio Kushi (Japan Publications, January I994) ISBN 0 87040878 X.

Massage

Having someone give you a massage is relaxing and pleasant but it won't burn off any calories or fat – except for the masseur. What massage can do is stimulate your lymph system, so that you will 'go to the loo' quite a lot afterwards, resulting in fluid elimination and, therefore, a little weight loss. It has also been demonstrated that vigorous massage with oils, cream, etc., can improve the appearance of cellulite a little.

■ Massage Therapy Institute of Great Britain; tel 0208 208 1607; or send SAE for list of practitioners to PO Box 2726 London NW2 4NR.

■ British Massage Therapy Council 01865 774123.

See also: Cellulite treatments, Salon treatments.

Mayo Clinic Diet

People have discussed the Mayo Clinic Diet for decades and yet it doesn't actually exist! The famous Mayo Clinic health centre and hospital in Rochester USA categorically states that it has never endorsed any diet plan. Rather, it has healthy eating and weight loss guidelines in line with those given by the USA and UK governments. The so-called 'Mayo Clinic Diet' appears in different guises throughout the world, though it often contains grapefruit at every meal and has a great deal of protein and salads, and little carbs. This kind of diet – said to help you lose up to 52 lb (23.5kg) in 10 weeks – is a fad/crash/high-protein diet and not to be recommended.
See also: Crash diets, Grapefruit Diet; High-protein diets.

Mediterranean Diet

Some diet plans base themselves on 'Mediterranean' style eating. This is really southern Med eating and consists of a lot of fruit and vegetables, salads dressed with olive oil, fish, bread, pasta and other grains, and small amounts of meat and poultry. This is a healthy way to eat and fairly much

in line with international advice. Olive oil has no special magic properties in helping you to lose weight so, if following the Mediterranean diet without counting calories, you would need to watch portion sizes of the higher-calorie elements in order to turn it into a slimming one.
See also: Low-fat diets.

Metabolic typing

The idea behind metabolic typing is that each of us has an individual metabolic pattern which governs the kind of foods that we should eat for optimum health and (if necessary) weight loss. The author of the metabolic typing book claims that even our digestive juices vary and asks you 65 questions to help you determine your type.

Nutritionists trained in the 'science' of metabolic typing give a personal consultation, which will look at nine body systems including your blood, endocrine system, electrolytes and so on. The two key areas are the autonomic nervous system and your 'oxidative' system, which covers the rate at which you convert food to energy. The process of determining your type (and the reasoning behind it) is all quite complicated and mainstream nutritionists mostly dismiss it as yet another example of pseudoscientific hogwash. However, as with many of these programmes, there is anecdotal evidence that they may work.

■ *The Metabolic Typing Diet* by William Linz Wolcott (Bantam Doubleday Dell Publishing, August 2000) ISBN 0 38549691 5.
■ Information on all aspects of metabolic typing from Wolcott's company www.healthexcel.com (email info@healthexcel.com; tel (00 1) 650 325 1840.

Metabolism booster diets

Several diets published over the past few years have claimed to work, at least in part, by boosting metabolic rate. Some (e.g., The Diet Cure) claim to boost thyroid function; others to 'fool' the metabolism so it doesn't slow when you lose weight (e.g., The Rotation Diet). Others offer breathing techniques (of little benefit) or include exercise – the only factor that definitely will help speed the metabolism. The sad truth is that weight loss and dieting are much more likely to slow down your metabolic rate than increase it (hence the need to reduce calorie intake in order to get slimmer), so take these claims with a pinch of salt. Section One explains the workings of your metabolism in detail.
See also: The Diet Cure, Fat Burning, The Rotation Diet.

Negative-calorie foods

For many years now people have eagerly talked about foods which are said to produce a 'negative calorie' effect in the body and thus help weight loss.

The hype is still going on – with one or two books selling well and various websites devoted to the 'negative calorie' concept. Interestingly, the information differs according to whom you listen to. Author Neal Barnard condemns animal produce and provides a list of vegetarian foods said to produce the negative calorie effect. For about $20 you can get another negative calorie book from a company which suggests that in eating a stick of celery (5 calories) you burn up 95 unwanted calories. They cite a weight loss of 14 lb (6.25kg) in seven days. Someone else says that fruits and veg are high in enzymes, some of which remain surplus to requirements after the digestive process and 'escape' into the bloodstream, speeding up the metabolic rate.

The truth is that all this is nonsense, and the negative calories concept is rubbish. All the plans offered will produce weight loss because they rely on reducing calorie intake down very low, usually on a high-fruit and -veg/low-fat/low-carbohydrate type of diet. There is no miracle to losing weight; you need to create a calorie deficit (see Q18).

■ www.negativecaloriediet.com
■ *Foods That Cause You to Lose Weight: The Negative Calorie Effect* by Neal Barnard (Wholecare April I999) ISBN 0 38080797 1 (USA); (Book Publishing Co, January 1995) ISBN 1 88233035 8 (UK).

Organic diets

Although many people prefer to eat organic foods because they feel they may be safer and/or taste better than mass-produced non-organic food, most organic foods contain almost the same number of calories as their non-organic counterparts. However, one or two points are worth raising. If organic food does taste better (and I am convinced that the organic veg and fruit I grow certainly do, and that the organic beef, pork, lamb and chicken I buy from neighbours are infinitely superior to cheap supermarket meat, although I couldn't claim that all organic food tastes better, because it doesn't), then it may mean that you're satisfied with less. There is also evidence that the basic organic foods (e.g. fruit, veg and meat) contain less water than non-organic, which would also make it more satisfying.

Often organically produced meat does, however, contain higher levels of fat than non-organic (because it is produced in the traditional way, whereas much modern supermarket meat is bred to be lean). This will mean that it contains more calories than non-organic, but smaller portions should satisfy you.

Lastly, deciding to have small amounts of top-quality food is a good way to watch calorie intake. I'd rather eat 75g of delicious wild salmon than 250g of mass market salmon quiche, and one square of organic dark chocolate than a whole bar of sugary confectionery.

■ The Soil Association; Bristol House, 40–56 Victoria Street, Bristol, BS1 6BY; tel 0117 929 0661; www.soilassociation.org, produces an *Organic Directory for the UK*, price £7.95 plus £1 p&p.
■ *Organic* by Sophie Grigson and William Black (Headline, May 2001) ISBN 0 74727220 4.

Overeaters Anonymous

Overeaters Anonymous isn't a slimming club – but its members often lose weight. It is an international nonprofitmaking fellowship started back in 1960, in California, when three people got together to try to help each other with their eating problems and followed the pattern of '12 steps to recovery' based on the Alcoholics Anonymous programme.

OA now has 7,500 meetings worldwide and there is no membership fee – the requirement for membership is a desire to stop compulsive eating. All members retain their anonymity, with first names only being used. A Gallup Poll survey found that their average member is a 44-year-old woman who has lost 40lb (18kg) and has found that her emotional and mental health has improved since joining OA.

There is a religious element to the organization and the '12 Steps' outlined frequently refer to God and a Greater Power. No dietary advice is offered, but the organization recommends that members develop their own 'plan of eating', perhaps with the help of a dietician.

■ Overeaters Anonymous World Service Office (head office), PO Box 44020, Rio Rancho, New Mexico 87174-4020, USA, tel (00 1) 505 891 2664; www.overeatersanonymous.org – the website has the facility to find your nearest meeting as well as plenty of other information – or you can phone 07626 984674 (South East England) or 07000 784985 (elsewhere in the UK) for the telephone number of your nearest meeting organizer.

See also: Internet slimming, Slimming clubs.

Personal trainers

If you have trouble motivating yourself to exercise, a personal trainer could be a good idea. With one-to-one help, you get an individual training programme, help with technique and motivation. A PT isn't inexpensive, though, and seeing one twice a week is better than once (plus you need to do your own sessions in between). Find a qualified trainer through the APT, who have a minimum standard, or through the FIA or the NRPT.

If a real personal trainer is not a possibility and you have access, the Internet offers many virtual PTs, many of which are free. You usually get a personal assessment by keying in personal and activity details, and you're then offered a variety of programmes to follow, including illustrated exercises, plus a diary record to fill in and monitor progress. Fitlinxx is one of the best (click on UK option) and Shape Up America is quite basic, but fun. You can also get an online personal diet and training programme with unlimited access to personal support from Fit-ness UK for £40 for a year.

■ Association of Personal Trainers, 0208 692 4023.

■ Fitness Industry Association, 0207 620 0700; www.fia.org.uk

■ National Register of Personal Trainers; 07971 954662; www.nrpt.co.uk

■ www.fitlinxx.com, www.fit-ness.co.uk, www.shapeup.org

See also: Exercise classes, Internet slimming.

Pilates

The eight basic principles of Pilates exercise (based on the teachings of Joseph Pilates, early in the 20th century) are relaxation, co-ordination, alignment, stamina, concentration, centring, breathing and flowing movements. The main benefits of Pilates, for people who want to enhance their body shape, are that it improves posture and gives a longer, leaner look to the muscles but, properly taught, there are many other benefits.

Anyone can set themselves up as a Pilates teacher, however, so when seeking out a class/studio/teacher, make sure they have done some appropriate training. www.pilates.co.uk has a list of certification centres.

■ Body Control Pilates Association information line: 0870 1690000; www.bodycontrol.co.uk for teachers near you, etc.

■ *The Official Body Control Pilates Manual* by Lynne Robinson and Helge Fisher (Macmillan, 2000) ISBN 0 33378202 X.

Postal/telephone slimming

If you can't get to a slimming class and don't use the Internet, you may find a postal slimming course helps keep you on track. With the independent courses listed below you will receive a weekly menu plan, other slimming advice, plus postal, e-mail or phone help. Cost, amount of choice in the menus, type of diet, and what exactly you get varies, from about £4 a week. Major slimming clubs also do packs for people who can't get to a class.

■ Shapes Slimming Clubs; FREEPOST (SCE6203), Melksham SN12 6SA; 01380 828372.

■ Pound Shedders; 01543 672690; www.pound-shedders.co.uk

■ Slimfit Home Membership; Slimfit Suite, Enterprise House, Valley St North, Darlington DL1 1GY; 01325 260060.

■ SlymRyte; 07050 177590; www.slymryte.co.uk

■ WeightWatchers 'At Home' programme, WeightWatchers UK Ltd, Ludlow Rd, Maidenhead, Berks SL6 2SL; 08457 123000.

■ Slimming World Postal Membership; PO Box 55, Alfreton, Derbyshire DE55 4UE; 01773 523860.

■ Rosemary Conley Postal Club; Quorn House, Meeting St., Quorn, Loughborough, Leics, LE12 8EX; 01509 620222.

■ Slimming Magazine Dietline Postal Service; Slimming Magazine Clubs, Broadway House, 112–134 The Broadway, London SW19 1RL.

See also: Diet coaches, Internet slimming, Slimming clubs.

The Pritikin Diet

Described as 'the world's most requested diet programme', the Pritikin programme was first published as a health-giving diet and fitness plan in 1979. The author, Nathan Pritikin, founder of the famous Pritikin Longevity Centre in California, advocated a very-low-fat, high-carb diet. Other books followed and in l991 his son Robert Pritikin devised the Pritikin Weight Loss Breakthrough, which still sells well. For an appraisal of very-low-fat diets and more information on the book, see Very-low-fat diets.

Protein Power

This book, first published in the USA in 1996, went on to become a bestseller worldwide. It follows in the tradition of the Atkins Diet, being high in protein, high in fat and low in carbohydrate. The authors, Michael and Mary Eades, claim that by following a low-carb diet you will reduce insulin levels and your health will improve via lower blood cholesterol and pressure (and a host of other benefits). Interestingly, the two famous diets at the other end of the spectrum (high-carb, low-fat Eat More, Weigh Less and the Pritikin programme, both reviewed under Very-low-fat diets) claim similar health benefits.

This is probably because losing weight in itself, by whatever method, tends to lower insulin resistance and decrease various health risks. The premise that a low-carb diet helps you lose weight by reducing circulating blood insulin is warped – reduction of food intake of any kind will achieve this.

My advice – until the benefits of a high-fat diet are proven beyond doubt – is that I'd stick with the current wisdom that high-carb, reduced-fat eating is healthiest, and choose a slimming diet accordingly. For a more detailed examination of a high-fat, high-protein diet similar to Protein Power, see the entry for the Atkins Diet.

■ *Protein Power* by Dr Michael R. Eades and Dr Mary Dan Eades (Thorsons, January 2000) ISBN 0 7225 3961 4.

See also: Atkins Diet, High-protein diets.

Raw food diets

There are several diet plans and organizations that advocate a raw-food, plant-based diet as the best way to good health, as well as weight loss and weight maintenance. Some of the most well known are listed at the end of this entry. Proponents of eating a raw, or high-percentage-raw, diet say that raw foods contain all the enzymes in the original plant which are lost in cooking, and that there are other advantages such as retention of vitamins and removal of 'toxins' from the body. The change in the balance of the type of food you can eat on a predominantly raw diet means that the amount of calories, protein, fat and carbohydrate it contains will almost certainly be vastly different from the typical Western diet.

The Diet

A typical plan advocates at least 75% of your food raw, perhaps with the addition of some whole cooked grains and pulses, good-quality fish, poultry and a few other things (though many raw fooders are strict vegans, and also try to avoid all cooked food). The raw foods are usually a choice of any veg, fruits, dried fruits and juices, nuts and seeds, sprouted seeds and grains, rolled or flaked grains, salad dressings, herbs and spices and more.

Typical calorie count for a day's eating: 1,250.

Promised weight loss: Slow and steady.

Typical day's eating:

■ ***Breakfast:*** Fresh fruit salad topped with chopped fresh almonds, wheatgerm and pumpkin seeds; sheep's milk bio yoghurt (preferably homemade) or coconut cream

■ ***Lunch:*** Mixed salad of various leaves, yellow peppers, tomatoes, red onions and parsley dressed with olive oil and balsamic vinegar dressing and topped with sprouted lentils.

■ ***Evening meal:*** Raw mixed vegetable soup (blended); homemade sunflower seed cheese; 1/2 avocado; raspberry and banana sorbet.

■ ***To drink:*** Water, juices, fruit smoothies, coconut milk.

Short-term effectiveness: Calorie and carbohydrate content automatically reduced on such a regime and weight loss will be almost certain for most people. ● **Score: 4**

Long-term effectiveness: If the regime is continued, weight loss will progress. However a raw, or nearly raw, regime is not easy to live with except for the totally committed and so for most people the chances of sticking with it for life are small. ● **Score: 3**

Ease of use: For most people this will be a very hard regime to get used to – it requires a complete rethink on shopping and meal preparation and makes a social life quite hard when mixing with people eating non-raw. However, time may be saved in respect of actual cooking and there is little need to calorie count. ● **Score: 2**

Cost: Doesn't need to be expensive as plants in season can be used; but unlikely to be very low-cost either. ● **Score: 3**

Palatability: A shock to the taste buds unless acclimatized gradually. However, eventually the diet should seem quite palatable. ● **Score: 2**

Satiety: High on bulk and very filling for few calories. The reasonable-to-high content of plant oils helps satiety. ● **Score: 5**

Health factor: The diet may contain a lot more fat than may be apparent, but the proportion of saturated fat should be low, with plenty of the good-for-you essential fats. There may be adequate protein (if enough pulses, nuts, seeds, etc. are eaten) but total carb content may be low. Obviously five fruit and vegetable portions a day won't be a problem, but a special effort needs to be made to eat enough carbohydrate, and adding some cooked grains, root veg, etc. to the diet would make it more balanced. Fibre content should be good.

With a completely raw diet based on plant foods alone, choices are limited and certain vitamins and minerals may be in short supply. The nutrients in some foods are better absorbed when cooked. ● **Score: 4**

Scientific basis: There is no special magic in raw foods that will help you to lose weight, other than that it is hard to overeat when much of your diet is raw and high in water and fibre. ● **Score: 4**

Total score 27

Percentage rating 67.5%

■ *The New Raw Energy* by Leslie Kenton (Vermilion, January 2001) ISBN 0 09185617 5.

■ *Living Foods for Health* by Dr Gillian McKeith (Piatkus, April 200) ISBN 0 74992074 2.

■ The Fresh Network – for raw eating news, information and products. PO Box 71, Ely, Cambs CB7 4GU; tel 0870 8007070; www.fresh-network.com

See also: Q92; Detox diets, Fit for Life, Food combining, Macrobiotic diets, Top 20 popular diets, Vegan diets, Wholefood diets.

Ready meals

Every supermarket stocks a variety of ready calorie- and fat-counted convenience meals, usually in single-portion sizes. These can be useful as a stand-by for busy people, but heavier people may find that the portion size and calorie content are too small for comfort. Most of these meals are best with a side salad or vegetable added for extra bulk, and/or a large portion of fruit afterwards, otherwise hunger may be a problem and total fibre and vitamin C content of your diet may also be low if you use ready meals frequently.

Some companies in the USA deliver ready-calorie- and fat-counted meals to your door. Nutri/System is probably the most famous – they will deliver all your meals for the day/week and there is a large choice of menus, but you have to add your own fruits, salads, drinks, vegetables and skimmed milk. Meals based on The Zone diet are also delivered in the USA, and are promised here soon. At the moment I can find only one company – Deliver a Diet (0870 774 7745) in the UK, which only delivers in the London area.

Although living largely on prepacked meals certainly won't suit everyone, it does approximate how a lot of people eat when they aren't dieting, and one two-year clinical study published in the *American Journal of Physiology* in 2000 found that women who lost weight (21lb/9.5kg on average over 16 weeks) on the Nutri/system had above average success in keeping the weight off.

Replacement meals

If you want to lose weight the idea is that you swap one or two meals a day for the meal replacement – usually a shake-type drink – which is all calorie-counted and nutrition-balanced for you. Then you eat one or two normal meals and watch the weight come off. Because there is little fuss or bother, many people do choose this way to slim and find it successful. The most well-known make now is probably SlimFast, though there are other brands with similar make-up, including the Cambridge Diet (see Very-low calorie diets) and you can also purchase meal replacement bars, soups etc.

The Diet

Most slimmers begin on two meal replacements a day plus one normal healthy meal. The replacement meals contain around 200–250 calories, the normal meal around 600 calories. Plus you have extras allowed, such as fruit and skimmed milk.

Typical calorie count for a day's eating: 1,200

Promised weight loss: Not specified.

Typical day's eating:

■ ***Breakfast:*** Milk Shake replacement meal

■ ***Snack:*** Apple

■ ***Lunch:*** Milk-shake replacement meal

■ ***Evening meal:*** Grilled chicken, baked potato, 2 servings of vegetables, gravy; banana.

■ ***To drink:*** 6–8 glasses water or calorie-free drinks.

Short-term effectiveness. Weight loss will begin quickly when two meals a day are replaced. Body fat/fluid/lean tissue loss will be similar to that on normal low-calorie diets. ● **Score: 4**

Long-term effectiveness: Two studies have shown that meal replacement dieting is effective. One, partially supported by SlimFast and reported at the European Congress on Obesity in 2001, showed that slimmers lost more weight than the control group when using meal-replacement drinks, and kept the weight off more successfully. Another, published in the *American Journal of Clinical Nutrition*, showed successful weight loss which was largely maintained after four years. However the studies were small. Most meal replacements suggest following a normal diet when you are down to target weight and for many people reverting to 'real food' may cause weight to return as new 'normal' eating habits haven't been learnt. ● **Score: 3**

Ease of use: Very easy and convenient – just mix up a shake or open the can or pack, and eat or drink. ● **Score: 5**

Cost: Reasonable when compared with the price of the meal you may otherwise have eaten. ● **Score: 4**

Palatability: Choice of flavours, etc. but you still can't get away from the fact that meal replacements are not everyone's milk shake. They are bought for the convenience, not their gourmet rating. This could be a problem, as one of the main reasons that people generally get overweight is because they love food. ● **Score: 2**

Satiety: Better than you might fear, but without much (or anything) to chew on, the mouth may feel deprived, and as the shakes go down so quickly it is easy to feel as though you haven't had any lunch after all, so psychological satiety is poor. ● **Score: 2**

Health factor: The four-year study already cited found that the meal-replacement slimmers had improved health profiles, including blood pressure, insulin levels and cholesterol counts. But that would probably be true for most people who have lost weight by whatever method Meal replacements' nutrient composition is covered by legislation so you won't go short of any vitamins, minerals or major nutrients on the diets but they are, in essence, not natural foodstuffs with all the many phytochemicals that 'real' foods such as fruits and vegetables contain, and it may be hard to get your 'five a day', although SlimFast suggest adding two pieces of fruit. ● **Score: 3**

Scientific basis: Replacement meals reduce calorie content of your diet and thus help you to create energy deficit, which will help you lose weight. This simple equation can't be argued with. ● **Score 5**

Total score 28

Percentage rating 70%

■ SlimFast, www.slim-fast.co.uk

See also: Q109, Crash diets, Top 20 popular diets, Very-low calorie diets.

The Rotation Diet

This was one of the biggest dieting phenomena of the l980s. The book (written by Martin Katahn in l986 after he lost five stones himself, so the story goes) is still in print today and works by rotating the number of calories per day that you are allowed. A complete rotation takes three weeks and this, according to Katahn, keeps the metabolic rate high.

The Diet

Women have a week on 600 (first 3 days) or 900 calories (next 4 days) a day, then a week on 1,200 calories a day, then a week back on 600 or 900. Men do 1,200/1,500 during weeks 1 and 3, with 1,800 on week 2. Then you take a break of at least a week eating normally, before returning to the diet as necessary. The diet is a typical low-cal, reduced-fat, reduced-portion diet.

Typical calorie count for a day's eating: 600–1,200 for women; 1,200–1,800 for men.

Promised weight loss: Average of 14lb (6.25kg) in the three weeks.

Typical day's eating (for women, 600 cals)

■ ***Breakfast:*** 1/2 banana; 28g high-fibre cereal, 225ml (8fl oz) skimmed milk.

■ ***Lunch:*** 110g low-fat cottage cheese; celery, cucumber, lettuce, slice of wholemeal bread.

■ ***Evening:*** Poached white fish fillet; broccoli, carrots; 1/2 grapefruit.

■ ***To drink:*** 8 glasses water, 2 cups coffee or tea, herb tea.

Short-term effectiveness: Very low calorie levels, especially for women, will result in immediate weight loss, much of which will be fluid. ● **Score: 4**

Long-term effectiveness: Used as Katahn suggests, weight loss will continue but the calorie count (for women) is too low for recommended long-term use. Studies show that weight lost quickly tend to return quickly. ● **Score: 1**

Ease of use: Three weeks' menus given, based on ordinary foods, but you need to weigh or measure a high proportion. ● **Score: 3**

Cost: Average. ● **Score: 3**

Palatability: Fairly old-fashioned type of 'cottage cheese and crispbreads' diet, although there are a few recipes which don't look too bad and make good use of herbs and spices. ● **Score: 3**

Satiety: Small portions, low calorie count (for women) and plenty of included foods which are high on the Glycaemic Index means that satiety is not likely to be good. ● **Score: 2**

Health factor: The women's diet averages out at just over 900 calories a day during the three-week cycle, which is too low for healthy slimming, may result in nutrient deficiencies and more severe loss of lean tissue than on a more moderate diet. This is a crash diet in effect – these are discussed elsewhere throughout the book. ● **Score: 1**

Scientific basis: Katahn claims that the rotation of the number of calories consumed prevents the drop in metabolism (which normally accompanies weight loss), which in turn helps speed up the rate at which you lose weight. In fact, weight loss is rapid because the calorie counts are low (very low for women) and because a fairly hefty amount of exercise is required on the plan (up to 45 minutes of aerobic exercise daily), which will also burn up extra calories – and help to maintain metabolic rate. Nothing new here – it's a low-cal diet and exercise plan, dressed up with a bit of pseudo-science to make it sound less boring. ● **Score: 2**

Total score 19

Percentage rating 47.5%

■ *The Rotation Diet* by Martin Katahn (Bantam Books, revised May 1987) ISBN 0 55327667 0.

See also: Crash diets, Top 20 popular diets.

Running

Running is one of the best calorie-burning aerobic exercises, but isn't for anyone who hasn't exercised in a while, who should start with walking, progress to gradient walking, jogging (very slow running) and then finally to running. It is also good for developing the muscles of the buttocks, thighs and calves, which will help to increase the metabolic rate even after exercise, and for bone density. Speed and distance monitors and heart rate monitors can be purchased from most of the suppliers listed under Exercise equipment.

■ UK Athletics; 0121 456 5098; www.ukathletics.org

■ Fell Runners Association; www.fellrunner.org.uk

■ Road Runners Association; www.roadrunnersclub.org.uk

■ www.runningmates.co.uk will help you find someone to run with.

■ www.onrunning.com for information on running.

Salon treatments

Various 'weight loss' and 'inch loss' treatments are available at beauty salons throughout the world. The main types are:

■ Wraps/bandaging, where most or all of the body is wrapped quite tightly in bandages or similar, soaked in minerals/herbs/seaweed, sometimes followed by massage. Examples: Frigithalgo, Universal Contour Wrap. Inch loss follows as the treatment promotes loss of fluid from the body.

■ Electrical stimulation, where electric current is passed through the fatty areas and the fat is said to split into free fatty acids which are transported out of the body via the lymph system. This is simply not true. Even if the body's fatty tissue were converted into free fatty acids by electrical stimulation, unless they were then used up for energy (via exercise or diet), they would simply end up as body fat again.

■ Electrical 'faradic' or 'galvanic' stimulation, sometimes in combination with oils or algae to 'boost metabolism'. The treatment is said to increase muscle tone, lose inches and improve skin tone. A course of a few sessions would make little difference to muscle tone; metabolism can hardly be boosted by external treatment such as this. Inches may be lost (if many measurements are taken from all over the worked-on areas) via fluid loss, and skin tone may well be better. Examples: ionithermie.

■ Lymphatic drainage via manual or machine massage, with or without treatment oils. This will result in weight loss via fluid loss, of a pound or two, which is a temporary effect.

All these salon treatments, and others like them, can help you to feel better and look better temporarily, but few if any have ever been proved actually to help you lose body fat, or even body weight, on a permanent basis. Most treatments are expensive, ranging from about £30 a session. *See also:* Cellulite treatments, Massage.

The Scarsdale Diet

Another hugely famous diet from the '70s, written by Dr Herman Tarnower, who ran a clinic in the town of the same name and created the diet for overweight patients. Now billed as 'the world's bestselling diet book', it is still selling well today.

The Diet

Interestingly, considering the number of diets published since, the Scarsdale is alone in its balance of the major nutrients. It contains 43% protein (the highest of all the diets, including Atkins), 22.5% fat (making it a low- to very-low-fat diet, unlike the other 'high-protein' diets which are, in fact, high-fat diets) and 34.5% carbohydrate. Tarnower claimed that even on this level of carbs, ketosis would happen (see Atkins diet), weight loss would be speedy and hunger not a problem. You are supposed to follow the weight-reducing diet for two weeks at a time only, followed by his keep-trim programme, higher in calories and choice but with a long list of banned foods.

Typical calorie count for a day's eating (basic diet): 1,000.

Promised weight loss: Much talk of people losing 20lb (9kg) in 14 days; average claimed is 1lb (0.5kg) per day.

Typical day's eating:

■ ***Breakfast:*** 1/2 grapefruit; slice of wholemeal toast (no butter or spread); coffee (no sugar or milk).

■ ***Lunch:*** Tuna fish well drained; salad with oil-free dressing; coffee.

■ ***Evening meal:*** Roast lamb, all visible fat removed; salad with lemon and vinegar dressing; coffee.

■ ***To drink:*** in addition: Water, diet drinks, tea, soda water.

Short-term effectiveness: Low in calories and quite low in carbohydrate, so will produce fat and fluid loss, as well as loss of lean tissue. ● **Score: 4**

Long-term effectiveness: The two weeks on, two weeks off approach is quite good and means that the overall calorie count of the plan isn't quite as low as it may seem, but the low palatability of the diet may mean it is hard to stick to. ● **Score: 3**

Ease of use: Tarnower was very strict about following the diet to the letter during the two weeks, so if you like being told what to do, with little room for choice, then it would be quite easy, although you may have trouble finding some of the items in the shops, depending on season. The recipes err on the complicated side. ● **Score: 3**

Cost: More expensive than some. ● **Score: 3**

Palatability: Meals suggested are not very appetizing. ● **Score: 2**

Satiety: High protein content would provide fairly good satiety, and plenty of side vegetables/salads allowed. ● **Score: 3**

Health factor: A little too low in calories for modern nutritionists and far too high in protein – high levels, especially of animal protein, may cause kidney problems or increase risk of osteoporosis. Weight loss claimed is far too rapid compared with official guidelines of 1–2lb (0.5–1kg) a week. ● **Score: 1**

Scientific basis: Tarnower claimed his balance of protein, carbohydrate and fat would produce optimum weight loss and satiety – exactly what all the diets of today claim (and each has a different balance!). The diet works because it is low in calories – and he recommends walking 2 miles a day as well, but the weight losses promised are probably optimistic. ● **Score: 2**

Total score 21

Percentage rating 52.5%

■ *The Complete Scarsdale Medical Diet* by Herman Tarnower and Samm Sinclair Baker (Bantam, December l985) ISBN 0 55317203 4.

See also: Top 20 popular diets

Size 8 Club

This club offers support to thin or small women and plenty of practical advice.

■ www.size8club.co.uk; 01689 842307.

See also: The Slenderella Syndrome: The Slim Woman's Survival Guide by Helena Fishlock-Lomax (Size 8 Club Ltd, 1999) ISBN 0 95356620 X.

Slimming clinics

There are hundreds of private slimming clinics all over the country, offering diet advice, which may or may not be in line with current official thinking. Many are quite liberal with their slimming pill prescriptions and researchers (posing as clients) often find they will prescribe even for people who have a normal body mass index. Charges are quite high, so think twice before attending such a clinic. You may be better off seeing your GP – who will possibly prescribe one of the better slimming pills if he/she really thinks you need it – or joining a slimming club.

■ *Yellow Pages* are a good source of clinics local to you; otherwise try the Internet or *Talking Pages* (0800 600900).

Slimming clubs

Since WeightWatchers was formed in the USA in 1963, millions of people have lost weight with the help of slimming clubs. Recent research suggests that by joining a club you may have more chance of reaching your target weight, and more chance of keeping the weight off, than by following other methods.

All clubs offer eating plans, motivational support, advice and companionship. Some, but not all, have a weekly weigh-in and exercise advice is usually given, though few clubs actually have the space or facilities to offer supervised exercise sessions. The exception to this is the Conley chain of clubs where there is a weekly 45-minute exercise session. There is usually a joining fee of a few pounds, plus a weekly attendance fee and, once you reach target weight, there is usually a different structure for weight maintenance.

The types of calorie-control on offer are usually based on recognized healthy eating principles, though the actual approaches vary (e.g. WeightWatchers has a 'points' system while Slimming World has 'free' foods and 'sin' foods), and the class leaders/advisers are trained by the companies involved.

The clubs listed below are probably the best, and/or have the most classes nationwide. The first three also have affiliated magazines with useful, motivation articles, recipes, success stories and so on.

■ WeightWatchers UK Ltd., Ludlow Road, Maidenhead, Berkshire, SL6 2SL; 08457 123000; www.weightwatchers.co.uk

■ Slimming World, Clover Nook Road, Somercotes, Alfreton, Derbyshire DE55 4RF; 08700 7546669; www.slimming-world.com

■ Rosemary Conley Diet and Fitness Clubs, Quorn House, Meeting St., Quorn, Loughborough, Leics LE12 8EX; 01509 620222; www.rosemary-conley.co.uk

■ Slimming Magazine Clubs, 112-134 The Broadway, London SW19 9RL; 0208 543 8989; 0500161 412 (freephone); www.slimmingmagazineclubs.co.uk

■ Lighten Up (not a club as such but offers an eight-week course all over the country); 46 Staines Road, Twickenham, TW2 5AH; 0845 603 3456; www.lightenup.co.uk

See also: Diet coaches, Internet slimming, Postal/telephone slimming.

Slimming patches

You may see a variety of 'slimming patches' advertised in the national and local newspapers, magazines and via mail drops or on the Internet. They are said to work by stimulating the thyroid to improve metabolism, or some are said to help control food cravings. Before you spend your money on these products I suggest you visit the www.healthwatch-uk.org website and see what this watchdog organization has to say about them. The same applies to diet pens, slimming soaps, and other amazing-sounding products. The general rule is – if it sounds too good to be true, it probably is.

See also: Cellulite treatments, Diet aromas, Slimming pills.

Slimming pills

For prescription pills, see Q37. Over-the-counter (OTC) pills of many kinds are available for the naive slimmer to purchase – at health food shops, chemists, by mail order or on the Internet. Few of these are of any real value. Many contain mixtures of several so-called slimming ingredients. Here is a selection of the most well-promoted:

■ ***Fat magnets/fat absorbers/fat blockers.*** These claim to absorb or attract fat so that it can no longer be absorbed. One common ingredient, chitosan, is a derivative of ground shell and is said to absorb 4–8 times its own weight in fat. Even taking 8 pills a day, this would average out at around 12g of fat not absorbed – or about a hundred calories saved. For the price, not of great benefit then, even if they do work, and side effects (lack of essential fat and vitamin absorption, for example) may be negative. No other fat-magnet-type products have been proved to work to help people lose weight without dieting, either, except for the prescription slimming pill orlistat (Xenical).

■ ***Starch blockers:*** Very popular a decade or so ago, these were supposed to block the calories in carbohydrate foods in the diet, but British research showed that they didn't work, and side effects such as stomach pains and diarrhoea were reported.

■ ***'Slim while you sleep' pills:*** These claim to help you to lose weight AND build muscle while you sleep. You take the pill before going to bed, after four hours without food, but tests have shown these pills to contain little more than collagen protein. They probably work to help weight loss (if they do) because you can't eat anything after around 7pm. In other words, diet alone will do the trick. But it isn't possible to build muscle without exercise so that claim is completely false.

■ ***Pyruvate:*** After one experiment in the US found that this substance may have a small effect in helping weight loss, sales of supplements boomed, but the case is yet to be proved – and most commercial supplements contain amounts of pyruvate much smaller than used in the successful research test.

■ ***Appetite suppressants:*** Some pills claim to alleviate hunger or make you feel 'full' more quickly – these are usually based on fibrous or gel-like substances, such as glucomannan (konjac). Guar gum, once sold on this basis, is now withdrawn as a supplement as it caused internal blockages and other problems.

Another much used substance in OTC slimming pills is hydroxycitrate which, one study published in the *International Journal of Obesity* showed, may help with the prevention of weight gain by helping satiety, but studies have failed to find it useful for weight loss. A high-fibre, low-GI diet will help you to feel full without any need for pills.

■ Metabolism boosters: See Ephedrine, Caffeine, Kelp.

■ Ephedrine: See Herbal diet supplements.

■ Kelp/fucus: See Herbal diet supplements.

■ Guarana: See Caffeine supplements.

■ Zotrim: See Herbal diet supplements.

See also: Caffeine supplements, Chromium picolinate, CLA, Co-enzyme Q10, Herbal diet supplements, Laxatives, Lecithin, Sports supplements.

Slimming surgery

There are three categories of 'slimming surgery': operations to help you eat less/absorb less food and therefore lose weight; liposuction to remove body fat mechanically; and skin tucks, to remove surplus skin left after weight loss.

Operations to help you lose weight

The two most frequently carried out are gastroplasty and gastric bypass. In gastroplasty, the stomach is stapled (vertical-banded gastroplasty) to divide it into two parts – the small top pouch holds only about 1–3 ounces (30–85g) of food so you can eat only tiny portions without feeling nausea or discomfort. The food slowly empties through a tiny opening into the rest of your stomach. The latest version of this operation is via keyhole surgery and the pouch may also be created by a doughnut-shaped silicone band which is inflated with saline. This is adjustable and fairly easily reversible.

Gastric bypass also involves stapling the stomach – all the way across – but in addition part of the small intestine is bypassed. A new outlet for food from the remaining stomach pouch is created by joining it to the intestine lower down, bypassing the duodenum and a small portion of the jejunum, which reduces the time that the food (both calories and nutrients) can be absorbed by the body.

With these two operations, international data shows that after one year patients had lost 53% and 72% of excess weight respectively, but the operations aren't without risk – abdominal hernias and gallstones are a common complication and to avoid nutritional deficiencies supplements need to be taken.

International selection criteria for these operations are a BMI of at least 35 if you have a disease treatable by weight loss, or 40 otherwise, plus various other requirements. Only 200 operations (many private) are carried out each year in the UK but 40,000 are done in the USA.

Jaw wiring

Jaw wiring – where the mouth can't open and so the only form of food that can be taken is liquid – was a common operation in the '70s and '80s, but the operations described above have largely superseded it as they are less inconvenient and have better long-term results. Few surgeons now carry out jaw wiring.

Liposuction

This is a serious surgical procedure that shouldn't be regarded as an alternative to conventional slimming in clinically overweight people – it is a cosmetic operation in which subcutaneous fat deposits (under the skin) are removed with a tiny vacuum and is used for 'spot reducing'. It is the most common cosmetic surgery performed in the USA with about 200,000 operations carried out each year.

The latest form – tumescent liposuction – includes injection of salt water containing local anaesthetic and hormones to control bleeding, bruising and swelling. There is also a fairly new ultrasound technique which ruptures the fat cells, making it easier to remove the contents.

Surgeons say that liposuction is best regarded as a body-contouring technique for people of normal or near-normal weight. The operation is not risk-free, recovery can be uncomfortable and take a long time; swelling may remain for some months. And while it is true that the removed fat cells cannot return, any fat cells left behind in the problem area can get bigger if calorie balance isn't maintained – and fat cells in other parts of the body will 'take on board' extra fat, meaning that you may end up with unsightly bulges in places you hadn't expected. So after liposuction, maintaining a sensible diet and exercise programme is very important.

Abdominoplasty

This is an operation to remove skin from areas where large weight loss (or pregnancy) has left a lot of surplus that can't be removed by exercise or dieting, as the skin is literally overstretched. This can be a problem particularly for older people who have been overweight a long time before slimming, as the skin loses its elasticity with age. The extra skin is cut away and restitched, leaving scars along the bikini line and sometimes the navel. Other procedures, including liposuction or repair to the muscles of the abdomen, may also be carried out at the same time.

■ For obesity surgery ask your GP for a referral to a consultant. You can also visit www.obesitysurgery.org.uk for more detailed information on these procedures.

■ For liposuction and abdominoplasty, contact The British Association of Aesthetic Plastic Surgeons (BAAPS), Royal College of Surgeons, 33-43 Lincoln's Inn Fields, London WC2A 3PN; 0207 405 2234.

Sports

For information about all official sports organizations, check out www.uksport.gov.uk. The website contains a full A–Z listing of all sports and contact details.
See also: Badminton, Cycling, Running, Swimming, Walking.

Sports supplements

Various supplements are used by exercisers and sportspeople to improve their performance/endurance/strength.

The most popular are:

■ ***Creatine:*** A nonessential amino acid which has been shown to enhance energy production in high-intensity exercise (e.g. sprint, weightlifting) but appears to do little for long-term aerobic energy. Creatine is one of the few performance enhancers still legal in the Olympics. For unfit people the advantage of taking a creatine supplement has been little researched – it may make it easier to improve in the gym, for example, but there are concerns about side effects, including cramp, dizziness and kidney problems in susceptible people. Creatine doesn't work if you take caffeine or caffeine-containing supplements at the same time.

■ ***L-carnitine:*** Another substance classed with the amino acids, which has been touted as an aid to exercise and fat-reduction. Research shows, however, that in healthy people, l-carnitine is of little use as a sports supplement or weight loss aid.

■ ***Protein bars or drinks:*** These are taken to augment protein intake via food, by people who want to build muscle. Protein per se won't work to build muscle – you need to exercise the muscles. Surplus protein will be converted to body fat.

Many sports supplements contain a cocktail of 'fat-burning' substances and herbs, discussed elsewhere in the book – including ephedrine, or a similar product, synephrine (citrus aurantium), hydroxycitric acid, another amino acid l-tyrosine, said to enhance the effect of fat-burning supplements, and chromium.

Before buying any supplements remember that they are not subject to the stringent testing and other regulations that apply to medicines and that there may be unwanted side effects. It would be sensible to discuss nutrition with a qualified Sports Nutritionist before purchasing these expensive products.

■ The British Dietetic Association can help you find a trained sports nutritionist; 0121 616 4900.

■ www.quackwatch.com has a fairly comprehensive non-hype library on supplements.

■ Reflex Nutrition Ltd is one of the better companies selling sports supplements; 0870757 3353.

See also: Caffeine/caffeine supplements, chromium picolinate, CLA, Co-enzyme Q10, Herbal diet supplements, Slimming pills, Vitamin and mineral supplements.

Sugar busters

Originally published in 1995, *Sugar Busters* was reissued in 1998 and became a worldwide hit. The authors believe that by avoiding all extrinsic sugar and foods high on the Glycaemic Index you'll lose weight and be healthier, because you will increase insulin sensitivity. They seem to believe that insulin resistance causes obesity and that sugar is toxic.

The Diet

The diet is similar to The Zone (which also avoids high-GI foods) but with a little more fat and a little less carbohydrate (Sugar Busters contains an estimated 30% protein, 40% fat and 30% carbohydrate).

You are allowed red meat and dairy produce as well as poultry and fish, olive oil, nuts and a selection of veg and fruits. Carbs such as sweet potatoes, wholemeal/grain breads, wholewheat pasta, brown rice and oats are allowed in small amounts, but you aren't allowed potatoes or refined carbohydrates like white bread, pasta, rice or carrots, and pulses don't figure at all. And of course, no refined sugar products.

Typical calorie count for a day's eating: approx 1,200.

Promised weight loss: Not specified but the main 'case history' in the book lost 3½lb (1.6kg) a week over a 5-month period.

Typical day's diet:

■ ***Breakfast:*** Orange juice; hot oat cereal with skimmed milk; coffee.

■ ***Lunch:*** Turkey on wholemeal bread with light mayonnaise and salad items.

■ ***Snack:*** 1 apple.

■ ***Evening meal:*** Grilled pork tenderloin slices, brown rice, sliced onions, green beans; 12 whole fresh nuts.

■ ***To drink:*** Low-cal diet drinks, water, tea, coffee.

Short-term effectiveness: Weight loss should soon be apparent if the 14-day diet is followed to the letter, although portion sizes are not specified, so it may be easy to eat extra calories if you feel like cheating. ● **Score: 3**

Long-term effectiveness: Weight loss may continue if the diet is followed, although few guidelines are given on portion sizes and calorie reduction will be based on avoiding the disallowed foods. ● **Score: 3**

Ease of use: Quite easy to follow and few out-of-the-ordinary foods are used. ● **Score: 4**

Cost: Moderate to high. ● **Score: 3**

Palatability: Good as there is plenty of variety and the fat content helps too. Some quite nice recipes offered. ● **Score: 4**

Satiety: Should be fairly good as high-GI foods are used and there is plenty of protein – but quantities of starchy carbs are quite small. ● **Score: 4**

Health factor: Despite the authors' plea to choose lean meat and moderate intake of high-fat dairy produce, the diet is still too high in fat to meet current recommendations, and too low in carbs and dietary fibre. It is also high in protein, which could be a health problem for some, especially over the long term (see High-protein diets). Ignoring pulses seems pointless as they are low-GI and sugar-free, and banning foods like potatoes and carrots is also of little health or slimming benefit. There is also little evidence that small amounts of extrinsic sugar in an overall balanced diet are bad for health. ● **Score: 3**

Scientific basis: A British study into the effects of sugar in weight-reducing diets published in 2001 in the *International Journal of Obesity* concluded that the practice of avoiding sugar in such diets is of questionable value – their participants lost similar amounts of weight on both sugar-free and 10% sugar diets. Other studies have shown that compliance (sticking to the diet) is higher if some sugar is allowed.

The premise that insulin causes weight gain is completely false – you need to create an energy surplus by overeating/underexercising (see Q18) for weight gain. What type of food those calories consists of is of little importance. Low-GI foods, though, do help to curb appetite and regulate blood sugars and are a helpful addition to a low-calorie diet. If you lose weight following Sugar Busters it will be because you have reduced the overall calorie content of your diet. ● **Score: 2**

Total score 26

Percentage rating 65%

■ *Sugar Busters!* by Sam S. Andrews, Luis A. Balart, Morrison C. Bethea and H. Leighton Steward (Vermilion, January l998) ISBN 0 09181687 4.

See also: Top 20 popular diets.

Swimming

Swimming is excellent exercise to help burn calories, increase muscle tone in arms, chest, back and legs, and increase suppleness slightly. As there is no impact, it is also good for people with joint problems – but because it is low-impact it is no good for increasing bone density.

■ The Amateur Swimming Federation of Great Britain has information about all local swimming clubs; 01509 618700; www.britishswimming.org

Vegetarian diets

If you are vegetarian and want to lose weight, or if you want to try vegetarianism as a way to lose weight, you need to watch the following points:

■ A vegetarian diet can be very healthy and low in saturated fat and calories – but not necessarily. You need to keep your intake of full-fat dairy produce (cheese, milk, cream) down quite low, instead choosing low- or moderate-fat versions and eating more of the plant sources of protein – seeds, nuts, pulses, tofu. These will also help keep calcium intake adequate (as will plenty of green leafy vegetables).

■ Keep sugar intake low – a veggie who lives on cakes, chocolate and biscuits isn't helping his/her health or waistline.

■ Some vegetarians fall short in selenium, iron and B vitamins. To ensure a full range of nutrients, get a varied diet including fruit, vegetables, salads, whole grains, pulses, nuts and seeds.

■ If going veggie for health reasons, consider keeping fish in your diet – oily fish is an important source of omega-3 essential fats. Otherwise, eat flaxseeds. Other sources of essential fats are nuts, seeds and plant oils.

■ The vegan (particularly the vegan slimmer) should take even more care to get all the nutrients – vitamin B12 is only found in animal products and seaweed (or supplements).

Popular diet books that can be easily followed by vegetarians or vegans include *Eat More, Weigh Less* (which is vegetarian with a lot of vegan choices), *The Glucose Revolution* and *Food Combining*. All these books are discussed elsewhere in the A–Z. A raw food diet also naturally leans towards veganism.

■ The Vegetarian Society, Parkdale, Dunham Rd., Altrincham, Cheshire WA14 4QG; 0161 925 2000; www.vegsoc.org

■ *Vegetarian Slimming* by Rose Elliot (Orion, January 1996) ISBN 0 75280173 2 – guidelines and recipes.

■ *Low Fat, Low Sugar* by Rose Elliot (HarperCollins, March 2000) ISBN 0 72253949 5 – healthy vegetarian cooking for slimmers and people with health problems such as diabetes and candida.

■ *Sue Kreitzman's Low-Fat Vegetarian Cookbook* (Piatkus, August l998) ISBN 0 74991910 8) – 100 recipes.

■ *The Vegetarian Society's Health and Vitality Cookbook* by Lyn Weller (HarperCollins, May 2000) ISBN 0 00414084 2 – 150 nutritionally analysed recipes.

■ *The Vegetarian Society's Simply Good Food* by Lyn Weller (HarperCollins, September 2000) ISBN 0 00710126 0 – practical dietary help as well as recipes suitable for entertaining.

■ *Judith Wills Virtually Vegetarian* (Piatkus, June l999) ISBN 0 74991974 4 – 100 nutritionally analysed vegetarian and fish recipes for health and weight loss.

Very-low-calorie diets (VLCDs)

VLCDs are diets which replace normal food with drinks, soups or bars and contain 800 calories a day or less but a complete range of nutrients. They may be high in fat and protein and low in carbohydrate, and produce ketosis which helps prevent hunger, and have been used privately and in the medical profession since the 80s as a guaranteed way to fast weight loss. The World Health Organization says that VLCDs should usually be reserved for achieving rapid short-term weight loss on medical grounds in patients with a body mass index over 30, and that they shouldn't be recommended for use without medical supervision. The WHO says that an acceptable minimum calorie level for such diets is 800 per day, and that going lower than this doesn't produce greater weight loss.

In the UK, the most famous VLCD is probably the Cambridge Diet, which can be obtained privately via a network of counsellors. The Cambridge 'sole source' diet is lower than the WHO recommended level, containing only 408 calories a day (for women under 5ft 8ins tall) or 544 calories a day (for taller women and all men) and is high in protein but low in fat as well as carbohydrates. The diet is recommended only for people with over a stone to lose. The company says it is not to be used for more than 4 weeks at a time, and will produce weight loss of a stone a month on average. For slower weight loss, the products can be used to replace just one or two meals a day, in which case see Replacement meals.

My advice? Follow the WHO recommendation and only embark on a VLCD if your doctor says it is wise and necessary. Otherwise, a normal diet of around 1,500 calories a day will produce steady weight loss with more chance of it staying off.

■ Cambridge Health Plan Ltd, Deben House, Old Kings Head Yard, Magdalen St., Norwich, NR3 1JE; 0800 161412 or 01603 626894; www.cambridge-diet.co.uk

See also: Q109; Crash diets, Replacement meals.

Very-low-fat diets

Low-fat eating, most health authorities worldwide agree, is a healthy way to eat and the best way of slimming and maintaining weight over a period of time. While most low-fat diets allow 20–30% of dietary calories as fat, some diets go much lower than this, attempting to remove all or almost all fat from the diet. As fat is present in small amounts in many foods, a completely fat-free diet isn't possible, but on a very-low-fat diet you may be eating around 10% of calories as fat, with a normal 10–20% of calories as protein and the remainder as carbohydrates. Two well-known diets adopt this way of eating – US doctor Dean Ornish's *Eat More, Weigh Less*, and *The Pritikin Weight Loss Breakthrough* by Robert Pritikin.

The Diet

Ornish's diet is basically vegetarian. Meat, poultry, game and fish aren't recommended and only a few very-low-fat dairy products such as fat-free yoghurt, skimmed milk, fat-free cheese and egg whites are allowed. On the Ornish diet, if you stick with the lists of 'eat freely', 'eat moderately' and 'banned' foods (which include not only all fats and oils, nuts, seeds, avocados and other fat-containing foods, but also refined carbohydrates including sugar, white flour and white rice), you can eat all you want without counting calories or portion sizes. Pritikin's diet allows lean meat three times a week but otherwise is similar in concept. The facts here refer to *Eat More, Weigh Less*.

Typical calorie count for a day's eating: 1,300 (based on female, eating until she feels full)

Promised weight loss: None specified, but Ornish patients lost on average 2 stones (12.6kg) over a year.

Typical day's eating:

■ ***Breakfast:*** Whole-grain cereal with fat-free yoghurt, fresh berries; orange juice

■ ***Lunch:*** Baked potatoes stuffed with a spiced spinach and fat-free cheese mixture; broccoli, potato and chickpea salad with fat-free dressing; green salad; fresh fruit.

■ ***Evening meal:*** Bruschetta with sun-dried tomatoes and capers; wholewheat pasta with dry-roast vegetables; green salad; peaches in wine

■ ***To drink:*** Water, tea coffee, skimmed milk, juices.

Short-term effectiveness: Not such rapid visible initial weight loss as with a high-protein, low-carb diet as more fluid will be retained; but fat loss will begin if the instructions are followed. ● **Score: 4**

Long-term effectiveness: If continued, the diet will work to help overweight people lose weight. Because satiety is good it may produce long-term compliance but on the other hand the sweeping changes needed may make it a hard diet to stick to for others and there is evidence that a more moderate low-fat diet will achieve more compliance long-term. ● **Score: 3**

Ease of use: While the lists of allowed and banned foods are straightforward and there is no need to count calories, in practice it is quite hard to make the allowed foods into inviting meals and a lot of new techniques need to be learnt, and sweeping changes made for people used to following a typical Western diet. ● **Score: 2**

Cost: Fairly low cost, although many of the recipes contain the more expensive fruits and vegetables. ● **Score: 4**

Palatability: Getting the fat content down this low means that for most people the diet will not be very palatable at least to begin with. The recipes show how to use herbs and spices to add flavour. ● **Score: 3**

Satiety: A diet very high in complex carbohydrates and with no limit on portion sizes should be filling and satisfying. ● **Score: 4**

Health factor: Very-low-fat diets may be short on essential fatty acids, found in oily fish, nuts, seeds and plant oils, and vegetarian low-fat diets may also be short in vitamin B12. There is currently much debate about the health of very-low-fat, high-carb diets as there is research to show that such diets actually lower 'good' HDL cholesterol and adversely affect the total blood fats profile in the body – but if the carbohydrates are 'complex', not refined, this may not be a problem. Lowered HDL levels may not be of concern if total cholesterol and LDL cholesterol also drop (which they do on an Ornish-type diet), and adding omega-3 fish oil supplements to a very-low-fat diet would probably get around the problem (if there is one!).

Plus points of the diet are that it is high in fruits, vegetables, whole grains and fibre, and low in saturated fat, sugar, refined carbs and salt. ● Score: 4

Scientific basis: A very-low-fat, high-carb diet will help you lose weight if, by using it, you create a calorie deficit. It is possible to overeat on carbohydrates alone, however, so some restraint needs to be used for the diet to work. Ornish doesn't peddle any silly ideas about why his diet works. ● Score: 4

Total score 28

Percentage rating 70%

■ *Eat More, Weigh Less* by Dean Ornish (Quill (HarperCollins), January 2001), ISBN 0 06095957 6.

■ *The Pritikin Weight Loss Breakthrough* by Robert Pritikin (Signet, January l999) ISBN 0 45119572 8.

See also: Hip-and-thigh Diet, Low-fat diets, Top 20 popular diets.

Vitamin and mineral supplements

Sometimes people on low-calorie diets are recommended to take a multivitamin and multimineral supplement – on healthy balanced diets that aren't too low in calories this may not be necessary, but a one-a-day supplement is unlikely to do any harm and may be a reasonable precaution to take.

Few vitamins or minerals actually directly influence your ability to lose weight on a slimming diet. A deficiency of iodine may make your thyroid gland sluggish, which may in turn affect your metabolic rate, but taking iodine supplements (in the form of kelp, for example) is not a good idea unless you know you are deficient. A deficiency of iron and/or B vitamins may make you feel tired and make exercising harder – but again, taking a supplement is a bad idea unless you know you are anaemic.

My advice – see your doctor if you think you need any supplements. Dosing yourself could do more harm than good, whereas a varied healthy diet does not.

Walking

Walking is the best all-round exercise for many people, particularly the unfit, slightly fit, and people who don't enjoy formal exercise or sport. To make walking more interesting and sociable, join a club such as the Ramblers Association, or try orienteering or racewalking.

■ Ramblers Association; 0207 339 8500; 01978 855148 (Wales); 01577 861222 (Scotland); www.ramblers.co.uk

■ British Orienteering Federation, 01629 734042; www.britishorienteering.org.uk

■ Racewalking Association, 01277 220687; www.racewalkingassociation.btinternet.co.uk

Weighted workouts

It is now recognized that weight training is as important a part of a slimming campaign as is aerobic exercise and diet. Working with weights burns calories while you do it, raises the metabolic rate after a workout, and builds muscle, which again burns more calories over time. The regime in Feature 30 is a beginner's weighted workout. There is information about weight training equipment for home use, and where to find weighted workouts outside the home, elsewhere in the A–Z.

■ British Amateur Weightlifting Association; 01865 200339; www.bawla.com

See also: Exercise classes, Exercise equipment, Gyms, Sports.

Whole food diets

Whole food is another way of saying 'a diet that is as natural as possible', avoiding refined foods such as white flour, white bread and white pasta, commercially made and highly processed foods, and eating mainly whole grains, pulses, fruit, vegetables, nuts, seeds and naturally reared meat, poultry and fish.

Such a diet may help you to lose weight – if you watch total fat intake (for natural fats from plants are just as calorific as any other), the diet becomes very similar to a healthy low-fat diet, discussed elsewhere in the A–Z. As it is also high in fibre and lots of bulky low-calorie or moderate-calorie foods, it will also help prevent you from overeating.

See also: Food combining, The F-Plan, Glycaemic Index diets, Low-fat diets, Macrobiotic diets, Mediterranean diet, Organic diets, Raw food diets, Vegetarian diets, Very-low-fat diets.

Yoga

Yoga is an excellent holistic exercise for almost all people – producing not only flexibility, a longer leaner look and better posture, but also benefits for the mind and health which may have a knock-on effect in helping improve your relationship with food. Depending on type, it can also burn a lot of calories.

There are various types of yoga. Hatha yoga is most commonly practised in the UK – you move into a pose (asana) and hold it, focusing on your breathing, then move on to another pose. This is a good all-round beginning class. Iyengar practises a precise form of yoga in which correct posture is the main goal. Ashtanta is the 'power' yoga, with swift moves from one pose to another, and is more akin to an aerobic workout.

■ British Wheel of Yoga, 1 Hamilton Place, Boston Road, Sleaford, Lincs NG34 7ES; 01529 306851; www.bwy.org.uk

See also: Alexander Technique, Book list, Exercise classes, Pilates.

The Zone

The original Zone diet – Enter The Zone – was written by US biochemist Barry Sears in I996, and since then several Zone diet books have together sold in their millions all over the world.

'The Zone' is a place where you go, apparently, if you eat a diet that contains precisely 40% carbs, 30% protein and 30% fat. Sears claims that eating this way will not only produce optimum fat burning and weight loss but will fight heart disease, cancer and more, by correctly balancing insulin and glucagon and the hormone-like compounds called eicosanoids.

The Diet

You work out how many grams of protein you need a day from the tables and then eat this much protein divided into 'blocks' of 7g each. Sears says you should eat no more and no less than this amount to stay in the Zone. The favoured protein foods are very-low-fat poultry, fish, dairy and vegetarian proteins. With each protein block you have to eat a carbohydrate block of 9g to keep in the Zone. The favoured carb foods are most fruits and veg and some pulses. The only favoured starch within this carb group is oatmeal – 'unfavourable' carbs are potatoes, pasta, rice, bread, some pulses, corn, sugar, and many more, as well as high-GI fruits and vegetables like carrots and bananas. With each protein and carb block you have a fat block equivalent to less than 2g. Olive oil and other monounsaturated fats are the favoured oils; saturates are unfavourable.

Typical calorie count for a day's eating: For an average sedentary woman needing 56g of protein a day (according to the Zone calculations) the calorie count would be approximately 536. For a mildly overweight active woman doing daily aerobic training, who would need, according to Zone calculations, 86g of protein a day, the calorie count would be approximately 800.

Promised weight loss: 1lb (0.5kg) a week is mentioned.

Short-term effectiveness: You would be almost bound to lose more than the pound a week mentioned in the book for the first few weeks – much of this loss would be fluid. ● **Score: 4**

Long-term effectiveness: The diet would be inadvisable for most people to follow for more than a short time as it is too low in calories. Some people who have followed it using the instructions in the book have reported feeling very hungry, dizzy and disheartened – the opposite of what the Zone says you will feel. ● **Score: 1**

Ease of use: A lot to remember; most people would need to be near the book at every meal. Even though you don't have to count calories, you do have to count blocks. And you have to weigh and measure to make sure your blocks contain the right amount of protein, carb or fat. ● **Score: 2**

Cost: Medium cost. ● **Score: 3**

Palatability: You can make quite normal meals, as 30% fat is allowed, but many people may not like the restriction on potatoes, rice, pasta and bread. Some quite nice recipes are given. ● **Score: 4**

Satiety: For many people the amount of food allowed is far too small – portion sizes will be little and the calorie count is ultra-low. As the diet doesn't produce a state of ketosis, which can kill appetite, many people will be hungry on this regime. ● **Score: 1**

Health factor: Although the overall balance of major nutrients isn't too bad compared with some other fad diets, such as high-fat, high-protein Atkins or very-low-fat Pritikin, and although most of the foods that you are allowed to eat are the ones we tend to think of as 'healthy', there just isn't enough to eat for most people. Avoiding a wide range of complex carbs, such as bread and potatoes, seems unnecessary, however. The health benefits cited would be apparent if any successful weight-reducing plan were followed. It has been shown that a diet higher in calories (a minimum of 1,200 is recommended by the World Health Organization) is better tolerated and more successful long-term than very-low-calorie regimes, unless done under medical supervision. ● **Score: 2**

Scientific basis: There is nothing special about the 40-30-30 food balance that will make you lose weight. Entering 'the Zone' entails a drastic reduction in calories for most people and this is what will cause the weight loss. Much of the 'science' in the book is a distortion of the facts as nutritional scientists know them. Eicosanoids don't cause disease and carbohydrates and insulin don't make you fat – unless you eat more calories than you need. ● **Score: 2**

Total score 19

Percentage rating 47.5%

■ *Enter The Zone* by Barry Sears and Bill Lawren (Regan Books, p/b November I996) ISBN 0 060987116 2; *The Zone Diet* (anglicized version) (HarperCollins January I999) ISBN 0 72253692 5. *The Soy Zone* (vegetarian) (Regan Books, May 2000) ISBN 0 06039310 6.

See also: Crash diets, Top 20 popular diets, Very-low-calorie diets.

The food value charts

Notes: * = foods high in extrinsic sugars tr = trace n/k = not known
Percentages shown are the percentage of total calories that the food contains in the form of fat, carbohydrate or protein, rather than percentage of the total weight of the food.

	Calories per listed portion	Total fat per listed portion (g)	Saturated fat per listed portion (g)	% of fat in item	% of carbohydrate in item	% of protein in item	Total fibre per listed portion (g)]
BISCUITS (all per biscuit)							
Digestive, 1 large	75	3.3	1.3	40	52*	8	0.4
Digestive, chocolate	85	4.1	2.0	44	50.5*	5.5	0.4
Ginger nut	45	5	0.7	30	65*	5	0.1
Rich Tea	35	5	0.7	38.5	56	5.5	0.1
Shortcake (oblong)	75	3.8	2.5	46.5	48.5	5	0.2
BREADS AND CRISPBREADS (all per 25g unless otherwise stated)							
Brown bread	56	0.5	0.1	9	75	16	1.0
Cream cracker, 1	40	5	0.6	33	58	9	0.1
French, white bread	62	0.6	0.1	1.2	83.3	15.5	0.3
Malt loaf	62	0.8	tr	12	74.5	12.5	1
Oatcake, 1	45	1.8	0.4	37	53.5	9.5	0.7
Pitta, white, 1	175	0.8	0.4	4	82.5	13.5	1.5
Pitta, wholemeal, 1	160	1.2	0.5	7	72	21	2.0
Rice cake, 1	24	0.2	tr	7	85.5	7.5	0.3
Dark rye crispbread, 1	25	0.2	tr	11.5	77.5	11	1.2
Wheatgerm bread	57	0.5	tr	8.5	74.5	17	0.8
White bread	58	0.5	0.1	6.5	80	13.5	0.4
Wholemeal bread	54	0.7	0.1	11	73	16	1.5
BREAKFAST CEREALS (all per 25g unless otherwise stated)							
All-Bran Plus	68	1.5	0.31	8.5	59	22.5	6.0
Branflakes	80	0.5	0.1	5.5	76	12.5	3.2
Cornflakes	92	0.4	tr	4	86.5	9.5	0.3
Fruit'n Fibre	90	1.2	0.7	12	78	10	1.7
Muesli (no-added-sugar)	82	1.7	0.3	19	71	10	3.1
Porridge oats, raw	94	2.2	0.4	22	63.5	14.5	1.7
Porridge (made up with water, per 100ml)	44	0.9	tr	18	70	12	0.8
Puffed Wheat	81	0.3	tr	3.5	79	17.5	1.6
Shredded Wheat, 1	80	0.7	tr	8.5	78.5	13	3.6
Special K	97	0.6	0.2	6	75.5	18.5	0.5
Weetabix, 1	65	0.7	0.1	9	77.5	13.5	1.5
CAKES AND BAKERY ITEMS (all per item or slice)							
Chocolate cake, 50g slice	230	13.6	6.5	53	42*	5	0.3
Croissant, 1 65g	280	16.5	5.2	54	38.5	7.5	1.0
Crumpet, 1 round	75	0.5	tr	3.5	83	13.5	0.7
Doughnut, jam, 1	260	12	3.5	41	52.5	6.5	0.5
Eclair, chocolate, 1	190	12	6.2	57.5	38*	4.5	0.3
Rich fruit cake, 50g slice	165	5.5	1.7	30	66*	4	0.9
Muffin, blueberry, 1	207	11.7	4.0	39	nk	nk	1.0
Scone, plain, 1	200	8	2.7	35.5	56.5*	8	0.9
Victoria sponge, 50g slice	230	13.2	4.2	51.5	43*	5.5	0.9

	Calories per listed portion	Total fat per listed portion (g)	Saturated fat per listed portion (g)	% of fat in item	% of carbohydrate in item	% of protein in item	Total fibre per listed portion (g)]
CHEESE (all per 25g unless otherwise stated)							
Brie or Camembert	75	5.8	3.6	69.5	tr	30.5	–
Cheddar	101	8.3	5.2	74.5	tr	25.5	–
Cheddar, half-fat	62	3.5	2.2	50.5	tr	49.5	–
Cheese spread	71	5.7	3.6	73	1	26	–
Cottage cheese, diet	20	0.4	0.2	18	tr	82	–
Cottage cheese, standard	24	1.0	0.6	37.5	5.5	57	–
Cream cheese, full-fat	110	12	7.5	97	tr	3	–
Danish Blue	89	7.3	4.6	74	tr	26	–
Edam	76	5.7	3.5	68	tr	32	–
Mozzarella	70	4.7	3.0	68	3	29	–
Soft cheese, low-fat	33	2.1	1.4	57	7.5	35.5	–
Stilton	103	9	6	78	tr	22	–
DRESSINGS, SAUCES AND PICKLES (all per tablespoon)							
Brown sauce	15	tr	–	tr	95.5*	4.5	tr
Burger relish	14	tr	–	tr	98*	2	tr
French dressing	69	7.4	0.6	100	tr	tr	–
Mayonnaise	104	11	1.6	99	tr	1	–
Salad cream	52	4.7	0.6	79	18*	3	–
Soya sauce	10	tr	–	6	71	23	–
Sweet pickle	21	tr	–	2	96*	2	tr
Tomato ketchup	17	tr	–	1	91*	8	–
HOT BEVERAGES							
Coffee, 200ml cup, black	2.5	–	–	–	41	59	–
Hot chocolate, 200ml cup made with semi-skimmed milk	142	3.8	2.4	24	57	19	–
Low-cal instant hot chocolate, per sachet	40	1.5	1.3	24	56*	20	–
Tea, 200ml cup, black	Tr	–	–	–	tr	tr	–
SOFT DRINKS							
Cola, 1 x 330ml can	135	–	–	–	100*	–	–
Lemonade, 1 x 200ml glass	50	–	–	–	100*	–	–
Orange squash, 1 x 200ml glass	60	–	–	–	100*	–	–
FRUIT JUICES (all per 125ml glass)							
Apple	50	–	–	–	97	3	tr
Grape	75	–	—	–	97	3	tr
Grapefruit, mixed citrus	50	–	–	–	96	4	tr
Mixed vegetable	25	–	–	–	85	15	tr

	Calories per listed portion	Total fat per listed portion (g)	Saturated fat per listed portion (g)	% of fat in item	% of carbohydrate in item	% of protein in item	Total fibre per listed portion (g)]
Orange	50	–	–	–	95	5	tr
Pineapple	55	–	–	–	97	3	tr
Fruit smoothie	163	0.6	tr	3.3	90.7	6	3.4
Tomato	25	–	–	–	83	17	0.6
EGGS							
Large, 1	98	7.2	2.1	67	tr	33	–
Medium, 1	84	6.1	1.8	67	tr	33	–
Small, 1	69	5.0	1.5	67	tr	33	–
Medium, fried, drained	120	10.5	3.1	78	tr	22	–
Medium, scrambled with low-fat spread and skimmed milk	115	9	2.7	64	4	32	–
FATS AND OILS (all per 25g)							
Butter	185	20.5	13.7	100	tr	tr	–
Corn oil	225	25	3.5	100	–	–	–
Low-fat spread	98	10	2.8	100	–	–	–
Olive oil	225	25	3.5	100	–	tr	–
Sunflower margarine	187	21	4.4	100	tr	tr	–
Suet, animal	224	25	14	100	–	tr	–
FISH (all per 100g unless otherwise stated)							
Cod, coley, haddock, monkfish fillet	76	0.7	0.1	8	–	92	–
Deep-fried fish in batter	200	10.3	0.9	47	14	39	tr
Fish finger, grilled, 1	50	2	2.8	38	34	28	tr
Haddock, smoked fillet	100	0.9	0.2	8	–	92	–
Herring fillet	234	18.5	3.7	71	–	29	–
Kipper, grilled fillet	205	11.4	1.8	50	–	50	–
Mackerel fillet	220	16	3.3	66	–	34	–
Pilchards in tomato sauce	126	5.4	1.1	38.5	2	59.5	–
Plaice fillet	93	1.9	0.1	18	–	82	–
Salmon fillet	197	13	2.3	59	–	41	–
Salmon, red, canned	155	8.2	1.5	47.5	–	52.5	–
Salmon, smoked	142	4.5	0.8	28.5	–	71.5	–
Scampi, deep-fried	316	17.6	1.7	50	34	16	tr
Trout, 1 average	200	6.7	2.2	30	–	70	–
Tuna in brine, drained weight	99	0.6	0.2	5.4	–	94.6	–
Tuna in oil, drained weight	189	9	1.4	42.8	–	57.2	–
Whitebait, deep-fried	525	47.5	4.4	81	4	15	tr
SEAFOOD (all per 100g)							
Crab meat, fresh	127	5.2	0.7	37	–	63	–
Crab meat, canned	81	0.9	0.1	10	–	90	–
Mussels, shelled weight	87	2	0.4	20.5	tr	79.5	–
Prawns, shelled	107	1.8	0.4	15	–	85	–
Scallops, shelled	105	1.4	0.4	12	tr	88	–
Squid	82	1.4	tr	15	tr	85	–
FRUIT (all per item, unless otherwise stated)							
Apple, dessert	45	tr	tr	tr	97	3	1.8
Apple, cooking, per 100g peeled and cored weight	35	tr	tr	tr	97	3	1.6

	Calories per listed portion	Total fat per listed portion (g)	Saturated fat per listed portion (g)	% of fat in item	% of carbohydrate in item	% of protein in item	Total fibre per listed portion (g)]
Apricot, fresh	10	tr	tr	tr	93	7	1.6
Apricot, dried, per 25g	45	tr	tr	tr	89.5	10.5	1.5
Banana, 1 medium	80	0.3	tr	3.5	91	5.5	1.0
Blackberries, per 25g	7	tr	tr	tr	83	17	0.7
Blackcurrants, per 25g	7	tr	tr	tr	88	12	0.9
Currants, dried, per 25g	60	tr	tr	tr	97	3	0.4
Cherries, per 25g	10	tr	tr	tr	95	5	0.2
Dates, each, fresh or dry	15	tr	tr	tr	96.5	3.5	0.2
Dates, stoned, per 25g	62	tr	tr	tr	96.5	3.5	1.0
Fig, dried, per 25g	57	tr	tr	tr	93	7	1.9
Fig, fresh, 1	10	tr	tr	tr	93	7	0.4
Gooseberries, cooking, per 25g	9	tr	tr	tr	93	7	0.6
Grapefruit, half	20	tr	tr	tr	90	10	1.0
Kiwi fruit	25	tr	tr	6	86	8	1.1
Lemon	15	tr	tr	tr	80	20	tr
Lime	10	tr	tr	tr	80	20	tr
Mango	100	tr	tr	tr	97	3	4.9
Melon, 200g slice	25	tr	tr	tr	90	10	1.4
Nectarine	50	tr	tr	tr	93	7	1.8
Orange	50	tr	tr	tr	92	8	2.7
Peach	50	tr	tr	tr	92	8	1.6
Pear, medium	50	tr	tr	tr	98	2	3.5
Pineapple, 1 ring	25	tr	tr	tr	95	5	0.6
Plum, 1 dessert	20	tr	tr	tr	94	6	0.7
Prunes, stoned, per 25g	35	tr	tr	tr	94	6	1.4
Raisins, per 25g	61	tr	tr	tr	98	2	0.5
Raspberries, per 25g	6	tr	tr	tr	84	16	0.6
Rhubarb, 1 large stick	6	tr	tr	tr	62.5	37.5	1.4
Satsuma, tangerine	20	tr	tr	tr	91	9	0.8
Strawberries, per 25g	6	tr	tr	tr	90	10	0.3
Sultanas, per 25g	62	tr	tr	tr	97	3	0.5
GRAINS (all per 25g unless otherwise stated)							
Couscous, dry weight	88	0.4	tr	4.5	83.5	12	0.5
Flour, white	87	0.3	tr	3	86	11	0.7
Flour, wholemeal	80	0.5	tr	6	77.5	16.5	2.2
Pasta, whole-wheat (cooked weight)	32	0.3	tr	8.5	72.5	18	0.8
Pasta, whole-wheat, dried (dry weight)	85	0.6	tr	7	78	15	2.1
Pasta, white (cooked weight)	29	tr	tr	3	83	14	0.3
Pasta, white, dried (dry weight)	95	0.2	tr	3	83	14	0.7
Pearl barley (dry weight)	90	0.4	tr	4	87	9	1.5
Rice, brown (cooked weight)	30	0.4	tr	7	86	7	0.1
Rice, brown (dry weight)	90	0.7	tr	7	85	6	0.4
Rice, white (cooked weight)	30	tr	tr	2	90	8	tr
Rice, white (dry weight)	90	0.2	tr	2.5	90	7.5	0.1
Spaghetti in tomato sauce, 1 x 213g can	127	1.5	0.2	10.5	77.5	12	1.5

	Calories per listed portion	Total fat per listed portion (g)	Saturated fat per listed portion (g)	% of fat in item	% of carbohydrate in item	% of protein in item	Total fibre per listed portion (g)]
MEAT AND POULTRY (all per 25g unless otherwise stated)							
Bacon, back, trimmed, grilled	73	4.7	1.8	58	–	42	–
Bacon, streaky, grilled	105	9	3.5	77	–	23	–
Beef, minced	57	3.8	1.7	60	–	40	–
Beef, minced, extra-lean	47	1.8	0.8	35	–	65	–
Beef, roast, fat removed	56	3.1	1.3	50.4	–	49.6	–
Beefburger, 50g, grilled	120	8.5	4.1	64	5	31	tr
Beef steak, lean only, grilled	42	1.5	0.6	32	–	68	
Chicken, average breast with skin, grilled	225	15	4.5	60	–	40	–
Chicken, average breast without skin, grilled	150	7	2.1	42	–	58	–
Chicken fillet, no skin, raw	30		0.3	30	–	70	–
Chicken, roast, meat only	37	1.3	0.4	33	–	67	–
Corned beef	54	3	1.6	50	–	50	–
Duck breast fillet (no skin)	31	1.2	0.3	36	–	64	–
Duck roast, meat and skin	85	7.2	2.0	77	–	23	–
Gammon steak, grilled, lean only	43	1.3	0.5	27	–	73	–
Ham, extra-lean	30	1.2	0.4	37.5	–	62.5	–
Kidneys, lambs'	22	0.7	0.2	27	–	73	–
Lamb, 1 average chop, trimmed	120	6.8	3.2	50	–	50	–
Lamb, leg, roast, lean only	48	2	1.0	38	–	62	–
Lamb, shoulder, roast	80	6.5	3.3	75	–	25	–
Liver, lambs'	45	2.5	0.7	52	3	45	–
Luncheon meat	78	6.7	2.5	77.5	6.5	16	–
Pheasant, roast, meat only	53	2.3	0.8	40	–	60	–
Pork fillet, raw	37	1.7	0.6	43	–	57	–
Pork, roast, lean only	46	1.7	0.6	34	–	66	–
Rabbit, meat only	31	1.0	0.4	29	–	71	–
Salami	122	11.3	5.0	83	1	16	–
Sausages, beef, grilled, per chipolata	70	4.5	1.6	59	21.5	19.5	–
Sausages, low-fat, grilled, per chipolata	50	2.4	1.2	43	23	34	–
Sausages, pork, grilled, per chipolata	75	5.8	2.4	70	13.5	16.5	–
Tongue	53	4	1.6	70	–	30	–
Turkey, dark meat, no skin	28	0.9	0.3	28	–	72	–
Turkey, light meat, no skin	26	0.3	tr	9.5	–	90.5	–
Veal fillet, raw	27	0.6	0.2	22	–	78	–
Venison fillet, roast	49	1.6	0.4	29	–	71	–
MILK AND CREAM (all per 25ml)							
Aerosol cream	16	1.5	1.0	87	10	3	–
Double cream	112	12	7.4	97	1.5	1.5	–
Single cream	53	5.3	3.3	90	5.5	4.5	–
Sour cream/crème fraîche	51	5	3.3	88	7	5	–
Milk, whole	16	1	0.6	52.5	27	20.5	–
Milk, semi-skimmed	11.5	0.4	0.3	31.5	39	29.5	
Milk, skimmed	8	tr	tr	2	57	41	–
Soya milk	8	0.5	tr	53.5	10	36.5	–

	Calories per listed portion	Total fat per listed portion (g)	Saturated fat per listed portion (g)	% of fat in item	% of carbohydrate in item	% of protein in item	Total fibre per listed portion (g)]
NUTS AND CRISPS (per 25g, all nuts shelled weight)							
Almonds	141	13.3	1.0	85	3	12	1.8
Brazils	155	15.3	3.6	89.5	2.5	8	1.1
Chestnuts	42	0.7	tr	14	81	5	1.0
Hazelnuts	95	9	0.6	85	7	8	1.6
Peanuts, fresh or dry-roasted	142	12.2	2.2	77.5	5.5	17	1.6
Walnuts	131	9	0.7	89	3	8	0.9
Crisps, standard	133	9	3.7	60.5	34.5	5	1.5
Crisps, lower-fat	105	6.5	2.8	56	36.5	7.5	1.6
PASTRY AND PIZZA							
Cornish pasty, 1 small	430	26.5	9.6	55.5	35	9.5	1.2
Filo pastry, per 25g	67	0.7	0.2	9.5	78	12.5	0.8
Jam tart, 1	150	5.8	2.1	35	61*	4	1.0
Mince pie, 1	200	9.5	3.4	43	53*	4	2.0
Pizza, 200g slice	475	24	10.0	t/c	t/c	t/c	2.8
Pork pie, one 140g	530	37.8	14.3	64.5	25	10.5	1.2
Puff pastry, per 25g	93	5.9	3.0	57	31.5	11.5	1.5
Quiche, 125g slice	390	28	12.8	65	20	15	0.8
Sausage roll, average 75g	358	27	10.0	68	26	6	1.0
Shortcrust pastry, per 25g	113	7	2.5	55	40	5	0.5
Steak and kidney pie, 1 individual 130g	480	31.5	12.5	59	30	11	1.0
PUDDINGS AND DESSERTS							
Blackcurrant cheesecake, 100g portion	240	10.6	5.6	39	51.5*	9.5	0.9
Custard, ready-made, 100ml	120	4.5	2.5	34	53*	13	–
Fruit pie, 100g portion	180	7.6	2.9	38	57.5*	4.5	1.7
Ice-cream, vanilla, 50g	83	3.3	2.0	35.5	55.5*	9	–
Trifle, per 100g portion	160	6.3	3.1	34	57*	9	0.5
PULSES (all per 25g)							
Baked beans in tomato sauce	16	0.1	tr	6	61	33	0.9
Butter beans, cannellini beans, canned or cooked weight	23	tr	tr	2.5	67.5	30	1.1
Chickpeas, canned or cooked weight	40	0.8	tr	18	60	22	1.0
Hummus	47	3.1	tr	60	24	16	0.6
Kidney beans, canned or cooked weight	25	0.1	tr	4.5	59.5	36	1.4
Lentils, canned or cooked weight	25	0.1	tr	4.5	64.5	31	1.0
Lentils, dry weight	76	0.2	tr	3	65.5	31.5	2.2
Split peas, canned or cooked weight	30	tr	tr	2.5	69.5	28	1.6
SEEDS (all per 25g)							
Pine nuts	172	17	1.1	89	2.9	8.1	0.4
Pumpkin seeds	142	11	1.7	71	12.2	16.8	1.2
Sesame seeds	150	14.5	2.1	87	1.0	12	2.0
Sunflower seeds	145	12	1.1	73.5	13	13.5	1.5
Tahini paste	152	14.7	2.1	87	0.5	12.5	2.0

	Calories per listed portion	Total fat per listed portion (g)	Saturated fat per listed portion (g)	% of fat in item	% of carbohydrate in item	% of protein in item	Total fibre per listed portion (g)]
SOUPS (per 300ml serving)							
Cream of chicken	175	11.5	1.8	59	29	12	0.3
Cream of tomato	173	8.7	0.9	45	46	9	1.2
Lentil	115	0.3	tr	2.5	72.5	25	3.0
Minestrone	90	2.9	0.9	29.5	55	15.5	2.1
Vegetable	110	1.8	tr	14.5	72.5	13	2.1
SPREADS AND CONSERVES (per 25g unless otherwise stated)							
Jam	65	–	–	–	99*	1	–
Liver pâté	80	6	2.1	67.5	1.5	31	–
Marmalade	65	–	–	–	100*	tr	tr
Marmite, per teaspoon	9	tr	–	3.5	4	92.5	–
Peanut butter	156	13.4	2.9	77.5	8	14.5	1.3
Taramasalata	110	11.5	0.8	94	3.5	2.5	–
SUGARS AND CONFECTIONERY (per 25g unless otherwise stated)							
Chocolate, milk or plain	132	7.5	4.5	51.5	42*	6.5	–
Honey	72	–	–	–	99.5*	0.5	–
Sugar, all kinds	98	–	–	–	100*	–	–
Sugar, per tsp	20	–	–	–	100*	–	–
Syrup	75	–	–	–	100*	–	–
Toffee	107	4.3	3.4	36	62*	2	–
VEGETABLES, (per 25g unless otherwise stated)							
Artichoke, globe,1 whole	15	tr	tr	1	70	29	1.0
Artichoke, Jerusalem	4.5	tr	tr	tr	64.5	35.5	0.9
Asparagus, 1 spear	4.5	tr	tr	0.5	24	75.5	0.8
Aubergine	3.5	tr	tr	tr	80	20	0.5
Avocado, 1/2 medium	145	14.4	2.6	89	3	8	2.2
Beans, broad	12	0.1	tr	10.5	55.5	34	1.5
Beans, French	10	tr	tr	tr	59	41	0.5
Beans, runner	5	tr	tr	7	53	40	0.5
Beansprouts	7	tr	tr	tr	29	71	0.2
Beetroot	11	tr	tr	tr	84	16	0.5
Broccoli	4.5	tr	tr	tr	31	69	0.6
Brussels sprouts	4.5	tr	tr	tr	36	62	1.0
Cabbage	5	tr	tr	tr	65	35	0.6
Carrots	6	tr	tr	tr	88	12	0.6
Cauliflower	2	tr	tr	tr	42	58	0.4
Celery	2	tr	tr	tr	61	39	0.3
Chicory	2	tr	tr	tr	62	38	0.2
Chinese leaves	3	tr	tr	tr	50	50	0.3
Corn on the cob, 1	80	1.5	0.2	17	70	13	2.6
Courgettes	5	0.1	tr	3.5	67.5	29	0.2
Cucumber	2	tr	tr	9	67	24	0.1
Leek	8	tr	tr	tr	72	28	0.6
Lettuce	3	0.1	tr	30	37.5	32.5	0.3
Mushrooms	3	0.1	tr	34.5	11.5	55	0.3
Mustard and cress, whole box	5	tr	tr	tr	34	64	0.4
Onions	6	tr	tr	tr	85	15	0.1
Parsnips	12	tr	tr	tr	86.5	13.5	1.2
Peas, shelled	13	0.1	tr	7	55	38	1.2
Peppers, green	4	0.1	tr	22.5	53.5	24	0.4
Peppers, other colours	8	0.1	tr	11	77	12	0.4
Potato, baked, 1 average (225g)	190	0.2	tr	1	89.5	9.5	3.3

	Calories per listed portion	Total fat per listed portion (g)	Saturated fat per listed portion (g)	% of fat in item	% of carbohydrate in item	% of protein in item	Total fibre per listed portion (g)]
Potato, boiled	20	tr	tr	1	92	7	0.3
Chips, average cut	65	3	0.3	41.5	55	3.5	0.6
Chips, oven	49	1.7	0.4	32	62.5	5.5	0.5
Potato mashed with milk and butter	30	1.2	0.7	38	57	5	0.3
Potato, roast, 50g chunk	80	2.4	0.3	27.5	65	7.5	0.9
Spinach	7	0.1	tr	14.5	17.5	68	0.5
Squash, butternut	9	tr	tr	tr	86.5	13.5	0.4
Swede	5	tr	tr	tr	77	13	0.5
Sweet potato	21	0.1	tr	6.5	88.5	5	0.6
Sweetcorn kernels	30	0.5	tr	15	69.5	15.5	0.5
Tomato, 1x 50g	7	tr	tr	tr	75	25	0.5
Tomatoes, canned	3	tr	tr	1	62.5	36.5	0.2
Turnip	4	0.1	tr	22	62	16	0.6
Watercress	3	tr	tr	tr	17	83	0.4
VEGETARIAN PRODUCTS							
Nut loaf, 100g slice	210	9.5	1.5	41	41	18	2
Quorn, per 25g	21	0.8	tr	34	8	58	1.2
Sosmix, 100g made-up weight	208	11	4.5	47.5	32	20.5	4
Tofu, 25g	17	1	0.1	53	3	44	tr
TVP mince, 25g, made-up weight	17	tr	tr	2.5	39	58.5	0.5
Vegeburger, 1 x 50g	81	4	0.8	45	22.5	32.5	2.1
YOGHURTS AND FROMAGE FRAIS (all per 25g unless otherwise stated)							
Fromage frais, diet fruit, per 100g pot	43	0.1	tr	2	39.5	58.5	–
Fromage frais, fruit	28	0.8	tr	27	48*	25	tr
Fromage frais, natural, 8% fat	28	2	1.1	64	9	27	–
Fromage frais, natural, very-low-fat	12	tr	tr	4	22	74	–
Yoghurt, diet fruit, per 125g pot	51	0.1	tr	2	54	44	tr
Yoghurt, natural, low-fat	13	0.2	tr	13.5	48	38.5	–
Yoghurt, natural, whole	17	1	0.2	52	25	23	–
Yoghurt, Greek	33	2.2	1.2	61	nk	nk	

Index

Bold page numbers refer to Features

Art Director: Mary Evans
Editor & Project Manager: Lewis Esson
Design: Sue Storey
Assistant Editor: Katie Ginn
Photography: Patrick McLeavey
Home Economist: Emma Patmore
Artwork: Lynne Robinson
Picture Research: Nadine Bazar
Production: Vincent Smith & Tracy Hart

First published in 2002 by
Quadrille Publishing Limited,
Alhambra House,
27-31 Charing Cross Road,
London WC2H OLS

This paperback edition first published in 2003

Cataloguing in Publication Data: a catalogue record for this book is available from the British Library

ISBN 1 84400 012 5

Printed and bound in Spain.
D.L. TO: 1168 - 2002

Book List

All books listed are recommended.

Cooking

■ *Good Housekeeping Eat Well, Stay Well* (Ebury Press, September 1999) ISBN 0 09186785 1
■ *Rosemary Conley's Low Fat Cookbook 2* (Century, October 2000) ISBN 0 71266977 9
■ *The Quick After Work Low Fat Cookbook* by Sue Kreitzman (Piatkus, March l998) ISBN 0 74991806 3
■ *The Sunday Times Vitality Cookbook by Susan Clark* (Collins, December 2000) ISBN 0 00711054 5
■ *Superfoods for Children* by Michael van Straten and Barbara Griggs (Dorling Kindersley, June 2001) ISBN 0 75131264 9
■ *Judith Wills Slimmer's Cookbook* (Piatkus, December l998) ISBN 0 74991881 0

Exercise

■ *The Complete Guide to Strength Training* by Anita Bean (A & C Black, August l997) ISBN 0 71364389 7
■ *The Complete Guide to Stretching* by Christopher Norris (A & C Black, February l999) ISBN 0 71364956 9
■ *The Complete Guide to Postnatal Fitness* by Judy DiFiore (A & C Black, September l998) ISBN 0 71364852 X
■ *Essentials of Exercise Physiology* (2nd edition) by William McArdle, Frank Katch, Victor Katch (Lippincott, Williams and Wilkins, February 2000) ISBN 0 68330507 7
■ *Yoga for Wimps* by Miriam Austin (Sterling Publishing Co, September 2000) ISBN 0 80694339 4

Natural health, fitness and weight control

■ *The Natural Health Bible* by Lisha Simester (Quadrille, January 2001) ISBN 1 90275766 1
■ *Live Well – the Ayurvedic Way to Health and Inner Bliss* by Jane Alexander (Thorsons, October 2001) ISBN 0 72254052 3
■ *Natural Health Handbook for Women* by Marilyn Glenville (Piatkus, March 2001) ISBN 0 74992191 9
■ *The Mind Body Workout – Pilates and The Alexander Technique* by Lynne Robinson and Helge Fisher (Pan, April l998) ISBN 0 33036946 6

Nutrition

■ *The Complete Guide to Sports Nutrition* by Anita Bean (A and C Black, 3rd edition, October 2000) ISBN 0 71365389 2
■ *Fats that Heal, Fats that Kill* by Udo Erasmus (Alive Books, 1993) ISBN 0 92047038 6
■ *Manual of Nutrition* (MAFF – published by The Stationery office, 10th Edition, 1995) ISBN 0 1124299 1
■ *Collins Gem Vegetarian Food* (HarperCollins l993) ISBN 0 00470117 8
■ *The Food Bible by Judith Wills* (Quadrille, January 2001) ISBN 1 90384546 7

Psychology of weight control

■ *Overcoming Overeating* by Hirschmann and Hunter (Ebury Press, January 2000) ISBN 0 09182561 X
■ *Slim for Life* by Judith Wills (Vermilion, May 2000) ISBN 0 09187799 7
■ *The Food and Mood Handbook* by Amanda Geary (Thorsons, May 2001) ISBN 0 00711423 0

Acknowledgements

12 Science Photo Library/Quest; 14 Gettyimages/John Lamb; 17 Getty images /Paul Redman; 19 Gettyimages / David Delossy; 20 Marie Claire Idées/François Deconicnk; 22 Patrick McLeavey; 26 Natural Visions/Colin Paterson-Jones; 28-29 Patrick McLeavey; 43 Ian Hooton; 44 Gettyimages/Lori Adamski Peek; 51 Gettyimages/Lori Adamski Peek; 57-97 Patrick McLeavey; 100-101 Photonica/Kazutomo Kawai; 104-118 Patrick McLeavey; 123 Retna/Michael Putland; 126-135 Patrick McLeavey; 136 Gettyimages/Dale Higgins; 137 Patrick McLeavey; 139 Corbis Stock Market/Dann Tardif; 140 Retna/Ewing Reeson; 142 Bubbles/Moose Azim; 144 Bubbles/Daniel Pangbourne; 145 Patrick McLeavey; 148 ImageState; 152 above Patrick McLeavey; 152 below Gettyimages /Yellow Dog Productions; 153 Patrick McLeavey; 158 ImageState; 159 Retna/Jenny Acheson; 160-161 Patrick McLeavey; 164 Retna/Ken Bank; 165 Patrick McLeavey; 173 Gettyimages/John Slater; 174 Photonica/James Gritz; 180 Collections/Kim Naylor; 181 Getty images/David Oliver; 183 Patrick McLeavey; 185 Bubbles/John Garrett; 186 Corbis Stock Market/Sharie Kennedy; 188 Gettyimages/Donna Day; 190-191 Patrick McLeavey; 198 Rex Features/Louisa Buller; 201 Gettyimages Images/Ben Edwards; 202 Patrick McLeavey; 207 Gettyimages/Third Age; 208 Patrick McLeavey; 212 Courtesy The Kobal Collection; 218 Gettyimages Images/Nick Dolding; 220 Corbis Stock Market/Cameron; 222 © Quadrille/page 13b from 10year for MEN; 224 Retna/Gavin Harrison; 225 Corbis Stock Market/Ariel Skelley; 228 ImageState; 231 Bubbles/Angela Hampton; 234 Patrick McLeavey.